Ovarian Stimulation

Second edition

Ovarian Stimulation

Edited by
Mohamed Aboulghar
Cairo University, Cairo, Egypt
Egyptian IVF ET Center
Botros Rizk
Elite IVF, Houston
University of Alabama, Alabama
Cairo University
King AbdelAziz University

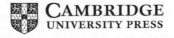

CAMBRIDGE
UNIVERSITY PRESS

CAMBRIDGE
UNIVERSITY PRESS

University Printing House, Cambridge CB2 8BS, United Kingdom

One Liberty Plaza, 20th Floor, New York, NY 10006, USA

477 Williamstown Road, Port Melbourne, VIC 3207, Australia

314–321, 3rd Floor, Plot 3, Splendor Forum, Jasola District Centre, New Delhi – 110025, India

103 Penang Road, #05–06/07, Visioncrest Commercial, Singapore 238467

Cambridge University Press is part of the University of Cambridge.

It furthers the University's mission by disseminating knowledge in the pursuit of education, learning, and research at the highest international levels of excellence.

www.cambridge.org
Information on this title: www.cambridge.org/9781107135970
DOI: 10.1017/9781316477021

First published 2011
This second edition 2022

Printed in the United Kingdom by TJ Books Limited, Padstow Cornwall

A catalogue record for this publication is available from the British Library.

Library of Congress Cataloging-in-Publication Data
Names: Aboulghar, Mohamed, editor. | Rizk, Botros, editor.
Title: Ovarian stimulation / edited by Mohamed Aboulghar, Botros Rizk.
Description: Second edition. | Cambridge, United Kingdom ; New York, NY : Cambridge University Press, 2022. | Includes bibliographical references and index.
Identifiers: LCCN 2021043512 (print) | LCCN 2021043513 (ebook) | ISBN 9781107135970 (hardback) | ISBN 9781316477021 (ebook other)
Subjects: MESH: Ovulation Induction – methods | Fertilization in Vitro – methods | Infertility – therapy |
BISAC: MEDICAL / Gynecology & Obstetrics
Classification: LCC RG135 (print) | LCC RG135 (ebook) | NLM WP 540 | DDC 618.1/780599–dc23
LC record available at https://lccn.loc.gov/2021043512
LC ebook record available at https://lccn.loc.gov/2021043513

ISBN 978-1-107-13597-0 Hardback

To a dear friend, an honorable man, a legendary scientist, a Nobel Prize winner and a world renowned leader.

To Professor Robert Geoffrey Edwards, the father of IVF and four million babies worldwide.

We dedicate this book to you in gratitude for your friendship, mentorship and leadership.

The world, East and West, has respected you, and we loved you and honored you.

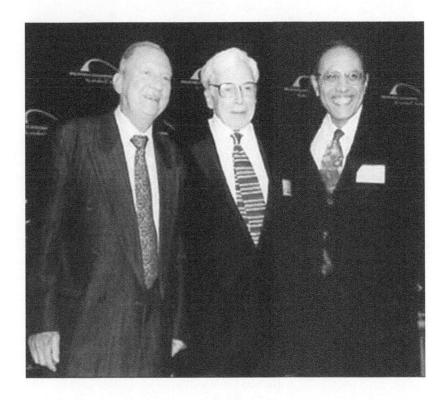

Contents

Section 1 Mild Forms of Ovarian Stimulation

Section 2 Ovarian Hyperstimulation for IVF

Section 3 Difficulties and Complications of Ovarian Stimulation and Implantation

Contributors

Mohamed Aboulghar
Faculty of Medicine
Cairo University
Cairo
Egypt
The Egyptian IVF-ET Center
Maadi
Cairo
Egypt

Mona M. Aboulghar
Department of Obstetrics and Gynecology
Egyptian IVF-ET Center
Cairo
Egypt

Pilar Alama
IVI Valencia
Valencia
Spain

Shima Elbakhit Albasha
Consultant of Obstetrics and gynecology and
Reproductive Medicine)
Fellowship program director
Department of reproductive medicine
(DORM)
Women wellness and research center
(WWRC)
Hamad medical corporation
Qatar

George Anifandis
Department of Obstetrics and Gynaecology
University of Thessaly
School of Health Sciences
Faculty of Medicine
Larissa
Greece

Jad Farid Assaf
American University of Beirut
Beirut
Lebanon

Nour Assaf
American University of Beirut
Beirut
Lebanon

Johnny Awwad
American University of Beirut
Beirut
Lebanon

Samira Barbara
Tiziri IVF center
Algiers
Algeria

Andrea Borini
9.baby
Family and Fertility Center
Bologna
Italy

Ernesto Bosch
IVI Valencia
Valencia
Spain

Ahmet Yigit Cakiroglu
Acibadem Mehmet Ali Aydinlar University
Department of Obstetrics and Gynaecology
Istanbul
Turkey

Stuart Campbell
St George's University of London, and Create
Fertility
London
UK

Astrid E. P. Cantineau
Department of Obstetrics and Gynaecology
University of Groningen
University Medical Center Groningen
Groningen
The Netherlands

Robert F. Casper
Division of Reproductive Sciences
Department of Obstetrics and Gynecology
Mount Sinai Hospital
Toronto, Ontario
Canada

Qiuju Chen
Shanghai Ninth People's Hospital
Shanghai
China

Ben J. Cohlen
Fertility Care Centre
Isala Clinics Zwolle
Location Sophia
The Netherlands

Alexandros Daponte
Department of Obstetrics and
Gynaecology
University of Thessaly
School of Health Sciences
Faculty of Medicine
Larissa
Greece

Adrija Kumar Datta
Create Fertility
Birmingham
UK

Panagiotis Drakopoulos
Centre for Reproductive Medicine
Universitair Ziekenhuis Brussel, and Faculty of
Medicine and Pharmacy
Vrije Universiteit Brussel
Brussels
Belgium
Department of Obstetrics and Gynecology
University of Alexandria
Egypt

Lina El-Taha
American University of Beirut Medical Center
American University of Beirut
Beirut
Lebanon

Sara Faour
Sodeco Eve Medical Center
Sodeco
Beirut
Lebanon

Chantal Farra
American University of Beirut
Beirut
Lebanon

Human Mousavi Fatemi
IVIRMA Middle-East
Abu Dhabi
United Arab Emirates

Bart C. J. M. Fauser
Division of Woman and Baby
University Medical Center
Utrecht
The Netherlands

Ahmed F. Galal
Department of Obstetrics and Gynecology
Alexandria University
Alexandria
Egypt

Suleiman Ghunaim
Department of Obstetrics and Gynecology
Division of Reproductive Endocrinology and
Infertility
Haifa Idriss-ART Unit
American University of Beirut Medical Center
Beirut
Lebanon

Shannon Gilmore
Elite IVF and Mobile Reproductive
Endocrinology and Infertility
Mobile
Alabama
USA

Eva Gómez
IGENOMIX
Valencia
Spain

Ahmet Helvacioglu
Elite IVF and Gynecology and Infertility
Associates
Fairhope
Alabama
USA

Yomna Islam
Egyptian IVF-ET Center
Cairo
Egypt

Dalia Khalife
Jumeirah American Clinic
Dubai
United Arab Emirates

Gabor T. Kovacs
Monash University
Victoria
Australia

Yanping Kuang
Department of Assisted Reproduction
Shanghai Ninth People's Hospital
Shanghai Jiao Tong University School of
Medicine
Shanghai
China

William Ledger
School of Women's & Children's Health
University of New South Wales
Sydney
Australia

Xuefeng Lu
Department of Assisted Reproduction
Shanghai Ninth People's Hospital
Shanghai Jiao Tong University School of Medicine
Shanghai
China

Antonis Makrigiannakis
Department of Obstetrics and Gynecology
University General Hospital of Heraklion
Medical School
University of Crete
Heraklion
Greece

David R. Meldrum
University of California
San Diego
USA

Christina I. Messini
Department of Obstetrics and Gynaecology
University of Thessaly
School of Health Sciences
Faculty of Medicine
Larissa
Greece

Ioannis E. Messinis
Department of Obstetrics and Gynaecology

University of Thessaly
School of Health Sciences
Faculty of Medicine
Larissa
Greece

Jose Miravet-Valenciano
IGENOMIX
Valencia
Spain

Mohamed F. Mitwally
Mitwally Fertility Clinic
San Antonio
Texas
USA

Monique Mochtar
Center for Reproductive Medicine
Department of Obstetrics and Gynaecology
Academic Medical Center
University of Amsterdam
Amsterdam
The Netherlands

Geeta Nargund
St Georges University Hospitals NHS Trust
London, and Create Fertility
London
UK

Amina Oumeziane
Tiziri IVF center
Alger
Algeria

Francesca Pennetta
9.baby
Family and Fertility Center
Bologna
Italy

Biljana Popovic-Todorovic
Centre for Reproductive Medicine
UZ Brussel
Brussels
Belgium

Alexander M. Quaas
University Hospital Basel
Reproductive Medicine and Gynecologic
Endocrinology (RME)
Department of Obstetrics and Gynecology
Basel
Switzerland

Abdel-Maguid Ramzy
Cairo University
Cairo
Egypt

Botros Rizk
Elite IVF
Houston
Texas
USA
Department of Obstetrics and Gynecology
Cairo University
Cairo
Egypt
Department of Obstetrics and Gynecology
King Abdulaziz University
Jeddah
Kingdom of Saudi Arabia

Anastasia Salameh

Hassan N. Sallam
Department of Obstetrics and Gynaecology
University of Alexandria
Alexandria
Egypt

Nooman H. Sallam
Assisted Reproduction Unit
Alexandria Fertility Clinic
Alexandria
Egypt

Raja Sayegh
Boston University School of Medicine
Boston, MA
USA

Natalie Shammas
Adventist health white memorial
medical center

Los angeles California
USA

Carlos Simón
University of Valencia
Valencia
Spain

Mehmet Cihat Unlu
Acibadem Mehmet Ali Aydinlar University
Department of Obstetrics and Gynaecology
Istanbul
Turkey

Diana Valbuena
IGENOMIX Foundation and IGENOMIX
Valencia
Spain

Evert J. P. van Santbrink
Division of Reproductive Medicine
Department of Obstetrics and Gynecology
Reinier de Graaf Gasthuis
Delft
The Netherlands

Madelon van Wely
Amsterdam UMC
Amsterdam
The Netherlands

Mohamed Youssef
Egyptian IVF-ET Center
Cairo
Egypt

Carlotta Zacà
9.Baby
Family and Fertility Center
Bologna
Italy

About the Editors

Mohamed Aboulghar

Mohamed Aboulghar, M.D. is Professor of Obstetrics and Gynecology, Faculty of Medicine, Cairo University and Clinical Director and founder of The Egyptian IVF-ET Center, Maadi, Cairo, Egypt, (the first IVF center in Egypt). He is also the founder and first president of the Middle East Fertility Society (MEFS) and Editorin-Chief and founder of the *Middle East Fertility Society Journal* (since 1996).

He has published over 200 papers in top international and regional medical journals, and over 20 chapters in international books.

He received the Egyptian National Award for Excellence in Medical Sciences in 2000, and the Egyptian State Merit Award in Medical Sciences in 2016. He received an Honorary Membership of the European Society of Human Reproduction and Embryology (Berlin 2004), and the Distinguished Service Medal of The Royal College of Obstetricians and Gynaecologists, in September 2018.

For several years, he has been an associate editor for *Human Reproduction and the American Journal of Obstetrics and Gynecology*. He is currently a member of the Editorial Board of *Fertility and Sterility*, and a reviewer for *Human Reproduction, Human Reproduction Update*, Fertility and Sterility and many more international journals.

He has organized 20 international conferences in the Middle East, and chaired 3 pre-congress courses in the American Society for Reproductive Medicine (ASRM) annual conference.

Botros Rizk

Botros Rizk is Medical Director, Elite IVF in Houston and Odessa Texas and former Professor and Head of Reproductive Endocrinology and Infertility and Medical and Scientific Director of USA In vitro fertilization and assisted reproduction at the University of South Alabama for 25 years from 1993 to 2019. Dr Rizk currently leads Elite IVF, Houston, Texas a premier assisted reproductive technology center in Texas.

Dr. Rizk is the President of the Middle East fertility Society. He currently serves as distinguished Adjunct Professor of Obstetrics and Gynecology in Cairo University, Egypt and served as Distinguished adjunct Professor of Reproductive medicine at King Abdulaziz University, Jeddah, Kingdom of Saudi Arabia. Dr. Rizk is distinguished Adjunct Scientific Director of IVF Michigan Rochester Hills. Dr Rizk is the scientific and Lab Director of Odessa Fertility Lab and Columbus Center for Reproductive Endocrinology and Infertility.

Mentored by Nobel Laureate Professor Robert Edwards, recipient of the Nobel prize in Medicine for achieving the first successful In Vitro fertilization in the world, Dr.Rizk started his career in Reproductive Medicine in London and Cambridge in the era of the legends where most of the current scientific developments and medical protocols where invented. He joined the prestigious University of Cambridge for three years from 1990 to 1993 as Clinical Lecturer and Senior Registrar. Dr. Rizk is board certified by the American Board of Obstetrics and Gynecology and the Royal College of Physicians and Surgeons of Canada and the Royal College of Obstetricians and Gynaecologist in England, as well as, the American Board of Bioanalysts in Embryology and Andrology.

Dr. Rizk's clinical and research interests have focused on ovarian stimulation including the development of the long agonist protocol which became the standard for two decades of IVF. He is internationally considered a leading authority on ovarian hyperstimulation syndrome and made original contributions to the pathophysiology and prevention of the syndrome. Dr. Rizk authored a book solely dedicated to ovarian hyperstimulation syndrome that is considered the standard reference for OHSS. Dr. Rizk is an authority on endometriosis; its novel medical management and robotic surgery. Dr Rizk is the principal investigator for tens of clinical trials for the FDA over the last three decades.

Professor Rizk edited and authored twenty eight medical textbooks and more than four hundred manuscripts embracing different aspects of international expert in infertility and assisted reproduction, as well as, ultrasonography and robotic surgery. Dr. Rizk is one of the early members of European Society for Human Reproduction and a founding member of Middle East Fertility Society. He chaired for several years many ASRM postgraduate courses teaching ART, ovarian stimulation, and ultrasonograhy.

Foreword

Alan H. DeCherney
National Institute of Child Health and HumM Development

Ovarian Stimulation is a text that is comprehensive, insightful, contains a great deal of new information, and is well organized, making it easy to read. The book is divided into 6 sections and 30 chapters and is authored by leaders in the field from the global community, with representatives from such places as Canada, Europe, the United States, Egypt, and Australia, to name a few.

The chapters evolve from ovarian stimulation through procedures before, during, and after stimulation. Oral and injectable agents for ovulation induction are discussed in great depth, incorporating a fair amount of new material. In addition, therapies, such as intrauterine insemination and laparoscopic ovarian drilling, are critically evaluated.

Ovarian Stimulation also addresses the utilization of GnRH, for both solitary use in ovarian stimulation and for use in combination with other agents. The occasionally serious adverse effect of ovulation induction (i.e., desecrated hyperstimulation syndrome) is looked at in terms of the diagnosis therapy and the use of novel agents in order to treat the entity, including early aspiration of ascites.

Individual patient scenarios are also addressed, including polycystic ovarian syndrome and the "poor responder." The discussion of the risk, benefits, and effectiveness of hCG versus LH is included. Of course, much of the data, application, and in-depth understanding come from the author's experience with in vitro fertilization (IVF), which is covered extensively by looking at natural cycle IVF, in vitro maturation of oocytes, as well as a more traditional approach.

Techniques for monitoring, such as ultrasound and serum estradiol levels, are also discussed in depth.

The text is a comprehensive approach for understanding ovarian stimulation. There is no lack of information as far as this topic is concerned. It is up to date with contemporary, excellent, and established references. The book is a monumental contribution that enriches our knowledge about a very important topic in reproductive endocrinology and infertility.

Foreword

Preface to the first edition

Ovarian stimulation has become an integral part of the management of infertility and assisted reproduction. A glance through scientific journals would demonstrate an explosion of publications related to ovarian stimulation. In every world congress and international infertility meeting the ovarian stimulation session is the most popular and lively session of the entire meeting.

This book was authored by the world leaders in infertility and reproductive endocrinology from the United States, Canada, Europe, Australia, the Middle East, and Africa. Each contributor has been the pioneer of the respective area of clinical research and practice.

The book covers in its different sections and chapters all aspects of ovarian stimulation: the different stimulation protocols from which to choose, the management of poor responders and hyper-responders, triggering ovulation and luteal phase support.

We have thoroughly enjoyed putting this book together and we take this opportunity to thank all the authors for their friendship and most valuable contributions.

To our readers, we put into your hands a concise and global book that we hope that you will thoroughly enjoy.

Preface to the second edition

Ovarian stimulation still occupies the central place in fertility management, particularly in assisted Reproduction. The second edition of this book has significant new contributions in addition to updates of the basic solid structure of the different sections in the first edition. The use of progestin primed stimulation, LH supplementation, freeze all embryos, GnRH agonist to trigger ovulation and luteal support different from progesterone are some of the new lines of treatment that became more widely used in the last decade. Endometrial receptivity and implantation failure are two areas that remain challenging today and are eloquently addressed. Difficult IVF cases and poor responders are some of the new highlights. Ovarian stimulation in PCOS patients have been divided into ovulation induction and controlled ovarian hyperstimulation for ART in two separate chapters. Many areas covered in this book are still being investigated such as freeze all embryos, and segregation of ART, as well as to the degree of mild stimulation. The advantages as well as the case against these controversial issues have been presented in the first section of the book.

We truly believe that ART has become much safer today because of the use of antagonist and GnRH agonist to trigger. The success and safety continue to move forward favorably. In your hands our beloved readers and colleagues we put a book that reflects today and perhaps tomorrow's contributions.

Chapter

1

Oral Agents for Ovarian Stimulation

Mohamed F. Mitwally and Robert F. Casper

Ovarian stimulation aims at the development of one or more of the ovarian follicles to reach the stage of maturity culminating in the release of one or more mature oocytes ready for fertilization. Ovarian follicular development is under the control of local factors inside the ovaries (most of it is poorly understood), as well as hormones produced from extraovarian sources, mainly pituitary gonadotropins. Other hormones may play a role in ovarian follicular development; the extent and details of such a role are not fully understood.

There are two mechanisms for ovarian stimulation: the first involves applying pharmacological agents that mimic endogenous gonadotropins (injectable gonadotropins) that directly stimulate ovarian follicular development through gonadotropin receptors. The second involves pharmacological agents that manipulate and moderate endogenous gonadotropin production. Those agents are oral ovulation induction agents that are believed to stimulate ovulation through moderating estrogen action, a major regulator of endogenous gonadotropin production. This chapter reviews those agents with a focus on the clinical aspects of their use.

Oral agents modulate estrogen action, and hence endogenous gonadotropin production through a direct effect on estrogen receptors, that is, selective estrogen receptor modulators (SERMs), or through modulation of estrogen production (inhibition), that is, aromatase inhibitors, or inhibitors of the estrogen synthesis enzyme (the aromatase enzyme). Clomiphene (clomifene) citrate (CC) is the most commonly used and known SERM and letrozole is the most commonly used and known aromatase inhibitor.

The first successful ovarian stimulation case was reported by Gemzell and his coworkers using human pituitary gonadotropins in 1958, and the first pregnancy was reported two years later [1;2]. One year later, in 1961, Bettendorf and his group reported a similar experience [3]. In the same year, Greenblatt and his coworkers published the first results of ovarian stimulation by an oral agent called at that time MRL/41, later known as CC [4]. Over the last two decades, insulin sensitizers have been introduced into clinical practice for ovulation induction in polycystic ovary syndrome (PCOS) patients with significant insulin resistance. The last decade introduced the success of a new group of oral agents for ovarian stimulation, the aromatase inhibitors. The aromatase inhibitor letrozole has been suggested as an alternative to CC as an agent for ovulation induction and to improve the outcome of controlled ovarian stimulation with gonadotropins. In 2000, we presented the first report in the literature on the success of letrozole in inducing ovulation in anovulatory women with PCOS [5].

Clomiphene Citrate

For more than half a century, CC has been the most commonly used agent for ovarian stimulation. Interestingly, since first reports in the early 1960s, results of CC treatment (ovulation and pregnancy rates) have not changed appreciably, despite the advent of modern immunoassays for steroid hormones, advances in ultrasound technology for cycle monitoring, and the introduction of commercial ovulation predictor kits that allow accurate identification of the midcycle luteinizing hormone (LH) surge. It has been puzzling that CC use has continued all those years as an ovarian stimulation agent despite the fact that CC is known as a pregnancy risk category X. This is particularly important when considering the relatively long half-life of about 5–21 days (depending on the isomer).

Moreover, CC can be stored in body fat. Those facts allow CC to accumulate in the body around crucial times of implantation, organogenesis, and embryogenesis [6–8].

Chemical Structure and Pharmacokinetics

Clomiphene citrate is a non-steroidal triphenylethylene derivative that exhibits both estrogen agonist and antagonist properties, that is, selective estrogen receptor modulator. Estrogen agonist properties are manifest only when endogenous estrogen levels are extremely low. Otherwise, CC acts mainly as an antiestrogen [6]. Clomiphene citrate is a racemic mixture of two distinct stereoisomers, enclomiphene and zuclomiphene, having different properties. Enclomiphene is the more potent antiestrogenic isomer and the one primarily responsible for the ovulation-stimulation actions of CC [6–8]. Enclomiphene has a half-life of few days, while the other isomer, zuclomiphene, is cleared far more slowly with levels detectable in the circulation for more than one month after treatment and may actually accumulate over consecutive treatment cycles [8]. Clomiphene citrate is cleared through the liver and excreted in the stool. About 85 percent of an administered dose is eliminated after approximately six days, although traces may remain in the circulation for much longer [7].

Mechanism of Action

Clomiphene citrate's structural similarity to estrogen allows it to bind to estrogen receptors (ER) throughout the body. Such binding lasts for an extended period of time, up to weeks rather than hours as is the case with natural estrogen. Such extended binding ultimately depletes ER concentrations by interfering with the normal process of ER replenishment [4].

It is believed that the hypothalamus is the main site of action because in normally ovulatory women, CC treatment was found to increase gonadotropin-releasing hormone (GnRH) pulse frequency [9]. However, actions at the pituitary level may also be involved since CC treatment increased pulse amplitude, but not frequency, in anovulatory women with polycystic ovarian syndrome, in whom the GnRH pulse frequency is already abnormally high [10]. The antiestrogenic effect on the hypothalamus, and possibly the pituitary, is believed to be the main mechanism of action for ovarian stimulation. Depletion of hypothalamic ER prevents correct interpretation of circulating estrogen levels, that is estrogen concentrations are falsely perceived as low leading to reduced estrogen negative feedback on GnRH

production by the hypothalamus and gonadotropins (follicle-stimulating hormone [FSH] and LH) by the pituitary. During CC treatment, levels of both LH and FSH rise, then fall again after the typical five-day course of therapy is completed. In successful treatment cycles, one or more dominant follicles emerge and mature, generating a rising tide of estrogen that ultimately triggers the midcycle LH surge and ovulation [9;10]. It is important to stress the two main prerequisites for the success of CC ovarian stimulation: presence of reasonable estrogen levels in the body and an intact hypothalamic/pituitary axis capable of producing endogenous gonadotropins.

Regimens of Clomiphene Citrate Administration for Ovarian Stimulation

Clomiphene citrate regimens for ovarian stimulation usually start on the second to fifth day after the onset of spontaneous or progestin-induced menses. Treatment typically begins with a single 50 mg tablet daily for five consecutive days, increasing by 50 mg increments in subsequent cycles until ovulation is induced. Once the effective dose of CC for ovarian stimulation is established, there is no indication for further increments unless the ovulatory response is lost, that is, higher doses will not improve the probability of pregnancy. The day of starting CC treatment has not been shown to affect the ovulation rates, conception rates, or pregnancy outcome in anovulatory women.

The dose required for achieving ovulation is correlated with body weight. However, there is no reliable way to predict what dose will be required in an individual woman. Although the effective dose of CC ranges from 50 to 250 mg/day, lower doses (e.g., 12.5 to 25 mg/day) may be tried in some women who are very sensitive to CC. Most women respond to treatment with 50 mg (52%) or 100 mg (22%). Although higher doses are sometimes required, the success rates are usually very low (150 mg, 12%; 200 mg, 7%; 250 mg, 5%). Most women who fail to respond to 150 mg of CC will ultimately require alternative or combination treatments [11;12].

Pregnancy rates are highest in the early cycles of CC treatment (first three cycles) with a significant decline in the chance of achieving pregnancy beyond the third treatment cycle down to a very low chance beyond the sixth treatment cycle. For that reason, it is not advisable to continue CC treatment beyond six treatment cycles [11]. It is important to mention here that the abovementioned data come from studies in anovulatory women when CC was used to induce ovulation. On the other hand, the value of CC treatment in enhancing the chance of achieving pregnancy in cases with ovulatory infertility has been questioned [12].

Outcome of Clomiphene Citrate Ovarian Stimulation

In anovulatory women with WHO Type II anovulation, CC has been reported to induce ovulation in 60–80 percent of patients with almost two-thirds responding to 50 mg or 100 mg dosage levels. After up to three ovulatory cycles, cumulative conception was encountered in a little less than two-thirds of patients (about 60 percent). Up to 85 percent pregnancy rate has been reported after five ovulatory cycles with fecundity of about 15 percent in ovulatory cycles [11]. It is important to realize that these figures were reported in anovulatory, young women in whom anovulation was the sole infertility factor. Interestingly, amenorrheic women are more likely to conceive than oligomenorrheic women after CC ovarian stimulation. This is probably because those who already ovulate, albeit inconsistently (oligomenorrheic), are more likely to have other coexisting infertility factors. Generally speaking, failure to conceive within six ovulatory cycles of CC treatment should be regarded as a clear indication to expand the diagnostic evaluation to exclude other infertility factors or to change the overall treatment strategy when evaluation is already complete [13].

Adverse Effects and Drawbacks of Clomiphene Citrate Treatment

Clomiphene citrate is in general a safe medication and usually well tolerated, with most of the side effects being relatively mild. Side effects are rarely severe enough to prevent continuation of treatment. Side effects are generally divided into those related to medication itself and other side effects that are related to ovarian stimulation in general, such as ovarian hyperstimulation syndrome and multiple gestation. Other serious long-term adverse effects of CC treatment have been suggested, including increased risk of ovarian cancer.

Hot flashes, the most common side effect occurring in about 10 percent of all women, is due to the antiestrogenic property of CC and seems to be dose-dependent. They are transient, rarely severe, and typically resolve soon after treatment ends. Other important side effects include visual disturbances; for example, blurred or double vision, scotomata, and light sensitivity are generally uncommon (< 2% prevalence) and reversible. However, there are isolated reports of persistent symptoms long after treatment is discontinued, with more severe complications such as optic neuropathy. Those visual side effects are contraindication for the use of CC that warrants stopping treatment and considering alternative methods of ovarian stimulation. Other fairly common but less serious side effects include breast tenderness, pelvic discomfort, and nausea, all observed in 2–5 percent of CC-treated women [14]. In addition, we have noted relatively common reports of premenstrual syndrome-type symptoms in women on CC [15].

Multiple-Gestation Pregnancy

With CC, ovarian stimulation multifollicular development is relatively common, which increases the risk of multiple gestation, reported to be approximately 8 percent. However, the overwhelming majority of multiple gestations that result from CC treatment are twins. Triplet and higher-order pregnancies are rare [16]. Several studies have shown that the number of multiple-gestation pregnancies can be decreased by the more judicious use of ovarian stimulation agents and by increased monitoring [17;18].

Severe Ovarian Hyperstimulation Syndrome

The incidence of severe ovarian hyperstimulation syndrome (OHSS) after CC treatment is difficult to determine, as definitions of the syndrome vary widely among studies. Mild OHSS (moderate ovarian enlargement) is relatively common, but also does not require active management. When CC induction of ovulation proceeds in the recommended incremental fashion designed to establish the minimum effective dosage, the risk of severe OHSS is remote [13].

Ovarian Cancer

There is an uncertain association of ovarian cancer with CC treatment that has been suggested by two epidemiological studies published early in the last decade. The first was a case–control study concluding that ovarian cancer risk was increased nearly threefold overall in women receiving various infertility treatments including CC [19]. The study methodology had several problems. The study compared infertile treated women to fertile women rather than to infertile untreated women, even though infertility and nulliparity have long been recognized as risk factors for ovarian cancer. In addition, there was no apparent increase in ovarian cancer risk in treated women who conceived. The second study was a cohort study concluding that risk of ovarian tumors was increased in women treated with CC [20]. Comparisons within the CC ovarian stimulation cohort showed no increase in risk with fewer than 12 cycles of treatment. This study too was widely criticized, primarily because it included cancers of varying types and tumors of low malignant potential (e.g., epithelial, germ cell, stromal), where the pathophysiology of each is likely very different.

The results of subsequent studies have been reassuring, but the question of whether treatment with ovulation-inducing drugs increases risk of ovarian tumors or cancer remains unsettled and cannot be summarily dismissed [21–28].

Congenital Anomalies

There is no consensus about evidence that CC treatment increases the overall risk of birth defects or of any specific malformation.

In a review by Scaparrotta *et al.* about potential teratogenic effects of CC, the authors concluded that there was some evidence for increased risk of fetal malformations, particularly neural tube defects and hypospadias, associated with CC exposure. The authors recommended that further investigations are needed to allow safe use of the drug [29].

The National Birth Defect Study (1997–2005) mentioned that several associations have been observed between CC exposure and birth defects. However, the study concluded that we should be careful when interpreting those associations because of the small number of cases, inconsistency of some findings, and inability to separate the effect of CC from the effect of subfertility [30].

Several large series have examined the question and have drawn the same conclusion [31;32]. Earlier suggestions that the incidence of neural tube defects might be higher in pregnancies conceived during CC treatment have not been confirmed by more recent studies [33]. A small study of pregnancy outcome in women inadvertently exposed to CC during the first trimester also found no increase in the prevalence of congenital anomalies [34]. However, most recently, an increase in the risk of congenital malformations of the heart has been suggested, though the study was not designed or powered to answer that question and further studies are needed to confirm or negate such a finding [35].

Pregnancy Loss

A fairly large study reviewed outcomes of 1744 CC pregnancies compared with outcomes of 3245 spontaneous pregnancies. Pregnancy loss was defined as clinical if a sac was seen on ultrasound or if it occurred after six weeks' gestation, and as preclinical if a quantitative human chorionic gonadotropin (hCG) was ≥ 25 IU/L and no sac was seen or pregnancy loss occurred earlier. The overall incidence of pregnancy loss was slightly higher, but not significant, for CC pregnancies (23.7%), compared with spontaneous pregnancies (20.4%). Preclinical pregnancy losses were increased by CC treatment (5.8% vs. 3.9%, $p < 0.01$) and for age ≥ 30 years (8.0% vs. 4.9%, $p < 0.001$), but not for age < 30 years (3.7% vs. 3.0%). Clinical miscarriages were increased by CC for women younger than 30 years (15.9% vs. 11.2%, $p < 0.01$), but not for age ≥ 30 years (20.1% vs. 22.3%) or overall (18.0% vs. 16.4%) [36].

A more recent study looking at rates of spontaneous miscarriage in 62 228 clinical pregnancies resulting from assisted reproductive technology procedures initiated in 1996–8 in US clinics also found that spontaneous miscarriage risk was increased among women who used CC [37]. However, the results of these studies are not definitive. Pregnancy loss after infertility treatment is a complex matter, influenced by several significant confounding factors such as insulin resistance and other genetic factors related to PCOS, the presence of endometriosis or unexplained infertility, and advancing maternal age [38].

Failure of Clomiphene Citrate Treatment

In anovulatory infertility, CC treatment failure is defined into two groups. The first group, ovulation failure (clomiphene resistance), includes patients who fail to ovulate in response to CC ovarian stimulation. The second group, clomiphene pregnancy failure, includes patients who ovulate in response to CC ovarian stimulation but fail to achieve pregnancy. This second group also includes women with ovulatory infertility who failed to achieve pregnancy after CC treatment.

Clomiphene citrate resistance (failure to achieve ovulation) is believed to be due to one of two main reasons: insulin resistance (women with PCOS) and inappropriate indication for CC treatment, for example, use in women with WHO Type I or III anovulation or women with ovulatory dysfunction due to medical disorders that require specific treatments such as thyroid disorders, congenital adrenal hyperplasia, and hyperprolactinemia.

The reasons for clomiphene pregnancy failure (women who ovulate in response to CC ovarian stimulation but do not achieve pregnancy) may be related to a wide variety of underlying infertility factors such as male factor, endometriosis, undiagnosed tubal factor, or endometrial receptivity factors. However, the success of many of these women in achieving pregnancy with alternative ovarian stimulation protocols using injectable gonadotropins or aromatase inhibitors supports the hypothesis that persistent antiestrogenic effects associated with CC might play a major role in the discrepancy between ovulatory rates and pregnancy rates [39–41].

Alternative Approaches for Clomiphene Resistance (Failure to Ovulate)

Longer duration or higher doses of CC treatment have been suggested, such as an eight-day treatment regimen or doses of 200 to 250 mg/day that can be effective when shorter courses of therapy fail. However, longer treatment and higher doses are expected to be associated with more antiestrogenic effects and reduced chances for achieving pregnancy even though ovulation is achieved [13]. Other suggestions included adjuvant treatments including the use of "insulin-sensitizing" agents (e.g., metformin and glitazones), exogenous hCG

and combinations (sequential treatment with CC and exogenous gonadotropins) and laparoscopic ovarian drilling, as well as corticosteroids to suppress adrenal androgens. The choice of adjuvant treatment should be based on the patient's history and the results of laboratory evaluation.

Antiestrogenic Effects: Probable Reason behind Clomiphene Citrate Treatment Failure

Clomiphene citrate exerts undesirable adverse antiestrogenic effects in the periphery (endocervix, endometrium, ovary, ovum, and embryo) that are unavoidable due to the long half-life of CC isomers. This could explain the "discrepancy" between the ovulation and conception rates observed in CC-treated patients, that is, explain the clomiphene treatment failure (ovulation but no pregnancy). Adverse effects on the quality or quantity of cervical mucus, endometrial growth and maturation, follicular or corpus luteum steroidogenesis, ovum fertilization, and embryo development have been reported by several studies [42–46]. The endometrium is believed to be one of the most important targets of the antiestrogenic effect of CC treatment. Successful implantation requires a receptive endometrium, with synchronous development of glands and stroma [47]. An interesting study has prospectively applied morphometric analysis of the endometrium, a quantitative and objective technique, to study the effect of CC on the endometrium in a group of normal women. In this study, CC caused a deleterious effect on the endometrium, demonstrated by a reduction in glandular density and an increase in the number of vacuolated cells [48]. In addition, a reduction in endometrial thickness below the level thought to be needed to sustain implantation was found in up to 30 percent of women receiving CC for ovulation induction or for unexplained infertility [44]. This observation has been confirmed by other studies [45;46].

Decreased uterine blood flow during the early luteal phase and the peri-implantation stage has been found with CC treatment [49]. Moreover, a direct negative effect of CC on fertilization and on early mouse and rabbit embryo development has been suggested [50].

Several investigators tried to reverse these antiestrogenic effects by administering estrogen concomitantly during CC treatment. Some studies reported increased endometrial thickness and improved pregnancy rates with this approach [51;52], while others have reported no benefit [43] or even a deleterious effect of estrogen administration [42]. Another approach has been to administer CC earlier during the menstrual cycle rather than starting on day 5 [53], to allow the antiestrogenic effect to wear off to some extent prior to ovulation and implantation. A third method has been to combine another SERM such as tamoxifen, which has more estrogen agonistic effect on the endometrium with CC, or to use tamoxifen as an alternative to CC [54]. However, none of these strategies have proved to be completely successful in avoiding the peripheral antiestrogenic effects of CC. A more recent publication has suggested that high-dose soy isoflavones may be able to overcome the antiestrogenic effect of CC on the endometrium [55]. This report remains to be confirmed by other investigators.

Aromatase Inhibitors

The aromatase enzyme is a microsomal member of the cytochrome P450 hemoprotein-containing enzyme complex superfamily (P450arom, the product of the CYP19 gene). It catalyzes the rate-limiting step in the production of estrogens, that is, the conversion of androgens (androstenedione and testosterone) into estrogens (estrone and estradiol, respectively) [56;57]. Aromatase activity is present in many normal tissues, such as the ovaries, the brain, adipose tissue, muscle, liver, and breast tissue, as well as in pathological tissues such as malignant breast tumors. The main sources of circulating estrogens are the ovaries in premenopausal women and adipose tissue in postmenopausal women [57].

Three generations of aromatase inhibitors have been developed (Table 1.1). The disadvantages of early generations (Box 1.1) as well as the advantages of third-generation aromatase inhibitors (Box 1.2) are presented (Table 1.1).

The third-generation aromatase inhibitors that are commercially available include two non-steroidal preparations, anastrozole and letrozole, and a steroidal agent, exemestane [58–60]. Anastrozole, ZN 1033 (Arimidex), and letrozole, CGS 20267 (Femara) are the most commonly used aromatase inhibitors in North America, Europe, and other parts of the world for treatment of post-menopausal breast cancer. They are completely absorbed after oral administration, with mean terminal half-life of approximately 45 hours (range, 30–60 hours) and clearance from the systemic circulation mainly by the liver. Mild gastro-intestinal disturbances account for most of the adverse events, although these have seldom limited continuation of clinical use. Other adverse effects are asthenia, hot flashes, headache, and back pain based on studies in postmenopausal women [58–60].

Along the last decade, the success of using aromatase inhibitors for ovarian stimulation has been reported, with letrozole the most commonly used aromatase inhibitor [61–68].

Hypotheses of the Mechanism of Ovarian Stimulation by Aromatase Inhibitors

Almost two decades now have passed since the first report of the use of aromatase inhibition for ovarian stimulation. Unfortunately, the underlying mechanisms behind the success of aromatase inhibition for ovarian stimulation have not been

Table 1.1 Different generations of aromatase inhibitors

Generation	Non-steroidal aromatase inhibitors; work by temporary (reversible) inactivation of the aromatase enzyme	Steroidal aromatase inhibitors (sometimes called suicidal inhibitors of the aromatase enzyme); work by permanent (irreversible) inactivation of the aromatase enzyme
First generation	Aminoglutethimide (Cytadren)	N/A
Second generation	Rogletimide Fadrozole (Afema)	Formestane
Third generation	Letrozole (Femara 2.5 mg/tablet) Anastrozole (Arimidex 1 mg/tablet) Vorozole (not marketed)	Exemestane (Aromasin 25 mg/tablet)

Box 1.1 Problems associated with early-generation aromatase inhibitors

Pharmacological disadvantages:

1. Low potency in inhibiting the aromatase enzyme, particularly in premenopausal women (very low potency)
2. Lack of specificity in inhibiting the aromatase enzyme with significant inhibition of other steroidogenesis enzymes, leading to medical adrenalectomy
3. Not all members are available orally (some require parenteral administration)
4. Variable bioavailability after oral administration
5. Variable half-life that changes with the period of administration due to induction of its metabolism

Clinical disadvantages:

1. Poorly tolerated on daily administration, with more than a third of patients discontinuing treatment due to adverse effects
2. Significant side effects related to the aromatase inhibitors, for example, drowsiness, morbilliform skin rash, nausea and anorexia, and dizziness, and side effects secondary to the steroids used for replacement therapy, for example, glucocorticoids
3. Interaction with alcohol with significant potentiation of its action
4. Significant interactions with other medications, for example, coumarin and warfarin
5. Need for replacement therapy due to medical adrenalectomy, for example, glucocorticoid and mineralocorticoid replacement
6. Long-term possible carcinogenesis (at least in animals)

Box 1.2 Advantages of third-generation aromatase inhibitors

Pharmacological advantages:

1. Extreme potency in inhibiting the aromatase enzyme (up to a thousand times the potency of the first-generation aminoglutethimide)
2. Very specific in inhibiting the aromatase enzyme without significant inhibition of the other steroidogenesis enzymes. This is true even at high doses
3. Absence of estrogen receptor depletion
4. Orally administered (other routes of administration are also possible, e.g., vaginal and rectal)
5. Almost 100 percent bioavailability after oral administration
6. Rapid clearance from the body due to short half-life (~ 8 hours for exemestane [Aromasin] to ~ 45 hours for letrozole [Femara] and anastrozole [Arimidex])
7. Absence of tissue accumulation of the medications or any of their metabolites
8. No significant active metabolites

Clinical advantages:

1. Well tolerated on daily administration for up to several years (in postmenopausal women with breast cancer), with few adverse effects
2. Few mild side effects
3. Very safe without significant contraindications
4. Absence of significant interactions with other medications
5. Very wide safety margin (toxic dose is several thousand times higher than recommended efficacious therapeutic dose)
6. Relatively inexpensive

completely elucidated. We believe that there are several mechanisms both centrally (at the level of the brain) and peripherally (at the level of the ovaries and the uterus) that work together.

Central Mechanism

By blocking estrogen synthesis in the brain, and by lowering circulating estrogens by reducing whole body estrogen synthesis, letrozole counteracts the negative feedback effect of estrogen on endogenous gonadotropin production (without depletion of ER as occurs with antiestrogens, e.g., CC). The resulting increase in endogenous gonadotropin secretion will stimulate the growth of the ovarian follicles. Withdrawal of estrogen centrally also increases activins, which are produced by a wide variety of tissues including the pituitary gland [69], and will stimulate synthesis of FSH by a direct action on the gonadotrophs [70].

Peripheral Mechanism

Peripherally, blocking the conversion of androgen substrates to estrogens by aromatase inhibition may increase ovarian follicular sensitivity to FSH stimulation. This is possibly due to the temporary accumulation of intraovarian androgens. There are data showing a stimulatory role for androgens in early follicular growth in primates [71], mediated directly through testosterone augmentation of follicular FSH receptor expression [72;73] and indirectly through androgen stimulation of insulin-like growth factor 1 (IGF-1), which may synergize with FSH to promote folliculogenesis [74;75].

Role of Aromatase Inhibitors in Ovarian Stimulation

Aromatase inhibitors may be used alone for ovarian stimulation, or as an adjuvant in conjunction with injectable gonadotropins. A major advantage of an aromatase inhibitor used *alone* is the ability to achieve restoration of monofollicular ovulation in anovulatory infertility, e.g., PCOS. Both multiple [61;62;64] and single-dose [63] regimens of aromatase inhibitor administered early in the menstrual cycle have shown efficacy in restoring ovulation in anovulatory women. A single dose regimen has the benefit of convenience, but the potential disadvantage of increasing side effects from administration of a larger dose. However, single doses that have been well tolerated were larger than the doses reported for ovarian stimulation [63;76].

The concomitant use of an aromatase inhibitor with injectable gonadotropins has been shown to improve the treatment outcome by reducing the total dose of gonadotropins required for optimum stimulation [64] and to improve the response to gonadotropins stimulation in poor responders [65]. The additional effect of aromatase inhibitors to reduce the supraphysiological levels of estrogen seen with the development of multiple ovarian follicles may also improve treatment outcome [77].

Women Who Might Benefit Most from Use of Aromatase Inhibitors for Ovarian Stimulation

Ovarian stimulation by aromatase inhibitors is associated with significantly lower estrogen production per follicle, hence overall lower estrogen levels. With multiple follicular development, such low estrogen production per developing follicle prevents the achievement of supraphysiological estradiol levels that are inevitable during ovarian stimulation. There are certain groups of women who might benefit from reducing estrogen levels during ovarian stimulation and ameliorating the supraphysiological estrogen levels attained during multiple follicular development. Examples include women who have estrogen-dependent disorders such as endometriosis or breast cancer, or those with an inherent clotting abnormality.

Polycystic Ovarian Syndrome

This group of patients is at particular risk of severe OHSS, particularly during intense stimulation with gonadotropins in assisted reproduction. Aromatase inhibitors may reduce the risk of OHSS in those patients, as discussed earlier, by lowering estrogen levels [78]. In our experience along the last 12 years, combining the aromatase inhibitor, letrozole, with the insulin sensitizer, rosiglitazone, during ovarian stimulation for assisted reproduction in women with PCOS has not resulted in any case of severe OHSS. Rosiglitazone might help in two ways, one by further reduction of estrogen levels through a direct inhibitory effect on the adipose cells' aromatase activity [79], and the other through a direct modulating effect on ovarian steroidogenesis, in particular reducing androgen production [80].

Letrozole may play a role at the level of the endometrium of PCOS women. Estrogen decreases the level of its own receptor by stimulating ubiquitination of ER (ERα). This results in rapid degradation of those receptors. Low estrogen levels decrease ubiquitination, which allows upregulation of the ER and increasing sensitivity to subsequent estrogen rise [81]. This could increase endometrial response to estrogen, resulting in faster proliferation of endometrial epithelium and stroma and improved blood flow to the uterus and endometrium, which might have a positive effect on implantation [82]. This might explain the normal endometrial development during letrozole stimulation despite the observed lower estrogen concentrations in these treated cycles.

Endometriosis

The expression of the aromatase enzyme in endometriotic tissues highlights the possible role played by locally produced estrogen in endometriosis progression [82]. Hence, aromatase inhibitors could be used for treating endometriosis [83]. The inhibition of local estrogen production in endometrial implants, and the lower estrogen levels associated with aromatase inhibition by aromatase inhibitors during ovarian stimulation, could possibly protect against progression of endometriosis during ovarian stimulation. This may improve the outcome of infertility treatment in this group of women. However, this idea still awaits confirmation by clinical trials.

Survivors of Estrogen-Dependent Malignancies Desiring Fertility

Recent advances in oncology including early detection and newer treatments have resulted in increasing numbers of patients surviving cancer following successful treatment. A significant proportion of estrogen-sensitive malignancies, such as breast cancer, affect women in the reproductive age group. Unfortunately, despite successful treatment, the majority of those women usually suffer from ovarian failure following chemotherapy. With the recent success of different fertility preservation options such as embryo and oocyte cryopreservation, some women may opt to freeze embryos or oocytes for later use by themselves or a gestational carrier. Oktay *et al.* reported the success of ovarian stimulation by aromatase inhibitors, letrozole and anastrozole, without a dramatic increase in serum estrogen concentrations, in women undergoing assisted reproduction before receiving cancer treatment. Patients were followed for almost two years after receiving ovarian stimulation with an aromatase inhibitor. During this follow-up period, the cancer recurrence rate was similar to that in patients who had no ovarian stimulation (control patients) [84].

Patients at High Risk of Coagulation Disorders

High estrogen states, both physiological such as during pregnancy or iatrogenic, for example, during estrogen treatment (hormone therapy or estrogen-containing contraceptives) and ovarian stimulation for fertility treatment, have been found to be associated with increased risk of thrombosis. This is particularly significant in women at high risk such as carriers of thrombophilia gene mutations, for example, antithrombin factors II and V [85]. Although it seems logical that those patients might benefit from lower estradiol levels when an aromatase inhibitor is used during ovarian stimulation, there are no data in the literature in support of this hypothesis.

Safety of Aromatase Inhibitors for Ovarian Stimulation

Almost all the data in the literature regarding pregnancy outcomes following the use of aromatase inhibitors for ovarian stimulation relate to the use of the aromatase inhibitor, letrozole. The accumulating data on outcome of babies delivered following letrozole use for ovarian stimulation support its safety. However, because of the short period of clinical experience with letrozole use for infertility treatment, patient understanding of the experimental use of letrozole for such indication is necessary.

Adverse Effects

Most of the data about clinical safety and adverse effects associated with the aromatase inhibitors come from clinical application in postmenopausal women with breast cancer. In this group of patients third-generation aromatase inhibitors were well tolerated, with most of the reported side effects being mild ones, including hot flashes, gastrointestinal events (nausea and vomiting), and leg cramps. Very few patients had to discontinue aromatase inhibitors due to drug-related adverse events, confirming the high clinical tolerability of aromatase inhibitors [86;87]. It is important to mention here that those reported adverse effects were observed in older women with advanced breast cancer who had received aromatase inhibitors daily over long periods of time, up to several years. Such treatment was obviously for much longer treatment periods than used for ovarian stimulation. In our clinical experience with letrozole use for ovarian stimulation, we have observed few adverse effects such as hot flashes and premenstrual syndrome-type symptoms. Interestingly, most of the patients who had a history of treatment with CC found letrozole better tolerated with fewer side effects. However, there are no clinical trials that have specifically looked at the adverse effects associated with the use of letrozole for ovarian stimulation.

Outcome of Pregnancies Achieved after Ovarian Stimulation with Letrozole

Although animal embryonic safety studies have found the aromatase inhibitor anastrozole to have no teratogenic or clastogenic effects, we do not have clinical data on the safety in babies delivered after its use for ovarian stimulation. On the other hand, there are reassuring data confirming the safety of the pregnancies achieved following the use of letrozole for ovarian stimulation.

We reported early pregnancy outcomes achieved after the use of letrozole for ovarian stimulation [88] compared with the outcome of pregnancies achieved with other ovarian stimulation treatments (gonadotropins and CC), as well as a control group of pregnancies spontaneously conceived without ovarian stimulation. Pregnancies conceived after letrozole treatment were associated with comparable miscarriage and ectopic pregnancy rates compared with all other groups, including the spontaneous conceptions. Later, a large multicenter study [89] that included 911 babies, 514 born after letrozole treatment and 397 after CC treatment, did not find any increase in the rates of major and minor malformations in babies conceived after letrozole treatment [90]. A more recent study that compared babies delivered after letrozole or CC stimulation protocols found a possible risk for low birth weight in the CC group. The babies in the letrozole group were the same percentile of birth

weights as the spontaneous conception controls [91]. The short half-life of letrozole and absence of ER antagonism result in a very favorable profile for infertility treatment compared with CC.

A recent Cochrane Database review about the use of aromatase inhibitors in subfertile women with PCOS concluded that the aromatase inhibitor letrozole appeared to improve live birth compared with CC [92].

A landmark multicenter, randomized trial comparing letrozole with CC for ovulation induction in 750 women with PCOS was published in 2014 by the Reproductive Medicine Network funded by the National Institutes of Health (NIH) in the United States [93]. The usual starting doses of letrozole (2.5 mg daily) or CC (50 mg daily) were given from day 3 to day 7 of the cycle for five days for up to five treatment cycles with the dose increased to a maximum of 7.5 mg for letrozole or 150 mg for CC if no ovulation occurred. The ovulation rate was higher in the letrozole group compared with the CC group (61.7% vs. 48.3%, respectively). The cumulative live birth rate was significantly higher in the letrozole group (25.5%) than in the CC group (19.1%; 95% CI 1.1–1.87) with no impact of body mass index on the results. In addition, the twin pregnancy rate was 3.4% in the letrozole group and 7.4% in the CC group [93].

References

1. Gemzell CA, Diczfalusy E, Tillinger KG. Clinical effects of human pituitary follicle stimulating hormone FSH. *J Clin Endocrinol Metab* 1958;**18**:138–148.

2. Gemzell CA, Diczfalusy E, Tillinger KG. Human pituitary follicle stimulating hormone. 1. Clinical effects of partly purified preparation. *Ciba F Coll Endocrin* 1960;**13**:191.

3. Bettendorf G, Apostolakis M, Voigt KD. Darstellung hochaktiver Gonadotropinfraktionen aus menschlichen Hypophysen und deren anwendung bei Menschen. *Proceedings, International Federation of Gynecology and Obstetrics*, Vienna 1961:76.

4. Greenblatt RB, Barfield WE, Jungck EC, Ray AW. Induction of ovulation with MRL/41. Preliminary report. *JAMA* 1961;**178**:101–104.

5. Mitwally MFM, Casper RF. Aromatase inhibition: a novel method of ovulation induction in women with polycystic ovarian syndrome. *Abstracts of the 16th Annual Meeting of the European Society for*

Human Reproduction and Embryology, 2000, Bologna, Italy.

6. Practice Committee of the American Society for Reproductive Medicine. American Society for Reproductive Medicine, Birmingham, Alabama, USA. Use of clomiphene citrate in women. *Fertil Steril* 2004;**82** Suppl 1:S90–S96.

7. Mikkelson TJ, Kroboth PD, Cameron WJ, *et al.* Single-dose pharmacokinetics of clomiphene citrate in normal volunteers. *Fertil Steril* 1986;**46**:392–396.

8. Young SL, Opsahl MS, Fritz MA. Serum concentrations of enclomiphene and zuclomiphene across consecutive cycles of clomiphene citrate therapy in anovulatory infertile women. *Fertil Steril* 1999;**71**:639–644.

9. Kerin JF, Liu JH, Phillipou G, Yen SS. Evidence for a hypothalamic site of action of clomiphene citrate in women. *J Clin Endocrinol Metab* 1985;**61**:265–268.

10. Kettel LM, Roseff SJ, Berga SL, Mortola JF, Yen SS. Hypothalamic-pituitary-ovarian response to clomiphene citrate in women with polycystic ovary syndrome. *Fertil Steril* 1993;**59**:532–538.

11. Garcia J, Jones GS, Wentz AC. The use of clomiphene citrate. *Fertil Steril* 1977;**28**:707–717.

12. Athaullah N, Proctor M, Johnson NP. Oral versus injectable ovulation induction agents for unexplained subfertility. *Cochrane Database Syst Rev* 2002;**3**:CD003052.

13. Usadi RS, Fritz MA. Induction of ovulation with clomiphene citrate. In: Sciarra JJ, ed. *Gynecology and Obstetrics*. Philadelphia: Harper & Row; 1986: Chapter 68.

14. Purvin VA. Visual disturbance secondary to clomiphene citrate. *Arch Ophthalmol* 1995;**113**:482–484.

15. Maruncic M, Casper RF. The effect of luteal phase estrogen antagonism on luteinizing hormone pulsatility and luteal function in women. *J Clin Endocrinol Metab* 1987;**64**:148–152.

16. Schenker JG, Yarkoni S, Granat M. Multiple pregnancies following induction of ovulation. *Fertil Steril* 1981;**35**:105–123.

17. Lipitz S, Reichman B, Paret G, *et al.* The improving outcome of triplet pregnancies. *Am J Obstet Gynecol* 1989;**161**:1279–1284.

18. Corson SL, Dickey RP, Gocial B, *et al.* Outcome in 242 in vitro fertilization-embryo replacement or gamete intrafallopian transfer-induced pregnancies. *Fertil Steril* 1989;**51**:644–650.

19. Whittemore AS, Harris R, Itnyre J. Characteristics relating to ovarian cancer risk: collaborative analysis of 12 US case-control studies. II. Invasive epithelial ovarian cancers in white women. Collaborative Ovarian Cancer Group. *Am J Epidemiol* 1992;**136**:1184–1203.

20. Rossing MA, Daling JR, Weiss NS, Moore DE, Self SG. Ovarian tumors in a cohort of infertile women. *N Engl J Med* 1994;**331**:771–776.

21. Venn A, Watson L, Lumley J, *et al.* Breast and ovarian cancer incidence after infertility and in vitro fertilisation. *Lancet* 1995;**346**:995–1000.

22. Modan B, Ron E, Lerner-Geva L, *et al.* Cancer incidence in a cohort of infertile women. *Am J Epidemiol* 1998;**147**:1038–1042.

23. Mosgaard BJ, Lidegaard O, Kjaer SK, Schou G, Andersen AN. Infertility, fertility drugs, and invasive ovarian cancer: a case-control study. *Fertil Steril* 1997;**67**:1005–1012.

24. Potashnik G, Lerner-Geva L, Genkin L, *et al.* Fertility drugs and the risk of breast and ovarian cancers: results of a long-term follow-up study. *Fertil Steril* 1999;**71**:653.

25. Pike MC, Pearce CL, Wu AH. Prevention of cancers of the breast, endometrium and ovary. *Oncogene* 2004;**23**:6379–6391.

26. Khoo SK. Cancer risks and the contraceptive pill. What is the evidence after nearly 25 years of use? *Med J Aust* 1986;**144**:185–190.

27. Fathalla MF. Factors in the causation and incidence of ovarian cancer. *Obstet Gynecol Surv* 1972;**27**:751–768.

28. Silva I dos S, Wark PA, McCormack VA, *et al.* Ovulation-stimulation drugs and cancer risks: a long-term follow-up of a British cohort. *Br J Cancer* 2009;**100**:1824–1831.

29. Scaparrotta A, Chiarelli F, Verrotti A. Potential teratogenic effects of clomiphene citrate. *Drug Saf* 2017; **40**(9):761–769. doi: 10.1007/s40264-017-0546-x.

30. Reefhuis J, Honein MA, Schieve LA, Rasmussen SA; National Birth Defects Prevention Study. Use of clomiphene citrate and birth defects, National Birth Defects Prevention Study, 1997–2005. *Hum Reprod* 2011; **26**(2):451–457. doi: 10.1093/humrep/deq313.

31. Hack M, Lunenfeld B. Influence of hormone induction of ovulation on the fetus and newborn. *Pediatr Adolesc Endocrinol* 1979;**5**:191.

32. Correy JF, Marsden DE, Schokman FC. The outcome of pregnancy resulting from clomiphene-induced ovulation. *Aust N Z J Obstet Gynaecol* 1982;**22**:18–21.

33. Whiteman D, Murphy M, Hey K, O'Donnell M, Goldacre M. Reproductive factors, subfertility, and risk of neural tube defects: a case-control

study based on the Oxford Record Linkage Study Register. *Am J Epidemiol* 2000;**152**:823–828.

34. Carlier P, Choulika S, Efthymiou ML. Clomiphene-exposed pregnancies–analysis of 39 information requests including 25 cases with known outcome. *Therapie* 1996;**51**:532–536.

35. Tulandi T, Martin J, Al-Fadhli R, et al. Congenital malformations among 911 newborns conceived after infertility treatment with letrozole or clomiphene citrate. *Fertil Steril* 2006;**85**:1761–1765.

36. Dickey RP, Taylor SN, Curole DN, et al. Incidence of spontaneous abortion in clomiphene pregnancies. *Hum Reprod* 1996;**11**:2642.

37. Schieve LA, Tatham L, Peterson HB, Toner J, Jeng G. Spontaneous abortion among pregnancies conceived using assisted reproductive technology in the United States. *Obstet Gynecol* 2003;**101**:959–967.

38. Hakim RB, Gray RH, Zacur H. Infertility and early pregnancy loss. *Am J Obstet Gynecol* 1995;**172**:1510–1517.

39. Franks S, Adams J, Mason H, Polson D. Ovulatory disorders in women with polycystic ovary syndrome. *Clin Obstet Gynaecol* 1985;**12**:605–632.

40. Hull MGR. The causes of infertility and relative effectiveness of treatment. In: Templeton AA, Drife JO, eds. *Infertility*. London: Springer-Verlag; 1992:33–62.

41. Wysowski DE. Use of fertility drugs in the United States, 1979 through 1991. *Fertil Steril* 1993;**60**:1096–1098.

42. Bateman BG, Nunley WC Jr, Kolp LA. Exogenous estrogen therapy for treatment of clomiphene citrate-induced cervical mucus abnormalities: is it effective? *Fertil Steril* 1990;**54**:577–579.

43. Ben-Ami M, Geslevich Y, Matilsky M, et al. Exogenous estrogen therapy concurrent with clomiphene citrate–lack of effect on serum sex hormone levels and endometrial thickness. *Gynecol Obstet Invest* 1994;**37**(3):180–182.

44. Gonen Y, Casper RF. Sonographic determination of a possible adverse effect of clomiphene citrate on endometrial growth. *Hum Reprod* 1990;**5**:670–674.

45. Nelson LM, Hershlag A, Kurl RS, Hall JL, Stillman RJ. Clomiphene citrate directly impairs endometrial receptivity in the mouse. *Fertil Steril* 1990;**53**:727–731.

46. Li TC, Warren MA, Murphy C, Sargeant S, Cooke ID. A prospective, randomised, cross-over study comparing the effects of clomiphene citrate and cyclofenil on endometrial morphology in the luteal phase of normal, fertile women. *Br J Obstet Gynaecol* 1992;**99**:1008–1013.

47. Hammond MG, Halme JK, Talbert LM. Factors affecting the pregnancy rate in clomiphene citrate induction of ovulation. *Obstet Gynecol* 1983;**62**:196–202.

48. Sereepapong W, Suwajanakorn S, Triratanachat S, et al. Effects of clomiphene citrate on the endometrium of regularly cycling women. *Fertil Steril* 2000;**73**:287–291.

49. Hsu CC, Kuo HC, Wang ST, Huang KE. Interference with uterine blood flow by clomiphene citrate in women with unexplained infertility. *Obstet Gynecol* 1995;**86**:917–921.

50. Yoshimura Y, Hosoi Y, Atlas SJ, Wallach EE. Effect of clomiphene citrate on in vitro ovulated ova. *Fertil Steril* 1986;**45**:800–804.

51. Shimoya K, Tomiyama T, Hashimoto K, et al. Endometrial development was improved by transdermal estradiol in patients treated with clomiphene citrate. *Gynecol Obstet Invest* 1999;**47**:251–254.

52. Gerli S, Gholami H, Manna C, et al. Use of ethinyl estradiol to reverse the antiestrogenic effects of clomiphene citrate in patients undergoing intrauterine insemination: a comparative, randomized study. *Fertil Steril* 2000;**73**:85–89.

53. Wu CH, Winkel CA. The effect of therapy initiation day on clomiphene citrate therapy. *Fertil Steril* 1989;**52**:564–568.

54. Saleh A, Biljan MM, Tan SSSL, Tulandi T. Effects of tamoxifen (Tx) on endometrial thickness and pregnancy rates in women undergoing superovulation with clomiphene citrate (CC) and intrauterine insemination (IUI). *Fertil Steril* 2000;**74**:S1–S90.

55. Unfer V, Casini ML, Costabile L, et al. High dose of phytoestrogens can reverse the antiestrogenic effects of clomiphene citrate on the endometrium in patients undergoing intrauterine insemination: a randomized trial. *J Soc Gynecol Investig* 2004;**11**:323–328.

56. Cole PA, Robinson CH. Mechanism and inhibition of cytochrome P-450 aromatase. *J Med Chem* 1990;**33**:2933–2942.

57. Santen RJ, Manni A, Harvey H, Redmond C. Endocrine treatment of breast cancer in women. *Endocrine Rev* 1990;**11**:1–45.

58. Winer EP, Hudis C, Burstein HJ, et al. American Society of Clinical Oncology technology assessment on the use of aromatase inhibitors as adjuvant therapy for women with hormone receptor-positive breast cancer: status report 2002. *J Clin Oncol* 2002;**20**:3317–3327.

59. Buzdar A, Jonat W, Howell A, *et al.* Anastrozole, a potent and selective aromatase inhibitor, versus megestrol acetate in postmenopausal women with advanced breast cancer: results of overview analysis of two phase III trials. Arimidex Study Group. *J Clin Oncol* 1996;**14**:2000–2011.

60. Marty M, Gershanovich M, Campos B, *et al.* Aromatase inhibitors, a new potent, selective aromatase inhibitor superior to aminoglutethimide (AG) in postmenopausal women with advanced breast cancer previously treated with antioestrogens. *Proc Am Soc Clin Oncol* 1997;**16**:156.

61. Mitwally MFM, Casper RF. Aromatase inhibition: a novel method of ovulation induction in women with polycystic ovarian syndrome. *Reprod Technol* 2000;**10**:244–247.

62. Mitwally MF, Casper RF. Use of an aromatase inhibitor for induction of ovulation in patients with an inadequate response to clomiphene citrate. *Fertil Steril* 2001;**75**:305–309.

63. Mitwally MF, Casper RF. Single-dose administration of an aromatase inhibitor for ovarian stimulation. *Fertil Steril* 2005;**83**:229–231.

64. Mitwally MF, Casper RF. Aromatase inhibition reduces the dose of gonadotropin required for controlled ovarian hyperstimulation. *J Soc Gynecol Investig* 2004;**11**:406–415.

65. Mitwally MF, Casper RF. Aromatase inhibition improves ovarian response to follicle-stimulating hormone in poor responders. *Fertil Steril* 2002;**77**:776–780.

66. Al-Omari WR, Sulaiman WR, Al-Hadithi N. Comparison of two aromatase inhibitors in women with clomiphene-resistant polycystic ovary syndrome. *Int J Gynaecol Obstet* 2004;**85**:289–291.

67. Fatemi HM, Kolibianakis E, Tournaye H, *et al.* Clomiphene citrate versus letrozole for ovarian stimulation: a pilot study. *Reprod Biomed Online* 2003;**7**:543–546.

68. Healey S, Tan SL, Tulandi T, Biljan MM. Effects of letrozole on superovulation with gonadotropins in women undergoing intrauterine insemination. *Fertil Steril* 2003;**80**:1325–1329.

69. Mason AJ, Berkemeier LM, Schmelzer CH, *et al.* Activin B: precursor sequences, genomic structure and in vitro activities. *Mol Endocrinol* 1989;**3**:1352–1358.

70. Roberts V, Meunier H, Vaughan J, *et al.* Production and regulation of inhibin subunits in pituitary gonadotropes. *Endocrinology* 1989;**124**:552–554.

71. Weil SJ, Vendola K, Zhou J, *et al.* Androgen receptor gene expression in the primate ovary: cellular localization, regulation, and functional correlations. *J Clin Endocrinol Metab* 1989;**837**:2479–2485.

72. Weil S, Vendola K, Zhou J, Bondy CA. Androgen and follicle-stimulating hormone interactions in primate ovarian follicle development. *J Clin Endocrinol Metab* 1999;**84**:2951–2956.

73. Vendola KA, Zhou J, Adesanya OO, Weil SJ, Bondy CA. Androgens stimulate early stages of follicular growth in the primate ovary. *J Clin Invest* 1998;**101**:2622–2629.

74. Vendola K, Zhou J, Wang J, *et al.* Androgens promote oocyte insulin-like growth factor I expression and initiation of follicle development in the primate ovary. *Biol Reprod* 1999;**61**:353–357.

75. Giudice LC. Insulin-like growth factors and ovarian follicular development. *Endocr Rev* 1992;**13**:641–669.

76. Package insert of letrozole Femara®.

77. Package insert of anastrozole Arimidex®.

78. Mitwally MF, Casper RF. Aromatase inhibitors in ovulation induction. *Semin Reprod Med* 2004;**22**:61–78.

79. Rubin GL, Zhao Y, Kalus AM, Simpson ER. Peroxisome proliferator-activated receptor gamma ligands inhibit estrogen biosynthesis in human breast adipose tissue: possible implications for breast cancer therapy. *Cancer Res* 2000;**60**:1604–1608.

80. Mitwally MF, Witchel SF, Casper RF. Troglitazone: a possible modulator of ovarian steroidogenesis. *J Soc Gynecol Investig* 2002;**9**:163–167.

81. Nirmala PB, Thampan RV. Ubiquitination of the rat uterine estrogen receptor: dependence on estradiol. *Biochem Biophys Res Commun* 1995;**213**:24–31.

82. Rosenfeld CR, Roy T, Cox BE. Mechanisms modulating estrogen-induced uterine vasodilation. *Vascul Pharmacol* 2002;**38**:115–125.

83. Vignali M, Infantino M, Matrone R, *et al.* Endometriosis: novel etiopathogenetic concepts and clinical perspectives. *Fertil Steril* 2002;**78**:665–678.

84. Oktay K, Buyuk E, Libertella N, Akar M, Rosenwaks Z. Fertility preservation in breast cancer patients: a prospective controlled comparison of ovarian stimulation with tamoxifen and letrozole for embryo cryopreservation. *J Clin Oncol* 2005;**23**:4347–4353.

85. Oktay K. Further evidence on the safety and success of ovarian stimulation with letrozole and tamoxifen in breast cancer patients undergoing in vitro fertilization to cryopreserve their embryos for fertility preservation. *J Clin Oncol* 2005;**23**:3858–3859.

86. Hamilton A, Piccart M. The third-generation non-steroidal aromatase inhibitors: a review of their clinical benefits in the second-line hormonal treatment of advanced breast cancer. *Ann Oncol* 1999;**10**:377–384.

87. Goss PE. Risks versus benefits in the clinical application of aromatase inhibitors. *Endocr Relat Cancer* 1999;**6**:325–332.

88. Mitwally MF, Biljan MM, Casper RF. Pregnancy outcome after the use of an aromatase inhibitor for ovarian stimulation. *Am J Obstet Gynecol* 2005;**192**:381–386.

89. Tulandi T, Al-Fadhli R, Kabli N, *et al.* Congenital malformations among 911 newborns conceived after infertility treatment with letrozole or clomiphene citrate. *Fertil Steril* 2006;**85**:1761–1765.

90. Hoffman JIE. Incidence of congenital heart disease: I. Postnatal incidence. *Pediatr Cardiol* 1995;**16**:103.

91. Badawy A, Shokeir T, Allam AF, Abdelhady H. Pregnancy outcome after ovulation induction with aromatase inhibitors or clomiphene citrate in unexplained infertility. *Acta Obstet Gynecol Scand* 2009;**88**:187–191.

92. Franik S, Eltrop SM, Kremer JA, Kiesel L, Farquhar C. Aromatase inhibitors (letrozole) for subfertile women with polycystic ovary syndrome. *Cochrane Database Syst Rev* 2018;**5**:CD010287. doi: 10.1002/14651858.CD010287.pub3.

93. Legro RS, Brzyski RG, Diamond MP, *et al.* Letrozole versus clomiphene for infertility in the polycystic ovary syndrome. *N Engl J Med* 2014;**371**:119–129.

Ovulation Induction for Anovulatory Patients

Evert J. P. van Santbrink and Bart C. J. M. Fauser

Introduction

The lack of ovulatory cycles may be considered as a major problem for women seeking pregnancy. This is reflected by the fact that about 20 percent of couples visiting a fertility clinic with an unfulfilled wish to conceive present with anovulation [1]. Clinical manifestation of anovulation is oligomenorrhea (intermenstrual period > 35 days) or amenorrhea (intermenstrual period > 6 months). Although ovulation may occur in oligomenorrhea, the longer the time period between menstruations the smaller the chance of that cycle being ovulatory. Classification of anovulatory patients may be performed using the criteria of the World Health Organization (WHO) as determined by Rowe et al. [2]. Criteria needed to classify patients are (1) serum prolactin in the normal range, (2) oligo- or amenorrhea, and (3) serum concentrations of follicle-stimulating hormone (FSH) and estradiol (E_2). In the near future, anti-Müllerian hormone (AMH) may be added.

In case of a hyperprolactinemia, a macroprolactinoma should be ruled out by a MRI scan of the sella turcica, and hyperprolactinemia should be treated with a dopamine agonist. In case of normoprolactinemia or when the oligo- or amenorrhea persists after correction of the hyperprolactinemia, these patients may be classified according to WHO criteria as follows: (WHO_1) hypogonadotropic, hypoestrogenic status; (WHO_2) normogonadotropic, normoestrogenic status; or (WHO_3) hypergonadotropic, hypoestrogenic status. The vast majority of these patients, the WHO_2 group, appear to be a very heterogeneous population in which – besides anovulation – obesity, biochemical, or clinical hyperandrogenism (alopecia, acne, or hirsutism) and insulin resistance play an important role. A large subgroup of the WHO_2 population fulfills criteria of polycystic ovary syndrome (PCOS). The prevalence of PCOS depends on the criteria used [3]. The syndrome was formerly known as the Stein–Leventhal syndrome [4] and more recently, criteria of the National Institute of Health (NIH) were replaced by criteria of the currently internationally accepted Rotterdam consensus meeting on PCOS [5–7]. According to this consensus, after exclusion of related disorders (Cushing syndrome, congenital adrenal hyperplasia, and hyperprolactinemia), PCOS is defined as having two out of three of the following disorders: (1) oligo- or anovulation, (2) clinical and/or biochemical signs of hyperandrogenemia, and (3) polycystic ovaries on ultrasound. It has to be noticed that the Rotterdam criteria, rather than replacing the NIH criteria, just broadened the definition of PCOS. Patients with hyperandrogenemia and polycystic ovaries (without ovulation disorders) and patients with polycystic ovaries and ovulation disorders (without hyperandrogenism) may also now be included in PCOS diagnosis (Figure 2.1). Debate is still going on about which phenotype belongs to PCOS and which phenotype does not [8;9]. This will possibly end when genotyping of PCOS becomes possible.

Interventions

Restoring normal physiology is the aim of primary treatment in patients presenting with infertility and chronic anovulation, that is, selection of a single dominant follicle followed by mono-ovulation [10]. This treatment process is generally referred to as "ovulation induction." Alternative protocols for ovarian stimulation used in fertility treatment are (controlled) ovarian hyperstimulation as used for intrauterine insemination (IUI) or in vitro fertilization (IVF). These treatment protocols are aiming at the development of multiple follicles instead of a single dominant follicle, and thereby intentionally result in a non-physiological condition.

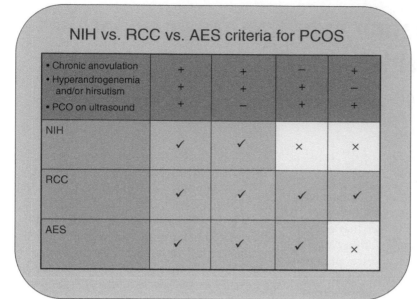

NIH vs. RCC vs. AES criteria for PCOS

• Chronic anovulation	+	+	–	+
• Hyperandrogenemia and/or hirsutism	+	+	+	–
• PCO on ultrasound	+	–	+	+
NIH	✓	✓	×	×
RCC	✓	✓	✓	✓
AES	✓	✓	✓	×

Figure 2.1 Comparison of possible combinations of patient characteristics (chronic anovulation, hyperandrogenemia and/or hirsutism, polycystic ovaries on ultrasound) defining polycystic ovary syndrome (PCOS) according to criteria of the NIH [5], the ASRM/ESHRE Rotterdam consensus criteria (RCC) [6;7], and the Androgen Excess Society (AES) taskforce [8]. A tick indicates the diagnosis of PCOS to be justified according to the definition, a cross not.

Anovulation may be considered an absolute factor to prevent pregnancy. Treatment results may be expected to be very good when normo-ovulatory cycles are restored, in the absence of concomitant fertility problems.

The majority of anovulatory patients (about 80%) will have normal serum concentrations of E_2 and FSH and a small proportion (approximately 10%) decreased concentrations of both hormones (WHO_2 and WHO_1, respectively according to the WHO classification) [2]. Treatment options in these two groups are different and will be discussed separately. The remaining group (approximately 10%) may be classified as WHO_3 and present with elevated FSH combined with decreased E_2 concentrations, resulting in anovulation caused by (imminent) ovarian failure. Whereas ovulation induction can be regarded as a useful treatment option in the WHO_1 (hypogonadotropic hypoestrogenic anovulatory patients) and WHO_2 (normogonadotropic normoestrogenic anovulatory patients) populations, treatment options in the WHO_3 group (hypergonadotropic hypoestrogenic anovulatory patients) are limited to oocyte donation combined with IVF or adoption programs.

Lifestyle Interventions

Individual risk identification in fertility patients with menstrual cycle disturbances may be performed before any treatment initiation by preconceptional counseling of the couple. This will make it possible to decrease individual risk factors prior to treatment initiation. Additional to the most well-known risk factor in the WHO_2 population (the largest subgroup in this population), that is, central obesity, other important issues for counseling may be smoking, exercise, and diet.

Overweight reduction – Besides chronic anovulation, the WHO_2 patient group may be characterized by chemical (increased serum concentrations of testosterone and androstenedione) or/and clinical (hirsutism, acne, and alopecia) hyperandrogenism, insulin resistance, and obesity. In particular central obesity is correlated with insulin resistance and hyperandrogenism, and approximately 50% of all PCOS patients have a body mass index (BMI = weight/length^2) above 25 kg/m^2 [11;12].

While the prevalence of obesity is rapidly increasing in all industrialized countries, this may be considered as a major and increasingly important problem. Obesity has been correlated not only with diminished chances (Figure 2.2) for both natural and assisted conception [13;14], but also with increased rates of miscarriage [15], congenital abnormalities, gestational diabetes, pregnancy-induced hypertension, stillbirth, and maternal mortality [16;17]. Apart from this,

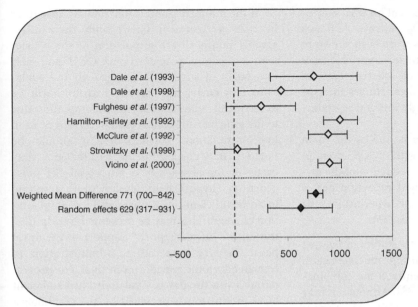

Figure 2.2 Association measure between obesity and total amount of gonadotrophins administered (IU) for ovulation induction in normogonadotrophic anovulatory infertility (median and 95% confidence interval). The weighted mean difference (WMD) was generated using inverse variance weighting. This material was originally published in [89], and has been reproduced by permission of Oxford University Press.

long-term health risks such as type 2 diabetes and cardiovascular disease may be increased [14;18].

Weight reduction in a lifestyle modification program has been reported to normalize the endocrine milieu and may result in improvement of insulin sensitivity and decreased androgen excess. Therefore, a limited but permanent weight reduction may not only lead to a return of regular spontaneous ovulation and pregnancy [19–21], but may also improve quality of life regarding long-term health risks. Many treatment strategies of obesity are recommended: behavioral counseling, lifestyle therapy, pharmacological treatment, and bariatric surgery [22]. Unfortunately, there are no properly designed studies supporting one strategy above the other in respect of infertility treatment. For long-term weight improvement, bariatric surgery may be preferable [23], but lifestyle modification combined with pharmacological intervention may also be very effective [24]. It should be considered that all these interventions may be potentially harmful for the pregnancy and therefore conducted prior to the pregnancy.

In the literature it is suggested that all obese women (BMI > 35 kg/m^2) seeking pregnancy should be denied any form of fertility treatment until limited (5–10 percent) weight reduction has been achieved. Non-hormonal contraception may be advised during the weight loss period until the

critical weight has been reached, because pregnancy would be unfavorable during this period [25;26].

Stop smoking – Although cumulative data on the influence of cigarette smoking on female fecundity generally conclude an adverse impact, these studies are observational cohort studies in diverse populations introducing potential bias. It is suggested that smoking induces accelerated follicular depletion, reflected by increased mean FSH serum concentrations in young smokers versus non-smokers [27–29]. This may result in early onset of menopause, which is supported by a large population-based cohort study [30]. Although the FSH requirement for ovarian stimulation in smokers may be increased, ovarian response to stimulation and pregnancy chances may not be impaired [31]. Smoking may also increase the risk of spontaneous abortion [32] and ectopic pregnancy [33]. In conclusion, there may be growing evidence for adverse effects of cigarette smoking on ovarian function and reproductive outcome, and this may justify healthcare professionals to encourage patients in this field to stop smoking before fertility treatment is started.

Diet restriction – Generally the focus of dietary intervention in studies with WHO$_2$ patients is energy restriction rather than dietary composition.

However, there is little agreement on what may be the optimal diet for WHO$_2$ patients. Although a range of dietary approaches has been shown to be effective, only two randomized controlled trials have compared the effect of different diets in WHO$_2$ patients [34;35]. In these studies the type of diet did not influence weight loss and reproductive outcome separately.

While insulin resistance is one of the main characteristics in women with PCOS, even in women with normal weight, reduction of the glycemic load rather than weight reduction per se may be beneficial in alleviating hyperinsulinemia and its metabolic consequences [36].

Exercise – There are not many studies evaluating the role of exercise alone on reproductive health but several studies have examined the combination of diet and exercise [37;38]. Although it may be clear that regular physical activity is important in weight loss programs because it is associated with better long-term weight loss maintenance [39], the contribution of exercise to weight loss alone in regaining menstrual cyclicity is still unclear.

Pharmacological Interventions

Hypogonadotropic Anovulation (WHO$_1$)

In hypogonadotropic hypoestrogenic patients anovulation results from a hypothalamic or pituitary problem. A gonadotropin-releasing hormone (GnRH) stimulation test may help to distinguish between the origin of the problem; administration of GnRH agonist will cause only an increase in serum gonadotropins if the pituitary gland is functional. In case the anovulation is caused by extreme weight loss, the primary goal will be to restore the normal weight that will most likely result in the return of a regular ovulatory cycle [40]. Alternatively, ovulation induction in the WHO$_1$ patient group with a functional pituitary gland may be achieved using a pulsatile GnRH-agonist pump. It is remarkable that continuous GnRH agonist administration results in pituitary "downregulation" as used in IVF procedures to prevent a premature luteinizing hormone (LH) rise [41], while pulsatile GnRH agonist administration may restore an ovulatory cycle leaving the physiological feedback loop intact.

If the pituitary gland is functionally absent, or in case of treatment failure with the GnRH-agonist pump, direct stimulation of the ovaries with exogenous gonadotropins (FSH and LH) may result in ongoing follicle growth and ovulation. Obviously, the only FSH around will be exogenously administered and accumulation due to the long half-life could result in serious ovarian hyperstimulation. Furthermore, it should be noted that a corpus luteum insufficiency may occur in the absence of a functional LH pulse generator (hypothalamic dysfunction), resulting in an insufficient luteal phase and low implantation chances. This may be prevented by administration of "luteal support." Support of the luteal phase may be achieved by administration of human chorionic gonadotropin (hCG) or progesterone from the day of ovulation until sufficient hCG production is provided by the trophoblast cells to rescue the corpus luteum [42].

Normogonadotropic Anovulation (WHO$_2$)
Aromatase Inhibitors

Aromatase inhibitors – Introduction: Aromatase inhibitors have been used over the past decades for the treatment of breast cancer and only recently they were introduced for ovulation induction [43]. The advantage over clomiphene (clomifene) citrate (CC) of this compound could be the lack of antiestrogenic effects on target organs such as the endometrium and cervical mucus. Compounds used for ovulation induction are merely letrozole but also less frequently anastrozole. Recommendation from the *2018 international evidence-based guideline on PCOS* proposes to consider letrozole as first-line treatment because significantly higher ovulation, pregnancy, and live birth rates were reported compared with CC [44]. Notably, differences in study population characteristics such as obesity (US population) and therapy naivety could have substantial impact on these outcomes.

Working mechanism: Inhibition of aromatase activity in the granulosa cells prevents conversion of androgens into estrogens and thereby inhibits negative feedback on the hypothalamic–pituitary level [45].

Treatment schedule: After a spontaneous or progestogen-induced withdrawal bleeding, letrozole is generally started on day 3 and continued for 5 days with a daily dose of 2.5 mg/day. In case of persistent anovulation the dose may be increased in two steps from 5 mg/day to a maximum of 7.5 mg/day.

Complications: Initially, potential fetal toxicity was reported for letrozole [46] resulting in an official warning by the producer (Novartis Pharmaceuticals) not to use letrozole for ovulation induction. Subsequently, these findings could not be reproduced in a larger patient group [47;48], a recent systemic review and meta-analysis failed to note an increased congenital anomaly rate either for letrozole or CC (prevalence < 5%) [49] in this specific population. Multiple pregnancy rates and ovarian hyperstimulation syndrome (OHSS) rates are reported to be comparable to those of CC [44]. Side effects reported are gastrointestinal disturbances, hot flushes, headaches, and back pain.

In conclusion, there is current evidence to recommend on the clinical use of aromatase inhibitors as routine first-line ovulation induction in WHO$_2$ patients [44]. Regarding to safety there is no evidence for increased potential fetal toxicity of letrozole compared with CC or the background risk in this population. It has to be noted that in many countries letrozole has no registration for use as an ovulation induction agent (off-label use) so patients should be informed before application.

Antiestrogens

Clomiphene citrate – Introduction: First-line treatment of WHO$_2$ anovulation has traditionally been performed with antiestrogens since the early 1960s [50] because these are effective, safe, patient friendly, and cheap. Meanwhile, there is evidence that letrozole may have better treatment outcome compared with CC as first-line treatment in WHO$_2$ anovulation [44] (Table 2.1).

Working mechanism: Clomiphene citrate is a non-selective E$_2$ receptor antagonist and interferes with endogenous estrogen feedback at the hypothalamic–pituitary level. This results in enhanced gonadotropin release by the pituitary gland and ovarian stimulation.

Treatment schedule: Clomiphene citrate is generally started on day 3 after a spontaneous or progestogen-induced withdrawal bleeding, and continued for 5 days with a dose of 50 mg/day. In case of persistent anovulation the dose may be increased in two steps to a maximum of 150 mg/day. Several studies reported effect of the chosen

starting day: when CC treatment was started on day 5 rather than day 1, this resulted in a decreased ovulation and pregnancy rate [51]. There is no additional value in adding metformin [52;53] or dexamethasone [54] as primary therapy to CC.

Treatment results: In approximately 80 percent of treated patients restoration of ovulation will occur and cumulative live birth rates reported vary between 40 and 60 percent [55;56]. Most pregnancies will occur in the first 6 ovulatory cycles and after 12 cycles pregnancy is unlikely [55]. Until now, CC is generally accepted as the most adequate first-line treatment in normogonadotropic anovulation.

Complications: Hot flushes and nausea are reported side effects. Development of multiple follicles has been reported, often resulting in a multiple pregnancy rate between 2 and 13 percent. Severe OHSS has not been reported following CC treatment [57]. The use of CC longer than 12 months has been reported as a possible increased risk factor for ovarian cancer and, combined with decreased pregnancy chances after this period, this may result in a recommendation not to use this drug for longer than 12 months [58].

Tamoxifen – Introduction: Tamoxifen (TMX) acts comparable to CC but is less popular in ovulation induction; a possible advantage over CC may be a less antiestrogenic effect on the endometrium and cervical mucus [59]. However, TMX is not licensed for the indication ovulation induction.

Working mechanism: Tamoxifen is a non-selective estrogen receptor modulator. Like CC it was initially developed for the treatment of breast cancer, but has been used for ovulation induction for many years.

Treatment schedule: Tamoxifen is generally started on day 3 after a spontaneous or progestogen-induced withdrawal bleeding, and continued for 5 days with a dose of 20 mg/day. In case of persistent anovulation the dose may be increased in two steps to a maximum of 60 mg/day.

Treatment results: Comparison of the efficacy of CC and TMX (prospective randomized trial) in 86 normogonadotropic anovulatory patients reported no significant differences in ovulation and pregnancy rates [60].

Complications: No specific complications are reported, but TMX may be comparable to CC.

Gonadotropins

Gonadotropins – Introduction: Patients remaining anovulatory or failing to conceive after being treated with first-line treatment modalities are generally treated with gonadotropins. The gonadotropins, LH and FSH, have been available for ovarian stimulation since the early 1960s. Initially, gonadotropins were extracted from urine of postmenopausal women (human menopausal gonadotropin [hMG]) in a 1:1 ratio of LH:FSH. Later on, non-active proteins were removed resulting in highly purified urinary preparations. Because this extraction process required enormous amounts of postmenopausal urine and the demands for gonadotropins were increasing, the possibilities to guarantee a consistent supply of the medication worldwide were compromised. This problem was solved in the 1990s, when recombinant DNA technology enabled the possibility to produce human FSH in Chinese hamster ovary cell lines. Moreover, these recombinant preparations offer improved purity and consistency. The batch-to-batch variation was also limited by using protein weight instead of bioactivity to determine the amount of active protein per unit. As a result, recombinant instead of urinary gonadotropins have been preferably used for ovulation induction during the last decade, although treatment results comparing urinary and recombinant FSH may be considered comparable [61].

Working mechanism: Direct stimulation of follicle growth in the ovary. In the ovarian theca cell, LH promotes conversion of cholesterol to androstenedione and testosterone, while subsequently FSH induces aromatization of these androgens in the ovarian granulosa cells to estrone and E_2. Both hormones are required for adequate follicle growth, although in WHO_2 patients small amounts of endogenous LH are sufficient to facilitate follicle development with exogenous FSH.

Treatment schedule: There are mainly two approaches in treatment regimens. The "step-up" protocol is aimed at increasing the initial low FSH dose (37.5–50.0 IU/day) by small increments (37.5–50.0 IU/day), until finally the FSH threshold is surpassed, resulting in ongoing follicle growth and ovulation. In contrast, the "step-down" protocol is aimed at a starting dose of FSH that equals the response dose and will thereby instantly cause ongoing follicle growth [62]. From that point, the daily FSH dose may be decreased (37.5–50.0 IU) every 3 days resulting in the development of a single dominant follicle.

While the step-down protocol mimics the physiological serum FSH profile more closely and dominant follicle growth is established more quickly, the step-up protocol results in less ovarian hyper-response and preliminary cancellation of stimulation [62;63]. To solve this dilemma and to determine the individual FSH response dose, a dose-finding step-up cycle can be used and consecutive treatment cycles may be performed according to the step-down protocol, unless the starting dose equals the response dose. In that case, a fixed-dose regimen can be used [64].

Urinary or recombinant hCG can be used to trigger ovulation when at least one follicle with a diameter of 16 mm is present. Stimulation may be canceled when more than three follicles > 12 mm in diameter are present.

Treatment results: Cumulative ovulation rate of 82%, ongoing pregnancy rate of 58%, single live birth rate of 43%, and multiple birth rate of 5% [65].

Complications: Although the overall multiple pregnancy rates after gonadotropin ovulation induction seem to be acceptable, the contribution of ovulation induction to higher-order multiple pregnancies is substantial [66]. Chances for OHSS and multiple pregnancy after gonadotropin ovulation induction are related to frequent monitoring and strict cancellation criteria [67]. To prevent multiple pregnancy, supernumerary follicles may be removed using transvaginal ultrasound-guided aspiration [68].

Insulin Sensitizers

Insulin sensitizers – Introduction: Available insulin sensitizers are metformin (a biguanide), pioglitazone/rosiglitazone (thiazolidinediones), and inositol (hydroxycyclohexane). Metformin reduces hepatic gluconeogenesis and insulin concentrations, while the thiazolidinediones enhance glucose uptake in adipose and muscle tissue and decrease hepatic glucose output, and inositol increases the insulin signal in the intracellular milieu. Insulin sensitizers are currently used to treat patients with diabetes, and, since it is generally accepted that insulin resistance plays an important role in the pathogenesis of normogonadotropic anovulation [6;7], there is considerable interest for their use in this group. The concomitant hyperandrogenism in PCOS patients may be explained by the fact that hyperinsulinemia increases ovarian androgen production and decreases sex hormone-binding globulin (SHBG) serum concentrations, resulting in an increased bioavailability of androgens [69]. Moreover, hyperinsulinemia promotes an estrogen hyper-response on ovarian FSH stimulation that induces an early FSH drop [70]. This may cause follicle growth arrest in the early follicular phase and the classic polycystic image of the ovaries on ultrasound. As obese patients benefit from insulin sensitizers most in ovulation induction, it may be important to realize that weight reduction by lifestyle modification is a primary solution for this problem and insulin sensitizers alone will not cause weight reduction [71;72].

Metformin – Working mechanism: Insulin sensitizers are reported to restore the endocrine milieu: lowering insulin resistance and hyperandrogenism may normalize ovarian FSH responsiveness and thereby promote restoration of ovulatory cycles [70].

Treatment schedule: Metformin is started in a daily dose of 2–3 × 500 mg to a maximum daily dose of 2000 mg.

Treatment results: First-line treatment with metformin is not superior to CC [52;53;71], neither is combined use of metformin and CC. In contrast, in second-line treatment of patients presenting with CC-resistant anovulation and especially when more overweight, additional metformin to CC is reported to result in increased ovulation rate [53;73]. In conclusion, metformin may be considered as second-line addition to CC, especially in patients with obesity. Therefore, the use of metformin should be restricted to patients with glucose intolerance or to specific patient subgroups that may benefit from its use in ovulation induction [73]. With regard to the thiazolidinediones, no conclusive data are available to suggest any advantage over metformin and therefore they should not be applied in this patient group to restore ovulatory cycles [73;74].

Complications: Common side effects are gastrointestinal complaints: nausea, vomiting, and diarrhea; these will diminish when metformin is used for a longer period. A very rare but more serious complication is lactic acidosis, only reported in patients with comorbidity (renal insufficiency, liver disease, or congestive heart failure). Metformin may reduce risk of gestational diabetes and it may be safe using it during pregnancy [75], but convincing evidence is lacking. Always discuss with patients that metformin is not licensed to be used for ovulation induction.

Pioglitazone/rosiglitazone: There is currently too little evidence to draw conclusions regarding the effectiveness of these compounds [73].

Inositol – Introduction: Inositol is a nutritional supplement that plays a role in insulin signaling. In this way it may be used to treat insulin resistance in PCOS patients.

Working mechanism: Inositol is a second messenger for insulin signal transduction; it enhances the intracellular insulin signal and may thereby decrease insulin resistance.

Treatment schedule: daily 2–4 g inositol (myo-inositol or D-chiro-inositol)

Treatment results: Although few published results there may be an advantage of inositol use in PCOS patients regarding hormonal profile, return of menstrual cyclicity and ovulation frequency, no data were reported on live birth and miscarriage rate [76].

Conclusion: There is currently insufficient evidence to use inositol as a regular treatment supplement in PCOS patients [73].

Surgical Intervention: Laparoscopic Electrocoagulation of the Ovaries (LEO)

The most classic intervention in the treatment of polycystic ovaries is ovarian wedge resection by laparotomy [77]. When, in the 1960s, ovulation-inducing drugs (i.e., CC and urinary gonadotropins) became available for clinical use [50;78] the laparotomic ovarian wedge resection became less popular, due to the serious adverse effects such as adhesions and loss of healthy ovarian tissue. As treatment results of ovulation induction with these drugs did not further improve, alternative treatment modalities were introduced. In the 1980s, this included a modern reintroduction of the wedge resection [79]: laparoscopic ovarian drilling of the ovarian surface. The ovarian surface is perforated using electrocautery or laser treatment [80]. By drilling small holes in the ovarian cortex the circulating serum androgen concentration is lowered and this may result in restoration of ovulation. Although the technique is theoretically not fully understood, it can be rather effective [81]. Recently, unilateral drilling has been demonstrated to be as successful as bilateral drilling but less time-consuming [82]. In CC-resistant PCOS patients cumulative pregnancy rate, live birth rate, and abortion rate with LEO are comparable with gonadotropin therapy, and multiple pregnancy rate was significantly decreased. Potential drawbacks regarding LEO are, besides the usual risks of laparoscopic surgery and general anesthesia, intra-abdominal adhesion formation [83] and potential accelerated decline of ovarian reserve [84].

Results

It should be recognized that ovulation induction is restricted to patients presenting with infertility and chronic anovulation while it aims at restoring physiology. Traditionally, ovulation induction treatment in normogonadotropic anovulation was started with an antiestrogen (CC), and, in case of treatment failure or absence of conception, this was followed by exogenous FSH. Treatment outcome of this sequence was rather successful: a cumulative pregnancy rate resulting in singleton live birth after 24 months of follow-up was 71 percent (Figure 2.3).

In recent years evidence built up that aromatase inhibitors are more effective as first-line treatment for ovulation induction compared to clomiphene with regard to ovulation and live birth rate (Table 2.1).

Over the years, the mechanism used for ovulation induction shifted from increasing the FSH serum concentration in order to "surpass the FSH threshold" (antiestrogens, aromatase inhibitors, exogenous FSH) to improvement of the preconceptional milieu resulting in enhanced ovarian responsiveness to FSH (lifestyle modification, insulin sensitizers, LEO) and a more optimal

Table 2.1 Comparison of letrozole and clomiphene treatment results, both as first-line ovulation induction agent in WHO_2 anovulation [90].

	Clomiphene	Letrozole	OR
Cum ovulation rate	77%	75%	NS
Cum pregnancy rate	26.4%	35.9%	1.56 (1.37–1.78)
Live birth rate	21.4%	31.4%	1.68 (1.42–1.99)
Miscarriage rate	20%	19%	0.94 (0.43–1.24)
Mult. pregnancy rate	1.7%	1.3%	0.73 (0.43–1.24)

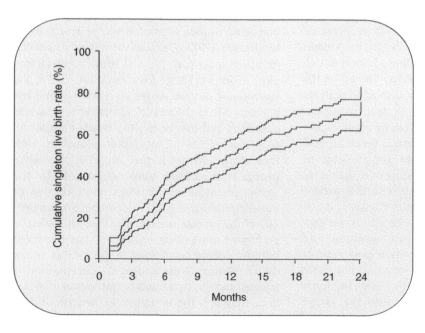

Figure 2.3 Cumulative singleton live birth rate of 71% with a 95% confidence interval after a 24-month follow-up period in the classical ovulation induction algorithm (clomiphene citrate followed by exogenous FSH in case of treatment failure) in 240 normogonadotropic anovulatory infertile patients. From Eijkemans et al. (2003), with permission [91].

environment for the embryo to implant and develop (pituitary downregulation in endometriosis, hydrosalpingectomy). Moreover, attempts to improve the treatment results were previously focused on modifying the compounds (CC vs. TMX, urinary vs. recombinant FSH) and improve treatment protocols (low-dose step-up vs. low-dose step-down protocols). Nowadays, this is more and more combined with attempts to improve local circumstances (the endocrine milieu) aiming at decreasing insulin resistance, hyperandrogenism, and embryotoxic factors.

This could enable an individualized treatment schedule in a patient-tailored way: for every patient an optimal effective treatment plan based on specific individual characteristics. Unfortunately, subgroups of patients that may benefit certain strategies have not clearly been identified yet [64]. Until recently, attempts to identify these subgroups were performed based on specific patient characteristics (Figure 2.4). Nowadays, the increased knowledge and availability of genetic profiles involved in ovulation induction may be helpful to accelerate the identification process and will improve the differentiation for individual patients [85].

Complications

The most serious complications resulting from ovulation induction are caused by the limited control of follicular development. In aromatase inhibitor and antiestrogen treatment, multifollicular development is regularly reported but reported multiple pregnancy rate is low, 2–13 percent. Severe OHSS has not been reported following CC treatment [57]. In FSH ovulation induction, the extended half-life of FSH makes it hard to predict how many follicles are actually reaching the dominant status, and sometimes daily ovarian ultrasound monitoring is

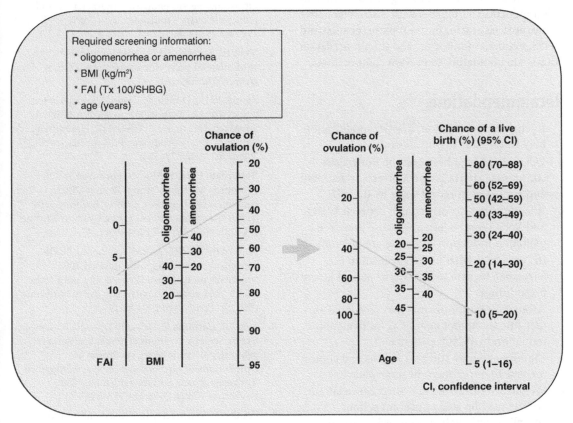

Figure 2.4 A nomogram predicting chances for ovulation and live birth after CC treatment based on initial screening parameters. Sloping lines are examples how to use this nomogram: patient 1 with an FAI of 7, amenorrhea and BMI of 40 kg/m² has a chance of ovulation during CC treatment of 36%. Patient 2, age 35 years has an 11% chance of live birth during CC treatment. From Imani *et al.* (2002), with permission [92].

required to adjust the treatment dosage before multifollicular development is a fact. This may result in daily hospital visits and increased patient inconvenience.

An alternative way to monitor follicle development during ovulation induction may be measurement of circulating E_2. The ASRM Practice Committee recommends caution when serum E_2 is rising rapidly or exceeds 2500 pg/ml [86]. However, in another publication a much lower threshold of 1000 pg/ml is recommended [87]. In regard to the aim of ovulation induction, that is, single follicle development, the 1000 pg/ml threshold may be a more realistic cancellation criterion.

In case of imminent ovarian hyperstimulation the treatment cycle is canceled. Advised criteria for cancellation to prevent multiple pregnancy and OHSS were in previous studies more than three follicles ≥ 16 mm [88]. Recently, criteria proposed were far more strict: no more than three follicles ≥ 10 mm [87].

It may be concluded that in gonadotropin ovulation induction all follicles with a diameter above 10 mm are a risk factor for multiple pregnancy, and OHSS, frequent monitoring, and strict cancellation criteria are mandatory to prevent complications.

Recommendations

- In chronic anovulation, lifestyle modification may be the first step to success
- PCOS diagnosed based on the Rotterdam consensus criteria is now universally accepted and endorsed in recent years by the NIH
- It is important to distinguish between WHO_1 and WHO_2 anovulation, because preferred ovulation induction strategies are different
- In case of off-label use of medication (i.e., letrozole), be sure to inform the patient before prescription
- Aromatase inhibitors may be considered as first-line treatment above CC for ovulation induction in WHO_2 patients
- Clomiphene may still be a safe second choice for first-line treatment in some patients
- Frequent monitoring and strict cancellation criteria may be able to prevent serious complications such as high-order multiple pregnancy and OHSS in ovulation induction, especially while using gonadotropins

- Attempts to improve outcome of ovulation induction have shifted from modification of the compound or treatment regimen to enhancement of local circumstances, aiming at decreasing insulin resistance, hyperandrogenism, and embryotoxic factors
- Increased availability of genetic profiles will be helpful to accomplish a more patient-tailored approach by identification of beneficial subgroups for certain interventions

References

1. Balen AH, Rutherford AJ. Managing anovulatory infertility and polycystic ovary syndrome. *BMJ* 2007;**335**:663–666.

2. Rowe PJ, Combaire FH, Hargreave TB, *et al.* *WHO Manual for the Standardized Investigation and Diagnosis of the Infertile Couple.* Cambridge, Mass.: Cambridge University Press; 2001.

3. Van Santbrink EJ, Hop WC, Fauser BC. Classification of nomogonadotrophic anovulatory infertility: polycystic ovaries diagnosed by ultrasound versus endocrine characteristics of polycystic ovary syndrome. *Fertil Steril* 1997;**67**:453–458.

4. Stein IF, Leventhal ML. Amenorrhea associated with bilateral polycystic ovaries. *Am J Obstet Gynecol* 1935;**29**:181–191.

5. Zawadski JK, Dunaif A. Diagnostic criteria for polycystic ovary syndrome: towards a rational approach. In: Dunaif A, Givens JR, Haseltine F, eds. *Polycystic Ovary Syndrome.* Boston: Blackwell Scientific; 1992:377–384.

6. Rotterdam ESHRE/ASRM-Sponsored PCOS consensus workshop group. Revised 2003 consensus on diagnostic criteria and long-term health risks related to polycystic ovary syndrome (PCOS). *Hum Reprod* 2004;**19**:41–47.

7. Rotterdam ESHRE/ASRM-Sponsored PCOS consensus workshop group. Revised 2003 consensus on diagnostic criteria and long-term health risks related to polycystic ovary syndrome (PCOS). *Fertil Steril* 2004;**81**:19–25.

8. Azziz R, Carmina E, Dewailly D, *et al.*; Androgen Excess Society. Positions statement: criteria for defining polycystic ovary syndrome as a predominantly hyperandrogenic syndrome: an Androgen Excess Society guideline. *J Clin Endocrinol Metab* 2006;**91**:4237–4245.

9. Franks S. Controversy in clinical endocrinology: diagnosis of polycystic ovarian syndrome: in defense of the Rotterdam criteria. *J Clin Endocrinol Metab* 2006;**91**:786–789.

10. ESHRE Capri Workshop Group. Mono-ovulatory cycles: a key goal in profertility programmes. *Hum Reprod Update* 2003;**9**:263–274.

11. Kiddy DS, Sharp PS, White DM, *et al.* Differences in clinical and endocrine features between obese and non-obese subjects with polycystic ovary syndrome: an analysis of 263 consecutive cases. *Clin Endocrinol (Oxf)* 1990;**32**:213–220.

12. Franks S, Kiddy D, Sharp P, *et al.* Obesity and polycystic ovary syndrome. *Ann N Y Acad Sci* 1991;**626**:201–206.

13. Rich-Edwards JW, Spiegelman D, Garland M, *et al.* Physical activity, body mass index, and ovulatory disorder infertility. *Epidemiology* 2002;**13**:184–190.

14. Norman RJ, Davies MJ, Lord J, Moran LJ. The role of lifestyle modification in polycystic ovary syndrome. *Trends Endocrinol Metab* 2002;**13**:251–257.

15. Wang JX, Davies MJ, Norman RJ. Obesity increases the risk of spontaneous abortion during infertility treatment. *Obes Res* 2002;**10**:551–554.

16. Dietl J. Maternal obesity and complications during pregnancy. *J Perinat Med* 2005;**33**:100–105.

17. Boomsma CM, Fauser BC, Macklon NS. Pregnancy complications in women with polycystic ovary syndrome. *Semin Reprod Med* 2008;**26**:72–84.

18. Valkenburg O, Steegers-Theunissen RP, Smedts HP, *et al.* A more atherogenic serum lipoprotein profile is present in women with polycystic ovary syndrome: a case-control study. *J Clin Endocrinol Metab* 2008;**93**:470–476.

19. Kiddy DS, Hamilton-Fairley D, Bush A, *et al.* Improvement in endocrine and ovarian function during dietary treatment of obese women with polycystic ovary syndrome. *Clin Endocrinol (Oxf)* 1992;**36**:105–111.

20. Clark AM, Thornley B, Tomlinson L, Galletley C, Norman RJ. Weight loss in obese infertile women results in improvement in reproductive outcome for all forms of fertility treatment. *Hum Reprod* 1998;**13**:1502–1505.

21. Hoeger KM. Role of lifestyle modification in the management of polycystic ovary syndrome. *Best Pract Res Clin Endocrinol Metab* 2006;**20**:293–310.

22. Yanovski SZ, Yanovski JA. Obesity. *N Engl J Med* 2002;**346**:591–602.

23. Sjöström L, Lindroos AK, Peltonen M, *et al.*; Swedish Obese Subjects Study Scientific Group. Lifestyle, diabetes, and cardiovascular risk factors 10 years after bariatric surgery. *N Engl J Med* 2004;**351**:2683–2693.

24. Wadden TA, Berkowitz RI, Womble LG, *et al.* Randomized trial of lifestyle modification and pharmacotherapy for obesity. *N Engl J Med* 2005;**353**:2111–2120.

25. Balen AH, Dresner M, Scott EM, *et al.* Should obese women with polycystic ovary syndrome receive treatment for infertility? *BMJ* 2006;**332**:434–435.

26. Nelson SM, Fleming RF. The preconceptual contraception paradigm: obesity and infertility. *Hum Reprod* 2007;**22**:912–915.

27. Cooper GS, Baird DD, Hulka BS, *et al.* Follicle-stimulating hormone concentrations in relation to active and passive smoking. *Obstet Gynecol* 1995;**85**:407–411.

28. El-Nemr A, Al-Shawaf T, Sabatini L, *et al.* Effect of smoking on ovarian reserve and ovarian stimulation in in-vitro fertilization and embryo transfer. *Hum Reprod* 1998;**13**:2192–2198.

29. Freour T, Masson D, Mirallie S, *et al.* Active smoking compromises IVF outcome and affects ovarian reserve. *Reprod Biomed Online* 2008;**16**:96–102.

30. Sammel MD, Freeman EW, Liu Z, Lin H, Guo W. Factors that influence entry into stages of the menopausal transition. *Menopause* 2009;**16**:1218–1227.

31. Sharara FI, Beatse SN, Leonardi MR, *et al.* Cigarette smoking accelerates the development of diminished ovarian reserve as evidenced by the CC challenge test. *Fertil Steril* 1995;**62**:257–262.

32. Winter E, Wang J, Davies MJ, Norman R. Early pregnancy loss following assisted reproductive technology treatment. *Hum Reprod* 2002;**17**:3220–3223.

33. Saraiya M, Berg CJ, Kendrick JS, *et al.* Cigarette smoking as a risk factor for ectopic pregnancy. *Am J Obstet Gynecol* 1998;**178**:493–498.

34. Moran LJ, Noakes M, Clifton PM, *et al.* Dietary composition in restoring reproductive and metabolic physiology in overweight women with polycystic ovary syndrome. *J Clin Endocrinol Metab* 2003;**88**:812–819.

35. Stamets K, Taylor DS, Kunselman A, *et al.* A randomized trial of the effects of two types of short-term hypocaloric diets on weight loss in women with polycystic ovary syndrome. *Fertil Steril* 2004;**81**:630–637.

36. Reaven GM. The insulin resistance syndrome: definition and dietary approaches to treatment. *Annu Rev Nutr* 2005;**25**:391–406.

37. Crosignani PG, Colombo M, Vegetti W, *et al.* Overweight and obese anovulatory patients with

polycystic ovaries: parallel improvements in anthropometric indices, ovarian physiology and fertility rate induced by diet. *Hum Reprod* 2003;**18**:1928–1932.

38. Moran LJ, Brinkworth G, Noakes M, Norman RJ. Effects of lifestyle modification in polycystic ovarian syndrome. *Reprod Biomed Online* 2006;**12**:569–578.

39. Knowler WC, Barrett-Connor E, Fowler SE, *et al.*; Diabetes Prevention Program Research Group. Reduction in the incidence of type 2 diabetes with lifestyle intervention or metformin. *N Engl J Med* 2002;**346**:393–403.

40. Wiksten-Almströmer M, Hirschberg AL, Hagenfeldt K. Prospective follow-up of menstrual disorders in adolescence and prognostic factors. *Acta Obstet Gynecol Scand* 2008;**87**:1162–1168.

41. Filicori M. Gonadotrophin-releasing hormone agonists. A guide to use and selection. *Drugs* 1994;**48**:41–58.

42. Beckers NG, Platteau P, Eijkemans MJ, *et al.* The early luteal phase administration of estrogen and progesterone does not induce premature luteolysis in normo-ovulatory women. *Eur J Endocrinol* 2006;**155**:355–363.

43. Mitwally MF, Casper RF. Use of an aromatase inhibitor for induction of ovulation in patients with an inadequate response to clomiphene citrate. *Fertil Steril* 2001;**75**:305–309.

44. Teede HJ, Misso ML, Costello MF, *et al.* Recommendations from the international evidence-based guideline for the assessment and management of polycystic ovary syndrome. *Fertil Steril* 2018;**110**:364–379.

45. Garcia-Velasco JA, Moreno L, Pacheco A, *et al.* The aromatase inhibitor letrozole increases the concentration of intraovarian androgens and improves in vitro fertilization outcome in low responder patients: a pilot study. *Fertil Steril* 2005;**84**:82–87.

46. Biljan MM, Hemmings R, Brassard N. The outcome of 150 babies following the treatment with letrozole or letrozole and gonadotropins. *Fertil Steril* 2005;**84**:O-231 abstract 1033.

47. Tulandi T, Martin J, Al-Fadhli R, *et al.* Congenital malformations among 911 newborns conceived after infertility treatment with letrozole or clomiphene citrate. *Fertil Steril* 2006;**85**:1761–1765.

48. Tatsumi T, Jwa SC, Kuwahara A, *et al.* No increased risk of major congenital anomalies or adverse pregnancy or neonatal outcomes following letrozole use in ART. *Hum Reprod* 2017;**32**:125–132.

49. Wang R, Kim BV, van Wely M, *et al.* Treatment strategies for women with WHO group II anovulation: systemic review and network meta-analysis. *BMJ* 2017;**356**:j138.

50. Pildes RB. Induction of ovulation with clomiphene. *Am J Obstet Gynecol* 1965;**91**:466–479.

51. Dehbashi S, Vafaei H, Parsanezhad MD, Alborzi S. Time of initiation of clomiphene citrate and pregnancy rate in polycystic ovarian syndrome. *Int J Gynaecol Obstet* 2006;**93**:44–48.

52. Moll E, Bossuyt PM, Korevaar JC, Lambalk CB, van der Veen F. Effect of clomifene citrate plus metformin and clomifene citrate plus placebo on induction of ovulation in women with newly diagnosed polycystic ovary syndrome: randomised double blind clinical trial. *BMJ* 2006;**332**:1485.

53. Legro RS, Barnhart HX, Schlaff WD, *et al.*; Cooperative Multicenter Reproductive Medicine Network. Clomiphene, metformin, or both for infertility in the polycystic ovary syndrome. *N Engl J Med* 2007;**356**:551–566.

54. Daly DC, Walters CA, Soto-Albors CE, Tohan N, Riddick DH. A randomized study of dexamethasone in ovulation induction with clomiphene citrate. *Fertil Steril* 1984;**41**:844–848.

55. Kousta E, White DM, Franks S. Modern use of clomiphene citrate in induction of ovulation. *Hum Reprod Update* 1997;**3**:359–365.

56. Imani B, Eijkemans MJ, te Velde ER, Habbema JD, Fauser BC. Predictors of patients remaining anovulatory during clomiphene citrate induction of ovulation in normogonadotropic oligoamenorrheic infertility. *J Clin Endocrinol Metab* 1998;**83**:2361–2365.

57. Homburg R. Clomiphene citrate–end of an era? A mini-review. *Hum Reprod* 2005;**20**:2043–2051.

58. Rossing MA, Daling JR, Weiss NS, Moore DE, Self SG. Ovarian tumors in a cohort of infertile women. *N Engl J Med* 1994;**331**:771–776.

59. Roumen FJ, Doesburg WH, Rolland R. Treatment of infertile women with a deficient postcoital test with two antiestrogens: clomiphene and tamoxifen. *Fertil Steril* 1984;**41**:237–243.

60. Boostanfar R. A prospective randomized trial comparing clomiphene citrate with tamoxifen citrate for ovulation induction. *Fertil Steril* 2001;**75**:1024–1026.

61. Bayram N, van Wely M, van Der Veen F. Recombinant FSH versus urinary gonadotrophins or recombinant FSH for ovulation induction in subfertility associated with polycystic ovary syndrome. *Cochrane Database Syst Rev* 2001;**2**: CD002121.

62. van Santbrink EJ, Fauser BC. Urinary follicle-stimulating hormone for normogonadotropic clomiphene-resistant anovulatory infertility: prospective, randomized comparison between low dose step-up and step-down dose regimens. *J Clin Endocrinol Metab* 1997;**82**:3597–3602.

63. Christin-Maitre S, Hugues JN; Recombinant FSH Study Group. A comparative randomized multicentric study comparing the step-up versus step-down protocol in polycystic ovary syndrome. *Hum Reprod* 2003;**18**:1626–1631.

64. van Santbrink EJ, Eijkemans MJ, Laven JS, Fauser BC. Patient-tailored conventional ovulation induction algorithms in anovulatory infertility. *Trends Endocrinol Metab* 2005;**16**:381–389.

65. Mulders AG, Eijkemans MJ, Imani B, *et al.* Prediction of chances for success or complications in gonadotrophin ovulation induction in normogonadotrophic anovulatory infertility. *Reprod Biomed Online* 2003;**7**:48–56.

66. Fauser BC, Devroey P, Macklon NS. Multiple birth resulting from ovarian stimulation for subfertility treatment. *Lancet* 2005;**365**:1807–1816.

67. Aboulghar MA, Mansour RT. Ovarian hyperstimulation syndrome: classifications and critical analysis of preventive measures. *Hum Reprod Update* 2003;**9**:275–289.

68. De Geyter C, De Geyter M, Castro E, *et al.* Experience with transvaginal ultrasound-guided aspiration of supernumerary follicles for the prevention of multiple pregnancies after ovulation induction and intrauterine insemination. *Fertil Steril* 1996;**65**:1163–1168.

69. la Marca A, Morgante G, Palumbo M, *et al.* Insulin-lowering treatment reduces aromatase activity in response to follicle-stimulating hormone in women with polycystic ovary syndrome. *Fertil Steril* 2002;**78**:1234–1239.

70. Coffler MS, Patel K, Dahan MH, *et al.* Enhanced granulosa cell responsiveness to follicle-stimulating hormone during insulin infusion in women with polycystic ovary syndrome treated with pioglitazone. *J Clin Endocrinol Metab* 2003;**88**:5624–5631.

71. Lord JM, Flight IH, Norman RJ. Metformin in polycystic ovary syndrome: systematic review and meta-analysis. *BMJ* 2003;**327**:951–953.

72. Palomba S, Orio F Jr., Nardo LG, *et al.* Metformin administration versus laparoscopic ovarian diathermy in clomiphene citrate-resistant women with polycystic ovary syndrome: a prospective parallel randomized double-blind

73. placebo-controlled trial. *J Clin Endocrinol Metab* 2004;**89**:4801–4809.

73. Morley LC, Tang T, Yasmin E, Norman RJ, Balen AH. Insulin-sensitising drugs (metformin, rosiglitazone, pioglitazone, D-chiro-inositol) for women with polycystic ovary syndrome, oligo amenorrhoea and subfertility. *Cochrane Database Syst Rev* 2017;**11**:CD003053.

74. Legro RS, Zaino RJ, Demers LM, *et al.* The effects of metformin and rosiglitazone, alone and in combination, on the ovary and endometrium in polycystic ovary syndrome. *Am J Obstet Gynecol* 2007;**196**:402.e1–402.e10; discussion 402.e10.

75. Glueck CJ, Goldenberg N, Pranikoff J, *et al.* Height, weight, and motor-social development during the first 18 months of life in 126 infants born to 109 mothers with polycystic ovary syndrome who conceived on and continued metformin through pregnancy. *Hum Reprod* 2004;**19**:1323–1330.

76. Pundir J, Psaroudakis D, Savnur P, *et al.* Inositol treatment of anovulation in women with polycystic ovary syndrome: a meta-analysis of randomised trials. *BJOG* 2018;**125**:299–308.

77. Stein IF, Cohen MR, Elson R. Results of bilateral ovarian wedge resection in 47 cases of sterility; 20 year end results; 75 cases of bilateral polycystic ovaries. *Am J Obstet Gynecol* 1949;**58**:267–274.

78. Mahesh VB, Greenblatt RB. Urinary steroid excretion patterns in hirsutism. II. Effect of ovarian stimulation with human pituitary FSH on urinary 17-ketosteroids. *J Clin Endocrinol Metab* 1964;**24**:1293–1302.

79. Gjönnaess H. Polycystic ovarian syndrome treated by ovarian electrocautery through the laparoscope. *Fertil Steril* 1984;**41**:20–25.

80. Greenblatt EM, Casper RF. Laparoscopic ovarian drilling in women with polycystic ovarian syndrome. *Prog Clin Biol Res* 1993;**381**:129–138.

81. Farquhar C, Lilford RJ, Marjoribanks J, *et al.* Laparoscopic 'drilling' by diathermy or laser for ovulation induction in anovulatory polycystic ovary syndrome. *Cochrane Database Syst Rev* 2007;**18**:CD001122.

82. Youssef H, Atallah MM. Unilateral ovarian drilling in polycystic ovarian syndrome: a prospective randomized study. *Reprod Biomed Online* 2007;**15**:457–462.

83. Saleh AM, Khalil HS. Review of nonsurgical and surgical treatment and the role of insulin-sensitizing agents in the management of infertile women with polycystic ovary syndrome. *Acta Obstet Gynecol Scand* 2004;**83**:614–621.

84. Seow KM, Juan CC, Hwang JL, Ho LT. Laparoscopic surgery in polycystic ovary syndrome: reproductive and metabolic effects. *Semin Reprod Med* 2008;**26**:101–110.

85. Overbeek A, Kuijper EA, Hendriks ML, *et al.* Clomiphene citrate resistance in relation to follicle-stimulating hormone receptor Ser680Ser-polymorphism in polycystic ovary syndrome. *Hum Reprod* 2009;**24**:2007–2013.

86. Practice Committee of the American Society of Reproductive Medicine. Ovarian hyperstimulation syndrome. *Fertil Steril* 2006;**86**:S178–S183.

87. Dickey RP, Taylor SN, Lu PY, *et al.* Risk factors for high-order multiple pregnancy and multiple birth after controlled ovarian hyperstimulation: results of 4,062 intrauterine insemination cycles. *Fertil Steril* 2005;**83**:671–683.

88. White DM, Polson DW, Kiddy D, *et al.* Induction of ovulation with low-dose gonadotropins in polycystic ovary syndrome: an analysis of 109 pregnancies in 225 women. *J Clin Endocrinol Metab* 1996;**81**:3821–3824.

89. Mulders AM, Laven JS, Eijkemans MJ, Hughes EG, Fauser BC. Patient predictors for outcome of gonadotrophin ovulation induction in women with normogonadotrophic anovulatory infertility: a meta-analysis. *Hum Reprod Update* 2003;**9** (5):429–449.

90. Franik S, Eltrop SM, Kremer JAM, Kiesel L, Farquhar C. Aromatase inhibitors for subfertile women with polycystic ovary syndrome. *Cochrane Database Syst Rev* 2018;**5**:CD010287.

91. Eijkemans MJ, Imani B, Mulders AG, Habbema JD, Fauser BC. High singleton live birth rate following classical ovulation induction in normogonadotrophic anovulatory infertility (WHO 2). *Hum Reprod* 2003;**18**:2357–2362.

92. Imani B, Eijkemans MJ, te Velde ER, Habbema JD, Fauser BC. A nomogram to predict the probability of live birth after clomiphene citrate induction of ovulation in normogonadotropic oligoamenorrheic infertility. *Fertil Steril* 2002;**77**:91–97.

Ovarian Hyperstimulation in Combination with Intrauterine Insemination

Ben J. Cohlen and Astrid E. P. Cantineau

Introduction

Worldwide intrauterine insemination (IUI) is still one of the most applied treatment options for couples with infertility for various reasons. The rationale for performing IUI is to increase the number of motile sperm with normal morphology at the site of fertilization at the right moment. With the use of sperm preparation techniques applied in in vitro fertilization (IVF), side effects such as severe cramping or infections hardly ever occur any more.

Besides increasing the number of spermatozoa, one can also increase the number of available oocytes by applying ovarian hyperstimulation (OH). With the use of hyperstimulation one might also overcome subtle cycle disturbances, and increase the accuracy of timing of the insemination [1]. On the other hand, applying hyperstimulation increases the probability of achieving multiple pregnancies [2;3]. Therefore, OH in IUI programs should be applied only when proven effective. Recently published large randomized trials support the use of IUI as a first-line treatment option [4;5] This chapter will focus on the indications for IUI in combination with (mild) OH, its methods and risks. The level of evidence (LOE) of important statements and conclusions will be added.

Indications

Intrauterine insemination is applied in couples with longstanding infertility caused by either a male factor, a hostile cervix, or by infertility without any detected explanation [1]. Often couples with mild endometriosis (grade I and II) are treated as couples with unexplained infertility, and IUI in combination with OH is offered [6]. In couples with anovulation, ovulation induction is advised and in these patients one should strive

after monofollicular growth. When anovulation is the sole problem, treatment could be combined with (timed) intercourse and there seems little place for IUI [7].

In couples with cervical hostility, it is advised to apply IUI in natural cycles, because the addition of OH does not further increase the probability of conception significantly (LOE 1b) [8]. One should bear in mind that to be able to detect a hostile cervix, one has to perform postcoital testing on a regular basis. More and more, postcoital testing is abandoned in the regular fertility workup making it impossible to detect cervical hostility. Performing postcoital testing in women with cystic fibrosis or cervical surgery might still be considered.

Whether or not to apply OH in couples with a male factor seems to be related to the average sperm quality expressed as total motile sperm count (TMSC) (LOE 1b) [9]. In couples with an average TMSC before processing of less than 10 million, the infertility of the couple might be explained by the infertility of the man, and IUI in natural cycles is advised. In couples with an average TMSC above 10 million, almost resembling unexplained infertility, a female factor might be present as well and OH is advised [10]. Recent randomized trials have used different cut-off levels of TMSC to apply OH, for instance the INeS trial [4] in which a TMSC of 3 million was applied. In couples with unexplained infertility, IUI in natural cycles does not increase the probability of conception (LOE 1a) [11;12], while it has been proven that the addition of OH significantly increases live birth rates (Figure 3.1) (LOE 1a) [11].

In general it is advised to apply IUI in combination with OH only when it clearly improves the probability of conception [5] and, therefore, to postpone this treatment option when the probability of

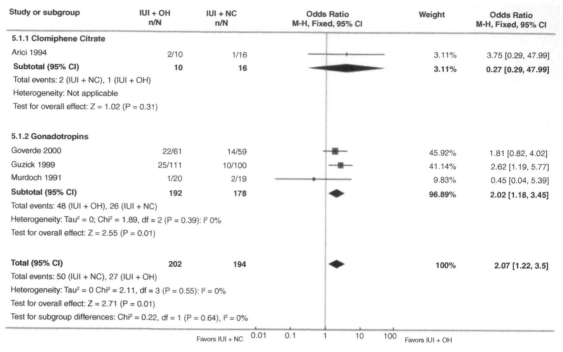

Study or subgroup	IUI + OH n/N	IUI + NC n/N	Odds Ratio M-H, Fixed, 95% CI	Weight	Odds Ratio M-H, Fixed, 95% CI
5.1.1 Clomiphene Citrate					
Arici 1994	2/10	1/16		3.11%	3.75 [0.29, 47.99]
Subtotal (95% CI)	**10**	**16**		**3.11%**	**0.27 [0.29, 47.99]**
Total events: 2 (IUI + NC), 1 (IUI + OH)					
Heterogeneity: Not applicable					
Test for overall effect: Z = 1.02 (P = 0.31)					
5.1.2 Gonadotropins					
Goverde 2000	22/61	14/59		45.92%	1.81 [0.82, 4.02]
Guzick 1999	25/111	10/100		41.14%	2.62 [1.19, 5.77]
Murdoch 1991	1/20	2/19		9.83%	0.45 [0.04, 5.39]
Subtotal (95% CI)	**192**	**178**		**96.89%**	**2.02 [1.18, 3.45]**
Total events: 48 (IUI + OH), 26 (IUI + NC)					
Heterogeneity: Tau² = 0; Chi² = 1.89, df = 2 (P = 0.39): I² 0%					
Test for overall effect: Z = 2.55 (P = 0.01)					
Total (95% CI)	**202**	**194**		**100%**	**2.07 [1.22, 3.5]**
Total events: 50 (IUI + NC), 27 (IUI + OH)					
Heterogeneity: Tau² = 0 Chi² = 2.11, df = 3 (P = 0.55): I² = 0%					
Test for overall effect: Z = 2.71 (P = 0.01)					
Test for subgroup differences: Chi² = 0.22, df = 1 (P = 0.64), I² = 0%					

Favors IUI + NC 0.01 0.1 1 10 100 Favors IUI + OH

Figure 3.1 IUI in natural cycle versus IUI in stimulated cycles. Outcome: live birth rate per couple [11].

achieving a spontaneous conception is still over 30–40 percent estimated with a prediction model (LOE 1b) [13].

Optimal Choice of Drug

Several drugs are available to achieve OH. Probably the oldest one is clomiphene citrate (CC), in dosages of 50–150 mg/day for 5 days. In contrast to couples with anovulation, where one should strive after monofollicular growth, the use of CC in OH programs aims at the growth of two to three follicles. Being an oral drug and relatively cheap it is a popular option, easy to apply although side effects, such as hot flushes, mood-swings, and headaches, are regularly present. Being an antiestrogen, its negative action on the endometrium should be monitored. Furthermore, also in CC-stimulated cycles multiple pregnancies occur [14;15].

Besides CC, gonadotropins are applied frequently. These drugs are more expensive, invasive, and potent compared with CC. A meta-analysis revealed that gonadotropins seems to be more effective compared with CC (Figure 3.2) (LOE 1a) [14]. An updated version of this review is due to be published shortly. In this study the risk of achieving a multiple pregnancy did not significantly differ between gonadotropins and CC.

Different types of gonadotropins are available, and several trials have compared urinary with recombinant gonadotropins. A meta-analysis of these trials did not show one type superior to the other [14]. Costs and other factors such as batch-to-batch consistency and the elimination of drugs co-extracted from urine should be taken into account when making a choice. Furthermore, there is an ongoing discussion regarding the optimal dose. Doubling the daily dose of gonadotropins from 75 IU to 150 IU does not result in improvement of treatment outcome, while it significantly increases the chances of achieving a multiple pregnancy (LOE 1a) [14]. When a very low-dose regimen is given on alternating days, very low pregnancy rates are seen, which makes it plausible that a minimum acquired dose of gonadotropins is needed.

Aromatase inhibitors have been introduced for OH in IUI programs since a while [16]. The rationale is that aromatase inhibitors do not have a negative effect on the endometrium and cervical mucus known from CC. However, compared with CC, these drugs do not seem to improve treatment outcome significantly while they are more expensive (LOE 1a) Figure 3.3 [14]. So far, there seems to be little place for aromatase inhibitors in IUI programs.

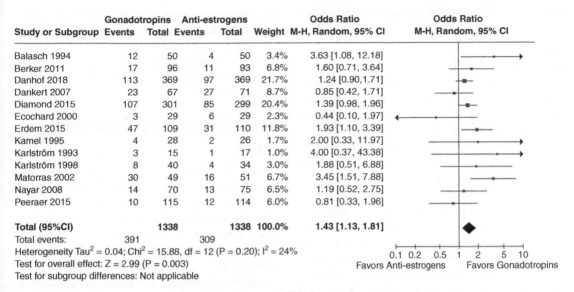

Figure 3.2 Pregnancy rate per couple gonadotropins versus CC [14].

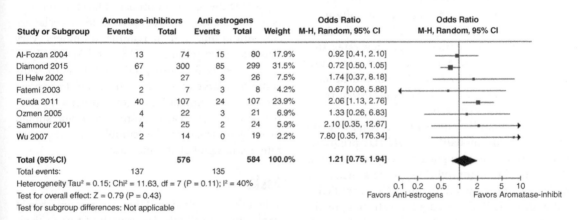

Figure 3.3 Pregnancy rate per couple AI versus CC (unpublished data).

It has been shown that in stimulated IUI cycles spontaneous luteinizing hormone (LH) surges occur frequently in up to one-third of all cycles [17]. When LH levels are not monitored, timing of the insemination might be influenced negatively (i.e., too late), resulting in significantly lower pregnancy rates (LOE 2) [9;17]. This might be one of the reasons that gonadotropin-releasing hormone (GnRH) agonists and antagonists were introduced in IUI programs. Up till now there seems no benefit of GnRH agonists, while they significantly increase the costs per treatment cycle (LOE 1a) [14]. Furthermore, the use of GnRH agonists might lead to more aggressive stimulation protocols, thus resulting in higher multiple pregnancy rates [14]. The use of a GnRH antagonist seemed promising; however, it has not been proven cost-effective until now [14].

A systematic review including one double-blinded randomized trial found a significant benefit of the use of luteal support with vaginally applied progesterone in IUI cycles stimulated with gonadotropins (LOE 1b) [18]. However, the randomized trial using double blinding was unable to detect a beneficial effect. Before this drug is introduced in IUI programs on a large scale, a multicenter placebo-controlled double-blinded trial with cost-effectiveness analyses seems mandatory to confirm these results.

Optimal Timing

Optimal timing of the insemination is a crucial factor in IUI programs. After ovulation oocytes should be fertilized within several hours. Inseminated sperm (bypassing the cervix, which acts as a reservoir for spermatozoa) has a limited period of survival, and sperm should therefore not be inseminated too early. Nevertheless there seems to be a window of optimal timing. Prospective studies comparing different time intervals after ovarian stimulation in IUI programs were analyzed [19]. The best available evidence comparing two time intervals of 24 hours and 34 hours after human chorionic gonadotropin (hCG) injection showed no significant difference in pregnancy rates per couple, suggesting a more flexible approach in timing. A randomized study of simultaneous hCG administration with IUI in stimulated cycles resulted in similar pregnancy rates suggesting a wider time interval than previously considered [20]. However, this should be confirmed with large prospective randomized trials, preferably multicentered.

There is hardly any evidence regarding the optimal timing modality. In OH/IUI programs, hCG is most often applied to induce ovulation. When the dominant follicle(s) reach a mean diameter of approximately 18 mm, hCG is applied in a dosage of 5000 IU. After administration, ovulation of the dominant follicles occurs between 34 and 46 hours later [21]. When IUI is timed by applying hCG at 18 mm, one should be aware of spontaneous LH surges and premature luteinization [17].

Another approach is to wait for a spontaneous LH surge and either inseminate 24 hours after detection of the spontaneous surge or augment the LH surge by applying hCG and inseminate 24 hours later [19]. The major disadvantage of this method is the high dropout level (up to 25 percent) due to failed detection of an LH surge with urinary detection kits [22].

One way to avoid the possibility of inaccurate timing is to inseminate more than once. However, a systematic review performed by Cantineau *et al.* clearly shows no benefit of a second insemination in couples with unexplained infertility (LOE 1a)

[23]. In couples with male infertility the discussion regarding a second insemination is still ongoing [23;24]. Another way is to inseminate when the dominant follicle is of a smaller size; however, this might result in the release of immature follicles [25].

Optimal Number of Treatment Cycles

How many treatment cycles of OH with IUI should be offered to couples with mild male and unexplained infertility? To answer this question, large, adequately powered prospective observational studies of 10–12 consecutive cycles should be performed in a well-defined population with clear description of the methods applied (ovarian stimulation, timing, semen preparation, etc.) to be able to draw firm conclusions. These studies do not exist. This might explain why different advice regarding the optimal number of treatment cycles is published. Everyone agrees that three cycles are the minimum, but maximum numbers vary between three and nine (LOE 2 and 3) [26;27].

It is advised to prospectively follow the outcome of a large cohort over time and to express the results as cumulative ongoing pregnancy rates per couple. After each additive cycle one should investigate whether the cumulative pregnancy rate is still significantly increased.

Risks

When OH is applied in IUI programs, one should strive after multifollicular growth of two to three dominant follicles to obtain the highest probability of conception with reasonable risks (LOE 1a) [28]. This way ovarian hyperstimulation syndrome (OHSS) hardly ever occurs. However, the chances to achieve a multiple pregnancy are significantly increased. It is very clear that when OH is applied, multiple pregnancies will occur. However, large randomized trials using mild stimulation protocols and strict cancellation criteria show acceptable multiple pregnancy rates of approximately 5 percent or lower [4;5;15]. Mild OH with 50–75 IU of follicle-stimulating hormone (FSH) per day in combination with strict cancellation criteria should minimize the risks. Trials that used more aggressive stimulation protocols, for instance 150 IU of FSH per day, show unacceptable high multiple pregnancy rates up to

25 percent [29]. It remains difficult to predict the occurrence of a multiple pregnancy. Large retrospective trials found correlation with a woman's age, the total number of follicles, and the number of follicles larger than 10–11 mm at the time of hCG administration [30]. It is therefore advised to monitor OH cycles with ultrasound and to measure all follicles with a mean diameter larger than 10 mm. The World Health Organization advises to abstain from IUI when more than two follicles larger than 15 mm or more than five follicles larger than 10 mm are present at the moment of hCG administration [10]. Alternatively, supernumerary follicles can be aspirated or one might convert the OH/IUI cycle to IVF. However, both these methods to avoid multiple pregnancies turn a relatively mild and non-invasive treatment into a more expensive and invasive treatment modality. Often couples are unprepared and uninformed for IVF, and therefore one should be careful in converting OH/IUI into these alternatives.

Nowadays IVF semen preparation techniques are used to prepare semen samples for IUI. There seems to be no significant difference in efficacy between gradient techniques and swim-up (LOE 1a) [31]. Both techniques apply wash and centrifuge, and therefore pelvic infections or uterine cramping are risks of the past.

Comparison with IVF

A recent large randomized trial from the Netherlands that compared OH/IUI with IVF with single embryo transfer or IVF in a modified natural cycle in couples with mild male or unexplained infertility and a Hunault score below 30 percent clearly shows OH/IUI to be the most cost-effective first-line treatment option with acceptable low multiple pregnancy rates [32]. This trial confirms the result of older trials such as the study by Goverde *et al.* [33] that revealed OH/IUI in couples with unexplained and mild male infertility to be more cost-effective compared with IVF (LOE 1b) [32]. The mean costs per couple were €7187 for IVF with single embryo transfer (IVF-SET) and €5070 for IUI with controlled OH (IUI-COH), which was significantly lower. For the birth of an additional healthy child the incremental cost-effectiveness ratios (ICER) for IVF-SET compared with IUI-COH was € 43 375, thus IUI-COH is the dominant

strategy, that is, more effective at lower costs. Of course, this seems the case only when the number of multiple pregnancies is kept to a minimum and high-order multiples are prevented [32].

Conclusion

Based upon the evidence provided above, we formulate the following grade A recommendations. IUI in combination with OH should be offered as a first-line treatment option to couples with long-standing mild male or unexplained infertility only. The probability of achieving a spontaneous pregnancy should be below 30 percent. When multiple pregnancies are kept to a minimum, OH/IUI is more cost-effective compared with IVF. Gonadotropins are the most effective drugs and should be offered in a low-dose, step-up protocol. There is no place for GnRH agonists or GnRH antagonists in IUI programs. Future randomized trials should investigate the cost-effectiveness of luteal support. Optimal timing can be achieved by either detection of a spontaneous LH surge or by administration of hCG. The window for optimal timing of insemination seems broad. A second insemination does not further improve the probability of conception, and the insemination should therefore be performed once. Strict monitoring of follicle growth and number by ultrasound is advised and cancel criteria (based upon level 3 evidence) are proposed. The optimal number of treatment cycles is not well established, nor the optimal method of semen preparation.

References

1. Cohlen BJ. Should we continue performing intrauterine inseminations in the year 2004? *Gynecol Obstet Invest* 2005;**59**:3–13.

2. Cohlen BJ, van Dop P. Prevention of multiple pregnancies after non-in vitro fertilization treatment. In: Gerris J, Olivennes F, de Sutter P, eds. *Assisted Reproductive Technologies. Quality and Safety*. London, UK: The Parthenon Publishing Group London; 2004:39–48.

3. Fauser BJCM, Devroey P, Macklon NS. Multiple birth resulting from ovarian stimulation for subfertility treatment. *Lancet* 2005;**365**:5000.

4. Bensdorp AJ, Tjon-Kon-Fat RI, Bossuyt PM, *et al.* Prevention of multiple pregnancies in couples with unexplained or mild male subfertility; randomised controlled trial of in vitro fertilisation with single embryo transfer or in vitro fertilisation in modified

natural cycle compared with intrauterine insemination with controlled ovarian hyperstimulation. *BMJ* 2015;**350**:g7771.

5. Farquhar CM, Liu E, Armstrong S, *et al.* Intrauterine insemination with ovarian stimulation versus expectant management for unexplained infertility (TUI): a pragmatic, open-label, randomized, controlled two-centre trial. *Lancet* 2018;**391** (10119):441–450.

6. Werbrouck E, Spiessens C, Meuleman C, D'Hooghe T. No difference in cycle pregnancy rate and in cumulative live-birth rate between women with surgically treated minimal to mild endometriosis and women with unexplained infertility after controlled ovarian hyperstimulation and intrauterine insemination. *Fertil Steril* 2006;**86**:566–571.

7. Weiss NS, Nahuis MJ, Bordewijk E, *et al.* Gonadotrophins versus clomiphene citrate with or without intrauterine insemination in women with normogonadotropic anovulation and clomifene failure (M-OVIN); a randomised, two-by-two factorial trial. *Lancet* 2018;**391**(10122):758–765.

8. Steures P, van der Steeg JW, Verhoeve HR, *et al.* Does ovarian hyperstimulation in intrauterine insemination for cervical factor subfertility improve pregnancy rates? *Hum Reprod* 2004;**19**:2263–2266.

9. Cohlen BJ, te Velde ER, van Kooij RJ, Looman CW, Habbema JD. Controlled ovarian hyperstimulation and intrauterine insemination for treating male subfertility: a controlled study. *Hum Reprod* 1998;**13**:1553–1558.

10. Cohlen B, Bijkerk A, Van der Poel S, Ombelet W. IUI: review and systematic assessment of evidence that supports global recommendations. *Hum Reprod Update* 2018;**24**(3):300–319.

11. Ayeleke RO, Asseler JD, Cohlen BJ, Veltman-Verhulst SM. Intra-uterine insemination for unexplained subfertility. *Cochrane Database Syst Rev* 2020;**3**:CD001838.

12. Bhattacharya S, Harrild K, Mollison J, *et al.* Clomifene citrate or unstimulated intrauterine insemination compared with expectant management for unexplained infertility: pragmatic randomised controlled trial. *BMJ* 2008;**337**:a716.

13. Steures P, van der Steeg JW, Hompes PG, *et al.*; Collaborative Effort on the Clinical Evaluation in Reproductive Medicine. Intrauterine insemination with controlled ovarian hyperstimulation versus expectant management for couples with unexplained subfertility and an intermediate

prognosis: a randomised clinical trial. *Lancet* 2006;**368**:216–221.

14. Cantineau AE, Cohlen BJ, Heineman MJ. Ovarian stimulation protocols (anti-oestrogens, gonadotrophins with and without GnRH agonists/antagonists) for intrauterine insemination (IUI) in women with subfertility. *Cochrane Database Syst Rev* 2007;**2**:CD005356.

15. Danhof NA, van Wely M, Repping S, *et al.*; SUPER study group. Follicle stimulating hormone versus clomiphene citrate in intrauterine insemination for unexplained subfertility: a randomized controlled trial. *Hum Reprod* 2018;**33** (10):1866–1874.

16. Requena A, Herrero J, Landeras J, *et al.*; Reproductive Endocrinology Interest Group of the Spanish Society of Fertility. Use of letrozole in assisted reproduction: a systematic review and meta-analysis. *Hum Reprod Update* 2008;**14**:571–582.

17. Cantineau AE, Cohlen BJ; Dutch IUI Study Group. The prevalence and influence of luteinizing hormone surges in stimulated cycles combined with intrauterine insemination during a prospective cohort study. *Fertil Steril* 2007;**88**:107–112.

18. Green K, Zolton JR, Schermerhorn SMV, *et al.* Progesterone luteal support after ovulation induction and intrauterine insemination: an updated systematic review and meta-analysis. *Fertil Steril* 2017;**107**(4):924–933.

19. Cantineau AEP, Janssen MJ, Cohlen BJ, Allersma T. Synchronised approach for intrauterine insemination in subfertile couples. *Cochrane Database Syst Rev* 2014;**12**:CD006942.

20. Aydin Y, Hassa H, Oge T, Tokgoz VY. A randomized study of simultaneous hCG administration with intrauterine insemination in stimulated cycles. *Eur J Obstet Gynaecol Reprod Biol* 2013;**170**(2):444–448.

21. Andersen AG, Als-Nielsen B, Hornnes PJ, Franch Andersen L. Time interval from human chorionic gonadotrophin (HCG) injection to follicular rupture. *Hum Reprod* 1995;**10**:3202–3205.

22. Lewis V, Queenan J Jr., Hoeger K, Stevens J, Guzick DS. Clomiphene citrate monitoring for intrauterine insemination timing: a randomized trial. *Fertil Steril* 2006;**85**:401–406.

23. Cantineau AE, Heineman MJ, Cohlen BJ. Single versus double intrauterine insemination (IUI) in stimulated cycles for subfertile couples. *Cochrane Database Syst Rev* 2007;**1**:CD003854.

24. Liu W, Gong F, Luo K, Lu G. Comparing the pregnancy rates of one versus two intrauterine

inseminations (IUIs) in male factor and idiopathic infertility. *J Assist Reprod Genet* 2006;2:75–79.

25. Martinez AR, Bernadus RE, Voorhorst FJ, Vermeiden JP, Schoemaker J. A controlled study of human chorionic gonadotrophin induced ovulation versus urinary luteinizing hormone surge for timing of intrauterine insemination. *Hum Reprod* 1991;6:1247–1251.

26. Aboulghar M, Mansour R, Serour G, *et al.* Controlled ovarian hyperstimulation and intrauterine insemination for treatment of unexplained infertility should be limited to a maximum of three trials. *Fertil Steril* 2001;75:88–91.

27. Custers IM, Steures P, Hompes P, *et al.* Intrauterine insemination: how many cycles should we perform? *Hum Reprod* 2008;23:885–888.

28. van Rumste MM, Custers IM, van der Veen F, *et al.* The influence of the number of follicles on pregnancy rates in intrauterine insemination with ovarian stimulation: a meta-analysis. *Hum Reprod Update* 2008;14:563–570.

29. Diamond MP, Legro RS, Coutifaris C, *et al.*; NICHD Reproductive Medicine Network. Letrozole, gonadotropin, or clomiphene for unexplained infertility. *N Engl J Med* 2015;373 (13):1230–1240.

30. Dickey RP, Taylor SN, Lu PY, *et al.* Risk factors for high-order multiple pregnancy and multiple birth after controlled ovarian hyperstimulation: results of 4,062 intrauterine insemination cycles. *Fertil Steril* 2005;83:671–683.

31. Boomsma CM, Heineman MJ, Cohlen BJ, Farquhar C. Semen preparation techniques for intrauterine insemination. *Cochrane Database Syst Rev* 2007;4:CD004507.

32. Tjon-Kon-Fat RI, Bensdorp AJ, Bossuyt PM, *et al.* Is IVF-served two different ways-more cost-effective than IUI with controlled ovarian hyperstimulation? *Hum Reprod* 2015;30 (10):2331–2339.

33. Goverde AJ, McDonnell J, Vermeiden JP, *et al.* Intrauterine insemination or in-vitro fertilisation in idiopathic subfertility and male subfertility: a randomised trial and cost-effectiveness analysis. *Lancet* 2000;355:13–18.

Chapter 4

Mild Approaches in Ovarian Stimulation

Adrija Kumar Datta, Stuart Campbell, and Geeta Nargund

Introduction

Conventional ovarian stimulation protocols intend to yield as many oocytes and embryos as possible to try to maximize the success of an in vitro fertilization (IVF) program. In reality, however, a series of studies over the last few years observed that live birth rates (LBRs) do not increase after a certain number of retrieved oocytes [1–3]; some studies even found a decline in LBRs when the number of oocytes was in excess of 18 [4] or blastocyst numbers above 5 [5]. Although the cumulative LBR keeps rising over and above the number of oocytes/embryos that maximizes per cycle live birth, the incidence of ovarian hyperstimulation syndrome (OHSS) and venous thromboembolism (VTE) also escalate in a parallel fashion [2;3;6]. A recent study, by restricting the stimulation dose to 150 IU/day, found only nine oocytes or four embryos optimizing the fresh cycle LBR [7]. In this study, the cumulative LBR was optimized with 15–20 oocytes in normal and high responders with no incidence of severe OHSS. This emerging evidence has now questioned

the fundamental concept of using intense ovarian stimulation that only raises treatment burden and risks with no apparent advantage in pregnancy outcome.

A mild approach to ovarian stimulation is not a new concept: following the birth of the first IVF baby through a completely unstimulated cycle, Natural and Mild IVF developed in parallel with conventional IVF (C-IVF). The aim is to develop safer and more "patient-friendly" protocols in which the risks of IVF treatment are minimized [8]. Mild approach IVF (MA-IVF) encompasses Natural cycle IVF, Natural modified IVF (NM-IVF), and Mild stimulation IVF (MS-IVF); the definition of each, as outlined by the International Society of Mild Approach Assisted Reproduction (ISMAAR) [9] and subsequently reflected in the glossary by the International Committee for Monitoring Assisted Reproductive Technology (ICMART)/World Health Organization (WHO) [10], has been summarized in Table 4.1. The basic principle and philosophy of Natural and Mild IVF are similar; the

Table 4.1 Terminologies (ICMART definition and ISMAAR consensus)

Protocol	Definition
Natural cycle IVF	An ART procedure in which one or more oocytes are collected from the ovaries during a menstrual cycle without the use of any pharmacological compound
Modified Natural IVF	An ART procedure in which one or more oocytes are collected from the ovaries during a spontaneous menstrual cycle. Pharmacological compounds are administered with the sole purpose of blocking the spontaneous LH surge and/or inducing final oocyte maturation *Modified Natural IVF with hCG:* The use of hCG to induce final oocyte maturation in a natural cycle *Modified Natural IVF with addition of GnRH antagonist:* The administration of GnRH antagonist to block the spontaneous LH surge with or without FSH or hMG as add-back therapy (ISMAAR)
Mild stimulation IVF	A protocol in which the ovaries are stimulated with gonadotropins, and/or other pharmacological compounds, with the intention of limiting the number of oocytes following stimulation for IVF (ICMART) A method when follicle FSH or hMG is administered at a lower dose and or for a shorter duration in GnRH antagonist co-treated cycle, or when oral compounds, antiestrogens or aromatase inhibitors, are used either alone or in combination with gonadotropins with an aim to collect a fewer number of oocytes (ISMAAR)

LH = luteinizing hormone; hCG = human chorionic gonadotropin; GnRH = gonadotropin-releasing hormone; FSH = follicle-stimulating hormone; hMG = human menopausal gonadotropin.

selection between the two strategies depends on individual patient circumstances.

Concerns with Conventional Ovarian Stimulation for IVF

Conventional protocols for ovarian stimulation take several weeks to complete. It often requires high-dose or prolonged course of gonadotropins, resulting in increased physical discomfort and emotional distress [11]. Indeed, treatment-related stress has been reported to be an important reason for dropping out of an IVF program [12]. High gonadotropin stimulation has also been found to raise the treatment cost (Table 4.2).

OHSS remains the greatest threat to IVF treatment; the current trend of intense ovarian stimulation followed by gonadotropin-releasing hormone (GnRH) agonist ovulation trigger and "freeze-all embryos" significantly reduces but does not completely eliminate the risk of OHSS [13]. A significant hyperestrogenic state also will put the patients at increased risk of VTE [6]. High circulating estrogen may be a potential risk to women with estrogen-sensitive conditions including breast cancer or thrombophilia.

High ovarian stimulation has been shown to have a negative impact on embryo development and endometrial receptivity [14]. Conventional stimulation appears to advance endometrial maturation, leading to embryo-endometrial asynchrony and reduced implantation rates [15]. Other mechanism includes disturbances of endometrial gene expression [16].

Advantages of MA-IVF

Safety profile: Both Mild and Natural IVF are well regarded for their safety profile. All systematic reviews with meta-analyses of randomized controlled trials (RCTs) where a low-dose gonadotropin was used alone or in combination with clomiphene (clomifene) citrate (CC) or letrozole in unselected populations identified significantly lower risk of OHSS compared with C-IVF (Table 4.3). No incidence of OHSS was observed in a large retrospective study of 20 244 cycles [17] as well as in a large RCT [18] by using a CC + gonadotropin with GnRH agonist trigger protocol. The incidence of VTE tends to be low due to only a modest increase in the level of serum estradiol with low-dose gonadotropin, particularly when combined with letrozole.

Many authorities including the American College of Obstetrics and Gynecology recommend this regimen in treating women with thrombogenic conditions (e.g., history of VTE or thrombophilia) (ACOG Committee Opinion No. 738). Mild gonadotropin stimulation combined with letrozole or tamoxifen has long been used in treating women with high risk of breast cancer.

Better patient tolerance, reduced stress: C-IVF, particularly when high gonadotropin doses are used due to poor ovarian reserve (POR), could be stressful to patients. At the other end, a high response leading to OHSS itself is a distressing condition. MS-IVF has been shown to be associated with less treatment-related stress [19]. A secondary analysis from a RCT reported fewer incidence of depression in MS-IVF cycles [11]; the same RCT observed more dropouts from treatment while undergoing C-IVF cycles.

Less expensive: Most RCTs that compared costs between mild and conventional IVF reported MS-IVF to be less expensive for women with normal or POR (Table 4.2). The mild stimulation protocol, which combines administration of CC and gonadotropin until the trigger for ovulation, avoids the use of a relatively expensive GnRH antagonist. A treatment cost between $675 and $725 has been reported by a single-arm study with this protocol [20]. Assisted conception remains a costly affair worldwide and MS-IVF may make it more accessible [21].

Treating older women or POR: IVF treatment of women over 40 or with POR remains a challenge. Incrementing gonadotropin dose has never been proved to improve the outcome. All systematic reviews that evaluated MS-IVF in poor responders found it to be as effective as C-IVF in terms of pregnancy success, with the added advantage of the former being less aggressive and less expensive. Acknowledging this benefit, the American Society of Reproductive Medicine (ASRM) recently recommended consideration of Mild IVF in treating poor responders [22]. The evidence of effectiveness of Natural/NM-IVF in this scenario is mainly limited to retrospective studies. There are only two related RCTs; both found Natural/NM-IVF to be associated with comparable pregnancy outcomes [23;24]. A retrospective study reported better LBR with NM-IVF, compared with high-dose antagonist regimen [25]. Repeated NM-IVF cycles followed by embryo transfer has been shown to

Table 4.2 Randomized controlled studies

Author (year)	Population	Mild	Conventional	Pregnancy outcomes MS-IVF vs. C-IVF	OHSS/ CCR MS-IVF vs. C-IVF	Other findings
Normal/high responders						
Baart et al. (2007) n = 111 [27]	Unselected	FSH 150 IU/d from D5 GnRH-ant	Long GnRHa DR, FSH 225 IU/d	OPRs/cycle: 19.0% vs. 17.1% (NS)	OHSS: 0% vs. 2% (NS)	Good-quality embryos: 51% vs. 35% ($p = 0.04$)
Blockeel et al. (2011) n = 76 [44]	Normal responders. First IVF/ICSI	FSH 150 IU/d from D5. GnRH-ant	Long GnRHa DR, FSH 225 IU/d	OPRs/cycle: 25% vs. 28% (NS)		#Oocyte: ↔
Casano et al. (2012) n = 412 [45]	High responders	FSH 150 IU/d from D4 (adjusted from D8). GnRH-ant	Long GnRHa DR, FSH 150 IU/d	LBR/cycle: 24.8% vs. 24.6% Cumulative LBR: 42.7% vs. 41.7% (NS)	OHSS: 1.6% vs. 2.0% CCRs: 1% vs. 0% (NS, both)	#Oocyte, embryo: ↔
Dhont et al. (1995) n = 303 [46]	Unselected	COCP pretreatment. CC 100 mg/d ×5 days, then hMG 150 IU/d. No GnRH-ant	COCP pretreatment. Long GnRHa DR, hMG 300 IU/d	LBRs/cycle: 18.5% vs. 25.7% (NS)	OHSS: 0% vs. 4.1% CCR: 25.5% vs. 2.6% ($p < 0.001$)	Embryo/ surplus embryos ↓MS-IVF
Elnashar et al. (2016) n = 80 [47]	Normal responders	Let 10 mg/d D3–7, FSH 75 IU/d from D5, GnRH-ant	Long GnRHa DR, FSH 150–225 IU/d	PRs/cycle: 12.5% vs. 42.5% ($p = 0.01$)		Good-quality embryo: ↔
Ghoshdastidar et al. (2010) n = 116 [48]	Good prognosis patients	CC 100 mg/d D2–6 + rFSH 100–150IU on D3, D5, daily from D7. GnRH-ant	Long GnRHa DR, rFSH 200–225 IU/d	PR/cycle: 35.7% vs. 40.0% Cumulative PRs: 60.0% vs. 58.0% (NS)		Top-quality embryo: 64% vs. 48% ($p < 0.05$) Dropout: 7.1% vs. 25.9% ($p < 0.05$)
Grochowski et al. (1999) n = 324 [49]	Normal responders first IVF/ICSI	CC 100 mg/d on D3–7 + hMG 150 IU on D4, 6, 8. No GnRH-ant	Long GnRHa DR, hMG 150–225 IU/d	PRs/ET: 29.7% vs. 25.5% (NS)	OHSS: 0% vs. 3.1% (NS)	Reduced cost with MS-IVF
Harrison et al. (1994) n = 150 [50]	Not specified	CC 100 mg/d on D3–7+ hMG 150 IU/d from D4. No GnRH-ant	Long-acting GnRH-a DR, hMG 225 IU/d	LBRs/cycle: 24% vs. 22% (NS)	CCR: 22% vs. 18% (NS)	#Oocytes/ embryos: ↔
Heijnen et al. (2007) n = 404 [34]	Normal responders first IVF/ICSI	FSH 150 IU/d from D5. GnRH-ant. SET	Long GnRHa DR, FSH 150 IU/d. DET	LBRs/cycle: 15.8% vs. 24.0% ($p < 0.05$). Cumulative LBRs: 43.4% vs. 44.7% (NS)	OHSS: 1.4% vs. 4% ($p = 0.04$) CCRs: 18% vs. 8% ($p < 0.001$)	Mean total costs: €8333 vs. €10 745 ($p = 0.006$). Dropout rates: ↓MS-IVF ($p = 0.001$)
Hohmann et al. (2003) n = 142 [51]	Normal response. < 3 prev. IVF	FSH fixed dose 150 IU/d from D5. GnRH-ant	Long GnRHa DR, fixed dose 150 IU/d FSH	OPRs/cycle: 16% vs. 18% (NS)	CCR: 2% vs. 0% (NS)	Grade 1 embryos: 61% vs. 29% ($p = 0.008$)
Karimzadeh et al. (2010) n = 200 [52]	Normal responders first IVF/ICSI	CC 100 mg D3–7. FSH 75 IU from D5; GnRH-ant + hMG 75 IU	Long GnRHa DR, FSH 150–225 IU/d	OPRs/ET: 32% vs. 26% (NS)	OHSS: 0% vs. 6% ($p = 0.02$) CCR: 4% vs. 0% (NS)	#Oocytes/ embryo. # Top-quality embryo: ↔

Study	Population	Protocol (MS-IVF)	Protocol (comparator)	Pregnancy/Live birth	CCR / OHSS	Other outcome
Long et al. (1992) $n = 70$ [53]	Normal responders. First IVF/ICSI	CC 50 mg/d on D2–6 + hMG 150 IU from D3, No GnRH-ant	GnRHa 0.25 mg/d from D2, hMG 150 IU/d	**LBR/cycle:** 11.8% vs. 8.3% (NS)	**CCR:** 17.6% vs. 16.7% (NS)	**#Oocytes/ embryos:** ↔
Lou et al. (2010) $n = 60$ [54]	Normal responders. First IVF/ICSI	hMG 150 IU/d (fixed) from D3. No GnRH-ant	Long GnRHa DR, rFSH 150–300 IU/d	**OPR/cycle:** 26.7% vs. 23.3% (NS)	**OHSS:** 0% vs. 6.7% (NS)	**Reduced cost** with MS-IVF
Mukherjee et al. (2012) $n = 94$ [55]	Normal responders	Let 5 mg/d D3–7, rFSH 75 from D3, GnRH-ant	rFSH 150–225 from D2, GnRH-ant	**PR/cycle:** 36% vs. 33% (NS)	**OHSS:** 0% vs. 13.5% ($p = 0.01$)	**Reduced cost** with MS-IVF
Oudshoorn et al. (2017) $n = 521$ [56]	High responder (not PCOS)	FSH fixed 100 IU/d in GnRH antagonist or agonist protocol	FSH fixed 150 IU/d, GnRH antagonist or agonist protocol	**LBR/cycle:** 25.7% vs. 25.2% (NS) **Cumulative LBRs:** 36% vs. 39.1% (NS)	**OHSS:** 4.7% vs. 14.7% ($p < 0.001$) **CCR:** 24.1% vs. 12.4% ($p = 0.001$)	**Cost:** ↔
Tummon et al. (1992) $n = 408$ [57]	Needed IVF except severe male factor	CC 100 mg/d on D5–9 + hMG 75 IU/d from D6. No GnRH-ant	Long GnRHa DR, then hMG dose adjusted with body weight	**PRs/cycle:** 10.7% vs. 9.2% (NS) **PRs/ET:** 19.2% vs. 17.5% (NS)	**CCR:** 30.8% vs. 10.1% ($p < 0.001$)	**# Oocytes/ embryo** ↓MS-IVF.
Zhang et al. (2016) $n = 564$ [18]	Normal responders first IVF/ICSI	COCP pre-Tx. CC 50 mg/d D3 till GnRHa trigger. FSH/hMG 75–150 IU/d. FET- SET	Long GnRHa DR, then FSH/hMG 150–300 IU/d. Fresh DET	**Cumulative LBR:** 49% vs. 63% (0.76; CI 0.64–0.89)	**OHSS:** 0% vs. 5.7% ($p < 0.001$)	**Multiple pregnancy:** ↑ with C-IVF
Poor responders						
Bastu et al. (2016) $n = 95$ [58]	POR (Bologna criteria)	Let 5 mg/d ×5 days, hMG 75+ rFSH 75 IU/d from D2. GnRH-ant	hMG 225 IU + rFSH 225 IU/d from D2, GnRH-ant	**CPR/cycle:** 15% vs. 13% (NS)	**CCR:** 24% vs. 29% (NS)	**#Oocytes/ embryos:** ↔
Goswami et al. (2004) $n = 38$ [59]	Prev. POR 1–3 long DR cycles	Let 2.5 mg/d from D3–7 + rFSH 75 IU/d D3 & 8. No GnRH-ant	Long GnRH-a DR, rFSH 300 IU/d	**CPR:** 23% vs. 24% (NS)	**CCR:** 7.7% vs. 4.0% (NS)	
Huang et al. (2015) $n = 105$ [60]	POR (Bologna criteria)	Let+ FSH 150 IU D4, 6, & 8.	GnRHa ("stop" protocol)	**CPR/cycle:** 26% vs. 25.5% (NS)		**Top-grade embryo:** ↔
Kim et al. (2009) $n = 90$ [24]	Previous cycle with < 4 follicles/ oocytes	rFSH 150 IU/d along with GnRH-ant	rFSH 225 IU from D3 GnRH-ant	**LBR/cycle:** 11.1% vs. 15.5 (NS)	**CCR:** 17.8% vs. 6.7% (NS)	**Grade 1/2 embryo:** ↓MS-IVF
Martinez et al. (2003) $n = 90$ [61]	Previous POR	CC 100 mg/d D4–8 + hMG 150 from D5	hMG 150 IU + FSH 150 IU from D2. Or, hMG 225 IU + FSH 225 IU from D2, GnRH-ant	**OPR/cycle:** 13.0% vs. 9.1% (NS)	**CCR:** 23.9% vs. 4.5% (NS)	

Table 4.2 (cont.)

Author (year)	Population	Mild	Conventional	Pregnancy outcomes MS-IVF vs. C-IVF	OHSS/ CCR MS-IVF vs. C-IVF	Other findings
Mohsen et al. (2013) $n = 60$ [62]	Previous 1 or more failed cycles.	Let 5 mg/d D2–6; hMG 150 IU/d from D7. GnRH-ant	GnRHa "short flare" from D2 hMG 300 IU	**CPR/cycle:** 13.3% vs. 16.6% (NS)	**CCR:** 20% vs. 16.6% (NS)	**Mean # of oocytes/ embryos:** ↔
Pilehvari et al. (2016) $n = 77$ [63]	POR (Bologna criteria)	CC 100 mg/d from D2–6; hMG 150 IU from D7. GnRH-ant	rFSH + hMG 300 IU/d from D2 GnRH-ant	**CPR/ET:** 4% vs. 5.6% (NS)	**CCR:** 28.6% vs. 31.4% (NS)	**Good-quality embryos:** ↔
Ragni et al. (2012) $n = 304$ [64]	FSH > 12 IU/L, prev. ≤ 3 oocyte	CC 150 mg/d on D3–7 No Gn/GnRH-ant	GnRHa "short flare," rFSH 450 IU/d	**LBR/ cycle:** 3% vs. 5%	**CCR:** 14% vs. 14%	**Lower cost** with CC
Revelli et al. (2014) $n = 640$ [65]	Age < 43 years, AMH 0.14–1.0 ng/ml AFC 4–10.	CC 100 mg/d, hMG/ Pergoveris 150 IU/d from D5. GnRH-ant	Long GnRHa DR, 300–450 IU/d	**OPR/ET:** 17.8% vs. 16.8% (NS)	**CCR:** 13% vs. 2.2% ($p < 0.01$)	**Top-grade embryo:** ↔
van Tilborg et al. (2018) $n = 511$ [66]	Age: < 43 years, FSH ≥ 15 IU/L, AMH < 1.5 ng/ml, AFC ≤ 8	rFSH 150 IU/d, GnRHa long DR or GnRH-ant protocol	rFSH 225 IU if AFC 8–10/ 450 IU/d if AFC < 8, GnRHa long/ GnRH-ant	**LBR/cycle:** 15.8% vs. 14.8% **Cumulative LBR:** 20% vs. 17.6% (NS)	**CCR:** 23.5% vs. 7.6% ($p < 0.001$)	**Cost:** €1099 less with MS-IVF
Youssef et al. (2017) $n = 39$ [67]	Age ≥ 35 years FSH> 10 IU/ AFC < 5/ prev. POR	COCP pretreatment; fixed FSH 150 IU/d from D5 of last pill; GnRH-ant	Long GnRHa DR, hMG 450 IU/d fixed dose	**OPR/ woman:** 12.8% vs. 13.6% (NS)	**CCR:** 26% vs. 18% (NS)	**Oocytes/ embryo** ↓ MS-IVF. **# Top-quality embryo:** ↔
Yu et al. (2018) $n = 116$ [68]	Age < 43 years, FSH ≥ 15 IU/L, AFC ≤ 8, AMH < 1.5 ng/ml	Letrozole 5 mg/d from D3 for 5 days. hMG 75 IU/d IM from D8	Long GnRHa DR from D3 of prev. cycle. hMG 225–330 IU/d	**LBR cycle:** 15.3% vs. 20.4% (NS)	**CCR:** 32.7% vs. 11.1% ($p < 0.05$)	**High-quality embryo:** ↔

DR = downregulation; GnRH-ant = GnRH antagonist; GnRHa = GnRH agonist; NS = not significant; ↔ = no difference; LBR = live birth rate; LET = letrozole; COCP = combined oral contraceptive pill; PREV. = previous; rFSH = recombinant FSH; SET = single embryo transfer; DET = double embryo transfer; ET = embryo transfer; AMH = anti-Müllerian hormone; AFC = antral follicle count; see text for other abbreviations. [RCTs that used ≤ 150 IU/d dose of gonadotropin ± oral agents as mild stimulation IVF] improve LBRs in women with POR [26]. The added advantage of selecting a NM protocol is to keep the course "patient's friendly" while undergoing multiple cycles of IVF.

Effectiveness of MA-IVF

Scientific Basis of Effectiveness

It is now apparent that the number of competent oocytes or embryos is not increased with higher stimulation doses. This concept was introduced more than 10 years ago in a RCT where the number of euploid embryo was found to be the same, whether conventional or mild dose was used for ovarian stimulation; a higher stimulation dose only helped to produce more aneuploid embryos [27]. The normal physiological endocrine or paracrine milieu inside a follicle is altered when exposed to a high level of exogenous hormones [28]. Indeed, a laboratory-based RCT found incremental dose of gonadotropin helped in increasing only the number of oocytes, with no increase in the number of good-quality embryos; the blastocyst–oocyte ratio actually correlated inversely with incremental stimulation [29]. Studies have revealed, in conventionally stimulated cycles, only 5 percent of oocytes will produce a baby [30]; in contrast, 25 percent of oocytes collected through Natural cycle IVF leads to a live birth [31].

Clinical Evidence of Effectiveness

Pregnancy outcomes: An analysis of 650 000 IVF cycles from the ASRM database found an inverse correlation between gonadotropin dose and LBR, regardless of women's age, prognosis, and number of oocytes retrieved [32]. However, despite this overwhelming evidence, Mild IVF has not gained wide acceptance among the IVF community mainly due to the doubt on its pregnancy outcome and the risk of cycle cancellation. The debate has been fueled by the evidence of lower ongoing pregnancy rates (OPRs) from older meta-analyses on unselected populations [33]. Since then, a series of RCTs have been published; apart from two trials [18;34], none proved C-IVF to be better in terms of LBRs. Interestingly, both the RCTs had a policy of single embryo transfer (SET) in the MS-IVF arm while double embryo transfer was carried out in the C-IVF arm, making

the comparison invalid. All the RCTs conducted on the poor-responder patients found comparable pregnancy outcomes with MS-IVF (Table 4.2).

All recent systematic reviews comparing MS-IVF and C-IVF found MS-IVF to yield comparable pregnancy success (Table 4.3). The ASRM Practice Committee recently performed a systematic review without meta-analysis and recommended consideration of MA-IVF to treat poor-responder women [22]. However, under-powered live-birth data, lack of evidence on the cumulative outcome, predominance of small RCTs with risk of bias, and considerable clinical heterogeneity among the trials were the main limitations acknowledged in all these reviews. Recently our group has conducted two updated systematic reviews comparing MS-IVF and C-IVF, adding more recent RCTs [35;36]; our meta-analysis from a pooled population adequately powered for live birth showed no difference in LBRs with a moderate quality of evidence.

Cumulative live birth is widely regarded as the yardstick of measuring the success of an IVF program. There is skepticism whether, by yielding fewer oocytes, MS-IVF holds the same cumulative success as C-IVF. Research on cumulative outcomes is limited; however, all studies that looked at this outcome did not find it better with C-IVF (Table 4.2), with one exception [18]. While per cycle LBRs are reported to be lower, Natural IVF cycles have been associated with high cumulative pregnancy rates and LBRs [37;38]. In unselected populations, a recent RCT found 51 percent cumulative LBR with up to six cycles of NM-IVF, compared with 59 percent following three cycles of C-IVF with SET [39].

Perinatal outcomes: A high number of retrieved oocytes have been associated with low-birth-weight babies and preterm delivery [40]. Several studies reported Natural IVF was associated with higher mean birth weight of the newborns and lower risk of preterm delivery, compared with those born through conventionally stimulated IVF cycles. On the contrary, an RCT comparing C-IVF with SET and NM-IVF did not find such difference [39]. A recent meta-analysis of related studies found higher prevalence of prematurity and low-birth-weight babies with conventionally stimulated IVF compared with Natural IVF [41]. A more physiological hormonal milieu in the endometrium has been implicated for this outcome.

Table 4.3 Systematic reviews comparing low-dose gonadotropin ± oral medications versus high-dose regimens

Systematic reviews	Interventions	LBR	CPR	OHSS	CCR	Comments
Unselected/normal responders						
Sterrenburg et al. 2011 [69]	Gn only low vs. high dose IVF	-	↔	↔	↔/↑	High CCR with 100 IU/d dose, not with 150 IU
Gibreel et al. 2012 [70]	CC + Gn vs. C-IVF	↔ •	↔ ••	↓ •	↑ •	CCR ↔ with antagonist
Matsaseng et al. 2013 [33]	Low Gn only/CC + Gn vs. C-IVF	↓#	-	↓	↑	5 RCTs, 4 with Gn only
Datta et al. 2021 [36]	Low Gn ± CC/Let vs. C-IVF	↔ **	↔ *	↓ **	↑ **	No difference in CLBR
Figueiredo et al. 2013 [71]	CC + Gn vs. C-IVF	↔ •	↔ ••	↓ •		7 RCTs
Unselected (poor responders as subgroup)						
Bechtejew et al. 2017 [72]	CC/Let + Gn vs. C-IVF	↔ •	↔ •••	↓ •		Imprecise evidence with Let
Fan et al. 2017 [73]	CC ± Gn vs. C-IVF	↔#	↔	↔	↑/↔	6 RCTs
Kamath et al. 2017 [74]	CC/Let ± Gn vs. C-IVF	↔ •	↔ •/••	↓ •	↑ •	Same findings – normal or poor responders
Poor responders only						
Song et al. 2016 [75]	Gn ± CC/Let vs. C-IVF	↔#	↔	-	↔	4 RCT/non-RCTs
ASRM 2018 [22]	Low Gn ± CC/Let vs. C-IVF		↔	-		Same findings, with or without CC/Let
Youssef et al. 2018 [76]	Lower vs. higher dose IVF	↔#	↔	-	↔/↑##	Same findings, with or without CC/Let, except for CCR
Datta et al. 2020 [35]	Low Gn ± CC/Let vs. C-IVF	↔ ••	↔ ••	-	↔ ••	No difference in CLBR
Montoya-Botero et al. 2021 [77]	Gn ± CC/Let vs. C-IVF	↔ •	↔ •	-	↑ •	No difference in CLBR
High responders only						
Datta et al. 2021 [36]	Gn only low vs. high-dose IVF	↔ ••	↔ ••	↓ ••	↔ ••	No difference in CLBR

CPR = clinical pregnancy rate; Let = letrozole; CLBR = cumulative live birth rate; see text for other abbreviations.

* Low, ** moderate, *** high quality of evidence. # Only one RCT; # No difference with Gn only protocol, high with oral medication; ## No difference with Gn only protocol, high with oral medication.

Criticism Surrounding MA-IVF

High risk of cycle cancellation: Earlier studies on Natural IVF were associated with high premature ovulation and cancellation rates [42]. However, recent systematic reviews observed no significant difference in the cycle cancellation rates (CCR) between NM-IVF and C-IVF cycles when a GnRH antagonist was used (Table 4.3). The use of indomethacin to prevent premature ovulation has been shown to be effective. The evidence is conflicting on MS-IVF: some RCTs found higher CCR with MS-IVF, while others did not find any

difference (Table 4.2). Adoption of different cancellation policy might have influenced the findings.

Fewer surplus embryos for cryopreservation: With the likelihood of creating fewer embryos through MS-IVF, there might not be many embryos for cryopreservation, which theoretically may lower cumulative live birth. Some studies reported fewer cryopreserved embryos in MS-IVF cycles compared with C-IVF, while others found the mean of total embryos in conventional-dose regimen not significantly higher. Most systematic reviews found lower (mean) number of embryos with MS-IVF; yet the mean or proportion of high-grade embryos has been found to be equivalent, if not better (Table 4.2), explaining why cumulative pregnancy tends to not compromise despite fewer embryos created.

Current Status and Future Developments

Notwithstanding skepticism and criticism MA-IVF is gaining more and more acceptance in the IVF community. Patients are also becoming more aware of this "patient-friendly" option. Recent recognition of Mild IVF by the ASRM as preferred approach for poor responders has been a landmark step [22]. A recent Cochrane review demonstrated that individualizing the stimulation doses according to ovarian reserve is no better than standard 150 IU, only a dose < 150 IU may decrease the risk of OHSS [43]. Mild/Natural IVF has secured a place in treating women with estrogen-sensitive conditions or women with multiple failed C-IVF cycles. Repeated NM-IVF with oocytes/embryo "banking" followed by transfer from a larger cohort of embryos has drawn attention in treating women with POR.

Research on Mild/Natural IVF has progressed with time. Our most recent systematic review with meta-analysis (Table 4.3) has produced moderate to high quality of evidence on the pregnancy outcomes, for the first time from an adequately powered population. Current data give assurance on the clinical effectiveness and safety (decreased risk of OHSS) of MS-IVF, which also reduces the treatment burden and cost. The presence of significant methodological variations between the studies remains a limiting factor in the evaluation of MA-IVF; it necessitates further well-designed RCTs to produce more robust evidence.

References

1. Sunkara SK, Rittenberg V, Raine-Fenning N, et al. Association between the number of eggs and live birth in IVF treatment: an analysis of 400 135 treatment cycles. Hum Reprod 2011;26(7):1768–1774.

2. Steward RG, Lan L, Shah AA, et al. Oocyte number as a predictor for ovarian hyperstimulation syndrome and live birth: an analysis of 256,381 in vitro fertilization cycles. Fertil Steril 2014;101(4):967–973.

3. Drakopoulos P, Blockeel C, Stoop D, et al. Conventional ovarian stimulation and single embryo transfer for IVF/ICSI. How many oocytes do we need to maximize cumulative live birth rates after utilization of all fresh and frozen embryos? Hum Reprod 2016;31(2):370–376.

4. Polyzos NP, Drakopoulos P, Parra J, et al. Cumulative live birth rates according to the number of oocytes retrieved after the first ovarian stimulation for in vitro fertilization/intracytoplasmic sperm injection: a multicenter multinational analysis including approximately 15,000 women. Fertil Steril 2018;110(4):661.e1–670.e1.

5. Smeltzer S, Acharya K, Truong T, Pieper C, Muasher S. Clinical pregnancy and live birth increase significantly with every additional blastocyst up to five and decline after that: an analysis of 16,666 first fresh single-blastocyst transfers from the Society for Assisted Reproductive Technology registry. Fertil Steril 2019;112(5):866.e1–873.e1.

6. Magnusson A, Wennerholm UB, Källén K, et al. The association between the number of oocytes retrieved for IVF, perinatal outcome and obstetric complications. Hum Reprod 2018;33(10):1939–1947.

7. Datta AK, Campbell S, Felix N, Singh JSH, Nargund G. Oocyte or embryo number needed to optimize live birth and cumulative live birth rates in mild stimulation IVF cycles. Reprod Biomed Online 2021;S1472-6483(21)00096-1. doi: 10.1016/j.rbmo.2021.02.010.

8. Nargund G, Chian RC. ISMAAR: leading the global agenda for a more physiological, patient-centred, accessible and safer approaches in ART. J Assist Reprod Genet 2013;30(2):155–156.

9. Nargund G, Fauser BC, Macklon NS, et al.; Rotterdam ISMAAR Consensus Group on Terminology for Ovarian Stimulation for IVF. The ISMAAR proposal on terminology for ovarian stimulation for IVF. Hum Reprod 2007;22(11):2801–2804.

10. Zegers-Hochschild F, Adamson GD, de Mouzon J, et al.; International Committee for Monitoring Assisted Reproductive Technology; World Health Organization. The International Committee for Monitoring Assisted Reproductive Technology (ICMART) and the World Health Organization (WHO) Revised Glossary on ART Terminology, 2009. Hum Reprod 2009;24(11):2683–2687.

11. de Klerk C, Macklon NS, Heijnen EM, et al. The psychological impact of IVF failure after two or more cycles of IVF with a mild versus standard treatment strategy. Hum Reprod 2007;22(9):2554–2558.

12. Verberg MF, Eijkemans MJ, Heijnen EM, et al. Why do couples drop-out from IVF treatment? A prospective cohort study. Hum Reprod 2008;23(9):2050–2055.

13. Seyhan A, Ata B, Polat M, et al. Severe early ovarian hyperstimulation syndrome following GnRH agonist trigger with the addition of 1500 IU hCG. Hum Reprod 2013;28(9):2522–2528.

14. Valbuena D, Martin J, de Pablo JL, *et al.* Increasing levels of estradiol are deleterious to embryonic implantation because they directly affect the embryo. *Fertil Steril* 2001;**76**(5):962–968.

15. Labarta E, Martínez-Conejero JA, Alamá P, *et al.* Endometrial receptivity is affected in women with high circulating progesterone levels at the end of the follicular phase: a functional genomics analysis. *Hum Reprod* 2011;**26**(7):1813–1825.

16. Haouzi D, Assou S, Dechanet C, *et al.* Controlled ovarian hyperstimulation for in vitro fertilization alters endometrial receptivity in humans: protocol effects. *Biol Reprod* 2010;**82**(4):679–686.

17. Kato K, Takehara Y, Segawa T, *et al.* Minimal ovarian stimulation combined with elective single embryo transfer policy: age-specific results of a large, single-centre, Japanese cohort. *Reprod Biol Endocrinol* 2012;**10**:35.

18. Zhang JJ, Merhi Z, Yang M, *et al.* Minimal stimulation IVF vs conventional IVF: a randomized controlled trial. *Am J Obstet Gynecol* 2016;**214**(1):96.e1–96.e8.

19. Hojgaard A, Ingerslev HJ, Dinesen J. Friendly IVF: patient opinions. *Hum Reprod* 2001;**16** (7):1391–1396.

20. Aleyamma TK, Kamath MS, Muthukumar K, Mangalaraj AM, George K. Affordable ART: a different perspective. *Hum Reprod* 2011;**26** (12):3312–3318.

21. Paulson RJ, Fauser BCJM, Vuong LTN, Doody K. Can we modify assisted reproductive technology practice to broaden reproductive care access? *Fertil Steril* 2016;**105**(5):1138–1143.

22. Practice Committee of the American Society for Reproductive Medicine. Electronic address: ASRM@asrm.org. Comparison of pregnancy rates for poor responders using IVF with mild ovarian stimulation versus conventional IVF: a guideline. *Fertil Steril* 2018;**109**(6):993–999.

23. Morgia F, Sbracia M, Schimberni M, *et al.* A controlled trial of natural cycle versus microdose gonadotropin-releasing hormone analog flare cycles in poor responders undergoing in vitro fertilization. *Fertil Steril* 2004;**81** (6):1542–1547.

24. Kim CH, Kim SR, Cheon YP, *et al.* Minimal stimulation using gonadotropin-releasing hormone (GnRH) antagonist and recombinant human follicle-stimulating hormone versus GnRH antagonist multiple-dose protocol in low responders undergoing in vitro fertilization/intracytoplasmic sperm injection. *Fertil Steril* 2009;**92**(6):2082–2084.

25. Lainas TG, Sfontouris IA, Venetis CA, *et al.* Live birth rates after modified natural cycle compared with high-dose FSH stimulation using GnRH antagonists in poor responders. *Hum Reprod* 2015;**30**(10):2321–2330.

26. Datta AK, Campbell S, Felix N, Nargund G. Accumulation of embryos over 3 natural modified IVF (ICSI) cycles followed by transfer to improve the outcome of poor responders. *Facts Views Vis Obgyn* 2019;**11**(1):77–84.

27. Baart EB, Martini E, Eijkemans MJ, *et al.* Milder ovarian stimulation for in-vitro fertilization reduces aneuploidy in the human preimplantation embryo: a randomized controlled trial. *Hum Reprod* 2007;**22**(4):980–988.

28. von Wolff M, Kollmann Z, Flück CE, *et al.* Gonadotrophin stimulation for in vitro fertilization significantly alters the hormone milieu in follicular fluid: a comparative study between natural cycle IVF and conventional IVF. *Hum Reprod* 2014;**29**(5):1049–1057.

29. Arce JC, Andersen AN, Fernández-Sánchez M, *et al.* Ovarian response to recombinant human follicle-stimulating hormone: a randomized, antimullerian hormone-stratified, dose-response trial in women undergoing in vitro fertilization/intracytoplasmic sperm injection. *Fertil Steril* 2014;**102**(6):1633.e5–1640.e5.

30. Patrizio P, Sakkas D. From oocyte to baby: a clinical evaluation of the biological efficiency of in vitro fertilization. *Fertil Steril* 2009;**91**(4):1061–1066.

31. Silber SJ, Kato K, Aoyama N, *et al.* Intrinsic fertility of human oocytes. *Fertil Steril* 2017;**107**(5):1232–1237.

32. Baker VL, Brown MB, Luke B, Smith GW, Ireland JJ. Gonadotropin dose is negatively correlated with live birth rate: analysis of more than 650,000 assisted reproductive technology cycles. *Fertil Steril* 2015;**104**(5):1145.e5–1152.e5.

33. Matsaseng T, Kruger T, Steyn W. Mild ovarian stimulation for in vitro fertilization: are we ready to change? A meta-analysis. *Gynecol Obstet Invest* 2013;**76**(4):233–240.

34. Heijnen EM, Eijkemans MJ, De Klerk C, *et al.* A mild treatment strategy for in-vitro fertilisation: a randomised non-inferiority trial. *Lancet* 2007;**369**(9563):743–749.

35. Datta AK, Maheshwari A, Felix N, Campbell S, Nargund G. Mild versus conventional ovarian stimulation for IVF in poor responders: a systematic review and meta-analysis. *Reprod Biomed Online* 2020;**41**:225–238.

36. Datta AK, Maheshwari A, Felix N, Campbell S, Nargund G. Mild versus conventional ovarian stimulation for IVF in poor, normal and hyper-responders: a systematic review and meta-analysis. *Hum Reprod Update* 2021;**27**:229–253.

37. Aboulghar MA, Mansour RT, Serour GA, *et al.* In vitro fertilization in a spontaneous cycle: a successful simple protocol. *J Obstet Gynaecol (Tokyo 1995)* 1995;**21**(4):337–340.

38. Nargund G, Waterstone J, Bland J, *et al.* Cumulative conception and live birth rates in natural (unstimulated) IVF cycles. *Hum Reprod* 2001;**16**(2):259–262.

39. Bensdorp AJ, Tjon-Kon-Fat RI, Bossuyt PM, *et al.* Prevention of multiple pregnancies in couples with unexplained or mild male subfertility: randomised controlled trial of in vitro fertilisation with single embryo transfer or in vitro fertilisation in modified natural cycle compared with intrauterine insemination with controlled ovarian hyperstimulation. *BMJ* 2015;**350**:g7771.

40. Sunkara SK, La Marca A, Seed PT, Khalaf Y. Increased risk of preterm birth and low birthweight with very high number of oocytes following IVF: an analysis of 65 868 singleton live birth outcomes. *Hum Reprod* 2015;**30**(6):1473–1480.

41. Kamath MS, Kirubakaran R, Mascarenhas M, Sunkara SK. Perinatal outcomes after stimulated versus natural cycle IVF: a systematic review and meta-analysis. *Reprod Biomed Online* 2018;**36**(1):94–101.

42. Pelinck MJ, Hoek A, Simons AH, Heineman MJ. Efficacy of natural cycle IVF: a review of the literature. *Hum Reprod Update* 2002;**8**(2):129–139.

43. Lensen SF, Wilkinson J, Leijdekkers JA, *et al.* Individualised gonadotropin dose selection using markers of ovarian reserve for women undergoing in vitro fertilisation plus intracytoplasmic sperm injection (IVF/ICSI). *Cochrane Database Syst Rev* 2018;**2**:CD012693.

44. Blockeel C, Sterrenburg MD, Broekmans FJ, *et al.* Follicular phase endocrine characteristics during ovarian stimulation and GnRH antagonist cotreatment for IVF: RCT comparing recFSH initiated on cycle day 2 or 5. *J Clin Endocrinol Metab* 2011;**96**:1122–1128.

45. Casano S, Guidetti D, Patriarca A, *et al.* MILD ovarian stimulation with GnRH-antagonist vs. long protocol with low dose FSH for non-PCO high responders undergoing IVF: a prospective, randomized study including thawing cycles. *J Assist Reprod Genet* 2012;**29**:1343–1351.

46. Dhont M, Onghena A, Coetsier T, De Sutter P. Prospective randomized study of clomiphene citrate and gonadotrophins versus goserelin and gonadotrophins for follicular stimulation in assisted reproduction. *Hum Reprod* 1995;**10**:791–796.

47. Elnashar I, Farghaly TA, Abdalbadie AS, *et al.* Low cost ovarian stimulation protocol is associated with lower pregnancy rate in normal responders in comparison to long protocol. *Fertil Steril* 2016;**106**(Suppl 3):e194–e195.

48. Ghoshdastidar S, Maity S, Ghoshdastidar B. Improved ICSI outcome in poor responders using a novel stimulation regime with micro-dose flare followed by GnRH antagonist in mid follicular phase. *Hum Reprod* 2010;**1**:i316.

49. Grochowski D, Wolczynski S, Kuczynski W, *et al.* Good results of milder form of ovarian stimulation in an in vitro fertilization/intracytoplasmic sperm injection program. *Gynecol Endocrinol* 1999;**13**:297–304.

50. Harrison RF, Kondaveeti U, Barry-Kinsella C, *et al.* Should gonadotropin-releasing hormone down-regulation therapy be routine in in vitro fertilization? *Fertil Steril* 1994;**62**:568–573.

51. Hohmann FP, Macklon NS, Fauser BC. A randomized comparison of two ovarian stimulation protocols with gonadotropin-releasing hormone (GnRH) antagonist cotreatment for in vitro fertilization commencing recombinant follicle-stimulating hormone on cycle day 2 or 5 with the standard long GnRH agonist protocol. *J Clin Endocrinol Metab* 2003;**88**:166–173.

52. Karimzadeh MA, Ahmadi S, Oskouian H, Rahmani E. Comparison of mild stimulation and conventional stimulation in ART outcome. *Arch Gynecol Obstet* 2010;**281**:741–746.

53. Long CA, Sopelak VM, Lincoln SR, Cowan BD. Luteal phase consequences of low-dose gonadotropin-releasing hormone agonist therapy in nonluteal-supported in vitro fertilization cycles. *Fertil Steril* 1995;**64**:573–576.

54. Lou HY, Huang XY. Modified natural cycle for in vitro fertilization and embryo transfer in normal ovarian responders. *J Int Med Res* 2010;**38**:2070–2076.

55. Mukherjee S, Sharma S, Chakravarty BN. Letrozole in a low-cost in vitro fertilization protocol in intracytoplasmic sperm injection cycles for male factor infertility: a randomized controlled trial. *J Hum Reprod Sci* 2012;**5**:170–174.

56. Oudshoorn SC, van Tilborg TC, Eijkemans MJC, *et al.* Individualized versus standard FSH dosing in women starting IVF/ICSI: an RCT. Part 2: The predicted hyper responder. *Hum Reprod* 2017;**32**:2506–2514.

57. Tummon IS, Daniel SA, Kaplan BR, Nisker JA, Yuzpe AA. Randomized, prospective comparison of luteal leuprolide acetate and gonadotropins versus clomiphene citrate and gonadotropins in 408 first cycles of in vitro fertilization. *Fertil Steril* 1992;**58**:563–568.

58. Bastu E, Buyru F, Ozsurmeli M, *et al.* A randomized, single-blind, prospective trial comparing three

different gonadotropin doses with or without addition of letrozole during ovulation stimulation in patients with poor ovarian response. *Eur J Obstet Gynecol Reprod Biol* 2016;**203**:30–34.

59. Goswami SK, Das T, Chattopadhyay R, *et al.* A randomized single-blind controlled trial of letrozole as a low-cost IVF protocol in women with poor ovarian response: a preliminary report. *Hum Reprod* 2004;**19**:2031–2035.

60. Huang R, Wang B, Yang X, Li TT, Liang XY. The comparison of mild stimulation vs. controlled ovarian hyperstimulation protocol in poor ovarian responders: a prospective randomized study. *Hum Reprod* 2015;**1**:i49–i50.

61. Martinez F, Coroleu B, Marques L, *et al.* Comparison of "short protocol" versus "antagonists" with or without clomiphene citrate for stimulation in IVF of patients with "low response". [Spanish]. *Rev Iberoam Fertil Reprod Hum* 2003;**20**:355–360.

62. Mohsen IA, El Din RE. Minimal stimulation protocol using letrozole versus microdose flare up GnRH agonist protocol in women with poor ovarian response undergoing ICSI. *Gynecol Endocrinol* 2013;**29**:105–108.

63. Pilehvari S, Shahrokh Tehraninejad E, Hosseinrashidi B, *et al.* Comparison pregnancy outcomes between minimal stimulation protocol and conventional GnRH antagonist protocols in poor ovarian responders. *J Family Reprod Health* 2016;**10**:35–42.

64. Ragni G, Levi-Setti PE, Fadini R, *et al.* Clomiphene citrate versus high doses of gonadotropins for in vitro fertilisation in women with compromised ovarian reserve: a randomised controlled non-inferiority trial. *Reprod Biol Endocrinol* 2012;**10**:114.

65. Revelli A, Chiadò A, Dalmasso P, *et al.* "Mild" vs. "long" protocol for controlled ovarian hyperstimulation in patients with expected poor ovarian responsiveness undergoing in vitro fertilization (IVF): a large prospective randomized trial. *J Assist Reprod Genet* 2014;**31**:809–815.

66. van Tilborg TC, Torrance HL, Oudshoorn SC, *et al.*; OPTIMIST study group. The end for individualized dosing in IVF ovarian stimulation? Reply to letters-to-the-editor regarding the OPTIMIST papers. *Hum Reprod* 2018;**33**:984–988.

67. Youssef MA, van Wely M, Al-Inany H, *et al.* A mild ovarian stimulation strategy in women with poor ovarian reserve undergoing IVF: a multicenter randomized non-inferiority trial. *Hum Reprod* 2017;**32**:112–118.

68. Yu R, Jin H, Huang X, Lin J, Wang P. Comparison of modified agonist, mild-stimulation and antagonist protocols for in vitro fertilization in

patients with diminished ovarian reserve. *J Int Med Res* 2018;**46**:2327–2337.

69. Sterrenburg MD, Veltman-Verhulst SM, Eijkemans MJ, *et al.* Clinical outcomes in relation to the daily dose of recombinant follicle-stimulating hormone for ovarian stimulation in in vitro fertilization in presumed normal responders younger than 39 years: a meta-analysis. *Hum Reprod Update* 2011;**17**:184–196.

70. Gibreel A, Maheshwari A, Bhattacharya S. Clomiphene citrate in combination with gonadotropins for controlled ovarian stimulation in women undergoing in vitro fertilization. *Cochrane Database Syst Rev* 2012;**11**:CD008528.

71. Figueiredo JB, Nastri CO, Vieira AD, Martins WP. Clomiphene combined with gonadotropins and GnRH antagonist versus conventional controlled ovarian hyperstimulation without clomiphene in women undergoing assisted reproductive techniques: systematic review and meta-analysis. *Arch Gynecol Obstet* 2013;**287**:779–790.

72. Bechtejew TN, Nadai MN, Nastri CO, Martins WP. Clomiphene citrate and letrozole to reduce follicle-stimulating hormone consumption during ovarian stimulation: systematic review and meta-analysis. *Ultrasound Obstet Gynecol* 2017;**50**:315–323.

73. Fan Y, Zhang X, Hao Z, *et al.* Effectiveness of mild ovarian stimulation versus GnRH agonist protocol in women undergoing assisted reproductive technology: a meta-analysis. *Gynecol Endocrinol* 2017;**33**:746–756.

74. Kamath MS, Maheshwari A, Bhattacharya S, Lor KY, Gibreel A. Oral medications including clomiphene citrate or aromatase inhibitors with gonadotropins for controlled ovarian stimulation in women undergoing in vitro fertilisation. *Cochrane Database Syst Rev* 2017;**11**:CD008528.

75. Song D, Shi Y, Zhong Y, *et al.* Efficiency of mild ovarian stimulation with clomiphene on poor ovarian responders during IVF\ICSI procedures: a meta-analysis. *Eur J Obstet Gynecol Reprod Biol* 2016;**204**:36–43.

76. Youssef MA, van Wely M, Mochtar M, *et al.* Low dosing of gonadotropins in in vitro fertilization cycles for women with poor ovarian reserve: systematic review and meta-analysis. *Fertil Steril* 2018;**109**:289–301.

77. Montoya-Botero P, Drakopoulos P, Gonzalez-Foruria I, Polyzos NP. Fresh and cumulative live birth rates in mild versus conventional stimulation for IVF cycles in poor ovarian responders: a systematic review and meta-analysis. *Hum Reprod Open* 2021;**2021**:hoaa066.

The Case against Mild Stimulation Protocols

Carlotta Zacà, Francesca Pennetta, and Andrea Borini

Introduction

The number of retrieved oocytes is one of the major parameters by which the intensity of ovarian stimulation is estimated. While conventional stimulation protocols in in vitro fertilization (IVF) are designed to obtain maximum oocytes yields, they have often been associated with increased risk of complications, increased costs derived from higher gonadotropin dosage, and lower embryo quality. For these reasons, physicians have introduced a milder approach to ovarian stimulation, focusing on a more patient-friendly and safe method, while attempting to improve IVF outcomes. Typically, the strengths of mild stimulation include: reduced mean number of days of stimulation, smaller total amount of gonadotropins, smaller mean number of oocytes retrieved balanced by possibly better embryo quality, decreased treatment discomfort, and reduced risk of complications. However, to date there are still unanswered questions about the possibility that a milder approach to ovarian stimulation is clinically superior to conventional regimens. In fact, larger prospective studies in different subgroups of patients are still needed to evaluate the impact of mild stimulation on cumulative pregnancy and live birth rates (LBRs). Moreover, widespread acceptance of mild stimulation is often limited by uncertainty among clinicians, as obtaining fewer oocytes/embryos may imply suboptimal results and increased chances of cycle cancellation.

Definition

There seems to be no consistency in terminology used by literature, media, and medical journals to define mild stimulation. In fact, different terms are often improperly used: such as "natural," "patient-friendly," "mild," "minimal," and "minimally stimulating" IVF. As a result, there is significant uncertainty among clinicians, scientists, and patients. The International Glossary on Infertility and Fertility Care published in 2017 refers to mild ovarian stimulation for IVF as a protocol in which the ovaries are stimulated with gonadotropins, and/or other pharmacological compounds, with the intention to limit the number of retrieved oocytes following stimulation for IVF [1].

A group of international experts with an interest on this subject founded the International Society for Mild Approaches in Assisted Reproduction (ISMAAR) and defined more specifically "mild-stimulation IVF" as "a method when follicle stimulating hormone (FSH) or human menopausal gonadotropin (hMG) is administered at a lower dose and or for a shorter duration in a gonadotropin releasing hormone (GnRH)-antagonist co-treated cycle, or when oral compounds, antiestrogens, or aromatase inhibitors (AIs) are used either alone or in combination with gonadotropins (Gn) with the aim of collecting fewer oocytes" [2]. In addition, some studies indicate the threshold of less than eight oocytes retrieved to identify mild stimulation cycles [3–5].

It is known, however, that even mild ovarian stimulation may be associated with a large number of oocytes retrieved in a proportion of women. In consideration of this, several studies [6] included improperly in the mild stimulation category cycles in which more than eight oocytes were retrieved, introducing a potential bias in the interpretation of results.

Mild stimulation is implemented through several strategies, using agents such as aromatase inhibitors, clomiphene (clomifene) citrate, low-dose exogenous gonadotropins, GnRH antagonists, and late follicular phase human chorionic gonadotropin/luteinizing hormone, employed as monotherapy or in combination.

To date, there is no consensus on drugs, regimens, and doses by which mild stimulation should be achieved, making this approach difficult to discriminate in comparison to standard ovarian stimulation [7].

More Oocytes Is Better

Ovarian stimulation to achieve multiple follicle development has been an integral part of IVF treatment. In the early 1980s, in order to increase IVF pregnancy rates, controlled ovarian hyperstimulation was introduced to stimulate multiple follicle development, thus retrieving multiple oocytes [8]. It is known that the number of oocytes retrieved is an important prognostic variable, a robust surrogate outcome measure for clinical success in IVF treatment. Therefore, over the years protocols have developed to optimize this outcome [9;10]. On the other hand, low numbers of retrieved oocytes have been associated with diminished outcomes, often attributed to ovarian aging [11]. It has been shown that the availability at retrieval of a good number of oocytes improves the chances to generate good-quality embryos and, consequently, to achieve a pregnancy and a live birth [12–15]. In order to maximize quality and quantity of both oocytes and embryos, the choice of the ovarian stimulation protocol is crucial. Nevertheless, in consideration of cost, complexity, effects, and stress associated with conventional ovarian stimulation regimens, some centers have adopted mild stimulation protocols in an attempt to make IVF treatment more patient-friendly, reduce the likelihood of complications (especially ovarian hyperstimulation syndrome [OHSS]), and limit the number of oocytes retrieved [6;16]. It is known that a low number of retrieved oocytes coincides with diminished outcomes [11]; indeed McAvey et al. demonstrated that, in cycles in which five or fewer metaphase II oocytes were obtained, a significantly lower likelihood of live birth was achieved [17]. A study published in 2017, aiming to determine the relationship between number of oocytes retrieved and LBR in fresh and cumulative IVF cycles in the latter case including outcomes from all cryopreserved oocytes and embryos generated by a single ovarian stimulation cycle, showed that patients with a low number of retrieved oocytes had poorer likelihoods in fresh cycles and a non-significant increase in the cumulative outcome [15]. In light of this, the optimization of oocyte yield appears crucial to maximize

the chances of success. Obtaining more embryos from a single oocyte collection, the chance of embryo cryopreservation and subsequent frozen embryo transfers is also increased, while the need of repeated ovarian stimulation [12] is reduced. Our data are consistent with this notion, confirming that by combining live births from fresh and frozen embryo transfer, there is a significant increase in the chances of success derived from a single ovarian stimulation cycle [15].

Two recent papers have investigated the relationship between cumulative LBRs and number of retrieved oocytes in younger and older patients. The significant progressive increase of cumulative LBR with the number of retrieved oocytes suggests that ovarian stimulation does not have detrimental effects on oocyte/embryo quality in both good-prognosis women younger than 40 [18] and in women with advanced reproductive age [19]. Regardless, ovarian stimulation remains a potential source of undesired side effects and every effort should be made to avoid excessive ovarian response to pharmacological treatment, to ensure patient convenience and safety above all to avoid OHSS and other iatrogenic complications.

Ovarian Stimulation and Ploidy

It has been postulated that ovarian stimulation may affect chromosome segregation in oocytes and therefore cause embryo aneuploidy. For this reason, conventional stimulation treatments have been replaced by protocols involving lower gonadotropin dosage.

The study of Baart and colleagues is one of the first and major investigations cited to support the hypothesis of an increase in aneuploidy rate caused by high gonadotropin doses [20]. In this study, the authors claimed that despite mild stimulation resulting in a lower oocyte recovery, the total number of euploid embryos obtained was the same as in cycles where ovarian stimulation was achieved with conventional protocols. However, the study has some limitations. First of all, embryo biopsy was performed on day 3 and chromosomal analysis was carried out by fluorescence in situ hybridization (FISH), factors that make chromosome analysis very unreliable. Furthermore, the mild controlled ovarian hyperstimulation group was affected by a high dropout (27/67), with important implications for the interpretation of outcome data; in addition, considering that female age was not high in the study groups, the percentage of aneuploid embryos was quite high (63% and 45% in the conventional and mild groups, respectively), which is indicative of the limits of the overall approach applied for chromosomal assessment.

On the other hand, several other studies have disputed the conclusions of Baart et al. [20]. For example, Verpoest et al. investigated the prevalence of aneuploidy in embryos of unstimulated women, concluding that numerical chromosomal abnormalities are also present in young women and in absence of ovarian stimulation [21].

Instead, although in a study in which biopsy was performed on day 3 and molecular analysis was achieved by FISH, in a group of fertile women Gleicher et al. reported a slight increase in aneuploidy parallel to gonadotropin dosage [22]. Nevertheless, this increase was compensated by an overall higher number of transferable euploid embryos, a factor that could lead to an overall higher cumulative outcome.

Labarta et al. conducted a prospective cohort study in donor women younger than 35 years old without previous history of ovarian stimulation treatments [23]. The study design excluded some important biases (such as influence of age on aneuploidy, infertility causes, interpatient variability, interlaboratory differences) because it involved the comparison of unstimulated and stimulated cycles. No differences were found between the two groups in terms of embryo quality, aneuploidy rate, and type of chromosomal abnormalities.

In another study, Rubio et al. investigated possible associations between gonadotropin dosage and embryo aneuploidy rates [24]. In particular, they compared the effect of two stimulation protocols: a standard dose of recombinant follicle-stimulating hormone (rFSH; 225 IU) and a reduced dose (150 IU rFSH) on the same group of patients (32 young donors). In donors who completed both treatments (22 women), a significant increase in fertilization and euploidy blastocyst rates was detected using the reduced dose protocol. On the other hand, however, no difference in pregnancy and implantation rates was reported between the two treatment groups.

In a more recent study Labarta et al. introduced the concept of ovarian sensitivity index (OSI) [25], referred to as dose of gonadotropins per obtained oocyte, observing that while gonadotropin doses are not positively related to the

aneuploidy rate, the OSI is negatively related to the number of euploid embryos. These data reinforce the idea that oocyte and embryo cohort quality depends on the ovarian response to a given dose of gonadotropins. Furthermore, the authors pointed out that a high ovarian response increases both the number of euploid and aneuploid embryos, while leaving unaltered the relative proportion. So a high ovarian response does not affect embryo quality.

The investigation of Sekhon et al. deserves attention, because it included a large sample size (828 patients that underwent 1122 IVF cycles) and, unlike other studies, the use of polymerase chain reaction to assess aneuploidy [26]. They concluded that in patients with normal ovarian response (no more than 12 days of stimulation) the odds of aneuploidy did not depend on the degree of exposure to exogenous gonadotropins.

In conclusion, to date, reliable evidence suggesting that more intense ovarian stimulation increases embryo aneuploidy rates is lacking.

Efficacy of IVF Treatment

Evaluation of the efficacy of IVF stimulation protocols is challenging. Current evidence suggests that outcomes derived from cryopreserved embryos are at least as high as those generated from fresh embryos [27]. Traditionally, IVF success rates have been reported in terms of live birth per fresh cycle or embryo transfer. More recently, with an increasing use of embryo cryopreservation, outcomes derived from fresh and cryopreserved embryos have become an important measure of clinical success [28]. Therefore, cumulative LBR is generally perceived as the most comprehensive outcome parameter to express the overall efficacy of an IVF treatment. The latter was closely correlated to the number of oocytes, which is moreover considered a surrogate of embryo quality. A greater number of oocytes retrieved correspond to higher chances to obtain one or two good-quality embryos suitable for fresh embryo transfer and to cryopreserve surplus embryos [17;29]. Therefore, unlike what is postulated in support of the mild stimulation approach, it is important to optimize the quantity of oocytes retrieved in order to maximize the chances of success. By obtaining more embryos from a single oocyte collection, the chances to cryopreserve embryos for later use are increased and the need of repeated ovarian stimulation [11] decreased. Cai *et al.* demonstrated that embryo quality and quantity are two of the most important predictors of fresh and cumulative outcome in IVF/intracytoplasmic sperm injection (ICSI) [30]. Several studies have found that higher oocyte yield results in an increased number of usable embryos/blastocysts [17;31]. Clearly, fewer cryopreserved embryos may give rise to fewer additional deliveries from frozen embryo transfers, thus reducing the overall efficacy of a single stimulated cycle [32]. Women undergoing controlled ovarian stimulation in their first IVF/ICSI cycle and single embryo transfer should be informed that, although the number of oocytes retrieved does not affect LBR in the fresh cycle, the higher the oocyte yield, the higher the probability to achieve a live birth from cryopreserved embryos. Cumulative LBR significantly increases with the number of oocytes retrieved [10;15;33]. Also in women classified as poor responders, it has been recently reported that with mild ovarian stimulation LBRs are extremely low [7]. Collectively, these studies argue against the notion that mild stimulation is more effective compared with more conventional stimulation regimens. Notably, in the majority of randomized studies the clinical outcome of the mild stimulation approach is reported to be as successful as that of standard treatments. Crucially, however, most of these studies do not include an overall analysis of efficacy, making a comprehensive comparison between mild and conventional stimulation impossible.

It would be interesting to compare the efficacy of the aggregation of embryos from multiple mild-stimulation cycles with a single conventional IVF cycle [7].

Costs

Some studies demonstrate that mild stimulation protocols are associated with a lower cost per fresh IVF cycle than conventional stimulation protocols [6;34]. However, an adequate and rational cost evaluation includes a cost-efficacy analysis. Some patients need, in fact, a greater average number of stimulated cycles to achieve a pregnancy, consequently cumulative costs may be higher. Compared with supernumerary frozen embryo transfers, repetitive fresh cycles are associated with higher cumulative costs, including injectable

medications, patient monitoring, anesthesia and surgical risks, patient stress, higher dropout rates, and other healthcare-related costs. It is necessary to consider that conventional stimulation compared with mild stimulation is associated with a higher number of oocytes retrieved that has an effect on the number of embryos available for freezing. A greater number of cryopreserved embryos may increase the chances of live birth in fewer stimulated cycles, resulting in a higher cumulative chance of pregnancy per retrieval and lower cumulative costs due to reduced number of additional stimulated cycles [3].

OHSS

OHSS is recognized as a major risk of assisted reproductive technology. This iatrogenic complication of ovarian stimulation has in moderate cases an incidence of 5 percent [35], while in severe cases it requires hospitalization in a proportion of 2 percent [36]. The meta-analysis by Matsaseng *et al.* from two randomized controlled trials (RCTs) found a significantly lower incidence of OHSS with mild stimulation compared with conventional stimulation [37]. This feature is often emphasized as a reason to prefer mild stimulation in the interest of patient safety. It has been shown that in patients with more than 15 retrieved oocytes the risk of OHSS is significantly increased [38]. However, it was also reported that, in order to prevent OHSS in these patients, final oocyte maturation can be achieved with GnRH agonist triggering, the fresh transfer can be avoided, and all embryos can be cryopreserved *and used in frozen embryo replacements* with excellent results [39]. This safe alternative for patients at risk for OHSS [40], referred to as freeze-all, was evaluated in a recent Cochrane review [41]. The review assessed the efficacy and safety of the freeze-all strategy compared with the conventional IVF/ICSI strategy, in terms of cumulative LBR and OHSS rate. The overall analysis showed that one strategy was not superior to the other in terms of cumulative LBR and that the choice to cancel a fresh transfer lowers the OHSS risk.

Time to Pregnancy

Time to pregnancy is an important outcome parameter that should be taken into account in the management of IVF treatment and in the counseling of couples.

It should be made clear that compared with conventional stimulation, mild stimulation protocols potentially involve higher number of stimulated cycles to achieve a pregnancy and consequently a longer time to pregnancy.

For this reason, many patients, especially if older, may not be prepared to accept a perspective of a longer time to pregnancy. Rather, they may prefer the option to generate more embryos for cryopreservation in one IVF treatment, thereby limiting the number of stimulations needed to achieve a live birth.

It is always of primary importance to consider the time factor, especially in older women. A variety of alternative stimulation protocols and ovulation triggers can be chosen on the basis of patients' characteristics, to achieve maximal stimulation while ensuring safety [3].

Conclusion

The ISMAAR defines specifically the mild stimulation approach. Regardless, there are some studies that, despite defining a specific range of recovered oocytes, still consider as treated with mild stimulation those cycles where more than eight oocytes are retrieved. This inconsistency calls for more differentiated definitions of mild stimulation, possibly relevant to specific protocols, cycle characteristics, and ovarian response. This would make easier the undertaking of efficacy studies. To date, approximately 20 RCTs compared one of the mild stimulation IVF protocols with one of conventional long downregulation or high-dose antagonist protocol [2]; most of them reported mild stimulation IVF to be equally successful in terms of pregnancy outcomes for embryo transfer. Unfortunately, the majority of RCTs do not correctly analyze the effectiveness of the treatments, not including cumulative results. As a consequence, in future studies there is a need to focus on cumulative results to achieve a comprehensive outcome analysis in traditional and mild stimulation protocols. Several studies also addressed potential benefits of mild stimulation in the light of lower incidence of OHSS. It has been widely demonstrated that cumulative LBR significantly increases with the number of oocytes retrieved [10;15;33] and that a recovery of more than 15 oocytes significantly increases the risk of

OHSS [38]. However, the trend toward the policy of freezing all, allows circumvention of OHSS risk associated with standard stimulation protocols. Patients undergoing mild IVF cycles should be made aware that on average, compared with standard stimulation, more fresh cycles are needed to achieve a live birth, with increased cumulative costs and risks. A higher number of stimulated cycles lead to a longer time to pregnancy too; this can represent a contraindication above all in older women, whose relative proportion is progressively increasing among IVF patients.

At present there is not solid evidence suggesting that aneuploidy rate in embryos may increase with higher gonadotropin dosages. To date, the lower cumulative results related to mild protocols and the high efficacy of vitrification protocols support the strategy to collect a high number of oocytes after GnRH analogue trigger in a one conventional IVF cycle and to freeze all embryos, to prevent OHSS, and to transfer cryopreserved embryos "one at a time" [2]. Further efficacy studies focusing on cumulative LBR, safety, comfort, and direct/indirect costs among different stimulation protocols are required to assess the relative performance of the different ovarian stimulation approaches.

References

1. Zegers-Hochschild F, Adamson D, Dyer S, et al. The International Glossary on Infertility and Fertility Care, 2017. *Hum Reprod* 2017;**32**(9):1786–1801.

2. Nargund G, Fauser BC, Macklon NS, et al. The ISMAAR proposal on terminology for ovarian stimulation for IVF. *Hum Reprod* 2007;**22**:2801–2804.

3. Alper MM, Fauser BC. Ovarian stimulation protocols for IVF: is more better than less? *Reprod Biomed Online* 2017;**34**(4):345–353.

4. Siristatidis C, Salamalekis G, Dafopoulos K, et al. Mild versus conventional ovarian stimulation for poor responders undergoing IVF/ICSI. *In Vivo* 2017;**31**(2):231–237.

5. Orvieto R, Vanni VS, Gleicher N. The myths surrounding mild stimulation in vitro fertilization (IVF). *Reprod Biol Endocrinol* 2017;**15**(1):48.

6. Verberg MFG, Eijkemans MJC, Machlon NS, et al. The clinical significance of the retrieval of a low number of oocytes following mild ovarian stimulation for IVF: a meta-analysis. *Hum Reprod Update* 2009;**15**:5–12.

7. Practice Committee of the American Society for Reproductive Medicine. Comparison of pregnancy rates for poor responders using IVF with mild ovarian stimulation versus conventional IVF: a guideline. *Fertil Steril* 2018;**109**(6):993–999.

8. Hillier SG, Afnan AM, Margara RA, Winston RM. Superovulation strategy before in vitro fertilization. *Clin Obstet Gynaecol* 1985;**12**(3):687–723.

9. Sunkara SK, Rittenberg V, Raine-Fenning N, *et al.* Association between the number of eggs and live birth in IVF treatment: an analysis of 400 135 treatment cycles. *Hum Reprod* 2011;**26**:1768–1774.

10. Ji J, Liu Y, Tong XH, *et al.* The optimum number of oocytes in IVF treatment: an analysis of 2455 cycles in China. *Hum Reprod* 2013;**28** (10):2728–2734.

11. Beckers NGM, Macklon NS, Eijkemans MJC, Fauser BCJM. Women with regular menstrual cycles and a poor response to ovarian hyperstimulation for in vitro fertilization exhibit follicular phase characteristics suggestive of ovarian aging. *Fertil Steril* 2002;**78**:291–297.

12. Briggs R, Kovacs G, MacLachlan V, Motteram C, Baker HW. Can you ever collect too many oocytes? *Hum Reprod* 2015;**30**(1):81–87.

13. Fauser BC, Devroey P, Macklon NS. Multiple birth resulting from ovarian stimulation for subfertility treatment. *Lancet* 2005;**365**:1807–1816.

14. Macklon NS, Stouffer RL, Giudice LC, Fauser BC. The science behind 25 years of ovarian stimulation for in vitro fertilization. *Endocr Rev* 2006;**27**:170–207.

15. Zacà C, Spadoni V, Patria G, *et al.* How do live birth and cumulative live birth rate in IVF cycles change with the number of oocytes retrieved? *EC Gynaecol* 2017;**20**:391–401.

16. Fauser BC, Devroey P, Yen SS, *et al.* Minimal ovarian stimulation for IVF: appraisal of potential benefits and drawbacks. *Hum Reprod* 1999;**14**:2681–2686.

17. McAvey B, Zapantis A, Jindal SK, Lieman HJ, Polotsky AJ. How many eggs are needed to produce an assisted reproductive technology baby: is more always better? *Fertil Steril* 2011;**96**:332–335.

18. Polyzos NP, Drakopoulos P, Parra J, *et al.* Cumulative live birth rates according to the number of oocytes retrieved after the first ovarian stimulation for in vitro fertilization/ intracytoplasmic sperm injection: a multicenter multinational analysis including 15,000 women. *Fertil Steril* 2018;**110**(4):661–670.

19. Devesa M, Tur R, Rodríguez I, *et al.* Cumulative live birth rates and number of oocytes retrieved in women of advanced age. A single centre analysis including 4500 women ≥38 years old. *Hum Reprod* 2018;**33**(11):2010–2017.

20. Baart EB, Martini E, Eijkemans MJ, *et al.* Milder ovarian stimulation for in-vitro fertilization reduces aneuploidy in the human preimplantation embryo: a randomized controlled trial. *Hum Reprod* 2007;**22**:980–988.

21. Verpoest W, Fauser BC, Papanikolaou E, *et al.* Chromosomal aneuploidy in embryos conceived with unstimulated cycle IVF. *Hum Reprod* 2008;**23** (10):2369–2371.

22. Gleicher N, Kim A, Weghofer A, Barad DH. Lessons from elective in vitro fertilization (IVF) in, principally, non-infertile women. *Reprod Biol Endocrinol* 2012;**10**:48.

23. Labarta E, Bosch E, Alama P, *et al.* Moderate ovarian stimulation does not increase the incidence of human embryo chromosomal abnormalities in in vitro fertilization cycles. *J Clin Endocrinol Metab* 2012;**97**:1987–1994.

24. Rubio C, Mercader A, Alamá P, *et al.* Prospective cohort study in high responder oocyte donors using two hormonal stimulation protocols: impact on embryo aneuploidy and development. *Hum Reprod* 2010;**25**:2290–2297.

25. Labarta E, Bosh E, Mercader A, *et al.* A higher ovarian response after stimulation for IVF is related to a higher number of euploid embryos. *Biomed Res Int* 2017;**2017**:5637923.

26. Sekhon L, Shaia K, Santistevan A, *et al.* The cumulative dose of gonadotropins used for controlled ovarian stimulation does not influence the odds of embryonic aneuploidy in patients with normal ovarian response. *J Assist Reprod Genet* 2017;**34**(6):749–758.

27. Roque M, Haahr T, Geber S, Esteves SC, Humaidan P. Fresh versus elective frozen embryo transfer in IVF/ICSI cycles: a systematic review and meta-analysis of reproductive outcomes. *Hum Reprod Update* 2019;**25**:2–14.

28. Maheshwari A, McLernon D, Bhattacharya S. Cumulative live birth rate: time for a consensus? *Hum Reprod* 2015;**30**(12):2703–2707.

29. Sunkara SK, Khalaf Y, Maheshwari A, Seed P, Coomarasamy A. Association between response to ovarian stimulation and miscarriage following IVF: an analysis of 124 351 IVF pregnancies. *Hum Reprod* 2014;**29**(6):1218–1224.

30. Cai QF, Wan F, Huang R, Zhang HW. Factors predicting the cumulative outcome of IVF/ICSI treatment: a multivariable analysis of 2450 patients. *Hum Reprod* 2011;**26** (9):2532–2540.

31. Vaughan DA, Leung A, Resetkova N, *et al.* How many oocytes are optimal to achieve multiple live births with one stimulation cycle? The one-and-done approach. *Fertil Steril* 2017;**107**(2):397–404.

32. Fauser BC, Nargund G, Andersen AN, *et al.* Mild ovarian stimulation for IVF: 10 years later. *Hum Reprod* 2010;**25**(11):2678–2684.

33. Drakopoulos P, Blockeel C, Stoop D, *et al.* Conventional ovarian stimulation and single embryo transfer for IVF/ICSI. How many oocytes do we need to maximize cumulative live birth rates after utilization of all fresh and frozen embryos? *Hum Reprod* 2016;**31**(2):370–376.

34. Baker VL. Mild ovarian stimulation for in vitro fertilization: one perspective from the USA. *J Assist Reprod Genet* 2013;**30**(2):197–202.

35. Delvigne A. Symposium: update on prediction and management of OHSS. Epidemiology of OHSS. *Reprod Biomed Online* 2009;**19**:8–13.

36. Papanikolaou EG, Tournaye H, Verpoest W, *et al.* Early and late ovarian hyperstimulation syndrome: early pregnancy outcome and profile. *Hum Reprod* 2005;**20**:636–641.

37. Matsaseng T, Kruger T, Steyn W. Mild ovarian stimulation for in vitro fertilization: are we ready to change? A meta-analysis. *Gynecol Obstet Invest* 2013;**76**:233–240.

38. Steward RG, Lan L, Shah AA, *et al.* Oocyte number as a predictor for ovarian hyperstimulation syndrome and live birth: an analysis of 256,381 in vitro fertilization cycles. *Fertil Steril* 2014;**101** (4):967–973.

39. Zacà C, Bazzocchi A, Pennetta F, *et al.* Cumulative live birth rate in freeze-all cycles is comparable to that of a conventional embryo transfer policy at the cleavage stage but superior at the blastocyst stage. *Fertil Steril* 2018;**110**(4):703–709.

40. Devroey P, Polyzos NP, Blockeel C. An OHSS-free clinic by segmentation of IVF treatment. *Hum Reprod* 2011;**26**:2593–7.

41. Wong KM, van Wely M, Mol F, Repping S, Mastenbroek S. Fresh versus frozen embryo transfers in assisted reproduction. *Cochrane Database Syst Rev* 2017;**3**: CD011184.

Chapter

6

GnRH Agonists for Ovarian Hyperstimulation

Lina El-Taha, Botros Rizk, Jad Farid Assaf, and Johnny Awwad

Historical Perspectives

Half a decade ago, we witnessed the culmination of much of what we comprehend today in classical ovarian endocrinology and physiology [1;2], human embryology [3] as well as clinical ovarian ultrasonography [4]. Much of the former was based upon the development of (radio-)immunoassays that could reliably detect low concentrations of hormones in body fluids, including the peripheral circulation. This meant that correlations of hormone concentrations and specific physiological events could be determined with precision, leading to many advances in clinical practice and drug development. The biological control of all these physiological elements is, of course, gonadotropin-releasing hormone (GnRH), whose decapeptide structure was elucidated by Andrew Schally and colleagues in 1971 [5], for which he was awarded his share of the Nobel prize in 1977. His co-prize winners were responsible for the pioneering of immunological competitive binding dilution assays, which underwrote all these developments.

Early in vitro fertilization (IVF) debates considered whether the natural cycle or multiple follicular development should be deployed for the best clinical benefit. It soon became clear that there were theoretical advantages to obtaining multiple oocytes for IVF. In reality and in the first instance, the full potential of the stimulated cycles was not achieved – mainly due to a single classical endocrine response. Multiple follicles, stimulated with human menopausal gonadotropin (hMG) or clomiphene (clomifene) citrate in combination with hMG, secrete estradiol to supraphysiological levels, attaining normal midcycle peak levels well in advance of the normal follicle midcycle size and maturity. The luteinizing hormone (LH) surge elicited by the prematurely elevated estrogen concentrations leads to a confusing array of responses

with consequent cycle cancellations on 15 percent to 40 percent of instances [6]. Exposure of follicles at different degrees of maturity to the signal to luteinize and "ovulate" elicits a range of responses, and a broad range of follicles may be present when the surge occurs. Follicles which are capable of ovulation undergo luteinization and ovulation, while less mature follicles respond unconventionally to the LH surge, with inhibition of the aromatase enzyme, and granulosa cell mitosis, probably without ovulation. This process, recorded in nonovulatory women as early as 1978 [7], became known as "premature luteinization." However, the full impact of the phenomenon in IVF took a considerable time to be elucidated, as measurements of LH in urine are imprecise, and the frequency of blood samples required to track all pulsatile changes with precision is impractically elevated.

The key to resolving the problem was published in 1980 [8], when it was shown that chronic application of a GnRH analogue in monkeys could reliably block the LH surge and ovulation for the duration of treatment. Application of the drug in humans, using multiple daily applications of a nasal spray of buserelin acetate, effectively blocked all spontaneous LH activity, allowing clinical control of follicular development with exogenous gonadotropins [9]. The method was then deployed in control of stimulated cycles for IVF [10–12] remarkably decreasing the cancellation rate of gonadotropin treated cycles to less than 2 percent [13].

The use of GnRH analogues, agonists, and antagonists, in the domain of assisted reproduction to block undesired spontaneous premature LH surges remains one of the cornerstone usages of these remarkable drugs, and a milestone in the success of controlled ovarian stimulation for assisted reproduction.

Mode of Action

GnRH is secreted physiologically in a pulsatile manner by the hypothalamus. It is transported via the portal circulation to orchestrate anterior pituitary gonadotroph secretion of follicle-stimulating hormone (FSH) and LH essential for timely follicular recruitment, development, and ovulation. Initial administration of GnRH agonists leads to a "flare" effect corresponding to an increase in endogenous LH and FSH secretion from pituitary gonadotrophs. However, continuous, non-pulsatile stimulation by GnRH analogues ultimately leads to pituitary downregulation/suppression through receptor-mediated phenomena [14]. A single dose of an agonist induces a rapid reduction in pituitary gonadotroph surface GnRH receptor-binding capacity, lasting for approximately 12 hours [15]. This downregulation process is mediated through the high-affinity binding of the agonist molecule to the membrane receptors. The stabilized receptor–hormone complexes are then internalized into the cell and slowly degraded by proteolysis, which upon prolonged GnRH agonist exposure is associated with a profound reduction in pituitary FSH and LH content and release [16], lasting at least a week following cessation of GnRH agonist administration [12].

Efficacy

The aim of GnRH agonist treatment is the elimination of the LH surge and fluctuating LH concentrations, which compromise outcome in cycles of ovarian stimulation for IVF [11;17]. In this regard, its efficacy appears uncontested, whether the treatment is administered using a multiuse nasal spray, daily injections, or depot formulation. The efficacy of GnRH agonist in pituitary suppression is a hallmark of modern ovarian stimulation treatment protocols irrespective of the particular GnRH agonist formulation used. It should be noted nonetheless that dose-finding studies are rare [18]. Available studies demonstrate the absence of any significant differences in reproductive outcomes between the different GnRH agonist formulations and different dosing regimens [19–22]. As a general rule, more potent agonists and more consistent application mechanisms induce a more powerful downregulation effect [23;24]. The largest available systematic review comparing the use of daily GnRH

agonist doses versus a single depot formulation included 16 randomized controlled trials (RCTs) [23]. Despite the wide heterogeneity in the characteristics of the daily formulations used and the non-uniformity in gonadotropin stimulation dosing, the review demonstrated no significant differences in clinical pregnancies (odds ratio [OR] 0.96, 95% CI 0.75–1.23; 11 studies, 1259 women) and in live birth/ongoing pregnancies (OR 0.95, 95% CI 0.70– 1.31; 7 studies, 873 women). Despite comparable reproductive outcomes, however, the use of the depot GnRH agonist was associated with a significantly higher consumption of gonadotropin units (standardized mean difference 0.26, 95% CI 0.08–0.43; 11 studies, 1143 women) and a significantly longer duration of stimulation (mean difference 0.65, 95% CI 0.46–0.84; 10 studies, 1033 women) compared with the daily GnRH agonist regimens [23].

Prior to the introduction of the GnRH antagonists, the long-suppression agonist protocol was considered the gold standard for conventional IVF treatment, because of the negligible incidence of premature LH rise and the good cycle control of follicular growth using exogenous gonadotropins. Indeed, complete "downregulation" deservedly meant that all follicular and endocrine events are highly controlled and managed throughout stimulation.

The alternative approach to prolonged downregulation would be to take advantage of the flare effect at the start of treatment in order to provoke the start of follicular growth. This approach is referred to as the "short-agonist" or "flare" protocol, and differs from the conventional long-suppression protocol, by the processes of follicular recruitment and selection.

This overview will address the characteristics of the GnRH agonist "long-suppression" and "flare" protocols.

The Conventional GnRH Agonist Long-Suppression Protocol

As described earlier, the consequence of continuous GnRH agonist administration is biphasic gonadotropin release with an initial "flare" effect lasting up to one week [14], followed by pituitary desensitization and suppression. In the long agonist protocol, it is common to initiate treatment in the midluteal phase of the preceding cycle to minimize the undesired effects of the "flare" observed in the first few days of treatment, or in the early follicular phase of the index cycle and continued until the ovulatory human chorionic gonadotropin (hCG) trigger [25]. The subsequent menstrual bleed denotes a reduced level of endogenous ovarian stimulation which may be subsequently confirmed by ultrasonography and a serum estradiol level. Gonadotropin administration is delayed until complete pituitary-ovarian suppression is achieved, and can usually be started conveniently thereafter.

Studies comparing the luteal start versus the follicular start failed to demonstrate any significant in-between group differences in the clinical pregnancy rates (OR 1.06, 95% CI 0.76–1.47; 5 RCTs, 750 women), the number of oocytes collected (mean difference [MD] -1.29, 95% CI -1.85 to 0.71; 4 RCTs, 527 women) and the amount of gonadotropin ampoules utilized (MD 1.12, 95% CI -0.73 to 2.97; 4 RCTs, 527 women) [26].

It is generally believed that starting ovarian stimulation following incomplete pituitary suppression may be associated with a poor reproductive outcome, as it may result in poorly synchronous follicle cohort and possibly less optimal endometrial receptivity. While the finding of elevated LH at the onset of stimulation remains of questionable significance, elevated or slowly declining estradiol levels after initial GnRH agonist administration appear to impact negatively treatment outcome. It is speculated that this estradiol rise may be driven by the presence of advanced follicles recruited in the luteal phase of the preceding cycle which became autonomous before significant agonist suppression could be achieved. Since achieving follicular synchronization at the beginning of ovarian stimulation is desirable, the strategy of prolonging agonist desensitization in women who do not achieve timely ovarian suppression has been evaluated and shown not to impact the outcome of the treatment cycle.

A consensus over the ideal gonadotropin dosing approach is far from settled. Lately, individualization of the gonadotropin dosage has gained favor as the best means to achieve optimal follicular growth, mature oocyte yield, and positive pregnancy outcomes while avoiding cycle cancellations due to poor and high response. Proposed algorithms are often guided by patient's age, body mass index, and measures of ovarian reserve with

adjustments of gonadotropin dose throughout stimulation according to observed response.

Although seemingly intuitive, this approach is particularly challenging in patients with poor ovarian response (POR), in whom increasing the gonadotropin dose may be appealing in order to enhance oocyte yield and pregnancy outcomes. Unfortunately, little evidence is available to support this contention. Data available to direct the choice of the gonadotropin dose in this particular population are limited by small sample size, lack of uniform stimulation protocol and universally used criteria to define POR. In general, several RCTs demonstrated the lack of additional benefit from the use of daily gonadotropin doses in excess of 300 IU to improve oocyte yield and pregnancy outcome [22;27]. More recently, a randomized trial compared the use of a fixed daily gonadotropin regimen of 450 IU versus 600 IU in 356 GnRH agonist suppressed women with POR. The study found no significant differences in measured outcomes between the two groups, namely duration of stimulation, cycle cancellations, number of mature oocytes retrieved, and pregnancy outcomes (biochemical pregnancy, clinical pregnancy, and implantation rate) [28]. Accordingly, the National Institute for Health and Care Excellence (NICE) recommended not to exceed 450 IU for the daily gonadotropin dose in women during ovarian stimulation [29].

On the other hand, the choice of the most suitable gonadotropin formulation for use with GnRH agonist suppressed cycles has not been determined. Both hMG and pure FSH preparations have been used interchangeably in this context. Yet, there is currently no strong evidence to show a clinically significant superiority of one preparation over the other [30;31] except in particular subpopulations of women such as in those with hypogonadotropic hypogonadism.

Traditionally, cycle control during ovarian stimulation is achieved via repeated serum estradiol levels and ultrasound monitoring of follicle development. The GnRH agonist is usually continued in parallel to gonadotropin stimulation until final follicle triggering using exogenous hCG. This is usually determined by the presence of at least two leading follicles with mean diameter greater than 17 mm. A highlight of the advantages associated with the long GnRH agonist protocol is the scheduling flexibility dictated by exogenous gonadotropin control of ovarian response. This was demonstrated in one of the earliest landmark randomized trials, whereby the precise timing of hCG triggering of ovulation in pituitary desensitized GnRH agonist cycles did not significantly influence final reproductive outcomes. Timing of the hCG trigger within one- to two-day intervals did not affect the number of oocytes retrieved, fertilization and cleavage rates, or pregnancy rates per initiated cycle and per embryo transfer [32;33].

The GnRH Agonist Flare Protocol

In women with reduced ovarian reserve, the long-suppression protocol may lead to long, arduous, and expensive drug treatment programs, with the yield of eggs dictated by the ovarian reserve. The limited egg yield is probably poorly influenced by any particular protocol adjustments, which has encouraged the quest for alternative options to boost response [34]. The use of the GnRH agonist in a flare protocol has been suggested in this context to achieve maximal ovarian stimulation during the early FSH-dependent oocyte recruitment phase.

In the flare protocol, the GnRH agonist is administered during the follicular phase of the treatment cycle from day 1 or 2, and continued until the day of hCG triggering. The "ultrashort" protocol, in contrast, differs in that the GnRH agonist is only administered for the first three days of the follicular phase, and then withdrawn thereafter. The flare effect is characterized by a rise in FSH and LH that lasts for three to six days and, although this can be exploited to elicit the start of follicular growth when GnRH agonist treatment is initiated in the early follicular phase, there are specific issues that can complicate this approach.

While it seems reasonable to take advantage of the flare output of LH and FSH to initiate follicular growth, the findings of comparative clinical studies have been disappointing. Poorer reproductive outcomes were associated with the short flare protocol compared with the standard long agonist protocol [35;36]. The short protocol was associated with 11 percent reduction of oocyte yield and 35 percent reduction in clinical pregnancies, a difference which persisted even after adjusting for possible confounding factors [36]. The reasons for these disappointing outcomes have been rarely addressed. Some studies suggested that the rise in serum androgens observed during the flare effect could have detrimental effects

on oocyte quality leading to low pregnancy outcomes [37;38].

Additional potential complications deriving from the flare effect at the start of the cycle include the rescue of a previous corpus luteum, the luteinization of advanced-stage follicles, and the inadvertent triggering of final maturation of a mature follicle when a midcycle bleeding episode is mistaken for menses.

Another physiological consequence of the flare protocol is the formation of functional ovarian cysts, which can be generated whenever the treatment is started. The incidence of these ovarian cysts varied between 5 percent and 30 percent in different studies [39–42]. The exact etiology of the formation of these functional cysts is not entirely elucidated; however, the flare effect is suggested to contribute by possible rescue of old corpus luteum. These cysts can disrupt the smooth approach to treatment, and poorly influence clinical outcome [42–44]. Aspiration of these functional cysts to evade compromising ovarian stimulation and pregnancy outcome has not been supported by available evidence [43;45]. Rather, when they do occur, follicular stimulation should be delayed when a fresh embryo transfer is planned.

Alternatively, these complications, which have been deemed responsible for a poorer outcome in IVF cycles, can be addressed and resolved by controlling the ovarian status before starting the flare treatment process using progestogens or oral contraceptives, so that there is no corpus luteum or responsive follicles present at the start of the treatment [46]. However, prolonged use of combined oral contraceptives may also suppress ovarian response to stimulation, leading to a higher gonadotropin consumption and prolongation of the duration of stimulation without altogether improving oocyte yield.

It should be noted that while the short protocol was promoted to enhance the follicle response, it failed to meet its aspired benefit in women with POR. Published literature comparing outcomes of various treatment protocols is generally limited to specific subpopulations, and most frequently to older women or those previously diagnosed as "poor responders" – without any accepted universal definition. In general, the clinical outcomes in these subgroups were shown to be overall inferior and in few instances at best similar to the long protocol [47].

It is important to emphasize that the management of POR is far from being well standardized. A Cochrane review in 2010 [48] demonstrated insufficient evidence to recommend the use of one particular protocol over the other and urged for more robust prospective RCTs. These have not been forthcoming as yet, although one report comparing agonist flare with GnRH antagonist protocols in poor-responder women achieved similar outcomes [49].

Despite low to moderate quality evidence, the latest Cochrane review showed significantly higher clinical pregnancy rates (OR 1.50, 95% CI 1.18– 1.92; 20 RCTs, 1643 women) in the general IVF population using the long agonist protocol compared with the flare regimen [26]. When considering only poor responders, subgroup analysis also supported the presence of a significant difference in clinical pregnancy rates (OR 3.12, 95% CI 1.39–7.02; 4 RCTs, 232 women) favoring the long protocol [26]. Ongoing pregnancy and live birth rates were nonetheless comparable for the long versus short agonist protocols (OR 1.30, 95% CI 0.94–1.81;12 RCTs including 976 women) despite a lack of universal definition for poor response, which has been the main limiting parameter influencing the interpretability and generalizability of these findings.

Subgroup analysis further showed evidence of a significantly higher number of oocytes in poor responders when the long GnRH agonist protocol was utilized compared with the short flare protocol (MD 1.40, 95% CI 0.75–2.06; 4 RCTs, 227 women) [26]. No differences were observed for the number of gonadotropin ampoules consumed (MD 1.10, 95% CI -1.81 to 4.01; one RCT, $n = 80$) or the cancellation rates (OR 1.11, 95% CI 0.40–3.05; one RCT, 150 women).

There have been a number of variations on the themes of GnRH agonist use discussed above, usually in patients who have failed to respond well to standard protocols. These include the "micro-dose flare" and "ultrashort" protocol in which the agonist use is discontinued some time prior to the end of the follicular phase. On the basis of a single RCT, the Cochrane review found no evidence of a difference in the clinical pregnancy rate when the short protocol was compared with the ultrashort protocol (OR 1.33, 95% CI 0.47–3.81; one RCT, 82 women) [26]. The ultrashort protocol did not offer any advantage in terms of number of oocytes recovered (MD 0.70, 95% CI -1.83 to 3.23; one RCT, 82 women), but was associated with a higher gonadotropin consumption (MD -13.85, 95% CI -21.49 to -6.21; one RCT, 82 women). Since these protocols failed to demonstrate superior ovarian stimulation and pregnancy outcomes, they have subsequently fallen out of practice.

Safety and Ovarian Hyperstimulation Syndrome

The safety record of GnRH agonists in the context of target organ specificity and fetal well-being is good. The only organ with high density-specific receptors binding GnRH agonists is the pituitary, and the drug's half-life in the circulation is short. Assurance on the safety of human embryonic exposure to GnRH is based on series of individual case reports in the early 1990s. Inadvertent GnRH agonist administration during the luteal phase did not compromise the continuation of pregnancy, but rather seemed to support implantation [50–54]. As such, when the agonist has been administered in the early stages of pregnancy, there appears to be no undesirable consequences [55].

On the other hand, the use of the standard long agonist protocol in women with a high ovarian reserve does result in ovarian hyperstimulation syndrome (OHSS) to an incidence and degree that can be excessively dangerous. The increase in incidence of OHSS has been reported to increase six times since the introduction of GnRH agonist in pituitary desensitization to prevent premature LH surge [56]. The risk of OHSS is particularly intensified in high-responder women [57].

Follicular Recruitment Dynamics in Long Agonist Cycles and Prediction of OHSS

When the patient is downregulated at the start of FSH treatment, subsequent follicular growth and recruitment is dictated by two elements: the ovarian reserve, which dictates the number of follicles available for recruitment, and the profile of circulating FSH concentrations. In most controlled ovarian stimulation cycles with GnRH agonist long suppression, FSH concentrations exceed the threshold values required for follicular recruitment. Because of the relatively long half-life of FSH (c. 30 hours),

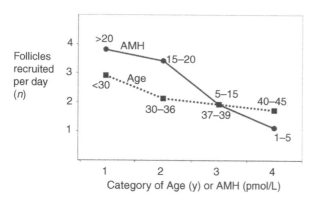

Figure 6.1 Numbers of follicles recruited each day during standard GnRH agonist long-course controlled ovarian stimulation, with categorization by age group (y) or by AMH evaluation (pmol/L).

serum FSH levels are maintained until sometime after the daily FSH dose is reduced. This fact has consequences in the stark reality rendering close control of recruitment and growth rather challenging, with steady-state circulating FSH taking considerable time to build up, and follicular response being slow to unfold. This combination normally results in maximal follicular recruitment way into the standard long-suppression controlled stimulation cycle. This phenomenon contrasts strongly with cycles controlled with GnRH antagonists, where endogenous control mechanisms of selection and de-selection influence follicular recruitment [58;59].

Critical to evaluation of responses to exogenous FSH in downregulated cycles is the study of follicular recruitment dynamics. This was evaluated for the purpose of determining factors that influence egg yields and outcomes, by analyzing observed follicular recruitment through two ultrasound scans in the mid–late follicular phase, in which the total number of follicles are identified, and the difference between the two scans used to calculate the numbers of follicles recruited per day earlier in the follicular phase [60]. It is no surprise that this calculated value (follicles recruited per day, fols/d) was shown to be strongly predictive of oocyte yield, but in fact it was found to be more predictive than the absolute number of follicles seen on stimulation day 8. The fols/d value correlated strongly with both oocyte yield and circulating anti-Müllerian hormone (AMH) concentrations taken prior to treatment. Figure 6.1 shows that the fols/d value was significantly influenced by patient age, but the slope of decline across the age bands was modest, and not strongly predictive of excessive responses.

On the other hand, Figure 6.1 also shows the profile of fols/d values in categories of patients determined by circulating AMH. The highest AMH category (> 20 pmol/L) showed that the stimulation protocol was recruiting in the region of four follicles each day. A simple calculation based upon an average of 12 days' stimulation indicates that in this category of patients, a sizeable proportion of cases will see a total recruitment in the region of 50 follicles. It is little surprise, therefore, that the administration of hCG to this number of highly vascular follicles results in a high incidence and degree of OHSS.

This single observation denotes that patients at risk of OHSS can be identified prior to treatment, simply through assessing their ovarian reserve with AMH. Furthermore, categorization of ovarian responses with AMH can be used to explore and define the ideal stimulation protocol for particular circumstances.

The Use of GnRH Agonists in Patients Selected According to Their Ovarian Reserve

Some advocate the universal application of GnRH antagonist control in all treatment cycles [61]. This is based upon an apparently reduced treatment burden in cycles controlled by GnRH antagonists, when compared with the standard long agonist, as the treatment cycles are shorter. It is also accepted that there is also a reduced risk of OHSS, and this phenomenon is intrinsic to the debate.

Nelson et al. [34;62] proposed an alternative approach, with individualization of treatment based upon the patient's ovarian reserve. In this model, the use of GnRH agonists was restricted to women with a "normal" ovarian reserve, which was defined as having a circulating AMH between 5 and 15 pmol/L. The role of AMH was highlighted by Anckaert *et al.* in a retrospective analysis of data from more than 700 normogonadotropic women undergoing controlled ovarian stimulation. AMH concentration showed a positive correlation with ovarian response in long agonist protocol in terms of number of oocytes retrieved. However, this was not mirrored in terms of embryo quality and pregnancy outcomes [63]. Flemming *et al.* concluded that more studies are needed to determine whether individualization of treatment protocols based on AMH serum concentration will result in improved clinical outcomes, increasing live birth rates and reducing cancellation rates and incidence of OHSS [64].

To optimize the choice of controlled ovarian stimulation protocol, ovarian response has been classically classified into high, normal, and poor response. The largest available meta-analysis comparing the long GnRH agonist or GnRH antagonist protocols showed an absolute risk reduction of 3.6 percent in ongoing pregnancy rates when a GnRH antagonist is used in the general IVF population for the prevention of premature luteinization (23.8% vs. 27.4%; relative risk [RR] 0.89, 95% CI 0.82–0.96) [65]. The number needed to harm was calculated to be 28, that is, one less ongoing pregnancy for every 28 women treated with the antagonist. The use of the antagonist protocol nonetheless was associated with a lower risk of OHSS (RR 0.63, 95% CI 0.50–0.81, 22 trials including 5598 women) and an absolute rate reduction by 2.5 percent. Stated differently, the number of women needed to prevent one case of OHSS was 40. It should be noted that a discrete choice analysis evaluating patients' preferences demonstrated that women were willing to trade-off a 2 percent increase in pregnancy outcome with a decrease in OHSS risk.

The higher ongoing pregnancy rates observed with the use of the long GnRH agonist protocol for pituitary suppression in the general IVF population may be explained by more consistently suppressed LH surges and better oocyte yield.

In women with polycystic ovary syndrome (PCOS), no differences in live and ongoing pregnancies were found between both protocols (RR 0.90, 95% CI 0.69–1.19; 3 RCTs including 363 women), albeit there was a significantly lower OHSS rate in the antagonist group (RR 0.53, 95% CI 0.30–0.95; 9 RCTs including 1294 women) [65]. The number needed to prevent one case of OHSS in the PCOS subpopulation was 14. Accordingly, the European Society of Human Reproduction and Embryology advocates the use of antagonist protocol in women predicted to have a high response, particularly in women with PCOS, due to its improved safety profile and comparable efficacy [66].

Luteal Support

Multiple follicular development results in an increase in ovarian output of factors with significant negative feedback effects on pituitary function. Correspondingly, LH activity is low during hyperstimulated cycles. When ovulation and luteinization is induced by exogenous hCG administration, the initial output of progesterone is considerable during the early luteal phase with abrupt loss of the natural midluteal progesterone peak. Consequently, if luteal support is not provided when the luteotropic effects of hCG are lost, then a defective luteal phase develops in coincidence with the window of implantation. This phenomenon may fail to provide sufficient support for implantation, and indicates that luteal support is mandatory irrespective of GnRH agonist pituitary suppression. The use of the GnRH agonist suppression protocol contributes further to lowering LH serum levels which remain persistently decreased into the luteal phase long after the agonist is discontinued. It has been established that progesterone supplementation alone is all that is required following hCG administration [67], and that estrogen is not required to improve reproductive outcomes [68].

Summary

The long GnRH agonist protocol remains the benchmark by which other protocols are measured. It eliminates interfering endocrine factors and maximizes follicular recruitment as endogenous control mechanisms are also obviated. These characteristics, although broadly uncomplicated and beneficial, can also bring risks and consequences. However, patients at risk of these consequences can now be reliably identified, leading to uncomplicated and successful treatment programs, with the standard long-course GnRH agonist as a major component providing reliable and safe IVF or intracytoplasmic sperm injection.

Acknowledgment

This chapter is based on the chapter from the first edition by Richard Fleming, with permission and acknowledgment.

References

1. Baird DT. Endocrinology of female infertility. *Br Med Bull* 1979;**35**:193–198.

2. Kerin JF, Edmonds DK, Warnes GM, *et al.* Morphological and functional relations of Graafian follicle growth to ovulation in women using ultrasonic, laparoscopic and biochemical measurements. *Br J Obstet Gynaecol* 1981;**88**:81–90.

3. Edwards RG, Steptoe PC. Current status of in-vitro fertilisation and implantation of human embryos. *Lancet* 1983;**2**:1265–1269.

4. Hackelöer BJ, Fleming R, Robinson HP, Adam AH, Coutts JR. Correlation of ultrasonic and endocrinologic assessment of human follicular development. *Am J Obstet Gynecol* 1979;**135**:122–128.

5. Schally AV, Arimura A, Baba Y, *et al.* Isolation and properties of the FSH and LH-releasing hormone. *Biochem Biophys Res Commun* 1971;**43**(2):393–399.

6. Smitz J, Devroey P, Braeckmans P, *et al.* Management of failed cycles in an IVF/GIFT programme with the combination of GnRH analogue and HMG. *Hum Reprod* 1987;**2**(4):309–314.

7. Gemzell CA, Kemman E, Jones JR. Premature ovulation during administration of human menopausal gonadotropins in non-ovulatory women. *Infertility* 1978;**1**:1–10.

8. Fraser HM, Laird NC, Blakeley DM. Decreased pituitary responsiveness and inhibition of the luteinizing hormone surge and ovulation in the stumptailed monkey (*Macaca arctoides*) by chronic treatment with an agonist of luteinizing hormone-releasing hormone. *Endocrinology* 1980;**106**:452–457.

9. Fleming R, Adam AH, Barlow DH, *et al.* A new systematic treatment for infertile women with abnormal hormone profiles. *Br J Obstet Gynaecol* 1982;**89**:80–83.

10. Porter RN, Smith W, Craft IL, Abdulwahid NA, Jacobs HS. Induction of ovulation for in-vitro fertilisation using buserelin and gonadotropins. *Lancet* 1984;**2**:1284–1285.

11. Fleming R, Haxton MJ, Hamilton MP, *et al.* Combined gonadotropin-releasing hormone analog and exogenous gonadotropins for ovulation induction in infertile women: efficacy related to ovarian function assessment. *Am J Obstet Gynecol* 1988;**159**:376–381.

12. Shalev E, Leung PC. Gonadotropin-releasing hormone and reproductive medicine. *J Obstet Gynaecol Can* 2003;**25**(2):98–113.

13. Diedrich K, Ludwig M, Felberbaum RE. The role of gonadotropin-releasing hormone antagonists in in vitro fertilization. *Semin Reprod Med* 2001;**19**(3):213–220.

14. Conn PM, Crowley WF Jr. Gonadotropin-releasing hormone and its analogues. *N Engl J Med* 1991;**324**(2):93–103.

15. Sandow J, Engelbart K, von Rechenberg W. The different mechanisms for suppression of pituitary and testicular function. *Med Biol* 1985;**63**:192–200.

16. Pelletier G, Dubé D, Guy J, Séguin C, Lefebvre FA. Binding and internalization of a luteinizing hormone-releasing hormone agonist by rat gonadotrophic cells. A radio autographic study. *Endocrinology* 1982;**111**:1068–1076.

17. Filicori M, Cognigni GE, Arnone R, *et al.* Role of different GnRH agonist regimens in pituitary suppression and the outcome of controlled ovarian hyperstimulation. *Hum Reprod* 1996;**11** Suppl 3:123–132.

18. Janssens RM, Lambalk CB, Vermeiden JP, *et al.* Dose-finding study of triptorelin acetate for prevention of a premature LH surge in IVF: a prospective, randomized, double-blind, placebo-controlled study. *Hum Reprod* 2000;**15**:2333–2340.

19. Dada T, Salha O, Baillie HS, Sharma V. A comparison of three gonadotrophin-releasing hormone analogues in an in-vitro fertilization programme: a prospective randomized study. *Hum Reprod* 1999;**14**(2):288–293.

20. El-Nemr A, Bhide M, Khalifa Y, *et al.* Clinical evaluation of three different gonadotrophin-releasing hormone analogues in an IVF programme: a prospective study. *Eur J Obstet Gynecol Reprod Biol* 2002;**103**(2):140–145.

21. Eftekhar M, Rahmani E, Mohammadian F. Comparison of pregnancy outcome in half-dose Triptorelin and short-acting Decapeptyl in long protocol in ART cycles: a randomized clinical trial. *Iran J Reprod Med* 2013;**11**(2):133–138.

22. Bastu E, Buyru F, Ozsurmeli M, *et al.* A randomized, single-blind, prospective trial comparing three different gonadotropin doses with or without addition of letrozole during ovulation stimulation in patients with poor ovarian response. *Eur J Obstet Gynecol Reprod Biol* 2016;**203**:30–34.

23. Albuquerque LE, Tso LO, Saconato H, Albuquerque MC, Macedo CR. Depot versus daily administration of gonadotrophin-releasing hormone agonist protocols for pituitary down regulation in assisted reproduction cycles. *Cochrane Database Syst Rev* 2013;**1**:CD002808.

24. Lockwood GM, Pinkerton SM, Barlow DH. A prospective randomized single-blind comparative trial of nafarelin acetate with buserelin in long-protocol gonadotrophin-releasing hormone analogue controlled in-vitro fertilization cycles. *Hum Reprod* 1995;**10**:293–298.

25. Meldrum DR, Wisot A, Hamilton F, *et al.* Timing of initiation and dose schedule of leuprolide influence the time course of ovarian suppression. *Fertil Steril* 1988;**50**(3):400–402.

26. Siristatidis CS, Gibreel A, Basios G, Maheshwari A, Bhattacharya S. Gonadotrophin-releasing hormone agonist protocols for pituitary suppression in assisted reproduction. *Cochrane Database Syst Rev* 2015;**11**:CD006919.

27. Berkkanoglu M, Ozgur K. What is the optimum maximal gonadotropin dosage used in microdose flare-up cycles in poor responders? *Fertil Steril* 2010;**94**(2):662–665.

28. Lefebvre J, Antaki R, Kadoch IJ, *et al.* 450 IU versus 600 IU gonadotropin for controlled ovarian stimulation in poor responders: a randomized controlled trial. *Fertil Steril* 2015;**104**(6):1419–1425.

29. National Institute for Health and Care Excellence. Fertility problems: assessment and treatment (CG156). 2017.

30. van Wely M, Westergaard LG, Bossuyt PM, van der Veen F. Effectiveness of human menopausal gonadotropin versus recombinant follicle-stimulating hormone for controlled ovarian hyperstimulation in assisted reproductive cycles: a meta-analysis. *Fertil Steril* 2003;**80**(5):1086–1093.

31. Coomarasamy A, Afnan M, Cheema D, *et al.* Urinary hMG versus recombinant FSH for controlled ovarian hyperstimulation following an agonist long down-regulation protocol in IVF or ICSI treatment: a systematic review and meta-analysis. *Hum Reprod* 2008;**23**(2):310–315.

32. Tan SL, Balen A, El Hussein E, *et al.* A prospective randomized study of the optimum timing of human chorionic gonadotropin administration after pituitary desensitization in in vitro fertilization. *Fertil Steril* 1992;**57**(6):1259–1264.

33. Youssef MA, Abou-Setta AM, Lam WS. Recombinant versus urinary human chorionic gonadotrophin for final oocyte maturation triggering in IVF and ICSI cycles. *Cochrane Database Syst Rev* 2016;**4**:CD003719.

34. Nelson SM, Yates RW, Lyall H, *et al.* Anti-Müllerian hormone-based approach to controlled ovarian stimulation for assisted conception. *Hum Reprod* 2009;**24**:867–875.

35. Frydman R, Belaisch-Allart J, Parneix I, *et al.* Comparison between flare up and down regulation effects of luteinizing hormone-releasing hormone agonists in an in vitro fertilization program. *Fertil Steril* 1988;**50**:471–475.

36. Cramer DW, Powers DR, Oskowitz SP, *et al.* Gonadotropin-releasing hormone agonist use in assisted reproduction cycles: the influence of long and short regimens on pregnancy rates. *Fertil Steril* 1999;**72**:83–89.

37. San Roman GA, Surrey ES, Judd HL, Kerin JF. A prospective randomized comparison of luteal phase versus concurrent follicular phase initiation of gonadotropin-releasing hormone agonist for in vitro fertilization. *Fertil Steril* 1992;**58**(4):744–749.

38. Gelety TJ, Pearlstone AC, Surrey ES. Short-term endocrine response to gonadotropin-releasing hormone agonist initiated in the early follicular, midluteal, or late luteal phase in normally cycling women. *Fertil Steril* 1995;**64**(6):1074–1080.

39. Keltz MD, Jones EE, Duleba AJ, *et al.* Baseline cyst formation after luteal phase gonadotropin-releasing hormone agonist administration is linked to poor in vitro fertilization outcome. *Fertil Steril* 1995;**64**(3):568–572.

40. Feldberg D, Ashkenazi J, Dicker D, *et al.* Ovarian cyst formation: a complication of gonadotropin-releasing hormone agonist therapy. *Fertil Steril* 1989;**51**(1):42–45.

41. Ron-El R, Herman A, Golan A, *et al.* Follicle cyst formation following long-acting gonadotropin-releasing hormone analog administration. *Fertil Steril* 1989;**52**(6):1063–1066.

42. Qublan HS, Amarin Z, Tahat YA, Smadi AZ, Kilani M. Ovarian cyst formation following GnRH agonist administration in IVF cycles: incidence and impact. *Hum Reprod* 2006;**21**(3):640–644.

43. Firouzabadi RD, Sekhavat L, Javedani M. The effect of ovarian cyst aspiration on IVF treatment with GnRH. *Arch Gynecol Obstet* 2010;**281**(3):545–549.

44. Segal S, Shifren JL, Isaacson KB, *et al.* Effect of a baseline ovarian cyst on the outcome of in vitro fertilization–embryo transfer. *Fertil Steril* 1999;**71**(2):274–277.

45. Rizk B, Tan SL, Kingsland C, *et al.* Ovarian cyst aspiration and the outcome of in vitro fertilization. *Fertil Steril* 1990;**54**(4):661–664.

46. Cédrin-Durnerin I, Bulwa S, Hervé F, *et al.* The hormonal flare-up following gonadotrophin-releasing hormone agonist administration is influenced by a progestogen pretreatment. *Hum Reprod* 1996;**11**:1859–1863.

47. Sbracia M, Farina A, Poverini R, *et al.* Short versus long gonadotropin-releasing hormone analogue suppression protocols for superovulation in patients > or = 40 years old undergoing intracytoplasmic sperm injection. *Fertil Steril* 2005;**84**:644–648.

48. Pandian Z, McTavish AR, Aucott L, Hamilton MP, Bhattacharya S. Interventions for 'poor responders' to controlled ovarian hyper stimulation (COH) in in-vitro fertilisation (IVF). *Cochrane Database Syst Rev* 2010;**1**:CD004379.

49. Berin I, Stein DE, Keltz MD. A comparison of gonadotropin-releasing hormone (GnRH) antagonist and GnRH agonist flare protocols for poor responders undergoing in vitro fertilization. *Fertil Steril* 2010;**93**:360–363.

50. Ron-El R, Golan A, Herman A, *et al.* Midluteal gonadotropin-releasing hormone analog administration in early pregnancy. *Fertil Steril* 1990;**53**(3):572–574.

51. Isherwood PJ, Ibrahim ZH, Matson PL, *et al.* Endocrine changes in women conceiving during treatment with an LHRH agonist. *Hum Reprod* 1990;**5**(4):409–412.

52. Smitz J, Camus M, Devroey P, Bollen N, Tournaye H, Van Steirteghem AC. CLINICAL REPORT: The influence of inadvertent intranasal buserelin administration in early pregnancy. *Hum Reprod* 1991;**6**(2):290–293.

53. Balasch J, Martinez F, Jové I, *et al.* Inadvertent gonadotrophin-releasing hormone agonist (GnRHa) administration in the luteal phase may improve fecundity in in-vitro fertilization patients. *Hum Reprod* 1993;**8**(7):1148–1151.

54. Weissman A, Shoham Z. Favourable pregnancy outcome after administration of a long-acting gonadotrophin-releasing hormone agonist in the mid-luteal phase. *Hum Reprod* 1993;**8**(3):496–497.

55. Janssens RM, Brus L, Cahill DJ, *et al.* Direct ovarian effects and safety aspects of GnRH agonists and antagonists. *Hum Reprod Update* 2000;**6**:505–518.

56. Delvigne A, Rozenberg S. Epidemiology and prevention of ovarian hyperstimulation syndrome (OHSS): a review. *Hum Reprod Update* 2002;**8**(6):559–577.

57. Ragni G, Vegetti W, Riccaboni A, *et al.* Comparison of GnRH agonists and antagonists in assisted reproduction cycles of patients at high risk of ovarian hyperstimulation syndrome. *Hum Reprod* 2005;**20**(9):2421–2425.

58. Fleming R. Recruitment prior to ovarian stimulation: ways of improving follicular recruitment. *RBM Online* 2005;**10** Suppl 3:55–59.

59. Huirne JA, Homburg R, Lambalk CB. Are GnRH antagonists comparable to agonists for use in IVF? *Hum Reprod* 2007;**22**:2805–2813.

60. Fleming R, Deshpande N, Traynor I, Yates RW. Dynamics of FSH-induced follicular growth in subfertile women: relationship with age, insulin resistance, oocyte yield and anti-Mullerian hormone. *Hum Reprod* 2006;**21**:1436–1441.

61. Devroey P, Aboulghar M, Garcia-Velasco J, *et al.* Improving the patient's experience of IVF/ICSI: a proposal for an ovarian stimulation protocol with GnRH antagonist co-treatment. *Hum Reprod* 2009;**24**:764–774.

62. Nelson SM, Yates RW, Fleming R. Serum anti-Müllerian hormone and FSH: prediction of live birth and extremes of response in stimulated cycles-implications for individualization of therapy. *Hum Reprod* 2007;**22**:2414–2421.

63. Anckaert E, Smitz J, Schiettecatte J, Klein BM, Arce JC. The value of anti-Müllerian hormone measurement in the long GnRH agonist protocol: association with ovarian response and gonadotrophin-dose adjustments. *Hum Reprod* 2012;**27**(6):1829–1839.

64. Fleming R, Broekmans F, Calhaz-Jorge C, *et al.* Can anti-Müllerian hormone concentrations be used to determine gonadotrophin dose and treatment protocol for ovarian stimulation? *Reprod Biomed Online* 2013;**26**(5):431–439.

65. Lambalk CB, Banga FR, Huirne JA, *et al.* GnRH antagonist versus long agonist protocols in IVF: a systematic review and meta-analysis accounting for patient type. *Hum Reprod Update* 2017;**23**(5):560–579.

66. The ESHRE Guideline Group on Ovarian Stimulation, Bosch E, Broer S, Griesinger G, *et al.* ESHRE guideline: ovarian stimulation for IVF/ICSI. *Hum Reprod Open* 2020;**2020**(2):hoaa009.

67. Aboulghar M. Luteal support in reproduction: when, what and how? *Curr Opin Obstet Gynecol* 2009;**21**:279–284.

68. Jee BC, Suh CS, Kim SH, Kim YB, Moon SY. Effects of estradiol supplementation during the luteal phase of in vitro fertilization cycles: a meta-analysis. *Fertil Steril* 2010;**93**(2):428–436.

Chapter

7

Role of GnRH Antagonist in Assisted Reproduction

Mohamed Aboulghar

Introduction

Induction of ovulation is one of the major advances in the treatment of subfertility in the last decades. One aspect of ovulation induction that required attention is the occurrence of a premature luteinizing hormone (LH) surge before the leading follicle reaches the optimum diameter for triggering ovulation by human chorionic gonadotrophin (hCG). It was reported that premature LH surge occurs in a significant number of patients undergoing ovulation induction [1]. Such premature LH surge prevents effective induction of multiple follicular maturation for in vitro fertilization (IVF) and resulted in a significant cancellation of IVF cycles [2].

Gonadotropin-releasing hormone agonists (GnRHa) have played an important role in reducing the incidence of premature LH surges. These agents had a high affinity to GnRH receptors, after an initial stimulating phase (flare up), downregulation occurs [3]. The resumption of pituitary gonadotropins secretion begins two weeks after stoppage of treatment. Full restoration of ovarian function takes place in six weeks or more [4]. Introduction of GnRHa in ovarian stimulation protocols for IVF prevented premature LH surge and resulted in an increased pregnancy rate in IVF treatment [5].

Gonadotropin-releasing hormone antagonists have emerged as an alternative in preventing LH surges [2].

The objective of this chapter is to review and analyze the role of GnRH antagonists in ovulation induction for IVF.

Development of GnRH Antagonists

Native GnRH is a small 10-amino acid peptide which is intermittently secreted by the hypothalamus, inducing pulsatile secretions of follicle-stimulating hormone (FSH) and LH from the anterior pituitary, by binding to a specific receptor in the pituitary cells to regulate the secretion and synthesis of LH and FSH. After binding with the receptor, the GnRH–receptor complex elicits several (calcium-dependent) reactions to release the pituitary hormones (LH and FSH); in addition, the number of GnRH receptors undergoes changes during certain physiological states such as lactation and old age [6].

The amino acids at position number 6 are involved in enzymatic splicing, those in position number 2 and 3 are involved in gonadotropin release, while residues 1, 6, and 10 are important for the three-dimensional structure and receptor binding [7].

Soon after the identification of the GnRH sequence, GnRHa were developed by substituting amino acids on residue 6 and 10 of the GnRH sequence [8].

The development of GnRH antagonists was more complex, the reasons being problems with solubility and histamine release [9].

The first generation of these compounds are characterized by modification on position number 1, 2, and 6 of the sequence of human GnRH.

The third-generation GnRH antagonists are characterized by modification on position numbers 1, 2, 3, 6, and 10 of the sequence of human GnRH; two of these compounds cetrorelix and ganirelix are devoid of the histamine-releasing property and the two drugs are now widely used in clinical medicine (Figure 7.1).

Mode of Action of GnRH Antagonists

Although the purpose of the development of GnRH antagonists was originally a non-steroid contraceptive drug [10], it was found that GnRH antagonists have potential benefit in assisted reproduction. The main objective of using GnRH antagonists in IVF is

Nal-Arg antagonist	Ac-DNal-DFpa-DTrp-Ser-Tyr-DArg-Leu-Arg-Pro-Gly-NH$_2$
Nal-Glu antagonist	Ac-DNal-DCpa-Dpal-Ser-Arg-DGlu(AA)-Leu-Arg-Pro-DAla-NH$_2$
Antide	Ac-DNal-DCpa-Dpal-Ser-Lys(Nic)-DLys(Nic)-Leu-ILys-Pro-DAla-NH$_2$
Cetrorelix	Ac-DNal-DCpa-Dpal-Ser-Tyr-DCit-Leu-Arg-Pro-DAla-NH$_2$
Ganirelix	Ac-DNal-DCpa-Dpal-Ser-Tyr-DHArg(Et$_2$)-Leu-HArg (Et$_2$)-Pro-DAla-NH$_2$

Figure 7.1 Selected structures of GnRH antagonist including cetrorelix and ganirelix, which are devoid of histamine-releasing properties and the only ones available for clinical use.

the avoidance of a premature LH surge. GnRH antagonists act by immediate suppression of pituitary gonadotropin release and rapid recovery of normal secretion of endogenous LH and FSH [9] after its stoppage. GnRH antagonists immediately block the GnRH receptor in a competitive fashion and hence reduce LH and FSH secretion within a period of 8 hours. The inhibition of LH secretion is more pronounced than that of FSH, this being most likely due to the different forms of gonadotropin regulation and the prolonged FSH half-life or the immunoactive and bioactive forms of FSH [11;12].

Dose-Finding Study for GnRH Antagonist (Ganirelix)

A multicenter, double-blind randomized dose-finding study of ganirelix was conducted in 333 women undergoing ovarian stimulation with recombinant FSH (rFSH) to establish the minimal effective dose preventing premature LH surges during ovarian stimulation. Recombinant FSH was given in a fixed daily dose of 150 IU for 5 days from days 2 to 6 of the menstrual cycles. From cycle day 7 onward, up to and including the day of hCG dosage, ganirelix 0.0625, 0.125, 0.25, 0.5, 1, and 2 mg were administered once daily by subcutaneous injection. The lowest (0.0625 mg) and highest (2 mg) dose groups were terminated prematurely on the advice of an external independent advisory committee. On the day of hCG, the number of follicles was similar in the six dose groups, whereas serum estradiol

(E$_2$) concentrations were highest in the 0.0625 mg group (1475 pg/ml) and lowest in the 2 mg group (430 pg/ml). The mean number of recovered oocytes and good-quality embryos was similar in all dose groups, and ranged from 8.6 to 10.0 and 2.5 to 3.8, respectively. The mean number of replaced embryos in the different dose groups ranged from 2.3 to 2.7. Progesterone was used for luteal phase support in all groups. The implantation rate was highest in the 0.25 mg group (21.9%) and lowest in the 2 mg group (1.5%). The early miscarriage rates (first 6 weeks after embryo transfer) were 11.9% and 13% in the 1 and 2 mg group, respectively, whereas in the other dose groups this incidence was zero up to a maximum of 3.7%. The vital pregnancy rate (with heart activity) at 5–6 weeks after embryo transfer was highest in the 0.25 mg group, that is, 36.8% per attempt and 40.3% per transfer, and resulted in an ongoing pregnancy rate 12–16 weeks after embryo transfer of 33.8% per attempt and 37.1% per transfer.

Based on this study, ganirelix was produced and marketed in a dose of 0.25 mg for use in assisted reproduction [13].

Single High-Dose Regimen (Cetrorelix)

In the single high-dose antagonist study, randomization was performed using a 3:1 ratio (antagonist/agonist). In this study a single dose of 3 mg antagonist was administered on day 7 of human menopausal gonadotropin (hMG) stimulation unless the E$_2$ level was below 400 pg/ml, in which case the injection was delayed. If triggering of ovulation was not done within four days of administration of the 3 mg dose of antagonist, a daily injection of 0.25 mg was given until hCG administration. The 3 mg dose was therefore selected as a safer choice for a protection period of at least four days [14]. The GnRHa reference treatment was started in the midluteal phase (cycle day 21–24) by administering the triptorelin depot formula and ovarian stimulation was started after 2 weeks if pituitary downregulation was established (serum E$_2$ level < 50 pg/ml). In both treatment groups, ovarian stimulation was started with a fixed daily dose of 150 or 225 IU hMG for the first four stimulation days. Thereafter, the dose of gonadotropin was adapted depending on the ovarian response.

Only 15.6 percent presented with LH rise on the day of starting cetrorelix injection. None of the patients in the cetrorelix group experienced a LH surge after cetrorelix administration. Triggering of ovulation was induced with hCG (10 000 IU) when at least one follicle > 18 mm was observed by ultrasound and the E_2 level was 1200 pg/ml. Thirty to 36 hours after triggering, oocyte pickup was performed. This was followed by IVF or intracytoplasmic sperm injection (ICSI) and no more than three embryos were to be replaced two to five days thereafter. The percentage of mature oocytes, fertilization rate, clinical and ongoing pregnancy rates, and miscarriage rates were not statistically different between the two groups [15]. Luteal phase support was given per the clinic's routine practice and was started no later than the day of embryo transfer [15].

GnRH Antagonist versus GnRH Agonist: Results of Randomized Trials and Meta-analyses

A Cochrane review to compare the IVF outcome between GnRHa versus GnRH antagonist was published in 2001 [16]. All five trials comparing the new fixed protocol of GnRH antagonist to the long protocol of GnRHa fulfilled the inclusion criteria. In four studies, the multiple low-dose (0.25 mg) antagonist regimen was applied and in one study, the single high-dose (3 mg) antagonist regimen was investigated. In all trials, reference treatment included a long protocol of GnRHa (buserelin, leuprorelin, or triptorelin) starting in the midluteal phase of the preceding cycle. In all five studies there was a small trend toward a higher clinical pregnancy rate in the GnRHa long protocol arm but the difference was not significant in any of the studies in the meta-analysis. There were significantly fewer clinical pregnancies in those treated with GnRH antagonist (odds ratio [OR] 0.79, 95% confidence interval [CI] 0.63–0.99). The absolute treatment effect was calculated to be 5 percent. The number needed to treat was 20. There was no statistically significant reduction in incidence of severe ovarian hyperstimulation syndrome (OHSS) (relative risk [RR] 0.51, 95% CI 0.22–1.18) using antagonist regimens compared with the long GnRHa protocol [16].

Over the years several randomized studies comparing GnRHa and GnRH antagonist for ovarian stimulation for IVF were published. Two new meta-analyses compared GnRH agonist versus GnRH antagonist. The first was published by Kolibianakis et al. in 2006 [17]. This meta-analysis aimed to answer the following clinical question: among patients treated for IVF with gonadotropins and GnRH analogues, is the probability of live birth per randomized patient dependent on the type of analogue used? Eligible studies were randomized controlled trials (RCTs), published as a full manuscript in a peer-reviewed journal. A literature search identified 22 RCTs comparing GnRH antagonists and GnRHa that involved 3176 subjects. Where live birth was not reported in a study that fulfilled the inclusion criteria, clinical pregnancy or ongoing pregnancy was converted to live birth in 12 studies using published data. No significant difference was present in the probability of live birth between the two GnRH analogues (OR 0.86, 95% CI 0.72–1.02]. The incidence of OHSS associated with hospital admission was significantly lower in the antagonist than the agonist protocol (OR 0.46, 95% CI 0.26–0.82, $p \leq 0.01$). In conclusion, the probability of live birth after ovarian stimulation for IVF does not depend on the type of analogue used for pituitary suppression [17].

Al-Inany et al. 2006 published an update to their Cochrane review [18] in the same year. Randomized controlled studies comparing different protocols of GnRH antagonists with GnRHa in assisted conception cycles were included in this review. Twenty seven RCTs comparing the GnRH antagonist with the long protocol of GnRHa fulfilled the inclusion criteria. Clinical pregnancy rate was significantly lower in the antagonist group (OR 0.84, 95% CI 0.72–0.97). The ongoing pregnancy/live birth rate showed the same significantly lower pregnancy rate in the antagonist group ($p = 0.03$; OR 0.82, 95% CI 0.69–0.98). However, there was a statistically significant reduction in the incidence of severe OHSS with the antagonist protocol ($p = 0.01$; RR 0.61, 95% CI 0.42–0.89). In addition, interventions to prevent OHSS (e.g., coasting, cycle cancellation) were administered more frequently in the agonist group ($p = 0.03$; OR 0.44, 95% CI 0.21–0.93). The authors concluded that the GnRH antagonist protocol is a short and simple protocol with good clinical outcome and significant reduction in the

Table 7.1 A comparison between GnRHa and GnRH antagonist in ovarian stimulation for IVF

	GnRH agonist	GnRH antagonist
Action	Downregulation of the pituitary	Immediate block of GnRH receptors
Period to block pituitary	2–4 weeks	8 hours
Recovery from effect	2–6 weeks	Immediate
Route of administration	Subcutaneous Intranasal	Subcutaneous Intramuscular
Dose	0.1 mg	0.25 mg
Duration of use	Around 4 weeks	Around 4–7 days
Cyst formation	Possible	No
OHSS	Higher incidence	Lower incidence
Consumption of gonadotropin	Higher	Lower
Pregnancy rate (results of meta-analyses)	Higher Higher Equal	Lower [16] Lower [18] Equal [17]
	Higher Equal	Lower [20] Equal [19]

incidence of severe OHSS and amount of gonadotropins, but the lower pregnancy rate compared with the GnRHa long protocol necessitates counseling subfertile couples before recommending change from GnRHa to GnRH antagonist [18].

One advantage of Kolibianakis' meta-analysis is that only fully peer-reviewed and published studies are included, but the study has two drawbacks. The first is that live birth rate is calculated indirectly in some patients and the second is that both long and short GnRHa protocols are included together.

Al-Inany's study has a drawback of including abstracts not published as full papers. Although this is acceptable by the regulations of Cochrane, these are not peer-reviewed full manuscripts. The advantages of the meta-analysis are that they only included the long GnRHa protocol and live birth was calculated from the studies directly.

In the updated Cochrane review (2016) [19], which included 73 RCTs and 12 212 patients, there was no conclusive evidence of a difference in the live birth rate between agonist and antagonist protocols (OR 1.02, 95% CI 0.85–1.23). Cycle cancellation due to poor ovarian response was higher in the antagonist protocol. Cycle cancellation due to high risk of OHSS was higher in the long GnRHa protocol.

Lambark *et al.* (2017) [20] included 50 studies in a meta-analysis, 34 randomized studies reported on general IVF patients, 10 studies on polycystic ovary syndrome (PCOS), and 6 studies on poor responders. They compared agonist versus antagonist protocols. In the general IVF patients, the ongoing pregnancy rate was significantly lower in the antagonist arm (RR 0.89, 95% CI 0.82–0.96). There was no significant difference in the ongoing pregnancy rate in the poor responders or the PCOS patients.

Long GnRHa protocol versus antagonist protocol versus short agonist protocol in IVF in a RCT showed that the short agonist regimen may be less effective [21].

In a randomized study, the cumulative live birth rate after one assisted reproductive technology (ART) cycle, including subsequent frozen-thawed cycles, in 1050 women showed that the chances of at least one live birth following utilization of all fresh and frozen embryos after the first ART cycle are similar in GnRH antagonist and GnRHa protocols [22].

Table 7.1 shows a comparison between GnRHa and GnRH antagonist in ovarian stimulation for IVF.

Different Options Suggested to Improve IVF Outcome in GnRH Antagonist Cycles

GnRH Antagonist Flexible Protocol

GnRH antagonists were used in a fixed regimen in the original phase III studies; subsequently the majority of clinical trials adopted this GnRH antagonist fixed protocol.

There was some evidence that tailoring the administration of the GnRH antagonist will lead to an improvement in the outcome of ovarian stimulation cycles [23]. The flexible protocol involves the administration of the GnRH antagonist according to the size of the leading follicle and not at a fixed date.

Ludwig et al., in a prospective randomized study to test the flexible antagonist protocol, found that tailoring of the GnRH antagonist protocol leads to optimization of ovarian stimulation, with more oocytes retrieved despite less FSH used [24].

Mansour et al., in a study comparing GnRH antagonist fixed versus flexible protocols, found that starting the antagonist according to the size of the follicle is effective as a fixed protocol, with a reduction in the dose of antagonist required [25].

In a non-randomized study, ongoing pregnancy rates were 37.5%, 34.7%, and 18.6% for days 4, 5, and 6 of starting the antagonist; consequently, it was found that delaying the onset of GnRH antagonist reduces the pregnancy rate [26].

A meta-analysis was conducted to compare fixed versus flexible protocols [27]. Eleven trials were identified, but only four RCTs met the inclusion criteria. There was no statistically significant difference in pregnancy rate per woman randomized, although there was a trend toward a higher pregnancy rate with the fixed protocol, especially with delayed administration beyond day 8 (OR 0.7, 95% CI 0.45–1.1). There was no premature LH surge in any participant in either protocol. However, there was a statistically significant reduction in both dose of antagonist (OR -1.2 95%, CI -1.26 to -1.15) and dose of gonadotropin (OR 95.5 IU, 95% CI 74.8–116.1) used in the flexible protocol.

Messinis et al., in a randomized study, found that administration of GnRH antagonist on alternate days or daily may prevent premature luteinization to a similar extent in IVF cycles [28]. However, the study was not powered to test differences in pregnancy rates.

Increasing the Dose of FSH with the Start of GnRH Antagonist

It was postulated that on the day of starting the GnRH antagonist, endogenous FSH suddenly stops and this will reduce the total FSH available for the growing follicles until the commencement of hCG. In an attempt to test this hypothesis, 151 subfertile couples undergoing IVF/ICSI were randomized on the day of starting the antagonist into two groups, with one continuing with the same dose of FSH, and the other group receiving an additional daily 75 IU of FSH. The results showed no statistically significant difference between the groups regarding the number of retrieved oocytes, or implantation or pregnancy rates [29]. The same conclusions were reached by another randomized study [30].

Clomiphene Citrate in GnRH Antagonist Protocol

Engel et al. studied ovarian stimulation for IVF using clomiphene (clomifene) citrate and rFSH or hMG, together with multiple doses of GnRH antagonist [31]. They found that the premature LH surge was 21.5 percent, which was considered unacceptable. In a non-randomized trial evaluating the cost-effectiveness of clomiphene citrate, the hMG protocol versus a long GnRHa/hMG protocol was evaluated [32]. The clinical pregnancy rate was 24 percent in the clomiphene citrate arm and 59 percent in the long GnRHa arm. The cost of medication was 1110 ± 492 Egyptian Pounds (LE) in the clomiphene citrate group and 1928 ± 458 LE in the long GnRHa protocol. However, the total cost per pregnancy was 19 653 LE in the clomiphene citrate group and 10 047 LE in the GnRHa group. The conclusion was that the use of clomiphene citrate in antagonist protocols is not cost-effective.

Oral Contraceptive Pills before IVF in GnRH Antagonist Cycles

A randomized prospective trial comparing GnRH antagonist/rFSH versus GnRHa/rFSH in women pretreated with oral contraceptives before IVF was performed [33]. Patient outcomes were similar for the days of stimulation, total dose of gonadotropin used, two-pronuclei embryos, clinical pregnancy rate (44.4% GnRH antagonist vs. 45.0% GnRHa, $p = 0.86$), and implantation rates (22.2% GnRH antagonist vs. 26.4% GnRHa, $p = 0.71$). Oral contraceptive cycle scheduling resulted in 78% and 90% of retrievals performed Monday through Friday for GnRH antagonist and GnRHa.

GnRH antagonist cycles with and without oral contraceptive pretreatment in potential poor-prognosis patients were compared [34]. In this retrospective study, 194 cycles of women with diminished ovarian reserve undergoing IVF with a protocol using GnRH antagonists were evaluated. Oral contraceptive pretreatment was used in 146 cycles; pregnancy rates were the same in both groups [34].

The effect of oral contraceptive pills (OCP) for cycle scheduling prior to GnRH antagonist protocol on IVF cycle parameters and pregnancy outcome was studied [35]. All OCP-pretreated cycles required significantly longer stimulation than non-pretreated cycles and higher total dose of FSH. Implantation and pregnancy rates were not affected by OCP pretreatment.

A prospective randomized study was performed to compare the efficacy of a GnRH antagonist multiple-dose protocol with or without OCP pretreatment and a GnRHa low-dose long protocol in 82 patients undergoing IVF/ICSI. GnRH antagonist with OCP pretreatment was at least as effective as the GnRHa low-dose long protocol in low responders, and can benefit the low responders by reducing the amount of FSH and the number of days of stimulation required for follicular maturation [36].

The effect of an OCP on follicular development in IVF/ICSI patients receiving a GnRH antagonist was evaluated in a randomized study [37]. OCP treatment resulted in significantly lower starting concentrations of FSH, LH, and E_2 ($p < 0.001$) and a thinner endometrium ($p < 0.0001$), extended stimulation period (11.6 vs. 8.7 days, $p < 0.0001$), and more oocytes retrieved (13.5 vs. 10.2, $p < 0.001$) compared with the control group. Ongoing pregnancy rates per started cycle in the non-OCP and OCP group were 27.5% and 22.9%, respectively (95% CI -3.7 to 12.8). Pregnancy loss was significantly increased in the OCP (36.4%) compared with the non-OCP group (21.6%) (95% CI of the difference: -28.4 to -2.3). It was concluded that pretreatment with OCP, compared with initiation of stimulation on day 2 of the cycle in patients treated with GnRH antagonist and rFSH, appears to be associated with a non-significant difference in ongoing pregnancy rates per started cycle and results in a significantly higher early pregnancy loss [38].

A systematic review and meta-analysis on OCP pretreatment in ovarian stimulation with GnRH antagonists for IVF showed that ongoing pregnancy rate per randomized woman was not significantly different between patients with and without OCP pretreatment (OR 0.74, 95% CI 0.53–1.03). Duration of gonadotropin stimulation (weighted mean difference [WMD] 1.41 days, 95% CI 1.13–1.68) and gonadotropin consumption (WMD 542 IU, 95% CI 127–956) were significantly increased after OCP pretreatment [39].

In a Cochrane review, Farquhar *et al.* evaluated the effect of precycle treatment by OCP in antagonist or agonist cycles on the outcome of IVF [40]. They included 29 RCTs (4701 women) in both agonist and antagonist cycles, comparing treatment with OCP versus no OCP. The rate of ongoing pregnancy and live birth rate was significantly lower in women pretreated with OCP (OR 0.74, 95% CI 0.58–0.95).

Other Options Used in Antagonist Protocol

In a non-randomized study comparing agonist versus antagonist protocols after supplementation of each arm with a small dose of recombinant hCG, there were no differences between the outcome in both arms [41].

In a randomized study using GnRH antagonist, patients received a starting dose of 150 IU rFSH or 150 IU rFSH plus 75 IU recombinant LH (rLH) for ovarian stimulation. Except for higher E_2 and LH levels on the day of hCG administration, no positive trend in favor of additional LH was found [42].

In a similar randomized study it was concluded that in an unselected group of patients, there is no evident benefit to support GnRH antagonist treated cycles with rLH [43].

Natural Cycle IVF and GnRH Antagonist

The administration of antagonist (cetrorelix) in the late follicular phase of natural cycles in patients undergoing IVF and ICSI has been investigated [44]. A total of 44 cycles from 33 healthy women were monitored, starting on day 8 by daily ultrasound and measurement of serum concentrations of E_2, LH, FSH, and progesterone. When plasma E_2 concentrations reached 100–150 pg/ml, with a lead follicle between 12 and 14 mm diameter, a single injection (subcutaneous) of 0.5 mg (19 cycles) or 1 mg (25 cycles) cetrorelix was administered. Human menopausal gonadotropin (150 IU) was administered daily at the time of the first injection of cetrorelix, and repeated thereafter until hCG administration. Four out of 44 cycles were canceled (9%). A total of 40 oocyte retrievals leading to 22 transfers (55%) was performed. In 10 cycles (25%), no oocyte was obtained. A total of seven clinical pregnancies was obtained (32.0% per transfer, 17.5% per retrieval), of which five are ongoing.

Modified natural cycle IVF was offered to 268 patients. Cumulative pregnancy rates were calculated. Ongoing pregnancy rate was 7.9% per started cycle and 20.7% per embryo transfer. The pregnancy rate after nine cycles was 44.4%. Pregnancy rate per cycle did not decline in higher cycle numbers, possibly due to selective dropout of poor-prognosis patients [45].

GnRH Agonist for Triggering Final Oocyte Maturation in the GnRH Antagonist Ovarian Hyperstimulation Protocol

With the introduction of the GnRH antagonist protocol for the prevention of a premature LH surge, it became possible to trigger ovulation with GnRHa. The GnRH antagonist occupies the GnRH receptor without causing downregulation, and by injecting a single bolus of GnRHa, the antagonist is displaced from the receptor. This activates the receptor, inducing a flare-up of gonadotropins (LH and FSH), which effectively stimulate the final oocyte maturation and ovulation. However, important differences exist regarding the profile and duration of the LH surge after triggering with GnRHa compared with that of the natural cycle. In the natural cycle, the LH surge is characterized by three phases with a total duration of ~48 hours. After GnRHa triggering, the surge consist of two phases, only, with a duration of ~24–36 hours leading to a significantly reduced amount of LH released [46].

After GnRHa trigger the circulating levels of progesterone and E_2 are significantly lower throughout the luteal phase compared with those obtained after hCG triggering due to the shorter half-life of LH (~60 minutes) compared with that of hCG (> 24 hours) [46]. The important clinical advantage of GnRHa triggering, however, is the

reported significant reduction in or even elimination of OHSS [46;47] caused by the shorter half-life of the endogenous LH surge compared with the continuous LH/hCG receptor stimulation after hCG triggering [46;48].

In a systematic review 3 publications out of 23 fulfilled the inclusion criteria for meta-analysis, which were (i) prospective, randomized controlled study design; (ii) stimulation with gonadotropins for induction of multifollicular development; (iii) suppression of endogenous LH by a GnRH antagonist; (iv) triggering of final oocyte maturation with a GnRHa; (v) control group randomized to receive hCG for final oocyte maturation, and (vi) any means of luteal phase support other than hCG. No OHSS occurred in two of the studies, whereas in one study OHSS incidence was not reported. In comparison to hCG, GnRHa administration is associated with a significantly reduced likelihood of achieving a clinical pregnancy (OR 0.21, 95% CI 0.05–0.84; $p = 0.03$). The odds of first-trimester pregnancy loss is increased after GnRHa triggering; however, the confidence interval crosses unity (OR 11.51, 95% 0.95–138.98; $p = 0.05$) [49].

In a prospective, randomized, controlled study, 305 IVF/ICSI patients were stimulated by a GnRH antagonist protocol. Triggering of ovulation was performed with either 10 000 IU hCG or 0.5 mg GnRHa (buserelin) supplemented with 1500 IU hCG on the day of oocyte retrieval. No significant differences were seen regarding positive βhCG/embryo transfer rate (48% and 48%), ongoing pregnancy rate (26% and 33%), delivery rate (24% and 31%), and rate of early pregnancy loss (21% and 17%) between the GnRHa and 10 000 IU hCG groups, respectively. However, a non-significant difference of 7% in delivery rates justifies further studies to refine the use of GnRHa for ovulation induction [50].

A Cochrane review evaluating GnRHa versus hCG for oocytes triggering in antagonist ART included 17 RCTs ($n = 1847$). GnRHa were associated with a lower live birth rate than was seen with hCG (OR 0.47, 95% CI 0.31–0.70). This suggests that for a woman with a 31% chance of achieving live birth with the use of hCG, the chance of a live birth with the use of a GnRHa would be between 12% and 24%. GnRHa were associated with a lower incidence of mild, moderate, or severe OHSS than was hCG (OR 0.15, 95% CI 0.05–0.47) [51].

GnRHa triggering possesses important advantages over hCG triggering, mainly in terms of a significant reduction in if not total elimination of OHSS. Although the modified luteal phase support has had a significant positive effect on the reproductive outcome after GnRHa triggering without increasing the risk of OHSS, the most optimal luteal phase support still has to be investigated.

Until the optimal luteal supplementation protocol has been defined an alternative option in patients with an extreme ovarian response or with a significant comorbidity is a freeze-all strategy and transfer in a subsequent natural or stimulated cycle [52].

In a randomized study including 190 participants at risk of OHSS, patients were divided into two groups, GnRHa trigger (Group A) and hCG trigger (Group B). The luteal phase support in Group A included 1500 IU of hCG at time of oocyte retrieval plus oral estrogen, and intramuscular progesterone. Group B was triggered by 5000 IU of hCG following by oral estrogen and vaginal progesterone. The ongoing pregnancy rate was not significantly different between the two groups. Moderate and severe OHSS was significantly higher in Group B [53].

GnRH Antagonist in Poor Responders

Two meta-analyses comparing GnRHa versus GnRH antagonist in poor responders were published in 2006. In the first meta-analysis, six RCTs fulfilled the inclusion criteria. There was no difference between GnRH antagonist and GnRHa (long and flare-up protocols) with respect to cycle cancellation rate, number of mature oocytes and clinical pregnancy rate per cycle initiated, per oocyte retrieval, and per embryo transfer. When the meta-analysis was applied to the two trials that had used GnRH antagonist versus long protocols of GnRHa, a significantly higher number of retrieved oocytes was observed in the GnRH antagonist protocols ($p = 0.018$; WMD 1.12, 95% CI 0.18–2.05). However, when the meta-analysis was applied to the four trials that had used GnRH antagonist versus flare-up protocols, a significantly higher number of retrieved oocytes ($p = 0.032$; WMD -0.51, 95% CI -0.99 to -0.04) was observed in the GnRHa protocols. Nevertheless, additional RCTs with better planning are needed to confirm these results [54].

The second meta-analysis on GnRH antagonist ovarian stimulation for poor responders included eight RCTs for poor response. No differences in clinical outcomes were found, except a significantly higher number of cumulus–oocyte complexes in the GnRH antagonist multiple-dose protocol compared with the GnRHa long protocol ($p = 0.05$) [49].

The use of aromatase inhibitors in poor-responder patients receiving GnRH antagonist protocol seems to restore an IVF cycle by decreasing the rate of cycle cancellation and seems to reduce the cost by reducing the total gonadotropin dosage [55].

Table 7.2 shows meta-analysis comparisons between GnRHa and GnRH antagonist.

Recombinant Luteinizing Hormone Supplementation for Controlled Ovarian Hyperstimulation in GnRH Antagonist Cycles

Studies which compared adding rLH during ovarian stimulation versus no rLH showed no evidence of a statistical difference in clinical pregnancy rates (one trial: OR 0.79, 95% CI 0.26–2.43) or in ongoing pregnancy rates (two trials: OR 0.83, 95% CI 0.39–1.80) comparing both groups. The pooled pregnancy estimates of trials including only poor responders showed a significant increase in pregnancy rate, in favor of co-administrating rLH (three trials: OR 1.85, 95% CI 1.10–3.11) [56].

In a randomized controlled study on 253 couples, rLH supplementation to the GnRH antagonist protocol in IVF/ICSI cycles has no effect on ongoing pregnancy rates in women 35 years or older [57].

Effect of GnRH Antagonist on LH Surge during Ovarian Stimulation

Tavaniotou *et al.* evaluated clomiphene/gonadotropin/GnRH antagonist protocol for IVF and concluded that sequential clomiphene citrate and gonadotropin administration is not recommended [58]. This protocol was associated with a high incidence of premature LH surges, which resulted in an adverse cycle outcome.

Lin *et al.* found out that in clomiphene/FSH stimulation for intrauterine insemination around

Table 7.2 Meta-analyses in GnRH antagonist and GNRHa for ovarian stimulation for IVF

Topic	Authors	Year	No. of studies	No. of cycles	Results
Agonist/antagonist	Al-Inany and Aboulghar [76]	2002	5	1796	Significantly higher clinical pregnancy rate in agonist (OR 0.79, 95% CI 0.63–0.99) No difference in OHSS rate
Agonist/antagonist	Kolibianakis et al. [17]	2006	22	3176	No significant difference in live birth rate (OR 0.82, 95% CI 0.7–1.02) OHSS lower in antagonist arm (OR 0.46, 95% CI 0.26–0.82)
Agonist/antagonist	Al-Inany et al. [18]	2006	27	3865	Significantly higher live birth rate with agonist (OR 0.84, 95% CI 0.69–0.97) OHSS significantly lower in antagonist (OR 0.61, 95% CI 0.42–0.89)
Fixed vs. flexible antagonist protocol	Al-Inany et al. [27]	2005	4	476	No significant difference between both drugs (OR 1.2, 95% CI 1.26–1.15)
Oral contraceptive pretreatment in GnRH antagonist	Griesinger et al. [39]	2008	4	847	No significant difference between OCP and no OCP (OR 0.74, 95% CI 0.53–1.03)
GnRHa vs. hCG for triggering ovulation with antagonist	Griesinger et al. [49]	2006	3	275	Triggering ovulation by GnRHa resulted in significantly lower pregnancy rate (OR 0.2, 95% CI 0.05–0.84)
GnRH antagonist vs. agonist in poor responders	Griesinger et al. [49]	2006	8	575	No significant difference (OR 1.28, 95% CI 0.84–1.96)

20% will have premature LH surge in the presence of GnRH antagonist even when they increased the dose from 0.25 mg to 0.5 mg [59].

Messinis *et al.* performed a study on a total of 73 women receiving ovulation stimulation IVF cycles with rFSH who were allocated randomly on cycle day 7 to the GnRH antagonist ganirelix in multiple doses (0.25 mg each), either daily ($n = 37$ women, group 1) or every other day ($n = 36$ women, group 2) until the day of hCG administration [28]. Serum FSH, LH, E_2, and progesterone values showed similar trends in the two groups. During FSH stimulation, 13 (35%) of the women in group 1 had premature LH rises (≥ 10 IU/L) of which 8 (22%) were after the start of antagonist administration. In group 2 there were 14 (39%) LH rises during FSH stimulation, of which 10 (28%) were after the start of antagonist administration. Luteinization (serum progesterone > 2 ng/ml) occurred in only one woman in each group overall (3%).

These data are consistent with the notion that an endogenous LH surge occurs invariably during superovulation induction in women [60;61] and suggest that the GnRH antagonist at the daily dose of 0.25 mg hardly prevents it. In fact, premature LH rises that could by definition belong to an LH surge [62] were seen in this study in 50 percent of the women during the administration of ganirelix.

However, these LH rises were followed by luteinization in only 2 out of 18 cases with LH ≥ 10 IU/L. The LH surge either is blocked or becomes abortive, that is, unable to induce luteinization in the vast majority of women. As a matter of fact, pregnancies after embryo transfer occurred in such cases in the present study. Whether the subtle increase in serum progesterone concentrations seen in the late follicular phase can affect endometrium maturation needs to be investigated.

GnRH Antagonists and OHSS

It has been reported that GnRH antagonist protocols are associated with a lower incidence of OHSS compared with GnRHa protocols [17;18].

Coasting can be used to prevent OHSS in antagonist cycles; however, prolongation of the follicular phase by delaying hCG administration results in a higher incidence of endometrial advancement on the day of oocyte retrieval in GnRH antagonist cycles [63].

A GnRH antagonist was also used to prevent OHSS in high-risk cycles stimulated by long GnRHa. A prospective randomized study in GnRHa long protocol cycles compared coasting and GnRH antagonist in patients at risk of OHSS. There were significantly more high-quality embryos

$(2.87 \pm 1.2$ vs. 2.21 ± 1.1; $p < 0.0001$), and more oocytes $(16.5 \pm 7.6$ vs. 14.06 ± 5.2; $p = 0.02$), in group B compared with group A. There were more days of coasting compared with days of antagonist administration $(2.82 \pm 0.97$ vs. 1.74 ± 0.91; $p < 0.0001$). In conclusion, the GnRH antagonist was superior to coasting in producing significantly more high-quality embryos and more oocytes as well as reducing the time until hCG administration. There was no significant difference in pregnancy rate between the two groups. No OHSS developed in either group [64].

Three patients with severe early OHSS, as diagnosed by analysis of hematocrit, white blood cell count, serum urea, and ultrasonographic assessment of ovarian size and ascitic fluid were treated by daily antagonist administration for one week, while resulting blastocysts were cryopreserved. Progression of severe early OHSS was inhibited in all three patients [65].

Six infertile patients who had been scheduled for embryo transfer and developed early-onset severe OHSS with ascites and hemoconcentration were chosen for treatment with 3 mg of a GnRH antagonist. The response of these patients was compared with that of five patients with severe early-onset OHSS who received support therapy alone. E_2 levels dropped significantly a few days after treatment. Peritoneal fluid regression measured by ultrasound was faster in the study group compared with controls. Hematocrit remained comparable in both groups during follow-up. In two cases a second bolus of GnRH antagonist was used due to clinical and biochemical findings during the four days of observation following the initial dose. None of the patients treated with GnRH antagonists required paracentesis. Treatment with high doses of GnRH antagonists seems to be effective in the management of severe OHSS but all embryos had to be frozen [66].

In a recent systematic review and meta-analysis which including 29 randomized studies (6399 patients), long GnRHa protocol was compared with the antagonist protocol. The incidence of OHSS was significantly lower in the antagonist protocol (OR 0.69, 95% CI 0.57–0.83; $p < 0.0001$) [67].

GnRH Antagonists in Older Patients

Cetrorelix protocol and GnRH analogue suppression long protocol for superovulation in ICSI patients older than 40 were compared.

Patients treated with the long protocol showed a significantly higher number of oocytes retrieved and a higher pregnancy rate for both the cycle and transfer with respect to the cetrorelix protocol patients. This study showed that the long protocol was more effective in older women than the cetrorelix protocol and that the GnRH antagonist may be detrimental in older women. Demirol and Gurgan, in a randomized prospective study, showed that the microdose flare-up protocol seemed to have a better outcome in poor-responder patients, with a significantly higher mean number of mature oocytes retrieved and higher implantation rate [68].

Psychosocial Well-Being during GnRH Antagonist Cycles

In a self-reported quality of life, psychosocial well-being, and physical well-being during ART treatment in 1023 women, women rated a short antagonist protocol better than a long agonist protocol [69].

IVF Babies in GnRH Antagonist Cycles

The health of 227 children born after controlled ovarian stimulation for IVF using the GnRH antagonist cetrorelix was studied. Outcome of pregnancy and, in deliveries, the date of birth, number and sex of children born, birth weight, body length, and abnormalities were recorded. At approximately one and two years of age, body weight and length and abnormalities in physical and mental development were recorded. Two hundred and nine and 18 children were born after fresh and frozen embryo transfers, respectively. Use of cetrorelix in controlled ovarian stimulation does not harm the children subsequently born [23].

Conclusions

An opinion article about a protocol for an ovarian stimulation protocol with GnRH antagonist co-treatment was published in 2009 [70]. The rationale was the need to improve the welfare and safety of patients undergoing IVF/ICSI, while maintaining a satisfactory pregnancy rate [71–73].

This opinion article stresses the importance of a shorter protocol of treatment as the GnRH antagonist causes a rapid suppression of gonado-tropin production [74] and this avoids the repeated daily injections of GnRHa for two or more weeks.

The GnRH antagonist treatment does not produce an initial flare-up of gonadotropins which may cause cyst formation [75]. Also the risk of OHSS is lower with the antagonist protocol [17;18]. On the other hand, it seems that the GnRHa long protocol is still the most widely used protocol worldwide, because of the possible higher pregnancy rate with this protocol and the stress of prolonged daily injections could be markedly diminished if the nasal spray of GnRHa is used to replace the injections.

The GnRH antagonist will continue to play an important role in ovarian stimulation for IVF; however, so far, it has not replaced the long GnRHa protocol and probably both protocols will continue to be used for ovarian stimulation for IVF.

References

1. Porter RN, Smith W, Craft IL, Abdulwahid NA, Jacobs HS. Induction of ovulation for in-vitro fertilization using buserelin and gonadotrophins. *Lancet* 1984;2:1284–1285.

2. Diedrich K, Diedrich C, Santos E, *et al.* Suppression of the endogenous luteinizing hormone surge by the gonadotrophin-releasing hormone antagonist cetrorelix during ovarian stimulation. *Hum Reprod* 1994;9(5):788–791.

3. Ron-El R, Raziel A, Schachter M, *et al.* Induction of ovulation after GnRH antagonists. *Hum Reprod Update* 2000;6(4):318–321.

4. Gordon K, Williams RF, Danforth DR, Hodgen GD. The combined use of GnRH antagonists with gonadotrophins or pulsatile GnRH in ovulation induction. In: Bouchard P, Caraty A, Coelingh-Bennink HJT, Pavlou SN, eds. *GnRH-analogs, Gonadotrophins and Gonadal Peptides.* London, UK Parthenon Publishing Group; 1992:239 pp.

5. Hughes EG, Fedorkow DM, Daya S, *et al.* The routine use of gonadotropin-releasing hormone agonists prior to in vitro fertilization and gamete intrafallopian transfer: a meta-analysis of randomized controlled trials. *Fertil Steril* 1992;58(5):888–896.

6. Clayton RN, Catt KJ. Gonadotrophin-releasing hormone receptors: characterization, physiological regulation, and relationship to reproductive function. *Endocr Rev* 1981;2:186–209.

7. Clayton RN, Catt KJ. Receptor-binding affinity of gonadotropin-releasing hormone analogs: analysis by radioligand-receptor assay. *Endocrinology* 1980;106(4):1154–1159.

8. Coy DH, Labrie F, Savary M, Coy EJ, Schally AV. LH-releasing activity of potent LH-RH analogs in vitro. *Biochem Biophys Res Commun* 1975;67(2):576–582.

9. Ditkoff EC, Cassidenti DL, Paulson RJ, *et al.* The gonadotropin-releasing hormone antagonist (Nal-Glu) acutely blocks the luteinizing hormone surge but allows for resumption of folliculogenesis in normal women. *Am J Obstet Gynecol* 1991;165:1811–1817

10. Kenigsberg D, Hodgen GD. Ovulation inhibition by administration of weekly gonadotropin-releasing hormone antagonist. *J Clin Endocrinol Metab* 1986;62(4):734–738.

11. Matikainen T, Ding YQ, Vergara M, *et al.* Differing responses of plasma bioactive and immunoreactive follicle-stimulating hormone and luteinizing hormone to gonadotropin-releasing hormone antagonist and agonist treatments in postmenopausal women. *J Clin Endocrinol Metab* 1992;75(3):820–825.

12. Bouchard PG, Charbonnel B, Caraty A, *et al.* The role of LHRH during the periovulatory period: a basis for the use of LHRH antagonists in ovulation induction. In: Filicori M, Flamigni C, eds. *Ovulation: Basic Science and Clinical Advances.* Elsevier Science BV International Congress series 1046. 1994.

13. The ganirelix dose-finding study group. A double-blind, randomized, dose-finding study to assess the efficacy of the gonadotrophin-releasing hormone antagonist ganirelix (Org 37462) to prevent premature luteinizing hormone surges in women undergoing ovarian stimulation with recombinant follicle stimulating hormone (Puregon). *Hum Reprod* 1998;13(11):3023–3031.

14. Olivennes F, Alvarez S, Bouchard P, *et al.* The use of a GnRH antagonist (cetrorelix) in a single dose protocol in IVF-embryo transfer: a dose finding study of 3 versus 2 mg. *Hum Reprod* 1998;13(9):2411–2414.

15. Olivennes F. Cunha-Filho JS, Fanchin R, Bouchard P, Frydman R. The use of GnRH antagonists in ovarian stimulation. *Hum Reprod Update* 2002;8:279–290.

16. Al-Inany H, Aboulghar M. Gonadotrophin-releasing hormone antagonist for assisted conception. *Cochrane Database Syst Rev* 2001;4:CD001750.

17. Kolibianakis EM, Collins J, Tarlatzis BC, *et al.* Among patients treated for IVF with

gonadotrophins and GnRH analogues, is the probability of live birth dependent on the type of analogue used? A systematic review and meta-analysis. *Hum Reprod Update* 2006;**12**(6):651–671.

18. Al-Inany HG, Abou-Setta AM, Aboulghar M. Gonadotrophin-releasing hormone antagonists for assisted conception. *Cochrane Database Syst Rev* 2006;**3**:CD001750.

19. Al-Inany HG, Youssef MA, Ayeleke RO, *et al.* Gonadotrophin-releasing hormone antagonists for assisted reproductive technology. *Cochrane Database Syst Rev* 2016;**4**:CD001750.

20. Lambalk BC, Banga FR, Huirne JA, *et al.* GnRH antagonist versus long agonist protocols in IVF: a systematic review and meta-analysis accounting for patient type. *Hum Reprod Update* 2017;**23**(5):560–579.

21. Sunkara SK, Coomarasamy A, Faris R, Braude P, Khalaf Y. Long gonadotropin-releasing hormone agonist versus short agonist versus antagonist regimens in poor responders undergoing in vitro fertilization: a randomized controlled trial. *Fertil Steril* 2014;**101**(1):147–153.

22. Toftager M, Bogstad J, Løssl K, *et al.* Cumulative live birth rates after one ART cycle including all subsequent frozen-thaw cycles in 1050 women: secondary outcome of an RCT comparing GnRH-antagonist and GnRH-agonist protocols. *Hum Reprod* 2017;**32**(3):556–567.

23. Ludwig M, Riethmüller-Winzen H, Felberbaum RE, *et al.* Health of 227 children born after controlled ovarian stimulation for in vitro fertilization using the luteinizing hormone-releasing hormone antagonist cetrorelix. *Fertil Steril* 2001;**75**(1):18–22.

24. Ludwig M, Katalinic A, Banz C, *et al.* Tailoring the GnRH antagonist cetrorelix acetate to individual patients' needs in ovarian stimulation for IVF: results of a prospective, randomized study. *Hum Reprod* 2002;**17**(11):2842–2845.

25. Mansour RT, Aboulghar MA, Serour GI, *et al.* The use of gonadotropin-releasing hormone antagonist in a flexible protocol: a pilot study. *Am J Obstet Gynecol* 2003;**189**(2):444–446.

26. Lainas T, Zorzovilis J, Petsas G, *et al.* In a flexible antagonist protocol, earlier, criteria-based initiation of GnRH antagonist is associated with increased pregnancy rates in IVF. *Hum Reprod* 2005;**20**(9):2426–2433.

27. Al-Inany H, Aboulghar MA, Mansour RT, Serour GI. Optimizing GnRH antagonist administration: meta-analysis of fixed versus flexible protocol. *Reprod Biomed Online* 2005;**10**(5):567 570.

28. Messinis IE, Loutradis D, Domali E, *et al.* Alternate day and daily administration of GnRH antagonist may prevent premature luteinization to a similar extent during FSH treatment. *Hum Reprod* 2005;**20**(11):3192–3197.

29. Aboulghar MA, Mansour RT, Serour GI, *et al.* Increasing the dose of human menopausal gonadotrophins on day of GnRH antagonist administration: randomized controlled trial. *Reprod Biomed Online* 2004;**8**(5):524–527.

30. Propst AM, Bates GW, Robinson RD, *et al.* A randomized controlled trial of increasing recombinant follicle-stimulating hormone after initiating a gonadotropin-releasing hormone antagonist for in vitro fertilization-embryo transfer. *Fertil Steril* 2006;**86**(1):58–63.

31. Engel JB, Ludwig M, Felberbaum R, *et al.* Use of cetrorelix in combination with clomiphene citrate and gonadotrophins: a suitable approach to 'friendly IVF'? *Hum Reprod* 2002;**17**(8):2022–2026.

32. Mansour R, Aboulghar M, Serour GI, *et al.* The use of clomiphene citrate/human menopausal gonadotrophins in conjunction with GnRH antagonist in an IVF/ICSI program is not a cost effective protocol. *Acta Obstet Gynecol Scand* 2003;**82**(1):48–52.

33. Barmat LI, Chantilis SJ, Hurst BS, Dickey RP. A randomized prospective trial comparing gonadotropin-releasing hormone (GnRH) antagonist/recombinant follicle-stimulating hormone (rFSH) versus GnRH-agonist/rFSH in women pretreated with oral contraceptives before in vitro fertilization. *Fertil Steril* 2005;**83**(2):321–330.

34. Bendikson K, Milki AA, Speck-Zulak A, Westphal LM. Comparison of GnRH antagonist cycles with and without oral contraceptive pretreatment in potential poor prognosis patients. *Clin Exp Obstet Gynecol* 2006;**33**(3):145–147.

35. Pinkas H, Sapir O, Avrech OM, *et al.* The effect of oral contraceptive pill for cycle scheduling prior to GnRH-antagonist protocol on IVF cycle parameters and pregnancy outcome. *J Assist Reprod Genet* 2008;**25**(1):29–33.

36. Kim CH, Jeon GH, Cheon YP, *et al.* Comparison of GnRH antagonist protocol with or without oral contraceptive pill pretreatment and GnRH agonist low-dose long protocol in low responders undergoing IVF/intracytoplasmic sperm injection. *Fertil Steril* 2009;**92**(5):1758–1760.

37. Huirne JA, van Loenen AC, Donnez J, *et al.* Effect of an oral contraceptive pill on follicular development in IVF/ICSI patients receiving

a GnRH antagonist: a ranmdomized study. *Reprod Biomed Online* 2006;**13**:235–245.

38. Kolibianakis EM, Papanikolaou EG, Camus M, *et al.* Effect of oral contraceptive pill pretreatment on ongoing pregnancy rates in patients stimulated with GnRH antagonists and recombinant FSH for IVF. A randomized controlled trial. *Hum Reprod* 2006;**21**(2):352–357.

39. Griesinger G, Venetis CA, Marx T, *et al.* Oral contraceptive pill pretreatment in ovarian stimulation with GnRH antagonists for IVF: a systematic review and meta-analysis. *Fertil Steril* 2008;**90**(4):1055–1063.

40. Farquhar C, Rombauts L, Kremer JA, Lethaby A, Ayeleke RO. Oral contraceptive pill, progestogen or oestrogen pretreatment for ovarian stimulation protocols for women undergoing assisted reproductive techniques. *Cochrane Database Syst Rev* 2017;**5**:CD006109.

41. Cavagna M, Louzada Maldonado LG, de Souza Bonetti TC, *et al.* Supplementation with a recombinant human chorionic gonadotropin microdose leads to similar outcomes in ovarian stimulation with recombinant follicle-stimulating hormone for intracytoplasmic sperm injection cycles using either a gonadotropin-releasing hormone agonist or antagonist for pituitary suppression. *Fertil Steril* 2010;**94**(1):167–172.

42. Griesinger G, Schultze-Mosgau A, Dafopoulos K, *et al.* Recombinant luteinizing hormone supplementation to recombinant follicle-stimulating hormone induced ovarian hyperstimulation in the GnRH-antagonist multiple-dose protocol. *Hum Reprod* 2005;**20** (5):1200–1206.

43. Cédrin-Durnerin I, Grange-Dujardin D, Laffy A, *et al.* Recombinant human LH supplementation during GnRH antagonist administration in IVF/ICSI cycles: a prospective randomized study. *Hum Reprod* 2004;**19**(9):1979–1984.

44. Rongières-Bertrand C, Olivennes F, Righini C, *et al.* Revival of the natural cycles in in-vitro fertilization with the use of a new gonadotrophin-releasing hormone antagonist (cetrorelix): a pilot study with minimal stimulation. *Hum Reprod* 1999;**14**(3):683–688.

45. Pelinck MJ, Vogel NE, Arts EG, *et al.* Cumulative pregnancy rates after a maximum of nine cycles of modified natural cycle IVF and analysis of patient drop-out: a cohort study. *Hum Reprod* 2007;**22** (9):2463–2470.

46. Humaidan P, Kol S, Papanikolaou EG. GnRH agonist for triggering of final oocyte maturation: time for a change of practice? *Hum Reprod Update* 2011;**17**(4):510–524.

47. Humaidan P, Papanikolaou EG, Kyrou D, *et al.* The luteal phase after GnRH-agonist triggering of ovulation: present and future perspectives. *Reprod Biomed Online* 2012;**24**(2):134–141.

48. Fauser BC, de Jong D, Olivennes F, *et al.* Endocrine profiles after triggering of final oocyte maturation with GnRH agonist after cotreatment with the GnRH antagonist ganirelix during ovarian hyperstimulation for in vitro fertilization. *J Clin Endocrinol Metab* 2002;**87**(2):709–715.

49. Griesinger G, Diedrich K, Devroey P, Kolibianakis EM. GnRH agonist for triggering final oocyte maturation in the GnRH antagonist ovarian hyperstimulation protocol: a systematic review and meta-analysis. *Hum Reprod Update* 2006;**12**(2):159–168.

50. Humaidan P, Bungum L, Bungum M, Yding Andersen C. Rescue of corpus luteum function with peri-ovulatory HCG supplementation in IVF/ICSI GnRH antagonist cycles in which ovulation was triggered with a GnRH agonist: a pilot study. *Reprod Biomed Online* 2006;**13**(2):173–178.

51. Youssef MA, Van der Veen F, Al-Inany HG, *et al.* Gonadotropin-releasing hormone agonist versus HCG for oocyte triggering in antagonist-assisted reproductive technology. *Cochrane Database Syst Rev* 2014;**10**:CD008046.

52. Leth-Moller K, Hammer Jagd S, Humaidan P. The luteal phase after GnRHa trigger-understanding an enigma. *Int J Fertil Steril* 2014;**8**(3):227–234.

53. Elgindy EA, Sibai H, Mostafa MI, *et al.* Towards an optimal luteal support modality in agonist triggered cycles: a randomized clinical trial. *Hum Reprod* 2018;**33**(6):1079–1086.

54. Franco JG Jr., Baruffi RL, Mauri AL, *et al.* GnRH agonist versus GnRH antagonist in poor ovarian responders: a meta-analysis. *Reprod Biomed Online* 2006;**13**(5):618–627.

55. Ozmen B, Sönmezer M, Atabekoglu CS, Olmus H. Use of aromatase inhibitors in poor-responder patients receiving GnRH antagonist protocols. *Reprod Biomed Online* 2009;**19**(4):478–485.

56. Baruffi RL, Mauri AL, Petersen CG, *et al.* Recombinant LH supplementation to recombinant FSH during induced ovarian stimulation in the GnRH-antagonist protocol: a meta-analysis. *Reprod Biomed Online* 2007;**14** (1):14–25.

57. König TE, van der Houwen LE, Overbeek A, *et al.* Recombinant LH supplementation to a standard GnRH antagonist protocol in women of 35 years or older undergoing IVF/ICSI: a randomized controlled multicentre study. *Hum Reprod* 2013;**28** (10):2804–2812.

58. Tavaniotou A, Albano C, Van Steirteghem A, Devroey P. The impact of LH serum concentration on the clinical outcome of IVF cycles in patients receiving two regimens of clomiphene citrate/gonadotrophin/0.25 mg cetrorelix. *Reprod Biomed Online* 2003;6(4):421–426.

59. Lin YH, Seow KM, Chen HJ, *et al*. Effect of cetrorelix dose on premature LH surge during ovarian stimulation. *Reprod Biomed Online* 2008;16(6):772–777.

60. Messinis IE, Templeton A. Effect of high dose exogenous oestrogen on midcycle luteinizing hormone surge in human spontaneous cycles. *Clin Endocrinol (Oxf)* 1987;27(4):453–459.

61. Glasier A, Thatcher SS, Wickings EJ, Hillier SG, Baird DT. Superovulation with exogenous gonadotropins does not inhibit the luteinizing hormone surge. *Fertil Steril* 1988;49(1):81–85.

62. Messinis IE, Templeton A, Baird DT. Endogenous luteinizing hormone surge during superovulation induction with sequential use of clomiphene citrate and pulsatile human menopausal gonadotropin. *J Clin Endocrinol Metab* 1985;61 (6):1076–1080.

63. Kolibianakis EM, Bourgain C, Papanikolaou EG, *et al*. Prolongation of follicular phase by delaying hCG administration results in a higher incidence of endometrial advancement on the day of oocyte retrieval in GnRH antagonist cycles. *Hum Reprod* 2005;20(9):2453–2456.

64. Aboulghar MA, Mansour RT, Amin YM, *et al*. A prospective randomized study comparing coasting with GnRH antagonist administration in patients at risk for severe OHSS. *Reprod Biomed Online* 2007;15(3):271–279.

65. Lainas TG, Sfontouris IA, Zorzovilis IZ, *et al*. Management of severe OHSS using GnRH antagonist and blastocyst cryopreservation in PCOS patients treated with long protocol. *Reprod Biomed Online* 2009;18(1):15–20.

66. Bonilla-Musoles FM, Raga F, Castillo JC, *et al*. High doses of GnRH antagonists are efficient in the management of severe ovarian hyperstimulation syndrome. *Clin Exp Obstet Gynecol* 2009;36(2):78–81.

67. Wang R, Lin S, Wang Y, Qian W, Zhou L. Comparisons of GnRH antagonist protocol versus GnRH agonist long protocol in patients with normal ovarian reserve: a systematic review and meta-analysis. *PLoS One* 2017;12(4):e0175985.

68. Demirol A, Gurgan T. Comparison of microdose flare-up and antagonist multiple-dose protocols for poor-responder patients: a randomized study. *Fertil Steril* 2009;92(2):481–485.

69. Toftager M, Sylvest R, Schmidt L, *et al*. Quality of life and psychosocial and physical well-being among 1,023 women during their first assisted reproductive technology treatment: secondary outcome to a randomized controlled trial comparing gonadotropin-releasing hormone (GnRH) antagonist and GnRH agonist protocols. *Fertil Steril* 2018;109(1):154–164.

70. Devroey P, Aboulghar M, Garcia-Velasco J, *et al*. Improving the patient's experience of IVF/ICSI: a proposal for an ovarian stimulation protocol with GnRH antagonist co-treatment. *Hum Reprod* 2009;24(4):764–774.

71. Fauser BC, Devroey P, Yen SS, *et al*. Minimal ovarian stimulation for IVF: appraisal of potential benefits and drawbacks. *Hum Reprod* 1999;14:2681–2686.

72. Ledger WL. Favourable outcomes from "mild" in-vitro fertilization. *Lancet* 2007;369:717–718.

73. Nargund G, Fauser BC, Macklon NS, *et al*. The ISMAAR proposal on terminology for ovarian stimulation for IVF. *Hum Reprod* 2007;22:2801–2804.

74. Lambalk CB, Leader A, Olivennes F, *et al*. Treatment with the GnRH antagonist ganirelix prevents premature LH rises and luteinization in stimulated intrauterine insemination: results of a double-blind, placebo-controlled, multicentre trial. *Hum Reprod* 2006;21(3):632–639.

75. Qublan HS, Amarin Z, Tahat YA, Smadi AZ, Kilani M. Ovarian cyst formation following GnRH agonist administration in IVF cycles: incidence and impact. *Hum Reprod* 2006;21:640–644.

76. Al-Inany H, Aboulghar M. GnRH antagonist in assisted reproduction: a Cochrane review. *Hum Reprod* 2002;17(4):874–885.

Chapter

8

Gonadotropins in Ovarian Stimulation

Madelon van Wely and Monique Mochtar

Introduction

Follicle-stimulating hormone (FSH)-containing gonadotropin preparations have been commercially available since the 1960s. Their first use was in ovulation induction in women with anovulatory disorders. Since 1978, however, after the first in vitro fertilization (IVF) baby was born, they have been used increasingly in assisted reproductive technologies (ART) such as IVF or intracytoplasmic sperm injection (ICSI) but also in intrauterine insemination (IUI) as ovarian stimulation to achieve multifollicular growth. Now, in many countries, ovulation induction stimulation comprises only 10% of gonadotropin usage, while 90% is used for ovarian (hyper) stimulation in ART, of which about half of the gonadotropin usage is for IVF and the other half is used for stimulated IUI cycles.

In the follicular phase of a normal menstrual cycle, a cohort of 10–20 antral follicles develops. Of this cohort only one follicle obtains dominance over the others and shows continued growth until ovulation takes place. In patients with hypogonadotropic anovulation (WHO type I), the aim of ovulation induction with a FSH-containing gonadotropin is to induce the growth of preferably no more than one dominant follicle – that is, mimicking the natural cycle – in order to prevent multiple pregnancies. In IVF, however, ovarian stimulation with FSH-containing gonadotropins is aimed to achieve the maturation of a much larger part of the antral follicle cohort, achieved by increasing the dosage. These large numbers of dominant follicles are accompanied with high serum estrogen levels, which can lead to a premature endogenous luteinizing hormone (LH) surge. In order to prevent this premature LH surge, pituitary desensitization is accomplished by the co-administration of either a gonadotropin-releasing hormone (GnRH) agonist or antagonist. A large part of the cohort of

follicles can then grow undisturbed until the preovulatory stage and will then be exposed to an exogenous midcycle LH activity, that is, human chorionic gonadotropin (hCG), in order to induce oocyte maturation and ovulation. However, just prior to actual ovulation, these, still unruptured, mature follicles will be punctured guided under transvaginal ultrasound in order to harvest the oocytes contained in the follicles (oocyte retrieval). In the laboratory the mature metaphase II oocytes will be fertilized. After in vitro culture of the zygote for three to five days it is transferred into the uterus, at which time the zygote is developed into embryos at the 8- to 64-cell stage (embryo or morula transfer).

History of Gonadotropins

In 1958 Carl Gemzell extracted gonadotropins from human pituitary glands [1]. From 1958 onwards, human pituitary gonadotropin preparations were successfully used for ovulation induction in the treatment of ovulation disturbances in several centers throughout the world [1;2]. However, it soon became clear that the reservoir of human pituitaries was too limited to cover the constantly growing demand for gonadotropin preparations. Moreover, more than 20 years after its commercial introduction, human pituitary gonadotropin made the headlines when cases of iatrogenic Creutzfeldt–Jakob disease (CJD) were discovered and linked to the use of human pituitary gonadotropin or human pituitary growth hormone – cases of CJD were identified in Australia, in France, and in the UK [3;4].

Human pituitary gonadotropin was followed up by human menopausal gonadotropin (hMG). Already by 1950 the first gonadotropin preparation extracted from the urine of menopausal women had been registered in Italy (a Pergonal formulation by Serono). But only in 1962, 10 years later, did the first report on successful ovulation induction followed by pregnancies in hypogona-dotropic anovulatory women appear [5;6]. Human menopausal gonadotropins consist of a purified preparation of gonadotropins extracted from the urine of postmenopausal women. The generic name is menotropins. Initially menotropins contained large quantities of potentially allergenic urinary proteins and had to be administered intramuscularly. Later on, when the preparations were purified it was possible to administer the compound subcutaneously. Lack of urinary proteins diminishes adverse skin reactions such as local allergy or hypersensitivity [7;8]. Menotropins contain an equal amount of FSH and LH.

Urofollitropins were the next group of gonadotropins. In urofollitropins, or FSH, many of the urinary proteins and the largest part of the LH were shed by using affinity processes. Consequently urofollitropins have low LH activity of less than 1 percent [9]. Still these urinary FSH (uFSH) preparations are contaminated with 95 percent non-gonadotropin-related proteins. Subsequently, highly purified uFSH preparations (highly purified urofollitropin or FSH-HP), containing less than 0.1 percent LH and virtually no contaminating urinary proteins, became available in the mid 1990s. These preparations were a result of applying immunochromatography with monoclonal antibodies against FSH.

One cycle of treatment with gonadotropins requires 20–30 liters of urine [10] and the demand for gonadotropins substantially increased over the years. In the early 1990s, this worldwide demand increased 100-fold. Meanwhile, the World Health Organization had announced the desirability of an international standard for quality control, and an International Unit for consistency was defined [11].

The advances in molecular technology enabled the production of recombinant FSH (rFSH) in 1992. Recombinant FSH is traditionally produced by transfecting a hamster cell line and has the advantage that it is homogeneous and free of contamination by proteins. The fear for infections, like with Creutzfeldt–Jakob, was a strong motivation to switch to rFSH [12–14], although no infectivity from the urine of humans has ever been detected in four decades of use. Theoretically, rFSH also bears a risk of introducing viruses into humans, although again this has never been described.

To date two recombinant preparations are available – follitropin alpha and follitropin beta.

Soon after the development of rFSH, recombinant DNA technology was used to develop a recombinant LH (rLH), on which the first clinical report was published in 1994 [15]. Most clinicians had switched to using recombinant products, when in 2000 a urinary-derived product reentered the market – highly purified hMG (HP-hMG or highly purified menotropin). HP-hMG contains an equal amount of FSH and LH activity, where the LH activity consists of added hCG.

A promising development is oral administration of gonadotropins, though no such product has entered the markets yet. The latest development is the development of follitropin epsilon, a rFSH variant produced by a human cell expression system (GlycoExpress), instead of a hamster cell line. Early development studies suggest follitropin epsilon might become a good alternative to follitropin alpha and beta [16].

Today the fertility doctor can choose from a wide spectrum of commercially available gonadotropin preparations that contain FSH alone or a combination of FSH and LH activity (i.e., presence of LH or hCG). All these products are recombinants or of purified urinary origin and can be administered subcutaneously. In the next section we go further into the difference between the FSH, LH, and hCG molecules.

Gonadotropin Molecules

The FSH Molecule and Its Isoforms

Follicle-stimulating hormone is composed of two non-covalently linked polypeptide chains, an α- and a β-subunit. Non-covalent means here that the α- and β-subunits are bound without any disulfide bridge linking them. Each subunit possesses two glycosylation sites to which oligosaccharides are normally attached. The α-subunit of FSH (14 000 daltons) contains 92 amino acids, and is similar in structure to the α-subunit of LH, thyroid-stimulating hormone (TSH), and hCG. The β-subunit is composed of 111 amino acids and different carbohydrates and provides the specific biological activity, again similar to the β-subunits of LH, TSH, and hCG.

The oligosaccharides on FSH are highly variable and the composition and complexity of the attached carbohydrate parts may differ. Each oligosaccharide may show single-branched, di-, tri-, and even tetra-branched structures, and each branch of the oligosaccharides may or may not terminate in a negatively charged sialic acid residue allowing FSH to exist as a number of isoforms, varying in acidity [17]. Consequently, there is not one single FSH protein but there are several isoforms of FSH. In humans 20 different FSH isoforms have been identified.

The more acidic isoforms contain a high number of sialic acid residues reflecting a more complex branching pattern, whereas less acidic isoforms have fewer sialic acid residues often reflecting lack of branching of the carbohydrates parts of the molecule [18–21]. The difference in acidity can be used to separate isoforms of FSH according to their electric charge. It has been shown that the isoelectric point can range from 3.5 to 7.0, where low isoelectric points represent more acidity [22].

Studies suggest that the more acidic isoforms possess a reduced in vitro bioactivity compared with the less acidic isoforms [23–25]. The amount of acidic FSH isoforms (isoelectric point below 4.0) is usually higher in urine-derived preparations compared with the recombinant products, which are more basic (alkaline) [26].

The isoform distribution of rFSH, however, resembles uFSH more closely than highly purified uFSH [26]. Taken together, the specific FSH isoform mixture may induce different and divergent biological effects [27;28].

The LH and HCG Molecules

As mentioned, the α-subunit of LH and hCG is identical to the α-subunit of FSH and again, as in FSH, the α- and β-subunits of LH and hCG are non-covalently bound. The difference between the three gonadotropins is determined by the β-subunit. The β-subunit of LH consists of 121 amino acids that confer its specific biological action and are responsible for the specificity of the LH receptor.

The β-subunit of hCG consists of 145 amino acids, 24 more than that of LH; however, a significant sequence is completely homologous to the β-subunit of LH. The two hormones differ in the composition of their carbohydrate moieties, which affects the bioactivity of the specific hormone and speed of degradation. Compared with the biological half-life of LH (20 minutes), hCG degrades much more slowly (24 hours). The half-life of FSH is 3–4 hours.

Gonadotropins and Their Effectiveness in IVF

In the natural cycle both FSH and LH are required for normal follicular growth and maturation. It is clear that in hypogonadotropic women, exogenous FSH and LH are necessary to stimulate follicle growth in IVF. The role of exogenous LH activity in the standard IVF population, however, is not so clear. Since it was suggested in the late 1980s that too high a concentration of LH might have a negative effect on fertilization and embryo quality, the idea arose that pure FSH preparations might be superior to hMG preparations. This hypothesis was tested in several clinical trials comparing uFSH with hMG with respect to pregnancy rates per IVF treatment cycle. Statistical significance was not reached in any of these individual studies. Subsequently, systematic reviews and meta-analyses were performed to combine the available data. A systematic review is a scientific tool that can be used to appraise, summarize, and communicate the results and implications of otherwise unmanageable quantities of research. In this way, healthcare providers can evaluate existing or new technologies and practices efficiently and consider the totality of available evidence. Systematic reviews are of particular value in bringing together a number of separately conducted studies, sometimes with conflicting findings, and synthesizing their results. Systematic reviews may or may not include a statistical synthesis called meta-analysis, depending on whether the studies are similar enough (testing for heterogeneity) so that combining their results is meaningful [29].

As mentioned, the data of the trials that compared uFSH and hMG have been pooled in several systematic reviews and meta-analyses. The first one suggested a difference in favor of uFSH [30]; the second one, however, including more trials and thus providing more evidence, no longer found a difference in pregnancy rates between these two products [31]. Be aware: the quality of a systematic review is as good as the quality of the included studies.

Recombinant preparations have batch-to-batch consistency, are free from urinary protein contaminants, and have the potential to be produced in limitless quantities. This seems advantageous; however, the question remains whether rFSH also leads to more live births per IVF cycle compared with urinary gonadotropins. Many randomized controlled trials have addressed this question, none of which reached statistical significance.

To combine all available evidence a Cochrane review was published on the effectiveness of rFSH with the three main types of urinary-derived gonadotropins (i.e., hMG, HP-hMG, FSH-P, and FSH-HP) for ovarian stimulation in women undergoing IVF or ICSI treatment cycles [32]. We included 41 randomized trials involving 9 472 couples. Overall, this review found no evidence of a difference in pregnancy outcomes when rFSH was compared with urinary-derived gonadotropins as a whole. The analysis ruled out a clinically relevant difference in live birth when comparing rFSH with FSH-P or with FSH-HP. Comparing rFSH with only hMG/HP-hMG resulted in a slightly lower live birth rate in the rFSH group. All studies overlapped in confidence boundary and as a result the inconsistency measure I^2 was 0% and we considered the evidence of moderate quality.

In a recent update focusing on dose used, there were no indications for a difference in live birth rate between rFSH and HP-FSH (12 trials, 2458 couples, relative risk [RR] 1.03, 95% confidence intervals [CI] 0.90–1.18, I^2 = 0%). Live birth rate was slightly lower with rFSH compared with HP-hMG (7 trials, 3393 couples, RR 0.88, 95% CI 0.78–0.99, I^2 = 0%). On the other hand no clinically relevant difference was observed for cumulative live birth including cryocycles. Besides the small differences in pregnancy outcomes, the difference in the required amount to reach a live birth in IVF/ICSI cycles was also small [33].

The main difference between the two compounds rFSH and HP-hMG is the presence of LH or LH-like ingredients. The question arose whether the lower pregnancy rates in the rFSH group were caused by a lack of LH activity in rFSH. We compared in a Cochrane review co-administration of rLH and rFSH versus rFSH alone for controlled ovarian hyperstimulation in downregulated IVF or ICSI cycles [34]. We included 36 trials (8128 women) that used a GnRH agonist for downregulation and 3 trials that used a GnRH antagonist. We found that the use of rLH combined with rFSH probably improves ongoing pregnancy rates, compared

with rFSH alone (19 trials, 3129 couples, RR 1.15, 95% CI 1.01–1.31; I^2 = 2%, moderate-quality evidence). There was however insufficient evidence for a difference in live birth rate. In view of the limited evidence in favor of co-administration of rLH and the associated extra costs, we considered there is no indication to start co-administration of rLH for IVF/ICSI cycles.

Gonadotropins and Their Adverse Effects in IVF

The main risk associated with the use of FSH-containing gonadotropin products is the development of ovarian hyperstimulation syndrome (OHSS). This is a serious condition characterized by increased vascular permeability and liquid accumulation in the peritoneal, pleural, and pericardial cavities, which occurs in 1 to 2 percent of cases. We found no evidence of a difference in OHSS for any of the gonadotropin comparisons [32]. OHSS can be easily prevented by starting with a relatively low dose of gonadotropin, especially in high-risk women such as young patients, those with polycystic ovary syndrome, and those with a low body mass index. A Cochrane review on individualized gonadotropin dosing found a low dose prevents OHSS in predicted high responders [35]. Current evidence does not suggest higher success rates when increasing the standard dose of 150 IU in the case of either poor or normal responders [35].

Summary

At present the fertility doctor can choose from a wide spectrum of commercially available gonadotropin preparations. The preparations that are mostly being used are HP-hMG, HP-FSH, and rFSH. The combination of rFSH plus rLH is usually only applied in trial settings.

In this chapter the different gonadotropin molecules were discussed. It was explained that there is not one single FSH protein but that there are several isoforms of FSH. In humans 20 different FSH isoforms have been identified, and it has been shown that in vitro the biopotency of these isoforms differs. Furthermore, gonadotropin preparations differ in purity and in the presence of LH activity. All these differences could be expected to have an impact on the main outcome of IVF and ICSI, that is, an ongoing pregnancy or live birth.

From the many randomized trials that have been performed it appears that all available gonadotropins are comparably effective and safe. The differences in isoform profile did not appear to have significant clinically significant effects in IVF or ICSI cycles. There appears to be some advantage of HP-hMG in terms of live birth, and addition of rLH may be beneficial in certain groups of women. However, differences were small.

The choice for one or the other product will depend upon the availability of the product, the convenience of its use, and the associated costs.

References

1. Gemzell CA, Diczfalusy E, Tillinger G. Clinical effect of human pituitary follicle-stimulating hormone (FSH). *J Clin Endocrinol Metab* 1958;**18**:1333–1348.

2. Bettendorf S. Human hypophyseal gonadotropin in hypophysectomized women. *Int J Fertil* 1963;**45**:799–809.

3. Cochius JI, Mack K, Burns RJ. Creutzfeld–Jakob disease in a recipient human pituitary derived gonadotrophin. *Aust N Z J Med* 1990;**20**:592–596.

4. Dumble LD, Klein RD. Creutzfeld-Jakob disease legacy for Australian women treated with human pituitary gonadotropins. *Lancet* 1992;**330**:848.

5. Lunenfeld B, Menzi A, Insler V. Effeti clinicci della gonadotropina umana della post-menopausa. *Rass Clin Terap* 1960;**59**:213–216.

6. Lunenfeld B. Treatment of anovulation by human gonadotrophins. *J Int Fedn Gynecol Obstet* 1963;**1**:153.

7. Biffoni M, Battaglia A, Borrelli F, *et al.* Allergenic potential of gonadotrophic preparations in experimental animals: relevance of purity. *Hum Reprod* 1994;**9**:1845–1848.

8. Biffoni M, Marcucci I, Ythier A, Eshkol A. Effects of urinary gonadotrophin preparations on human in-vitro immune function. *Hum Reprod* 1998;**13**:2430–2434.

9. Lunenfeld B, Eshkol A. Immunology of follicle stimulating hormone and luteinizing hormone. *Vitam Horm* 1970;**27**:131–159.

10. Balen AH, Hayden CJ, Rutherford AJ. What are the clinical benefits of recombinant gonadotrophins? Clinical efficacy of recombinant gonadotrophins. *Hum Reprod* 1999;**14**:1411–1417.

11. World Health Organization. Agents stimulating gonadal function in human. Report of a WHO scientific group. World Health Organization Tech Rep Ser 514. Geneva: World Health Organization; 1973.

12. Reichl H, Balen A, Jansen CA. Prion transmission in blood and urine: what are the implications for recombinant and urinary-derived gonadotrophins? *Hum Reprod* 2002;**17**:2501–2508.

13. Serban A, Legname G, Hansen K, Kovaleva N, Prusiner SB. Immunoglobulins in urine of hamsters with scrapie. *J Biol Chem* 2004;**279**:48817–48820.

14. Shaked GM, Shaked Y, Kariv-Inbal Z, *et al.* A protease-resistant prion protein isoform is present in urine of animals and humans affected with prion diseases. *J Biol Chem* 2001;**276**:31479–31482.

15. Hull M, Corrigan E, Piazzi A, Loumaye E. Recombinant human luteinising hormone: an effective new gonadotropin preparation. *Lancet* 1994;**344**:334–335.

16. Abd-Elaziz K, Duijkers I, Stöckl L, *et al.* A new fully human recombinant FSH (follitropin epsilon): two phase I randomized placebo and comparator-controlled pharmacokinetic and pharmacodynamic trials. *Hum Reprod* 2017;**32** (8):1639–1647.

17. Hård K, Mekking A, Damm JB, *et al.* Isolation and structure determination of the intact sialylated N-linked carbohydrate chains of recombinant human follitropin expressed in Chinese hamster ovary cells. *Eur J Biochem* 1990;**193**:263–271.

18. Creus S, Chaia Z, Pellizzari EH, *et al.* Human FSH isoforms: carbohydrate complexity as determinant of in-vitro bioactivity. *Mol Cell Endocrinol* 2001;**174**:41–49.

19. Timossi CM, Barrios-de-Tomasi J, González-Suárez R, *et al.* Differential effects of the charge variants of human follicle-stimulating hormone. *J Endocrinol* 2000;**165**:193–205.

20. Ulloa-Aguirre A, Timossi C. Biochemical and functional aspects of gonadotrophin-releasing hormone and gonadotrophins. *Reprod Biomed Online* 2000;**1**:48–62.

21. Ulloa-Aguirre A, Timossi C, Barrios-de-Tomasi J, Maldonado A, Nayudu P. Impact of carbohydrate heterogeneity in function of follicle-stimulating hormone: studies derived from in vitro and in vivo models. *Biol Reprod* 2003;**69**:379–389.

22. Ulloa-Aguirre A, Zambrano E, Timossi C, *et al.* On the nature of the follicle-stimulating signal delivered to the ovary during exogenously controlled follicular maturation. A search into the immunological and biological attributes and the molecular composition of two preparations of urofollitropin. *Arch Med Res* 1995;**26 Spec No**:S219–S230.

23. Yding Andersen C, Leonardsen L, Ulloa-Aguirre A, *et al.* FSH-induced resumption of meiosis in mouse oocytes: effect of different isoforms. *Mol Hum Reprod* 1999;5:726–731.

24. Yding Andersen CY, Leonardsen L, Ulloa-Aguirre A, *et al.* Effect of different FSH isoforms on cyclic-AMP production by mouse cumulus-oocyte-complexes: a time course study. *Mol Hum Reprod* 2001;7:129–135.

25. Yding Andersen C. Effect of FSH and its different isoforms on maturation of oocytes from pre-ovulatory follicles. *Reprod Biomed Online* 2002;5:232–239.

26. Lambert A, Rodgers M, Mitchell R, *et al.* In-vitro biopotency and glycoform distribution of recombinant human follicle stimulating hormone (Org 32489), Metrodin and Metrodin-HP *Hum Reprod* 1995;10:1928–1935.

27. Andersen CY, Westergaard LG, van Wely M. FSH isoform composition of commercial gonadotrophin preparations: a neglected aspect? *Reprod Biomed Online* 2004;9:231–236.

28. Dias JA, Ulloa-Aguirre A. New human follitropin preparations: how glycan structural differences may affect biochemical and biological function and clinical effect. *Front Endocrinol (Lausanne)* 2021;12:636038. doi: 10.3389/fendo.2021.636038.

29. Deeks JJ, Higgins JPT, Altman DG (eds.). Chapter 10: Analysing data and undertaking meta-analyses. In: Higgins JPT, Thomas J, Chandler J, *et al.*, eds. *Cochrane Handbook for Systematic Reviews of Interventions*, version 6.2 (updated February 2021). Cochrane; 2021.

30. Daya S, Gunby J, Hughes EG, Collins JA, Sagle MA. Follicle-stimulating hormone versus human menopausal gonadotropin for in vitro fertilization cycles: a meta-analysis. *Fertil Steril* 1995;64:347–354.

31. Agrawal R, Holmes J, Jacobs HS. Follicle-stimulating hormone or human menopausal gonadotropin for ovarian stimulation in in vitro fertilization cycles: a meta-analysis. *Fertil Steril* 2000;73:338–343.

32. van Wely M, Kwan I, van der Veen F, *et al.* Recombinant FSH versus urinary gonadotrophins for ovarian hyperstimulation in IVF or ICSI cycles. A systematic review and meta-analysis. *Hum Reprod* 2009;24:S1, i134.

33. Bordewijk EM, Mol F, van der Veen F, van Wely M. Required amount of rFSH, HP-hMG and HP-FSH to reach a live birth. A systematic review and meta-analysis. *Hum Reprod Open* 2019; **2019** (3): hoz008. https://doi.org/10.1093/hropen/hoz008.

34. Mochtar MH, Danhof NA, Ayeleke RO, Van der Veen F, van Wely M. Recombinant luteinizing hormone (rLH) and recombinant follicle stimulating hormone (rFSH) for ovarian stimulation in IVF/ ICSI cycles. *Cochrane Database Syst Rev* 2017;5: CD005070.

35. Lensen SF, Wilkinson J, Leijdekkers JA, *et al.* Individualised gonadotropin dose selection using markers of ovarian reserve for women undergoing in vitro fertilisation plus intracytoplasmic sperm injection (IVF/ICSI). *Cochrane Database Syst Rev* 2018;2:CD012693.

Egg Donation: Implications for Counseling Donor and Recipient, Donor Preparation, and Recipient Preparation

Ernesto Bosch and Pilar Alama

Introduction

Oocyte donation (OD) is defined as the assisted reproduction technique (ART) in which a different woman than the one that will receive the resulting embryo provides the female gamete. Its diffusion has grown progressively due to both its excellent results and the increase of its indications [1]. According to the last European registers by the European Society of Human Reproduction and Embryology (ESHRE) in 2011, about half of the cycles of OD reported had been performed in Spain [2].

Spanish Assisted Reproduction Law is based on legislation that was passed in November 1988 (Law 35/1988). Although some countries already had regulations or recommendations for ART at that time, Spain was the first country to create a specific law to cover this area of medicine. Royal Decree 412/1996 and Ministerial Order of 25 March 1996 establish donor requirements, as well as mandatory standard screening procedures, to rule out the transmission of genetic, hereditary, or infectious diseases. In 2006, a new Spanish Law on Assisted Reproduction was approved (Law 14/2006), which determined requirements for gamete and embryo use, and regulations on financial compensation. These are the most important topics included in Spanish Law on Egg Donation:

- Donation of human gametes is a formal confidential contract between the donor and the reproductive medicine center
- Identity of donors must remain anonymous
- The maximum number of children generated from a single donor's gametes should not exceed six in Spain
- It is the responsibility of the institution to match donors and recipients as much as possible, according to blood groups, phenotype, and physical characteristics in general

Implications for Counseling Donor and Recipient

Counseling Donors

To be accepted as an oocyte donor, women must be aged between 18 and 35 years old and be healthy. The following steps are necessary to be admitted as an oocyte donor in our centers:

- *Medical history*: During the first visit, an interview is conducted to complete the familiar and personal history. In it, the potential donor is informed in detail of the steps of the procedure, as well as the possibility, prevention, incidence, management, and consequences of complications, with special reference to ovarian hyperstimulation syndrome (OHSS).

- *Psychological screening*: Psychological evaluation and counseling is carried out by a qualified mental health professional. The donor will be asked to speak with a psychologist to ensure that she fully understands the benefits and risks of OD, and is properly motivated to become a donor.

- *Gynecological examination*: The donor's menstrual cycles are evaluated and a vaginal ultrasound is performed to examine ovaries, to count antral follicles, and to ensure there is no pathology in her ovaries. At the same time, body mass index (BMI) is calculated. Women are not accepted as donors if BMI is lower than 18 kg/m^2 or higher than 28 kg/m^2 or if the antral follicle count is less than 10 or higher than 35.

- *Medical screening*: This involves testing for blood type, Rh factor, antibody screening, complete blood count, hemostasis, biochemistry, and infectious disease screening, such as HIV, CHV, and syphilis.

- *Genetic screening*: Blood tests for karyotype and for carrier screening tests for severe recessive and X-linked childhood diseases based on next-generation sequencing (NGS; 549 genes implicated in 623 disease phenotypes) are performed. All donors with abnormal karyotype or who are carriers of X-linked diseases will be excluded from our Oocyte Donation Program. This aspect will be discussed further in the section Counseling for Genetic Matching.

Donor Management

Before starting the OD cycle, an oral contraceptive pill (OCP) is administered for a maximum of 21 days, starting on day 1 or 2 of the menses of the previous cycle. Nevertheless, most donors are usually taking OCP for birth control. After a five-day wash-out period from taking the last pill, donors start their stimulation protocol with follicle-stimulating hormone (FSH), highly purified human menopausal gonadotropin (HP-hMG), or FSH plus HP-hMG. The medication is self-administered. There are no differences in term of results according to the type of gonadotropin used [3].

The gonadotropin doses for the stimulation depend on the age of the donor, the antral follicle count, BMI, and the background of the donor in previous ovarian stimulation cycles.

Oocyte donors are monitored regularly across the stimulation to determine follicle growth and to ensure it is within an appropriate healthy range. Centers use vaginal ultrasound and blood tests to monitor follicle growth. Daily doses of 0.25 mg gonadotropin-releasing hormone (GnRH) antagonist (ganirelix or cetrorelix) start when the biggest follicle reaches 14 mm in mean diameter. Once there are three follicles larger than 17.5 mm or one of them is greater than 20.5 mm, oocyte pickup is scheduled. To trigger final oocyte maturation, 0.2 mg of GnRH agonist is administered in all cases. The cycle is canceled if expected oocyte yield is below eight.

Transvaginal oocyte retrieval takes place 36 hours after triggering. Donors receive light IV sedation for the retrieval procedure to ensure their comfort, and they rest for 2 hours at the clinic before they are discharged. In some cases, a post-retrieval vaginal scan is scheduled two to three days following egg retrieval.

One of the controversies regarding ovarian stimulation for in vitro fertilization (IVF) regards the impact that successive cycles could have on oocyte recovery in terms of quality and quantity of the obtained oocytes. In this sense, our group evaluated the effect of successive ovarian stimulation cycles in oocyte donors on the number of obtained oocytes, fertilization rate, embryo development, and implantation and pregnancy rates [4]. No significant differences were observed in any of these variables, depending on the ordinal cycle evaluated [4].

Counseling Recipients

Oocyte recipients enter our egg donation program for one of the following main diagnoses: advanced age (more than 40 years), low response during IVF, premature ovarian insufficiency, failure to achieve pregnancy after at least three cycles of ART, endometriosis, poor oocyte quality, natural menopause, genetic or chromosomal disorders (Turner's syndrome, etc.), unexplained recurrent miscarriage, surgical menopause, and mixed causes [5]. Figure 9.1 shows the main indication of OD in our center during 2015.

Before treatment begins, the recipient undergoes preliminary testing. This assessment phase includes infectious disease screening (e.g., HIV, CHV, syphilis) and blood type, and Rh factor for both parents. In women older than 45 years old, a recent mammogram, full blood count, coagulation tests, and blood biochemistry may also be required.

To help the donor team select an oocyte donor for matching, recipients will be asked to complete a list with their physical characteristics, such as hair color, weight and height, and eye color. The recipients are offered the opportunity to receive emotional support by the psychologist of our Unit. Among all ART procedures, gamete donation and especially OD are usually those with more psychological implications. Counseling regarding the degree of motherhood and disclosure to the children is usually provided under request.

Oocyte Recipient Management

The vast majority of oocyte recipients undergo hormone replacement therapy (HRT).

- In patients with ovarian function, a depot GnRH agonist is administered in the midluteal

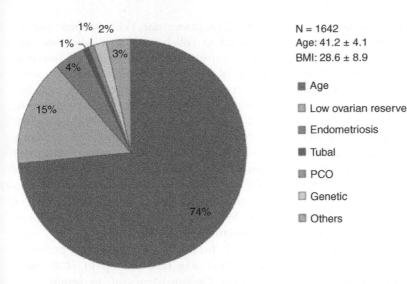

N = 1642
Age: 41.2 ± 4.1
BMI: 28.6 ± 8.9

Figure 9.1 Main indication of oocyte donation in IVI Valencia in 2015. PCO = polycystic ovary.

■ Age

▤ Low ovarian reserve

▨ Endometriosis

▧ Tubal

▦ PCO

▢ Genetic

▨ Others

phase of their cycle, or a GnRH antagonist is administered daily with menstruation for five days. This allows for pituitary suppression, which avoids spontaneous ovulations during the endometrial preparation.

- Recipients without ovarian function are submitted to the same endometrial preparation protocol, but do not undergo pituitary suppression.

When exogenously administered, estrogens are supplied either orally or transdermally from day 1 to day 3 of the menstrual cycle in which the embryo transfer will be performed; estrogens can be administered either in an increasing dose (regularly 2 to 6 mg/day of valerianate of estradiol [EV]) or a constant dose from the beginning of the menstrual cycle (6 mg/day).

On day 15 or day 16 of HRT, a transvaginal ultrasound is performed to measure endometrial thickness, and serum estradiol and progesterone levels are tested. Most recipients are ready to receive embryos within two weeks after starting HRT, although administration of EV can be maintained if needed for a maximum of 49 days, until a suitable donation becomes available, without affecting cycle outcome [6]. In case of vaginal spotting or bleeding in the recipient during HRT administration, the cycle is canceled.

Micronized progesterone (800 mg/day, vaginally) is initiated on the day of OD. Embryo transfers are always performed under ultrasound guidance at the blastocyst stage. The regimen of

HRT is maintained until 12 days after embryo transfer. If pregnancy is achieved, it is continued with the same dose until 12 weeks of pregnancy.

Counseling for Genetic Matching

Population-based carrier screening for single-gene disorders has been proposed since the 1960s. In the last two decades close to 1150 recessive genes that cause Mendelian diseases have been identified (www.ncbi.nlm.nih.gov/omim). Although rare individually, in developed countries these diseases collectively account for 20 percent of infant mortality and approximately 10 percent of pediatric hospitalizations [7]. Now, the advent of high-throughput NGS makes a comprehensive preconception screening panel more feasible, allowing for the possibility of affordable testing for a wide range of conditions that a family history will never detect. Taking advantage of this technology, we have created a preconception carrier genetic screening test (CGT) for severe recessive and X-linked childhood diseases. Its use allows for a blind-matching program between donors and recipients that avoids both ethical issues and the unnecessary discarding of donors beyond those that carry an X-linked pathogenic variant [8].

Our initial experience has been recently reported [8]. The analyses comprised 1170 gamete donors (926 females [79%] and 244 males [21%]), corresponding to 45.5% of the tests performed. Another 1400 patients (54.5%) were screened, of whom 1124 (80.3%) were the partners of the patients receiving gametes. Gamete donors who tested microbiologically negative were subjected simultaneously to karyotype analysis and fragile X (females only) investigation, resulting in an abnormal karyotype in 6 percent of them, who were then rejected as donors. The rest underwent CGT, starting with fragile X. Eighteen female donors were additionally excluded from the program because they carried a pathogenic or likely pathogenic variant in an X chromosome gene, representing 1.94 percent of the total tests requested.

They received information on the adverse finding, including genetic counseling and discouragement from entering the donation program. The remaining donors (1162 of 1170 initially screened) were included in a blind-matching, computerized controlled database. By request, the match system always displayed a set of donors genetically compatible with the patient requesting gamete donation.

Counseling for Embryo Transfer

Some authors have suggested that elective single embryo transfer (eSET) should be the gold standard in OD as the cumulative pregnancy rate achieved after transferring fresh or cryopreserved embryos is similar between single and double embryo transfers (DET), but with the obvious reduction in the twin pregnancy rate [9] and, therefore, a lower risk of obstetric and perinatal complications. However, widespread eSET utilization is still a matter of debate because, nowadays, the pregnancy rate after one single procedure diminishes significantly when eSET is performed, compared with DET [10]. While twin pregnancies are generally considered an adverse effect of IVF procedures, it is obvious that a negative pregnancy test is also undesirable. Furthermore, the reasons that patients usually argue when requesting DET, such as their age, impact of previous failed procedures and, in particular, the economical and psychological cost of making more attempts to achieve success, are present more in daily OD practice. Given this context, the real challenge is to avoid, or at least to significantly reduce, occurrence of twin pregnancies without compromising the overall pregnancy rate.

In order to significantly lower the twin pregnancy rate in donor oocyte cycles without affecting

the overall pregnancy rate, IVI developed a predictive model in collaboration with the Valencian (Spain) company Veratech. This model allows estimations of the probability of pregnancy when transferring a single embryo, the probability of pregnancy when transferring two embryos, and the probability of twin pregnancy when transferring two embryos and accomplishing pregnancy. The multiple pregnancy risk was obtained by constructing a logistic regression model. A total of 3189 cycles in which two embryos were transferred were included; of those, 2392 were randomly selected and used to construct the model, while 797 were employed for internal validation purposes. This process was repeated up to 1000 times to increase the consistency of the results.

The twin pregnancy rate in our population included in the analysis was 42.7%, with a 15–80% range. In 81.8% of cases, the probability of a twin pregnancy was between 30% and 50%. Only 1.3% of the cycles gave a probability below 30%, and probability was equal to or over 50% in 16.8% of the cases (Figure 9.2).

The variables that were closely associated with the multiple pregnancy risk were day of transfer and embryo cohort quality, defined as the number of embryos with 8 cells on day 3. The number of patient's cycle and endometrial preparation treatment duration related inversely with the twin pregnancy risk.

The resulting AUC-ROC was 0.59 (0.56–0.62) and the accuracy rate was 0.59 (0.57–0.60). In accordance with these data, if all the patients with an estimated twin pregnancy risk that

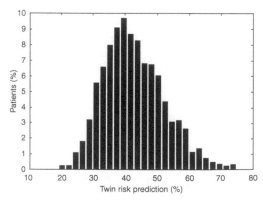

Figure 9.2 Distribution of the twin pregnancy probability estimation for all patients having double embryo transfer.

exceeded 40% had a single embryo transferred, the twin pregnancy rate would lower by half. If this measure was applied to a risk over 35%, the risk of twins would reduce by two-thirds. If it was applied to a risk over 30%, two embryos would be transferred in only 7% of the cycles, which would lead to the practical elimination of twin pregnancies.

Since this predictive model has been applied, a highly significant reduction in the twin rate has been achieved in our donor oocyte program, which currently lies at about 15–20%. If its use continues, user trust (both doctors and patients) will grow, and it will lead to a progressive reduction in twin pregnancy rates without lowering pregnancy rates.

Oocyte Donation Synchronization

We consider many different factors during donor selection such as race, reproductive history, physical characteristics of the woman and her partner, blood type, and genetic carrier screening. We call matching the time when we select a donor for a recipient after taking into account all the above-mentioned factors.

The time at which the donor and recipients are matched has changed in the last six years thanks to the improvement in the oocyte vitrification technique and the creation of an Egg Donor Bank. However, it is important to note that in our current practice, we conduct donations both with fresh and vitrified oocytes depending on different circumstances related to the availability of oocytes and the needs of the recipient.

Before introducing vitrification, the number of donors and recipients in the clinic determined the time of matching: if there were many donors, the matching was done the day of the donor's pickup. This means that sometimes recipients were on the waiting list for so many days that they may bleed. If, however, the clinic eventually had very few donors needed for special features, then donors and recipients were synchronized. This means that recipients and donors start with ovarian stimulation (donors) and HRT (recipients) at the same time. The limitation of this situation is that in case of an issue with the donor's stimulation (cancellations, fewer oocytes than expected) the recipient's cycle had to be canceled, and the donation time was only indicative and could

not be officially scheduled. The likelihood for this to happen underlines the importance of having a large Egg Donor Bank with the availability of a large and varied number of stored oocytes that meet different characteristics [11].

In addition to this, about 65 percent of our recipients come from foreign countries. So we need to consider compatibility issues from a medical viewpoint and we must take into account the logistics of the process. As our usual medical practice now has an Egg Bank, the time of matching the donor and the recipient depends on different aspects: if recipients need specific characteristics or have a specific date for embryo transfer.

❖ Recipients who need specific characteristics: infrequent blood type (0 negative, AB negative), specific race, screening specific genetic diseases, or partners who would like to have another baby with the same donor as they had before

➤ First, we use our donor selection database and select one donor or two with the required characteristics. Sometimes there will be donors under stimulation with the required characteristics, and sometimes we call them to return to our clinic

➤ Second, all the oocytes obtained during pickup are vitrified for the recipient

➤ Finally, the recipient chooses the best time to schedule embryo transfer, and we provide them with instructions to begin HRT depending on the date of embryo transfer

❖ Recipients who do not need specific characteristics

➤ Recipients who have a date for embryo transfer

• First, we reserve oocytes from our Egg Donor Bank

• Second, the recipient begins HRT depending on embryo transfer date

• Finally, we have two options:

1. We use fresh oocytes when we have a donor pickup scheduled on the same date as the donation (with the same characteristics as the partner). The reservation is canceled in this case

2. We use vitrified oocytes

➤ Recipients who do not have a date for embryo transfer

- The recipient begins with HRT and remains on the waiting list
- If on these dates an egg donor with the same characteristics as the recipient undergoes pickup, we use fresh oocytes for the egg donation
- If the recipient stays on the waiting list longer than 20–25 days, we use oocytes from the Egg Donor Bank

The OD Program is managed given an application, which allows us to know the relevant egg donor data. This application includes number of donors under stimulation, donors with vitrified oocytes, and vitrified oocytes that are located at other IVI clinics. We have developed a matching application for our software in which a list of best possible donors is supplied after the introduction of recipients' characteristics including phenotype, blood type, and other special features.

Optimization of an Oocyte Donation Cycle

The relatively high aneuploidy rate observed in human embryos after an IVF/ICSI cycle has been classically attributed to the technique itself, and assuming that this prevalence might be lower in natural conceptions. Two main hypotheses have been proposed to contribute to these findings: (1) exogenous factors related to the IVF technique, such us controlled ovarian stimulation (COS) treatments or lab conditions; (2) a high ovarian response after using gonadotropins.

This concept relates directly to OD, as donors have a good ovarian reserve that allows modulating the ovarian response by adjusting the doses of gonadotropins.

A positive relationship between ovarian response and the embryo aneuploidy rate has been described when mild COS is performed in infertile patients, but this is not observed in patients who undergo conventional COS treatments with higher doses [12]. It has recently been suggested that a threshold level for gonadotropin doses may exist, and that no more competent oocytes can be obtained if it is exceeded [13]. Conversely, other recent studies have indicated that high ovarian response to gonadotropins is not so detrimental to embryo quality. In fact, it has been shown that high ovarian response to

conventional ovarian stimulation does not increase embryo aneuploidy rates in preimplantation genetic screening by array comparative genomic hybridization [14]. Besides, the larger the number of available euploid blastocysts, the higher the clinical pregnancy rate observed [15].

In order to analyze the number of euploid blastocysts (i.e., viable embryos) that are obtained after a donor ovarian stimulation cycle according to ovarian response, and therefore estimate its reproductive potential, we performed a post hoc analysis of a subset of data generated during a prospective cohort study carried out in our center that was previously reported [16]. Forty-six oocyte donors subjected to ovarian stimulation with 150 IU of recombinant FSH and 75 IU of HP-hMG in a GnRH agonist long protocol were included. Preimplantation genetic screening was performed in all viable embryos. Mean number of euploid embryos per cycle was calculated according to ovarian response and gonadotropin doses.

A positive relationship between ovarian response and the number of euploid embryos was observed (Figure 9.3). When ovarian response was above the median ($\geq$ 17 oocytes), the mean number of euploid embryos per donor was 5.0 ± 2.4, while when < 17 oocytes were obtained the mean number of euploid embryos was 2.7 ± 1.4 ($p = 0.000$). Aneuploidy rate was not related to ovarian response or gonadotropin doses. Cumulative live birth rate, according to being above or below the median of total number of oocytes obtained, was 70.8% versus 50.0% ($p = 0.15$), respectively.

Therefore, according to these data, the number of euploid embryos available for embryo transfer increases as the number of oocytes obtained does. Aneuploidy rate did not increase with ovarian response or gonadotropin doses. Considering the total number of euploid embryos seems more relevant than the aneuploidy rate.

References

1. Remohi J, Gartner B, Gallardo E, *et al.* Pregnancy and birth rates after oocyte donation. *Fertil Steril* 1997;**67**:717–723.

2. The European IVF-Monitoring Consortium (EIM), for the European Society of Human Reproduction and Embryology (ESHRE), Kupka MS, D'Hooghe T, Ferraretti AP, *et al.* Assisted reproductive technology in Europe, 2011: results generated from European registers by ESHRE. *Hum Reprod* 2016;**31**:233–248.

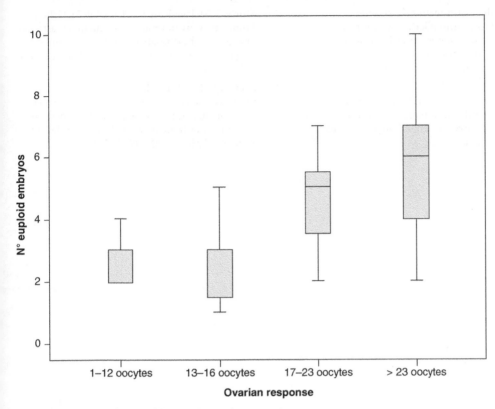

Figure 9.3 Number of euploid blastocysts according to ovarian response.

3. van Wely M, Kwan I, Burt AL, *et al.* Recombinant versus urinary gonadotrophin for ovarian stimulation in assisted reproductive technology cycles. *Cochrane Database Syst Rev* 2011;**2**: CD005354.

4. Caligara C, Navarro J, Vargas G, *et al.* The effect of repeated controlled ovarian stimulation in donors. *Hum Reprod* 2001;**16**:2320–2323.

5. Budak E, Garrido N, Soares SR, *et al.* Improvements achieved in an oocyte donation program over a 10-year period: sequential increase in implantation and pregnancy rates and decrease in high-order multiple pregnancies. *Fertil Steril* 2007;**88**:342–349.

6. Soares SR, Troncoso C, Bosch E, *et al.* Age and uterine receptiveness: predicting the outcome of oocyte donation cycles. *J Clin Endocrinol Metab* 2005;**90**:4399–4404.

7. Kumar P, Radhakrishnan J, Chowdhary MA, Giampietro PF. Prevalence and patterns of presentation of genetic disorders in a pediatric emergency department. *Mayo Clin Proc* 2001;**76**:777–783.

8. Martin J, Asan, Yi Y, *et al.* Comprehensive carrier genetic test using next-generation deoxyribonucleic acid sequencing in infertile couples wishing to conceive through assisted reproductive technology. *Fertil Steril* 2015;**104**:1286–1293.

9. Clua E, Tur R, Coroleu B, *et al.* Elective single-embryo transfer in oocyte donation programmes: should it be the rule? *Reprod Biomed Online* 2012;**25**:642–648.

10. Pandian Z, Marjoribanks J, Ozturk O, Serour G, Bhattacharya S. Number of embryos for transfer following in vitro fertilisation or intra-cytoplasmic sperm injection. *Cochrane Database Syst Rev* 2013;**7**:CD003416.

11. Cobo A, Garrido N, Pellicer A, Remohí J. Six years' experience in ovum donation using vitrified oocytes: report of cumulative outcomes, impact of storage time, and development of a predictive model for oocyte survival rate. *Fertil Steril* 2015;**104**:1426–1434.

12. Baart EB, Martini E, Eijkemans MJ, *et al.* Milder ovarian stimulation for in-vitro fertilization reduces aneuploidy in the human preimplantation embryo: a randomized controlled trial. *Hum Reprod* 2007;**22**:980–988.

13. Arce JC, Andersen AN, Fernández-Sánchez M, *et al.* Ovarian response to recombinant

human follicle-stimulating hormone: a randomized, antimüllerian hormone-stratified, dose-response trial in women undergoing in vitro fertilization/intracytoplasmic sperm injection. *Fertil Steril* 2014;**102**:1633–1640.

14. Ata B, Kaplan B, Danzer H, *et al.* Array CGH analysis shows that aneuploidy is not related to the number of embryos generated. *Reprod Biomed Online* 2012;**24**:614–620.

15. Morin S, Melzer-Ross K, McCulloh D, Grifo J, Munne S. A greater number of euploid blastocysts in a given cohort predicts excellent outcomes in single embryo transfer cycles. *J Assist Reprod Genet* 2014;**31**:667–673.

16. Labarta E, Bosch E, Alamá P, *et al.* Moderate ovarian stimulation does not increase the incidence of human embryo chromosomal abnormalities in in vitro fertilization cycles. *J Clin Endocrinol Metab* 2012;**97**:1987–1994.

Chapter 10

Progestin-Primed Ovarian Stimulation

Xuefeng Lu and Yanping Kuang

Introduction

The reproductive cycle requires complex interactions and feedback between gonadotropin-releasing hormone (GnRH), the gonadotropins follicle-stimulating hormone (FSH) and luteinizing hormone (LH), and the ovarian sex steroid hormones estrogen and progesterone. To improve the success rate of in vitro fertilization-embryo transfer (IVF-ET) by optimizing oocyte retrieval, controlled ovarian stimulation (COS) has been widely performed. Exogenous gonadotropins were used to achieve supraphysiological levels during the follicular phase to override the process of dominant follicle selection and enable multiple follicular recruitment, which lead to a rapidly increasing serum estradiol level and induce a premature LH surge. GnRH agonist (GnRHa) and GnRH antagonist were used to prevent the premature LH surge and premature ovulation [1]. In 2003, based on ultrasonographic studies, Baerwald et al. demonstrated that multiple cohorts or "waves" of 2–5 mm follicles were recruited continuously during a menstrual cycle, including in the luteal phase [2;3]. This finding suggested that follicles developing during the menstrual cycle might have the potential to develop, offering new possibilities for ovarian stimulation. Based on the improvement in the vitrification techniques, luteal phase ovarian stimulation was found feasible for producing competent oocytes in women undergoing IVF, and progesterone was a new regimen for preventing the premature ovulation. These findings made the ovarian stimulation more flexible and the starting of ovarian stimulation could be at follicular phase or luteal phase (Figure 10.1).

Luteal Phase Ovarian Stimulation

The competence of the antral follicles in normal human ovaries during the luteal phase was not distinguishable from antral follicles during the early stage of the follicular phase in terms of the number, size range, and steroidogenic activities [4]. However, in the luteal phase, physiological plasma FSH and LH levels are being held down to a very low level and insufficient to maintain antral follicle development, and follicles undergo atresia. Ovarian stimulation during the luteal phase was originally used for fertility preservation of cancer patients [5–7]. Mature oocytes and embryos were reported to be obtained by COS during the luteal phase. However, all the oocytes and embryos obtained were for cryopreservation and no pregnancy data were available. In 2009, our group reported the first live birth of embryos developed from oocytes retrieved following luteal phase stimulation [8]. A 40-year-old woman with a 10-year history of primary infertility received ovarian stimulation initiating from menstrual cycle day 3 (MC3) with the use of human menopausal gonadotropin (hMG) 150 IU and letrozole 2.5 mg. Her therapy cycle spontaneously transitioned into the luteal phase beginning on MC10 but the follicles continued to develop with hMG and letrozole stimulation. Ovulation was triggered with 0.1 mg triptorelin. Four mature oocytes were obtained and two high-quality embryos developed for vitrified cryopreservation in this IVF treatment cycle. Two months later, the two embryos were transferred in a natural cycle, creating a twin pregnancy and a favorable delivery. Three-year follow-up showed that the physical and psychomotor development of the twin babies were in the normal range of children conceived naturally. This case report documents favorable outcomes of oocyte development competence following luteal phase ovarian stimulation and opens the door to generalize the successful outcome from luteal phase stimulation into a routine setting.

After this study, we attempted to stimulate the luteal phase existing antral follicles in patients

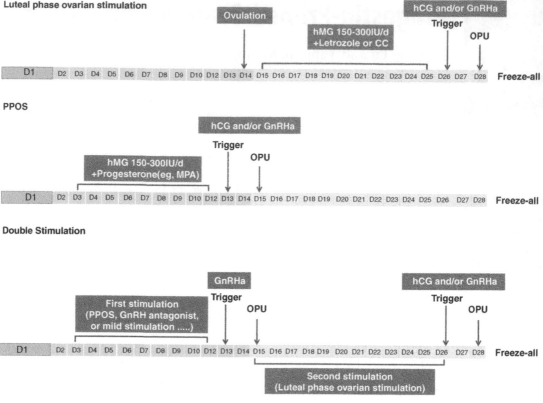

Figure 10.1 Schematic representation of the endogenous and exogenous progesterone-primed ovarian stimulation. CC = clomiphene (clomifene) citrate; hCG = human chorionic gonadotropin; hMG = human menopausal gonadotropin; MPA = medroxyprogesterone acetate; OPU = ovum pickup; PPOS = progestin-primed ovarian stimulation.

with poor ovarian response or with diminished ovarian reserve (DOR). However, we found the antral follicles in the luteal phase were not sensitive to exogenous gonadotropin stimulation compared with ovarian stimulation during the follicular phase, the duration of hMG stimulation was as long as 20.6 days. Actually, in 2013, Buendgen *et al.* had conducted a study on the efficacy of luteal phase ovarian stimulation. They reported that a higher dose of FSH was required as well as a longer duration of ovarian stimulation in cycles initiated in the luteal phase, compared with stimulation started in the follicular phase, and therefore was not feasible for routine use [9]. Then from our previous reported case, we noticed that initiating ovarian stimulation with hMG and letrozole during the luteal phase might lead to a satisfactory ovarian response and pregnancy outcome. To extend the luteal phase stimulation to a routine IVF setting that can be used

independently of menstruation, a prospective controlled cohort study including 242 women with normal ovarian reserve was conducted to explore the efficacy of luteal phase stimulation with hMG and letrozole [10]. All participants succeeded in producing oocytes, and 227 women had high-quality embryos to cryopreserve (93.8%). The average number of oocytes retrieved was 13.1, producing an average of 4.8 good embryos. The mean duration of ovarian stimulation was 10.2 days, with a mean dose of hMG of 2211.3 IU. So adjuvant administration of letrozole in luteal phase ovarian stimulation appeared to increase the sensitivity of follicles to gonadotropins and shorten the duration of ovarian stimulation, but the detailed mechanism should be further investigated. As there was asynchrony between the endometrium and embryos in this study, all developed embryos had to be cryopreserved for frozen embryo transfers (FETs). In FET cycles, the clinical pregnancy rate, ongoing pregnancy rate, and implantation rate were 55.46% (127/229), 48.91% (112/229), and 40.37% (174/431), respectively [10]. Our further study found clomiphene (clomifene) citrate was as effective as letrozole in improving the ovarian response in luteal phase ovarian stimulation [11], that were confirmed by a study from another center [12].

Interestingly, the average serum LH was only 1.9 mIU/ml (range 0.1–11.0 mIU/ml) on the trigger day in these 242 women, and no incidence of premature LH surge happened in the luteal phase ovarian stimulation IVF cycles. The endogenous increased estrogen levels did not induce LH surge, but LH surge could be induced by GnRHa trigger, which provided sound evidence of modest-extent pituitary suppression during the luteal phase stimulation and indicated the GnRHa could be used for the ovulation trigger in luteal phase stimulation. Consistent with our finding, previous experiments in rhesus macaque had showed progesterone could block the positive feedback effect of estradiol on gonadotropin release [13;14]. The physiological plasma levels of progesterone, whether achieved by normally functioning corpora lutea or the artificial imposture by progestin implant during the follicular phase of the cycle, prevent the estrogen-induced gonadotropin discharge in intact rhesus macaque [14;15]. The same blocking effect of progesterone was observed when progesterone was simultaneously administered with estradiol benzoate to castrated women of fertile age with uninterrupted estradiol replacement [16].

Recently, studies from other IVF centers confirmed our results and showed that use of GnRHa or GnRH antagonist was not necessary for blocking an endogenous LH surge in the luteal phase. Wu et al. reported that compared with the GnRH antagonist protocol, the luteal phase stimulation without GnRH antagonist being used did not show any difference regarding the number of oocytes, the number of high-quality embryos, and the clinical pregnancy and implantation rates [17]. Zhang et al. recently performed a retrospective study to compare the clinical outcomes of luteal phase ovarian stimulation versus follicular ovarian stimulation in women with poor ovarian response. They reported more oocytes retrieved and higher metaphase II (MII) oocyte rates in luteal phase ovarian stimulation but clinical pregnancy rate, and live birth rate were not statistically different between the luteal phase and follicular phase ovarian stimulation groups. The more oocytes retrieved in luteal phase stimulation might be due to a different protocol being used [18]. Ubaldi et al. further reported a similar number of MII oocytes were obtained from follicular and luteal phase stimulation when an identical protocol was used for both the follicular and luteal phase stimulations [19]. Even though it was not evident that luteal phase stimulation provides a benefit to a population with a good ovarian response, luteal phase stimulation might be a promising protocol to treat women with poor ovarian response, particularly for patients unable to yield enough viable embryos through follicular phase ovarian stimulation or other protocols.

As a new ovarian stimulation, the safety of the luteal phase stimulation was also further analyzed. The incidence of live-birth defects in the luteal phase ovarian stimulation group (1.02%) was slightly higher than in the GnRHa short protocol group (0.64%) and the mild ovarian stimulation group (0.46%) [20]. However, none of these differences reached statistical significance. Further analysis with a large number of patients showed that no statistical differences were observed for gestational age, birth weight, neonatal anomalies, or number of malformations among luteal phase ovarian stimulation, GnRHa short protocol, and mild ovarian stimulation group [11].

One reassuring argument for the competence of oocytes obtained in the luteal phase was the absence of an increased risk of aneuploidy in 43 patients with a genetic diagnosis of aneuploidy by trophectoderm biopsy. The rate of euploid blastocysts biopsied was 46.9% in the follicular phase ovarian stimulation compared to 44.8% in the luteal phase ovarian stimulation [21].

Progestin-Primed Ovarian Stimulation

During ovarian stimulation, the LH surge in response to rapidly rising estradiol triggers ovulation and luteinization of the follicle. Premature LH surge was a major cause for cycle cancellation in women undergoing IVF treatment. Efforts to minimize the occurrence of premature LH surge have mainly relied on the use of GnRHa and GnRH antagonist in conventional protocols [1]. In previous studies, progesterone secreted by the corpus luteum strongly blocked the LH surge in luteal phase stimulation independent of GnRH antagonist. The LH surge suppression effect of progesterone and the freeze-all protocol's efficacy suggest that progestins might be used as an alternative to GnRH antagonist for suppressing premature LH surge in follicular phase ovarian stimulation and a progestin-primed ovarian stimulation (PPOS) protocol was developed.

In 2015, we reported the first prospective study of the PPOS protocol, and 10 mg/day medroxyprogesterone acetate (MPA) was used as the progestin in this study for its unique advantage. MPA has moderate to strong progestin action and fewer androgenic properties and does not interfere with the measurement of endogenous progestogen production. The results showed that the duration of stimulation was significantly longer by one day, and the total dose of hMG was higher with the PPOS protocol, but the numbers of mature oocytes and viable embryos were not significantly different in a population of normal responders (9.9 vs. 9.0; 4.3 vs. 3.7, respectively), compared with a GnRHa short protocol. Moreover, the rates for implantation, pregnancy, and miscarriage were not different between PPOS and the GnRHa short protocol [22]. Consistent with the results in luteal phase ovarian stimulation, oral MPA was efficient in terms of LH suppression and no incidence of LH surge happened in the PPOS group. Oocyte yield and pregnancy outcomes were comparable with the GnRHa short protocol. Ovulation could be triggered by the LH surge induced by GnRHa in most of the patients. However, similar to a GnRH antagonist protocol, about 2.71 percent of women had a suboptimal LH response after trigger by GnRHa in the PPOS protocol, and a dual trigger consisting of GnRHa with a low dose of hCG was recommended for triggering ovulation in PPOS [23].

To investigate the efficacy of PPOS using a lower dose of MPA, a randomized controlled study including 300 infertile women was designed to compare the clinical outcome and endocrinological characteristics of PPOS using different doses of MPA (4 or 10 mg/day) in patients undergoing IVF. hMG 225 IU/day and MPA (group A, 10 mg/day; group B, 4 mg/day) were started simultaneously from MC3. The results indicated PPOS using 4 or 10 mg of MPA per day was comparable in terms of the number of oocytes retrieved and pregnancy outcome after FET [24].

The PPOS protocol has the advantage of using GnRHa for triggering to reduce the dose of exogenous hCG for oocyte maturation triggering and might benefit patients with polycystic ovary syndrome (PCOS) who are at high risk for ovarian hyperstimulation syndrome (OHSS). We further performed a randomized study to demonstrate the efficacy of the hMG+MPA protocol in PCOS patients [25]. In this study, hMG and MPA (10 mg/day) were administered simultaneously beginning on MC3 in the study group; a GnRHa short protocol was used as a control. Ovulation was triggered by GnRHa and hCG (1000 IU) in the hMG+MPA protocol, and by 2000 IU hCG in the GnRHa short protocol when dominant follicles matured. LH suppression persisted during ovarian stimulation and no incidence of premature LH surge was seen in both groups. The number of oocytes retrieved and mature oocytes, clinical pregnancy rates per transfer, implantation rates, and cumulative pregnancy rates per patient were comparable between the hMG+MPA group and the GnRHa short protocol group. No significant difference was found in the fertilization rate and the ongoing pregnancy rate between the two groups. However, a higher total dose of hMG was used in the hMG+MPA protocol. No OHSS occurred in the hMG+MPA group, but there were two cases of OHSS in the GnRHa short protocol group. As the incidence of OHSS was low in both groups, no significant difference was found. Recently, Xiao et al. compared the efficacy of the PPOS protocol with that of the traditional GnRH antagonist protocol in patients with PCOS. The PPOS group had a longer gonadotropin duration (10.40 vs. 9.11 days) and a higher dose of gonadotrophin (1971 vs. 1719.75 IU) than the GnRH antagonist group. There was no significant difference in the number of good-quality embryos between the two groups. The number of cryopreserved embryos was slightly greater in the GnRH antagonist group than in the PPOS group (7.91 vs. 6.45, respectively). The cycle cancellation rate due to no viable embryos was similar between these two groups. Remarkably, no patients experienced mild to moderate OHSS in the PPOS group, but six patients in the GnRH antagonist group developed moderate OHSS. The difference was significant (0% vs. 6.67%, $p = 0.038$) [26].

In addition to PCOS patients, poor-responder patients might be another group to benefit from the PPOS protocol. Recently, we reported a randomized study with PPOS in poor responders. A total of 340 poor responders who met with Bologna criteria were randomly allocated into the PPOS group and GnRH antagonist group. The results showed that the incidence of premature LH surge in the PPOS group was significantly lower than that in the GnRH antagonist group (0% vs. 5.88%). However, the average number of oocytes, viable embryos, and the live birth rate in the PPOS group were comparable to those in the GnRH antagonist group. This study demonstrated that PPOS had a more robust control for preventing premature LH rise than GnRH antagonist in poor responders, but PPOS in combination with freeze-all did not significantly increase the probability of pregnancy for poor responders compared with the GnRH antagonist protocol [27].

In addition to MPA, micronized progesterone and dydrogesterone could be applied in the PPOS protocol, and efficiently block the premature LH surge [28;29]. Studies from another center confirmed the efficacy of progestin on the blockage of the LH surge [30]. It was noteworthy that even though progestin could block the LH surge, the effects of the progesterone was totally different from the GnRH antagonist. The GnRH antagonist can immediately suppress LH levels, but the LH suppression by progestin was slowly and dependent on the initiating estradiol level and timing. The LH surge was regulated by GnRH secretion, which was regulated by the central positive and negative feedback actions of the ovarian steroid hormones, estrogen and progesterone. Progesterone had divergent effects on the regulation of GnRH which drive the LH surge. Firstly, the high plasma concentration of progesterone can enhance the negative feedback effects of estradiol. As observed in the luteal phase, FSH and LH secretion are being held down to a very low level [31]. Secondly, progesterone blocks the positive feedback effect of estradiol on gonadotropin release. The physiological plasma levels of progesterone, either achieved by normally functioning corpora lutea or addition of exogenous progesterone during the follicular phase of the cycle, prevented the estrogen-induced gonadotropin discharge in intact rhesus monkeys [13–15]. The same blocking effect of progesterone was observed when progesterone was simultaneously administered with estradiol benzoate to castrated

women of fertile age with uninterrupted estradiol replacement [16]. Thirdly, progesterone plays a facilitatory role in the initiation of the gonadotropin surge after a period of estrogen priming in female rhesus monkey, rat, and human [32]. When serum progesterone levels rose after an increase in serum estradiol concentrations had occurred, the LH surge occurred earlier and was accompanied by an FSH peak [32;33]. So a sufficient amount of progesterone and a sufficient duration of the progesterone increment was necessary to block the estrogen-induced gonadotropin surges. The facilitation and inhibition of the GnRH surge by progesterone appear to be regulated via different effects on the GnRH neurosecretory system. The negative effects of progesterone on the positive feedback actions of estradiol require an intact hypothalamus, as the physiological levels of progesterone fail to block the positive feedback in monkeys with hypothalamic lesions on a replacement regimen of exogenous GnRH [34;35].

Because of the divergent effects of progesterone on the regulation of gonadotropin secretion, the initiating use of exogenous progesterone should be at the early stage of the follicular phase with comparatively low estradiol level. Even Yildiz et al. reported no premature ovulations were found in a flexible PPOS protocol with the MPA added on stimulation day 7 and concluded the flexible PPOS protocol was effective [36]. However, this was a small-sized retrospective study. Moreover, the estrogen level on the stimulation day 7 and LH level on the trigger day were not reported, and ovulation was triggered when three or more follicles reached a diameter of > 17 mm, which was earlier than our previous report on triggering ovulation when follicles reached a diameter of > 18 mm. The efficacy of flexible PPOS should be confirmed in further studies.

To confirm the safety of the PPOS protocol, a retrospective cohort study was conducted to investigate neonatal outcomes and congenital malformations in children born after IVF and vitrified embryo transfer cycles using PPOS treatment [37]. Prevalence of congenital malformations in live borns following PPOS treatment was comparable with the rate after conventional stimulation protocols for both singletons and twins.

Double Stimulation

The luteal phase ovarian stimulation made it possible to design the protocol for double stimulation: first in the follicle phase, then second in the luteal phase. We firstly tested the efficacy of double stimulations (Shanghai protocol) during the follicular and luteal phases in 38 women with poor ovarian response [38]. A second ovarian stimulation started immediately after the first oocyte retrieval; hMG and letrozole were administrated to stimulate follicle development, and oocyte retrieval was carried out a second time when dominant follicles had matured. For both the first and second stimulations, final oocyte maturation was triggered with 0.1 mg triptorelin. The primary outcome measured was the number of oocytes retrieved: stage 1, 1.7 ± 1.0; stage 2, 3.5 ± 3.2. In total, 167 oocytes were collected and 26 out of 38 (68.4%) produced one to six viable embryos cryopreserved for later embryo transfer. Twenty-one women underwent 23 cryopreserved embryo transfers, resulting in 13 clinical pregnancies. The good implantation and pregnancy rate indicated that embryos derived from double stimulation have similar development potential. These results showed double ovarian stimulations provide more opportunities for retrieving and might serve as a useful strategy for patients with poor ovarian response. Moreover, this study provides clear evidence that a second ovarian stimulation could be conducted immediately after a first stimulation and oocyte retrieval.

Recently, Ubaldi et al. conducted a prospective study on double stimulation in a cohort of patients with DOR [19]. The follicular and luteal phase stimulation started on MC2 and five days after the first oocyte retrieval, respectively. An identical protocol (300 IU rFSH + 75 IU rLH + GnRH antagonist) was used for both the follicular and luteal phase stimulations, and the euploid blastocyst formation rates per MII oocyte were compared as the primary outcome. This study revealed a similar number of MII oocytes after both follicular and luteal phase stimulation. The in vitro developmental competence to blastocyst stage was also similar, and with preimplantation genetic diagnosis for aneuploidy no statistically significant difference in the proportion of euploid blastocysts derived from the two stimulation phases was found. These results confirm the feasibility of double stimulation in a single menstrual cycle for poor responders.

To assess the efficacy and safety of the double stimulation protocol, Cimadomo et al. defined the mean number of blastocysts produced per oocyte retrieval in 188 poor prognosis patients undergoing double stimulation and preimplantation genetic testing for aneuploidies. Significantly fewer blastocysts were obtained after follicular phase stimulation than luteal phase stimulation (1.2 vs. 1.6), due to fewer oocytes collected (3.6 vs. 4.3) and a similar mean blastocyst rates per retrieval. The mean euploidy rates per retrieval were similar between follicular phase stimulation and luteal phase stimulation derived cohorts of oocytes [21]. Double stimulation was further tested in oncological patients [39]. The results showed a similar number of mature oocytes were retrieved in the first stimulation and second stimulation, and cancer treatment was not delayed for any of these patients.

Although various stimulation protocols and alternative approaches have been suggested for dual stimulation, however, the non-downregulation protocols such as the natural cycle, minimal/mild stimulation, GnRH antagonist protocols, and PPOS have the potential to continue stimulation after first oocyte retrieval in a single menstrual cycle. All the downregulation protocols were not ready for the second stimulation in a single cycle, in which GnRHa receptor inaction results in the over-suppression of the ovary, and the recovery of the pituitary from downregulation during the luteal phase was slow [40]. Moreover, in the downregulation protocol, hCG was necessary for ovulation trigger. hCG has a relative longer half-life, and ovulation triggering with hCG might also luteinize the subsequent dominant follicles [41].

In conclusion, both endogenous and exogenous progesterone were effective in inhibiting the premature LH surge during ovarian stimulation and did not compromise the quantity and quality of oocytes retrieved in IVF cycles. Progesterone could be applied in a variety of ovarian stimulation protocols – luteal phase stimulation with endogenous progesterone, progestin-primed follicular phase stimulation, double stimulation in follicular and luteal phase of the same cycle. These protocols were cheap, friendly and convenient and make ovarian stimulation more flexible.

References

1. Macklon NS, Stouffer RL, Giudice LC, Fauser BC. The science behind 25 years of ovarian stimulation for in vitro fertilization. *Endocr Rev* 2006;**27**:170–207.

2. Baerwald AR, Adams GP, Pierson RA. Characterization of ovarian follicular wave dynamics in women. *Biol Reprod* 2003;**69**:1023–1031.

3. Baerwald AR, Adams GP, Pierson RA. A new model for ovarian follicular development during the human menstrual cycle. *Fertil Steril* 2003;**80**:116–122.

4. McNatty KP, Hillier SG, van den Boogaard AM, *et al.* Follicular development during the luteal phase of the human menstrual cycle. *J Clin Endocrinol Metab* 1983;**56**:1022–1031.

5. von Wolff M, Thaler CJ, Frambach T, *et al.* Ovarian stimulation to cryopreserve fertilized oocytes in cancer patients can be started in the luteal phase. *Fertil Steril* 2009;**92**:1360–1365.

6. Bedoschi GM, de Albuquerque FO, Ferriani RA, Navarro PA. Ovarian stimulation during the luteal phase for fertility preservation of cancer patients: case reports and review of the literature. *J Assist Reprod Genet* 2010;**27**:491–494.

7. Sonmezer M, Turkcuoglu I, Coskun U, Oktay K. Random-start controlled ovarian hyperstimulation for emergency fertility preservation in letrozole cycles. *Fertil Steril* 2011;**95**(2125):e9–e11.

8. Kuang YP, Chen QJ, Hong QQ, *et al.* Luteal-phase ovarian stimulation case report: three-year follow-up of a twin birth. *J IVF Reprod Med Genet* 2013;**1**(2):1000106.

9. Buendgen NK, Schultze-Mosgau A, Cordes T, Diedrich K, Griesinger G. Initiation of ovarian stimulation independent of the menstrual cycle: a case-control study. *Arch Gynecol Obstet* 2013;**288**:901–904.

10. Kuang Y, Hong Q, Chen Q, *et al.* Luteal-phase ovarian stimulation is feasible for producing competent oocytes in women undergoing in vitro fertilization/intracytoplasmic sperm injection treatment, with optimal pregnancy outcomes in frozen-thawed embryo transfer cycles. *Fertil Steril* 2014;**101**:105–111.

11. Wang N, Wang Y, Chen Q, *et al.* Luteal-phase ovarian stimulation vs conventional ovarian stimulation in patients with normal ovarian reserve treated for IVF: a large retrospective cohort study. *Clin Endocrinol* 2016;**84**:720–728.

12. Li Y, Yang W, Chen X, *et al.* Comparison between follicular stimulation and luteal stimulation protocols with clomiphene and HMG in women with poor ovarian response. *Gynecol Endocrinol* 2016;**32**:74–77.

13. Spies HG, Niswender GD. Blockade of the surge of preovulatory serum luteinizing hormone and ovulation with exogenous progesterone in cycling rhesus (*Macaca mulatta*) monkeys. *J Clin Endocrinol Metab* 1971;**32**:309–316.

14. Dierschke DJ, Yamaji T, Karsch FJ, *et al.* Blockade by progesterone of estrogen-induced LH and FSH release in the rhesus monkey. *Endocrinology* 1973;**92**:1496–1501.

15. Pohl CR, Knobil E. The role of the central nervous system in the control of ovarian function in higher primates. *Annu Rev Physiol* 1982;**44**:583–593.

16. March CM, Goebelsmann U, Nakamura RM, Mishell DR, Jr. Roles of estradiol and progesterone in eliciting the midcycle luteinizing hormone and follicle-stimulating hormone surges. *J Clin Endocrinol Metabol* 1979;**49**:507–513.

17. Wu Y, Zhao FC, Sun Y, Liu PS. Luteal-phase protocol in poor ovarian response: a comparative study with an antagonist protocol. *J Int Med Res* 2017;**45**:1731–1738.

18. Zhang W, Wang M, Wang S, *et al.* Luteal phase ovarian stimulation for poor ovarian responders. *JBRA Assist Reprod* 2018;**22**:193–198.

19. Ubaldi FM, Capalbo A, Vaiarelli A, *et al.* Follicular versus luteal phase ovarian stimulation during the same menstrual cycle (DuoStim) in a reduced ovarian reserve population results in a similar euploid blastocyst formation rate: new insight in ovarian reserve exploitation. *Fertil Steril* 2016;**105**:1488.e1–1495.e1.

20. Chen H, Wang Y, Lyu Q, *et al.* Comparison of live-birth defects after luteal-phase ovarian stimulation vs. conventional ovarian stimulation for in vitro fertilization and vitrified embryo transfer cycles. *Fertil Steril* 2015;**103**:1194.e2–1201.e2.

21. Cimadomo D, Vaiarelli A, Colamaria S, *et al.* Luteal phase anovulatory follicles result in the production of competent oocytes: intra-patient paired case-control study comparing follicular versus luteal phase stimulations in the same ovarian cycle. *Hum Reprod* 2018;**33**:1442–1448.

22. Kuang Y, Chen Q, Fu Y, *et al.* Medroxyprogesterone acetate is an effective oral alternative for preventing premature luteinizing hormone surges in women undergoing controlled ovarian hyperstimulation for in vitro fertilization. *Fertil Steril* 2015;**104**:62.e3–70.e3.

23. Lu X, Hong Q, Sun L, *et al.* Dual trigger for final oocyte maturation improves the oocyte retrieval rate of suboptimal responders to

gonadotropin-releasing hormone agonist. *Fertil Steril* 2016;**106**:1356–1362.

24. Dong J, Wang Y, Chai WR, *et al.* The pregnancy outcome of progestin-primed ovarian stimulation using 4 versus 10 mg of medroxyprogesterone acetate per day in infertile women undergoing in vitro fertilisation: a randomised controlled trial. *BJOG* 2017;**124**:1048–1055.

25. Wang Y, Chen Q, Wang N, *et al.* Controlled ovarian stimulation using medroxyprogesterone acetate and hMG in patients with polycystic ovary syndrome treated for IVF: a double-blind randomized crossover clinical trial. *Medicine* 2016;**95**:e2939.

26. Xiao ZN, Peng JL, Yang J, Xu WM. Flexible GnRH antagonist protocol versus progestin-primed ovarian stimulation (PPOS) protocol in patients with polycystic ovary syndrome: comparison of clinical outcomes and ovarian response. *Curr Med Sci* 2019;**39**:431–436.

27. Chen Q, Chai W, Wang Y, *et al.* Progestin vs. gonadotropin-releasing hormone antagonist for the prevention of premature luteinizing hormone surges in poor responders undergoing in vitro fertilization treatment: a randomized controlled trial. *Front Endocrinol (Lausanne)* 2019;**10**:796.

28. Yu S, Long H, Chang HY, *et al.* New application of dydrogesterone as a part of a progestin-primed ovarian stimulation protocol for IVF: a randomized controlled trial including 516 first IVF/ICSI cycles. *Hum Reprod* 2018;**33**:229–237.

29. Zhu X, Zhang X, Fu Y. Utrogestan as an effective oral alternative for preventing premature luteinizing hormone surges in women undergoing controlled ovarian hyperstimulation for in vitro fertilization. *Medicine* 2015;**94**:e909.

30. Crha I, Ventruba P, Filipinska E, *et al.* [Medroxyprogesterone acetate use to block LH surge in oocyte donor stimulation]. *Ceska gynekologie* 2018;**83**:11–16.

31. diZerega GS, Hodgen GD. Cessation of folliculogenesis during the primate luteal phase. *J Clin Endocrinol Metab* 1980;**51**:158–160.

32. Helmond FA, Simons PA, Hein PR. Strength and duration characteristics of the facilitory and inhibitory effects of progesterone on the estrogen-induced gonadotropin surge in the female rhesus monkey. *Endocrinology* 1981;**108**:1837–1842.

33. Helmond FA, Simons PA, Hein PR. The effects of progesterone on estrogen-induced luteinizing hormone and follicle-stimulating hormone release in the female rhesus monkey. *Endocrinology* 1980;**107**:478–485.

34. Gougeon A. Regulation of ovarian follicular development in primates: facts and hypotheses. *Endocr Rev* 1996;**17**:121–155.

35. Richter TA, Robinson JE, Lozano JM, Evans NP. Progesterone can block the preovulatory gonadotropin-releasing hormone/luteinising hormone surge in the ewe by a direct inhibitory action on oestradiol-responsive cells within the hypothalamus. *J Neuroendocrinol* 2005;**17**:161–169.

36. Yildiz S, Turkgeldi E, Angun B, *et al.* Comparison of a novel flexible progestin primed ovarian stimulation protocol and the flexible gonadotropin-releasing hormone antagonist protocol for assisted reproductive technology. *Fertil Steril* 2019;**112**:677–683.

37. Zhang J, Mao X, Wang Y, *et al.* Neonatal outcomes and congenital malformations in children born after human menopausal gonadotropin and medroxyprogesterone acetate treatment cycles. *Arch Gynecol Obstet* 2017;**296**:1207–17.

38. Kuang Y, Chen Q, Hong Q, *et al.* Double stimulations during the follicular and luteal phases of poor responders in IVF/ICSI programmes (Shanghai protocol). *Reprod Biomed Online* 2014;**29**:684–91.

39. Tsampras N, Gould D, Fitzgerald CT. Double ovarian stimulation (DuoStim) protocol for fertility preservation in female oncology patients. *Hum Fertil* 2017;**20**:248–253.

40. Smitz J, Van Den Abbeel E, Bollen N, *et al.* The effect of gonadotrophin-releasing hormone (GnRH) agonist in the follicular phase on in-vitro fertilization outcome in normo-ovulatory women. *Hum Reprod* 1992;**7**:1098–1102.

41. Niederberger C, Pellicer A, Cohen J, *et al.* Forty years of IVF. *Fertil Steril* 2018;**110**:185.e5–324.e5.

Ovarian Stimulation in Poor Responders

Qiuju Chen and Yanping Kuang

Controlled ovarian stimulation (COS) is an important step during in vitro fertilization (IVF) treatment that aims to produce sufficient follicles and oocytes to achieve pregnancy. Despite recent progresses in assisted reproductive technology (ART), a poor ovarian response (POR) remains one of the most challenging issues for reproductive clinicians [1]. The incidence of POR during COS has been reported to range from 5.6 percent to 35.1 percent depending on differences in the definition of poor response [1–4]. Patients with POR have higher cycle cancellation rates, lower pregnancy rates, and heavier financial burden [4–6]. In this chapter, we discuss the classification and treatments of POR.

The Classification of Poor Responders

Bologna Criteria

There has been a lack of consensus regarding the definition of POR until the Europe Society of Human Reproduction and Embryology (ESHRE) proposed the Bologna criteria in 2011 [7]. Bologna criteria are based on three conditions: (1) advanced maternal age (> 40 years) or any other POR risk factor; (2) a previous incident of POR; and (3) a low ovarian reserve test in terms of anti-Müllerian hormone (AMH) and antral follicle count (AFC). Two of these three criteria are required for a POR diagnosis. In addition, two cycles with POR after maximal stimulation are sufficient to classify a patient as a poor responder even in the absence of the other criteria mentioned.

These criteria were adopted as the definition of POR in nearly half of the interventional trials registered in clinicaltrials.gov since 2011. This definition of POR makes it possible to compare results and draw reliable conclusions. However, this classification model described a very heterogeneous group of patients with highly different success rates after ART, which limited the values in decision-making regarding continuation of treatments [5–10]. These debates led to the recent development of the Poseidon criteria for POR, stratifying patients into more homogeneous subgroups.

Poseidon Criteria

The Poseidon (Patient-Oriented Strategies Encompassing IndividualizeD Oocyte Number) criteria were used for "low prognosis" patients undergoing ART in 2016 [11]. The Poseidon criteria propose a shift from the terminology of POR to the concept of low prognosis. The low-prognosis patients are classified into four groups according to the female age, ovarian reserve markers (AMH and/or AFC), and the number of oocytes retrieved in previous stimulation cycles [11;12]. Table 11.1 shows the comparison between Bologna criteria and Poseidon criteria's stratification. Poseidon criteria combine "qualitative" (age and the expected aneuploidy rate) and "quantitative" parameters (AMH and/or AFC) and ovarian response – if a previous stimulation was performed. Moreover, the following groups of patients with different degree of low prognosis require specific evidence-based clinical treatment strategy.

The Poseidon criteria have some advantages. They emphasize the association of age and euploid embryos. Although 35 years is defined as the threshold of aged for the increasing ratio of aneuploid oocytes, it is not closely associated with ovarian response to gonadotropin (Gn), some aged women still have good response to Gn, meaning the compensatory action of the ovarian function, or the oocyte aging is more advanced than the granulosa cell aging. Secondly, the Poseidon criteria introduce a new measure for

Table 11.1 Comparison between Bologna criteria and Poseidon's stratification

	Poseidon criteria (2016)		Bologna criteria (2011)	
	Pre-stimulation	Post-stimulation	Pre-stimulation	Post-stimulation
Unexpected	Group 1: Age < 35 years + Sufficient ovarian reserve	1a: poor (< 4 oocytes) 1b: suboptimal (4–9 oocytes)		(5) 2 previous POR
	Group 2: Age ≥ 35 years + Sufficient ovarian reserve	2a: poor (< 4 oocytes) 2b: suboptimal (4–9 oocytes)		
Expected	Group 3: Age < 35 years + DOR		(1) Age ≥ 40 years + DOR	(2) Age ≥ 40 years + A previous POR (3) DOR + A previous POR (4) Age ≥ 40 years + DOR + A previous POR
	Group 4: Age ≥ 35 years + DOR			

Diminished ovarian reserve (DOR): AFC < 5 and/or AMH < 1.2 ng/ml; sufficient ovarian reserve: AFC ≥ 5 and/or AMH ≥ 1.2 ng/ml. POR: A previous poor response (< 4 oocytes with a conventional stimulation protocol).

successful treatment, namely, the ability to retrieve the number of oocytes necessary to obtain at least one euploid embryo for transfer. The success measurement is more practical and precise for the low-prognosis population [11–13].

Nearly half of IVF/intracytoplasmic sperm injection (ICSI) patients match the Poseidon condition, its cumulative live birth rate (CLBR) is 56 percent over 18 months of IVF/ICSI treatment and varies between the Poseidon groups, which is primarily attributable to the impact of female age [14]. The CLBR was highest in group 1, followed by group 3 and group 2, and lowest in group 4 (44.6%, 35.5%, 24.5%, and 12.7%, respectively) in another large retrospective study in Poseidon population [15].

Treatment Strategy for Poor Responders

Sufficient Ovarian Reserve of Poseidon Criteria (Group 1 and 2)

Poseidon groups 1 and 2 encompass good reserve patients, the poor response is sometimes an unexpected event, and doctors should review the stimulation process and find a distinct diagnostic and therapeutic approach in relation to patients' characteristics.

Monitor Follicular Growth

Gn starting dose is targeted for the antral follicle cohort and tailored on the relevant factors of female age, body mass index (BMI), and basal ovarian status. Gn dose is commonly 150–225 IU/day and maintains the serum follicle-stimulating hormone (FSH) values at no less than 10–15 IU/ml during stimulation. Gn starting dose should be increased for cases with high BMI. Multiple protocols of luteinizing hormone (LH) suppression are suitable for this population. GnRH agonist long protocol has the most strength grade for pituitary suppression. GnRH antagonist protocol is more popular for the advantages of short-term stimulation and high safety [3;16;17]. Progestin-primed ovarian stimulation (PPOS) in combination with freeze-all is also a potential choice for the groups 1 and 2, especially for refractory low responders [18;19].

The dynamic follicular activity during stimulation is closely monitored. The follicle stagnation, slow growth, or smaller cohort of growing follicles indicates the follicle resistant or ovarian insensitivity, mainly due to the relative or absolute Gn insufficiency during COS, and increasing Gn dose would be the first choice of treatments [20]. Indices such as FORT (follicle output rate, ≥ 80%) and FOI (follicle-to-oocyte index, ≥ 50%) are used to determine if the ovarian reserve is properly explored during a previous ovarian stimulation [21;22].

Secondly, the extent of pituitary suppression should be carefully monitored, low LH levels on the trigger day are associated with a low mature oocyte yield in GnRH antagonist cycles [23;24]. The over-suppressed LH levels may interfere with follicle growth at the mid- and later-follicular phase, and result in slow follicular development or reduced pregnancy outcomes [23]. Previous evidence reported that a late-follicular-phase LH threshold existed to predict reproductive outcomes and it was about 1.60 mIU/ml in GnRH agonist trigger cycles or 0.5–1.2 mIU/ml in human chorionic gonadotropin (hCG) trigger cycles [23;24]. Add-back recombinant LH or 100–200 IU daily of hCG may be effective for the cases of over-suppressed LH. Human menopausal gonadotropin is prefer to purified FSH for the ovarian stimulation in over-suppressed-LH cases.

For the cases of asynchronous follicle development during COS, the follicle sizes on the trigger day are more disparate, the lead follicle performs less reliably as a representation of all follicles, resulting in less oocyte yield when triggered according to the lead follicle size. Our clinic attempts to shift the stimulation target to the subdominant follicle cohorts and trigger until the subdominant follicles reach the appropriate size, in order to harvest more oocytes. GnRH agonist long protocol or pretreatment by estrogen/progestin may be an alternative to control the synchronism of antral follicles before stimulation.

Trigger Efficacy

Trigger is a critical step to induce oocyte maturation in preparation for oocyte retrieval when follicles grow to an appropriate size. Ovarian follicles that are "too small" are less likely to yield mature oocytes following LH-like exposure [25] and once ovarian follicles grow too large, follicles may contain "post-mature" oocytes and are also not competent for fertilization [26]. The decision on timing of trigger in relation to follicle size is multifactorial, taking into account the size of the growing follicle cohort, the hormonal data, duration of stimulation, and experience of previous cycles. Most often, final oocyte maturation is triggered at sizes of two or three lead follicles > 17 to 18 mm in diameter, with most follicles ≥ 14 mm [27;28].

The drugs for trigger are commonly hCG 5000 IU and/or GnRH agonist 0.1–0.2 mg. Insufficient trigger results in the increased incidence of empty follicles, unexpected less oocyte recovery, or immature oocytes at the 36-hour oocyte retrieval [28]. Trigger efficacy can be accurately assessed by the incidence of oocyte recovery (ratio of oocytes divided by punctuated preovulatory follicles, > 80%) and mature oocyte yield (the proportion of mature oocytes retrieved from follicles of 12–19 mm on the day of trigger, > 60%) [28]. Few cases (2–5%) present a suboptimal pituitary response after GnRH agonist trigger (posttrigger LH < 15 mIU/ml), especially in the cases of extremely low LH values on the trigger day [29]. Prolonging the interval of trigger and oocyte retrieval and double trigger are helpful for these cases by overcoming any impairments in granulosa cell function, oocyte meiotic maturation, or cumulus expansion, resulting in successful aspiration of mature oocytes and delivery [28;30]. In our clinic, when the unexpected low oocyte yield and few granulosa cells in follicular fluid after unilateral puncture occur in the process of oocyte retrieval, we attempt to delay operation by 1–3 hours; mostly the cases could get better results than with the scheduled time.

Genetic Factor for Poor Response

A genetic screening test is advisable for patients with sufficient reserve and repeated poor response after excluding the above iatrogenic factors. The genetic variants of Gn and their receptors are associated with abnormal ovarian response. In particular, FSHR polymorphisms (e.g., Ser680Asn and Thr307Ala), LH β-subunit variant, and LH polymorphisms have been associated with reduced sensitivity to Gn and inadequate response following ovarian stimulation [31–33]. They actually required higher Gn consumption to compensate for the Gn receptor defects in normal gonadotropic women [34;35].

Our research group reported two live births by women harboring pathogenic LHCGR variants using their own oocytes. These patients always presented empty follicle syndrome using the routine IVF procedure, but harvested autologous oocytes by dual trigger with a high dose of hCG and delaying the retrieval time (40–50 hours after trigger). Their mutant LHCGR, which presumably loses its membrane localization capacity, disrupts ovulation but has no effect on fertilization or embryo development. The function of LHCGR variants retains partial activity in vivo and more time is needed to promote oocyte maturation [36].

All the technical details, for examples, abnormal follicle development, Gn insufficiency, and improper trigger, as well as problems in retrieval time, can contribute, alone or combined, to reduced oocyte outputs, so treatments targeted for the different pathogenesis are necessary.

Diminished Ovarian Reserve of Poseidon Criteria (Group 3 and 4)

For DOR patients, the first step is to evaluate the epibiotic ovarian function and make a reasonable expectation for ovarian stimulation and pregnancy. The aim of ovarian stimulation is to get approximately 50–90 percent follicle outputs from antral follicles (3–8 mm) and harvest at least one euploid blastocyst. The follicles in DOR patients are characterized by high variation in growth and maturation, which add difficulty for the treatments [37;38].

Monitor Follicular Growth

The commonly used dose of Gn is 75–225 IU/day, adjusting on the basal FSH levels, AFC, BMI, and previous response to Gn. Increasing Gn dose may not contribute much to the increase of oocyte yield in the population with few FSH-sensitive follicles. Previous evidence indicated that more exogenous FSH administration did not increase the possibility of live birth compared with modified natural cycle in Bologna poor responders [39]. Clomiphene (clomifene) and letrozole are also used to increase ovarian response, but they are not recommended for the cases with elevated basal FSH values.

GnRH analogues and progestin have been used to suppress premature LH surge during COS for the DOR. The guideline of ESHRE in 2019 equally recommended GnRH antagonist and agonist for the predicted poor responders for the comparable safety and efficacy [16]. The GnRH antagonist protocol is associated with less suppression in the early follicular phase and short-term injection, so the GnRH antagonist protocol is listed as the first choice in an IVF worldwide survey of treatments for poor responders [40]. PPOS in combination with freeze-all is an alternative approach for the DOR cases [37;38]. Non-conventional start of ovarian stimulation including flexible-start ovarian stimulation, double stimulation, even the retrieval of preovulatory follicle in the menstrual period, is mandatory to freeze embryos, although the quality of evidence is low and controversial.

It is more difficult to control LH levels during the stimulation in DOR patients than in those with sufficient ovarian reserve. The transient LH suppression by GnRH antagonist is accomplished by competitive blockage of GnRH receptor, the ability of endogenous estrogen-induced GnRH release is still preserved, and a small proportion of antagonist cycles fail to control spontaneous LH surge, especially in older women, and those with DOR and poor response to Gn. A recent randomized controlled trial (RCT) of Bologna poor responders indicated that the incidence of premature LH surge in PPOS was lower than in GnRH antagonist cycles (0% vs. 5.88%), PPOS showed a stronger pituitary suppression, but the oocyte competence and pregnancy outcomes did not obviously improve compared with the GnRH antagonist protocol [38].

Trigger Efficacy

The reports about the criteria of trigger in DOR patients are very limited, mostly studies still use the trigger criteria of treatments with sufficient ovarian reserve. Several studies showed the double trigger using GnRH agonist and hCG may be better than GnRH agonist or hCG alone for DOR responders [19;30].

The follicles in DOR patients are prone to ovulate at a relative smaller diameter, the older (above age 43) women's follicles to significant degrees demonstrated premature luteinization and harvested atretic oocytes if allowed to mature to traditional follicle sizes. Early oocyte retrieval, with hCG trigger at approximately 16 mm lead follicle sizes, in such patients, avoided oocyte exposure to premature luteinization, thereby significantly improving clinical pregnancy rates [41]. Another pilot study showed that a lead follicle range of approximately 16.0–18.0 mm appeared the best size to trigger ovulation in the DOR women, whether due to advanced female age or premature ovarian insufficiency [42]. The evidence still needs to be confirmed by large RCTs.

Oocyte Retrieval and Embryo Culture

The interval of oocyte retrieval and trigger is commonly 36 hours in normal responders. Follicular flushing is recommended to increase oocyte yields and pregnancy rates in DOR patients although it is still controversial [43]. For the cases of older women, with history of previous premature ovulation, the serum hormone fluctuation should be closely monitored, the presence of untimely serum LH rise and significant estradiol decrease during stimulation is considered as a warning signal for clinicians to make an optimal schedule timely. Our clinic recommends to carry out retrival 1–2 hours sooner than the standard schedule for the group of older women, DOR, and with the high risk of premature ovulation.

The oocyte yield of this group depends on the number of FSH-sensitive antral follicles, FOI should be more than 50 percent in a successful ovarian stimulation cycle. The reduced oocyte quantity may be accompanied with a certain extent of decline of oocyte quality in the DOR patients, some patients need multiple retrievals and embryo transfers to increase the possibility of pregnancy.

Treatment for the Cases of Extremely Low Ovarian Reserve

The degree of ovarian failure is classified into biochemical failure, transient ovarian failure, and premature ovarian insufficiency based on age, ovarian reserve, and menstrual cycle. Extremely low ovarian reserve (LOR) represents a true difficult population of transient ovarian failure and premature ovarian insufficiency. This population has common characteristics of elevated basal FSH level (> 20 mIU/ml), low AMH (< 0.4 ng/ml), absence of or few AFCs, and with irregular menstrual cycle or amenorrhea. Different from the ovarian follicle depletion of normal menopause, the young LOR women are characterized by intermittent ovarian function. Someone may think oocyte donation is more effective for the low prognosis, but for the couples of young, highly desiring parenthood, it is worth attempting the autologous oocyte IVF [44;45].

The ovarian stimulation in LOR women is aimed to promote one available follicle to mature and retrieve. In our clinic, ethinyl estradiol (EE, 12.5–50 μg/day) and medroxyprogesterone acetate (MPA, 10 mg/day) are used to suppress FSH/LH for the cases with elevated FSH (> 20 mIU/ml). For the cases with endogenous estradiol > 20 pg/ml, a growing follicle will present in one or two weeks, but for the difficult cases with hypergonadotropic and estrogen deficiency (estradiol < 20 pg/ml), a follicle might need a longer time to develop.

A low dose of Gn is administrated until the serum FSH falls into approximately normal range and the growing sign of follicle presents. The final stage of oocyte maturation is induced using a GnRH agonist and/or hCG. The oral contraceptive pill (OCP) is stronger at inhibiting the hypergonadotropic hormones than the composite of EE/MPA. One tablet of OCP enables serum FSH levels to decrease from 50 mIU/ml to 15 mIU/ml in a week, then the reduced dose of OCP (0.5 tablet) continues to prevent premature LH surge and a low dose of Gn is added to promote follicle growth if necessary.

The decline of oocyte quantity and quality is obvious in the population of LOR women, about one-third of LOR does not harvest good-quality embryos; however, the implantation rate and pregnancy outcome in LOR patients who could shift to the step of embryo transfer are similar, or slightly lower than others in poor responders. Given the irreversible process of ovarian failure, accumulating embryos through multiple attempts is beneficial for the older LOR women.

Adjuvant Drugs for Poor Responders

Adjuvant therapy is defined as any additional treatment used other than GnRH analogues and gonadotropins during the IVF/ICSI cycle with the aim of increasing pregnancy success, especially in women with POR. Currently, the most frequently proposed adjuvant therapies include dehydroepiandrosterone (DHEA), growth hormone (GH), coenzyme Q10 (CoQ10), metformin, and aspirin [2;16;46]. A recent meta-analysis synthesized the data of 19 RCTs and indicated that DHEA, CoQ10, and GH were the top three agents that improved the probability of achieving pregnancy and had lower cycle cancellation rates among the adjuvant treatments for POR patients [46]. However, the use of adjuvant DHEA, GH, and CoQ10 before and/or during ovarian stimulation is probably not recommended for poor responders in the guideline of ESHRE in 2019 [16]. The addition of adjuvants in ovarian stimulation is still in debate in terms of efficacy and safety.

Summary

POR is extremely heterogeneous, and individualized treatment is the key to achieving a better outcome for the low prognosis population. Making a proper evaluation before stimulation and monitoring the process of tailoring FSH dose, controlling LH levels, sufficient trigger, and correcting retrieval time are all important factors. Detecting genetic variants of gonadotropins and their receptors is of benefit for the repeated unexpected poor responders. Small follicle ovulation occasionally presents in the older DOR group, early oocyte retrieval may be one of the rescue treatments for this population. Pretreatment by estrogen and progesterone and accumulating embryos provide an opportunity to achieve biological parenthood for the cases with extremely low reserve. In all, all the technical details can contribute, alone or combined, to reduced oocyte output; the individualized treatments targeted for the different pathogenesis are the key to a better outcome for the low prognosis population.

References

1. Oudendijk JF, Yarde F, Eijkemans MJ, Broekmans FJ, Broer SL. The poor responder in IVF: is the prognosis always poor? a systematic review. *Hum Reprod Update* 2012;**18**:1–11.

2. Bosdou JK, Venetis CA, Kolibianakis EM, *et al.* The use of androgens or androgen modulating agents in poor responders undergoing in vitro fertilization: a systematic review and meta-analysis. *Hum Reprod Update* 2012;**18**:127–145.

3. Papathanasiou A, Searle BJ, King NM, Bhattacharya S. Trends in 'poor responder' research: lessons learned from RCTs in assisted conception. *Hum Reprod Update* 2016;**22**:306–319.

4. Surrey ES, Schoolcraft WB. Evaluating strategies for improving ovarian response of the poor responder undergoing assisted reproductive techniques. *Fertil Steril* 2000;**73**:667–676.

5. Papathanasiou A. Implementing the ESHRE "poor responder" criteria in research studies: methodological implications. *Hum Reprod* 2014;**29**:1835–1838.

6. Polyzos NP, Devroey P. A systematic review of randomized trials for the treatment of poor ovarian responders: is there any light at the end of the tunnel? *Fertil Steril* 2011;**96**:1058–1061.

7. Ferraretti AP, La Marca A, Fauser BC, *et al.* ESHRE consensus on the definition of 'poor response' to ovarian stimulation for in vitro fertilization: the Bologna criteria. *Hum Reprod* 2011;**26**:1616–1624.

8. Ferraretti AP, Gianaroli L. The Bologna criteria for the definition of poor ovarian responders: is there a need for revision? *Hum Reprod* 2014;**29**:1842–1845.

9. Venetis CA. The Bologna criteria for poor ovarian response: the good, the bad and the way forward. *Hum Reprod* 2014;**29**:1839–1841.

10. Younis JS. The Bologna criteria for poor ovarian response; has the job been accomplished. *Hum Reprod* 2012;**27**:1874–1875.

11. Poseidon Group (Patient-Oriented Strategies Encompassing IndividualizeD Oocyte Number); Alviggi C, Andersen CY, Buehler K, *et al.* A new more detailed stratification of low responders to ovarian stimulation: from a poor ovarian response to a low prognosis concept. *Fertil Steril* 2016;**105**:1452–1453.

12. Esteves SC, Alviggi C, Humaidan P, *et al.* The POSEIDON criteria and its measure of success through the eyes of clinicians and embryologists. *Front Endocrinol (Lausanne)* 2019;**10**:814.

13. Humaidan P, La Marca A, Alviggi C, Esteves SC, Haahr T. Future perspectives of POSEIDON stratification for clinical practice and research. *Front Endocrinol (Lausanne)* 2019;**10**:439.

14. Leijdekkers JA, Eijkemans MJC, van Tilborg TC, *et al.* Cumulative live birth rates in low-prognosis women. *Hum Reprod* 2019;**34**:1030–1041.

15. Shi W, Zhou H, Tian L, *et al.* Cumulative live birth rates of good and low prognosis patients according to POSEIDON criteria: a single center analysis of 18,455 treatment cycles. *Front Endocrinol (Lausanne)* 2019;**10**:409.

16. ESHRE Reproductive Endocrinology Guideline Group. Ovarian stimulation for IVF/ICSI: guideline of the European Society of Human Reproduction and Embryology. https://www.eshre.eu/Guidelines-and-Legal/Guidelines/Ovarian-Stimulation-in-IVF-ICSI.

17. Al-Inany HG, Youssef MA, Ayeleke RO, *et al.* Gonadotrophin-releasing hormone antagonists for assisted reproductive technology. *Cochrane Database Syst Rev* 2016;**4**:CD001750.

18. Kuang Y, Chen Q, Fu Y, *et al.* Medroxy progesterone acetate is an effective oral alternative for preventing premature luteinizing hormone surges in women undergoing controlled ovarian hyperstimulation for in vitro fertilization. *Fertil Steril* 2015;**104**:62–70.

19. Zhang J, Wang Y, Mao X, *et al.* Dual trigger of final oocyte maturation in poor ovarian responders undergoing IVF/ICSI cycles. *Reprod Biomed Online* 2017;**35**:701–707.

20. Sunkara SK, Ramaraju GA, Kamath MS. Management strategies for POSEIDON group 2. *Front Endocrinol (Lausanne)* 2020;**11**:105.

21. Gallot V, Berwanger da Silva AL, Genro V, *et al.* Antral follicle responsiveness to

follicle-stimulating hormone administration assessed by the follicular output RaTe (FORT) may predict in vitro fertilization-embryo transfer outcome. *Hum Reprod* 2012;27:1066–1072.

22. Alviggi C, Conforti A, Esteves SC, *et al.* Understanding ovarian hypo-response to exogenous gonadotropin in ovarian stimulation and its new proposed marker-the follicle-to-oocyte (FOI) index. *Front Endocrinol (Lausanne)* 2018;9:589.

23. Benmachiche A, Benbouhedja S, Zoghmar A, Humaidan P. Low LH level on the day of GnRH agonist trigger is associated with reduced ongoing pregnancy and live birth rates and increased early miscarriage rates following IVF/ICSI treatment and fresh embryo transfer. *Front Endocrinol (Lausanne)* 2019;10:639.

24. Propst AM, Hill MJ, Bates GW, *et al.* Low dose human chorionic gonadotropin may improve in vitro fertilization cycle outcomes in patients with low luteinizing hormone levels after gonadotropin-releasing hormone antagonist administration. *Fertil Steril* 2011;96:898–904.

25. Revelli A, Martiny G, Delle Piane L, *et al.* A critical review of bi-dimensional and three-dimensional ultrasound techniques to monitor follicle growth: do they help improving IVF outcome? *Reprod Biol Endocrinol* 2014;12:107.

26. Ectors FJ, Vanderzwalmen P, Van Hoeck J, *et al.* Relationship of human follicular diameter with oocyte fertilization and development after in-vitro fertilization or intracytoplasmic sperm injection. *Hum Reprod* 1997;12:2002–2005.

27. Kolibianakis EM, Albano C, Camus M, *et al.* Prolongation of the follicular phase in in vitro fertilization results in a lower ongoing pregnancy rate in cycles stimulated with recombinant follicle-stimulating hormone and gonadotropin-releasing hormone antagonists. *Fertil Steril* 2004;82:102–107.

28. Abbara A, Clarke SA, Dhillo WS. Novel concepts for inducing final oocyte maturation in in vitro fertilization treatment. *Endocr Rev* 2018;39:593–628.

29. Meyer L, Murphy LA, Gumer A, *et al.* Risk factors for a suboptimal response to gonadotropin-releasing hormone agonist trigger during in vitro fertilization cycles. *Fertil Steril* 2015;104:637–642.

30. Griffin D, Feinn R, Engmann L, *et al.* Dual trigger with gonadotropin releasing hormone agonist and standard dose human chorionic gonadotropin to improve oocyte maturity rates. *Fertil Steril* 2014;102:405–409.

31. Perez Mayorga M, Gromoll J, Behre HM, *et al.* Ovarian response to follicle-stimulating hormone (FSH) stimulation depends on the FSH receptor genotype. *J Clin Endocrinol Metab* 2000;85:3365–3369.

32. Simoni M, Nieschlag E, Gromoll J. Isoforms and single nucleotide polymorphisms of the FSH receptor gene: implications for human reproduction. *Hum Reprod Update* 2002;8:413–421.

33. Mohiyiddeen L, Newman WG, McBurney H, *et al.* Follicle-stimulating hormone receptor gene polymorphisms are not associated with ovarian reserve markers. *Fertil Steril* 2012;97:677–681.

34. Alviggi C, Clarizia R, Pettersson K, *et al.* Suboptimal response to GnRHa long protocol is associated with a common LH polymorphism. *Reprod Biomed Online* 2009;18:9–14.

35. Alviggi C, Pettersson K, Longobardi S, *et al.* A common polymorphic allele of the LH beta-subunit gene is associated with higher exogenous FSH consumption during controlled ovarian stimulation for assisted reproductive technology. *Reprod Biol Endocrinol* 2013;1:51.

36. Lu X, Yan Z, Cai R, *et al.* Pregnancy and live birth in women with pathogenic LHCGR variants using their own oocytes. *J Clin Endocrinol Metab* 2019;104:5877–5892.

37. Chen Q, Wang Y, Sun L, *et al.* Controlled ovulation of the dominant follicle using progestin in minimal stimulation in poor responders. *Reprod Biol Endocrinol* 2017;15:71.

38. Chen Q, Chai W, Wang Y, *et al.* Progestin vs. gonadotropin-releasing hormone antagonist for the prevention of premature luteinizing hormone surges in poor responders undergoing in vitro fertilization treatment: a randomized controlled trial. *Front Endocrinol (Lausanne)* 2019;10:796.

39. Lainas TG, Sfontouris IA, Venetis CA, *et al.* Live birth rates after modified natural cycle compared with high-dose FSH stimulation using GnRH antagonists in poor responders. *Hum Reprod* 2015;30:2321–2330.

40. Patrizio P, Vaiarelli A, Levi Setti PE, *et al.* How to define, diagnose and treat poor responders? Responses from a worldwide survey of IVF clinics. *Reprod Biomed Online* 2015;30:581–592.

41. Wu YG, Barad DH, Kushnir VA, *et al.* Aging-related premature luteinization of granulosa cells is avoided by early oocyte retrieval. *J Endocrinol* 2015;226:167–180.

42. Wu YG, Barad DH, Kushnir VA, *et al.* With low ovarian reserve, highly individualized egg retrieval (HIER) improves IVF results by avoiding premature luteinization. *J Ovarian Res* 2018;11:23.

43. Souza ALM, Sampaio M, Noronha GB, *et al.* Effect of follicular flushing on reproductive outcomes in patients with poor ovarian response undergoing assisted reproductive technology. *J Assist Reprod Genet* 2017;**34**:1353–1357.

44. Koning CH, Popp-Snijders C, Schoemaker J, Lambalk CB. Elevated FSH concentrations in imminent ovarian failure are associated with higher FSH and LH pulse amplitude and response to GnRH. *Hum Reprod* 2000;**15**:1452–1456.

45. Lukaszuk K, Kunicki M, Liss J, Bednarowska A, Jakiel G. Probability of live birth in women with extremely low anti-Müllerian hormone concentrations. *Reprod Biomed Online* 2014;**28**:64–69.

46. Zhang Y, Zhang C, Shu J, *et al.* Adjuvant treatment strategies in ovarian stimulation for poor responders undergoing IVF: a systematic review and network meta-analysis. *Hum Reprod Update* 2020;**26**:247–263.

Chapter

12

Ovarian Stimulation in Difficult IVF Cases

Amina Oumeziane and Samira Barbara

Introduction

Poor ovarian responders (PORs) are the most challenging patients in assisted reproductive technology (ART) and account for 9 to 24 percent of in vitro fertilization (IVF) patients [1]. The difficulties to classify these patients are due to the lack of clear definition, 47 randomized controlled trials (RCTs) and 41 different definitions were reported [2].

In 2011, an ESHRE consensus on the definition of poor response to ovarian stimulation for IVF was published to standardize the definition known as the Bologna criteria and a consensus was reached on the minimal criteria needed to define poor ovarian response (POR) [3].

At least two of the following three features must be present:

1. Advanced maternal age (≥ 40 years) or any other risk factor for POR
2. A previous POR (≤ 3 oocytes with a conventional stimulation protocol)
3. An abnormal ovarian reserve test (ORT); antral follicle count (AFC), 5–7 follicles; or

anti-Müllerian hormone (AMH), 0.5–1.1 ng/ml

Two episodes of poor ovarian response after maximal stimulation are sufficient to define a patient as poor responder in the absence of advanced maternal age or abnormal ORT.

PORs based on Bologna criteria have low pregnancy outcomes, which are independent of the age of patients (< 40 years or ≥ 40years); the live birth rate per cycle was 7.1% versus 5.2% (odds ratio [OR] 1.38, 95% confidence intervals [CI] 0.77–2.46) and the live birth rate per patient was 11.6% versus 8.8% (OR 1.36, 95% CI 0.75–2.46) [2].

Later, the Bologna criteria paper was questioned and different authors proposed its revision [4;5].

In 2016, a group of reproductive endocrinologists and scientists described another approach to stratify patients with poor ovarian response. The POSEIDON (Patient-Oriented Strategies Encompassing IndividualizeD Oocyte Number) criteria have been defined [6] (Figure 12.1).

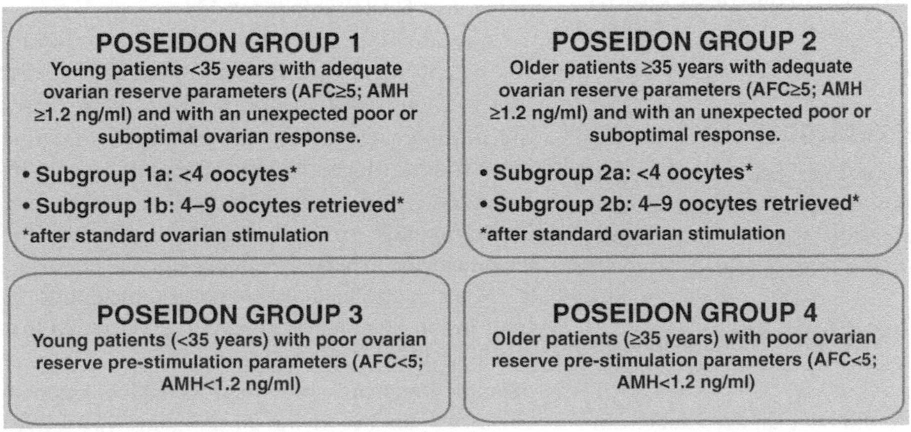

POSEIDON GROUP 1
Young patients <35 years with adequate ovarian reserve parameters (AFC≥5; AMH ≥1.2 ng/ml) and with an unexpected poor or suboptimal ovarian response.

• Subgroup 1a: <4 oocytes*
• Subgroup 1b: 4–9 oocytes retrieved*
*after standard ovarian stimulation

POSEIDON GROUP 2
Older patients ≥35 years with adequate ovarian reserve parameters (AFC≥5; AMH ≥1.2 ng/ml) and with an unexpected poor or suboptimal response.

• Subgroup 2a: <4 oocytes*
• Subgroup 2b: 4–9 oocytes retrieved*
*after standard ovarian stimulation

POSEIDON GROUP 3
Young patients (<35 years) with poor ovarian reserve pre-stimulation parameters (AFC<5; AMH<1.2 ng/ml)

POSEIDON GROUP 4
Older patients (≥35 years) with poor ovarian reserve pre-stimulation parameters (AFC<5; AMH<1.2 ng/ml)

Figure 12.1 POSEIDON classification. Haahr et al. [70].

Risk Factors of Poor Ovarian Responder Patients

The screening of POR patients remains an important step to optimize the management. Confusion exists between real poor ovarian response to treatment and potential causes of poor ovarian response. Many factors can lead to PORs, some of them are well established others are still controversial. The risk factors for ovarian aging have been determined and classified into: medical, life style, genetic, autoimmune, and idiopathic [7]. Iatrogenic factors such as surgery of endometrioma and ovarian cystectomy may be involved in ovarian aging and early menopause [8;9], as well as chemotherapy and radiotherapy, while uterine artery embolization is controversial [10]. It has been reported that endometrioma cyst could reduce the ovarian reserve [11]. More recently, low ovarian reserve was related to other risk factors such as diabetes mellitus type I [12] and transfusion-dependent beta-thalassemia [13]. It is also considered that family history of premature menopause, X chromosome derangement (i.e., mosaics deletions and translocation), fragile X mental retardation [14;15], and premature ovarian failure are responsible for low ovarian reserve [16]. Short menstrual cycle length, single ovary, chronic smoking, and unexplained infertility are also known as factors of poor ovarian reserve [14;15].

Predictive Markers of Ovarian Response

It has been demonstrated that AFC and AMH levels are the most important markers to predict ovarian response; these markers combined with women's age are correlated to outcomes. Ovarian reserve tests have to be assessed prior to ovarian stimulation [17;18].

Different Interventions

A variety of regimens have been employed to optimize the ovarian response of these women with disappointing results [19]. In this chapter different interventions will be reviewed.

GnRH Agonist and GnRH Antagonist Protocols

The best protocol should have an acceptable cancellation rate of cycle, and yield the maximum number possible of mature good-quality oocytes with a satisfactory pregnancy rate [20].

Both gonadotropin-releasing hormone (GnRH) agonists and GnRH antagonist aim to suppress luteinizing hormone (LH). In poor responders GnRH agonist may lead to over-suppression of the pituitary, requiring a high dose of gonadotropin; however, follicles are well synchronized [21]. GnRH antagonist avoids suppression of endogenous gonadotropin secretion at the stage of follicle recruitment. Otherwise, in poor responders follicles are often heterogeneous [22].

A Cochrane review was conducted to evaluate numerous interventions aiming to improve the controlled ovarian hyperstimulation (COH) and pregnancy outcomes in PORs; one of these interventions was to evaluate different regimens of pituitary downregulation.

GnRH agonist long protocol, long GnRH agonist stop protocol, mini-dose long agonist protocol, GnRH flare-up protocol, multidose GnRH antagonist protocol, in IVF cycles, were compared. The authors showed that there is insufficient evidence to identify a particular pituitary suppression regimen to improve outcomes due to the lack of definition of PORs, and to the incomplete data and heterogeneity of the trials [23].

In a meta-analysis including 1127 POR patients in 14 studies, the effectiveness of GnRH agonist and GnRH antagonist has been evaluated. The authors demonstrated that there is no significant difference in the number of oocytes retrieved, the number of mature oocytes, cancellation rate, and the clinical pregnancy rate, but there was a significant difference in duration of stimulation in favor of GnRH antagonist [24].

A randomized controlled trial (RCT) enrolling 37 patients who met Bologna criteria reported that the long GnRH agonist protocol increases the number of oocytes and estimated that one more oocyte increases the live birth rate by 5 percent. The study indicated that the long GnRH agonist protocol should be the first-line treatment for expected PORs [25].

More recently, a meta-analysis including 26 trials in the general IVF population concluded that the long GnRH agonist protocol showed higher ongoing pregnancy rate than GnRH antagonist, but in 6 trials out of the 26 including 780 PORs, there was no difference in ongoing pregnancy rate (relative risk 0.87, 95% CI 0.65–1.17) for GnRH antagonist versus GnRH agonist [26].

Gonadotropins and Oral Compounds

Maximizing gonadotropin dose in the COH aims to increase the oocyte number leading to higher live birth rate in fresh transfer [27]. It has been demonstrated that the increase in live birth rate is related to the oocyte number [28].

In expected PORs, there are few eggs to retrieve. To evaluate the effectiveness of low dose of gonadotropin with or without oral compounds (clomiphene (clomifene) citrate or letrozole) compared with high dose of gonadotropin, a systematic review was performed; 2104 POR patients were enrolled in 14 RCTs. No evidence of a difference in pregnancy outcomes, duration of stimulation, cancellation rate of the cycle, and number of embryos obtained was noted when low dose of gonadotropin alone was compared with high dose of gonadotropin. When low doses of gonadotropin with oral compounds were compared to gonadotropin alone, there were fewer metaphase II (MII) oocytes obtained, shorter duration of stimulation, lower total dose of gonadotropin used, and higher cancellation rate [29].

In 2018, the Practice Committee of the American Society for Reproductive Medicine recommended that in patients who are classified as poor responders and pursuing IVF cycles, strong consideration should be given to a mild ovarian stimulation protocol (low-dose gonadotropin with or without oral agents) due to lower costs and comparable low pregnancy rates compared with traditional IVF stimulation protocols [30].

LH Supplementation

Regarding the two-cell–two-gonadotropin theory, addition of LH to follicle-stimulating hormone (FSH) increases androgens in theca cells and induces follicular growth. Androgens stimulate FSH receptor expression in granulosa cells, growth factor, and increase the number of antral follicles to be recruited. In the midfollicular phase, LH binding to LH receptors in granulosa cells sustains FSH-dependent granulosa activities including aromatase induction and growth factor release and regulates final oocyte maturation [31].

In a systematic review concerning PORs, Lehert et al. showed that the number of oocytes retrieved and clinical pregnancy rate (CPR) were significantly higher in the group treated by recombinant LH (rLH) combined with recombinant FSH (rFSH) versus rFSH alone, it was suggested there was an increase in CPR of 30 percent for the patients who received rLH + rFSH [32].

The Cochrane review update in 2017 evaluated the effectiveness and safety of rLH combined with rFSH for ovarian stimulation compared with rFSH alone in women undergoing IVF cycles and suggested a higher ongoing pregnancy rate in PORs treated with GnRH analogue downregulation with rLH combined to rFSH compared with rFSH alone.

The ongoing pregnancy rate was higher in studies of low responder women when compared with studies not restricted to low responder women; this finding requires very cautious interpretation, as the subgroup of low responders was very small [33].

Conversely, in the ESPART study, a large RCT conducted by Humaidan et al. evaluated the efficacy and safety of follitropin alfa/lutropin alfa in ART. There were 939 POR women who were randomized using selection criteria that incorporate Bologna criteria. There was no statistically significant difference in the number of oocytes retrieved following COH between patients who received rFSH/rLH and those who received rFSH alone. The live birth rate was similar in both groups (10.6% and 11.7%, respectively with rFSH/rLH and rFSH alone) [34].

Otherwise, in a systematic review, Alviggi et al. evaluated the rLH supplementation in ART and concluded that rLH can be proposed for hyporesponders and women 36–39 years of age undergoing COH in IVF cycles [35].

Long-Acting Recombinant FSH (Corifollitropin Alfa)

Corifollitropin alfa is composed of FSH and carboxy-terminal peptide with a long elimination; half-life of 68 hours. Corifollitropin alfa reaches a peak serum concentration 24–45 hours after injection, while rFSH reaches its peak serum concentration after five days of stimulation. PORs may benefit from the particularity of corifollitropin alfa that allows small antral follicles to be exposed to high level of FSH in the early follicular phase thus securing recruitment and growth of these follicles [36].

The first study using corifollitropin alfa in PORs, published by Polyzos et al., showed that this molecule does not appear to significantly increase pregnancy rate [37]. Similar results were published by Kolibianakis *et al.* in a RCT, the burden of treatment and cost are reduced [38].

Adjuvants to Controlled Ovarian Hyperstimulation

Many adjuvants have been used in COH to enhance the success in IVF [39].

Androgens

Dehydroepiandrosterone (DHEA) is a steroid hormone produced in the ovarian theca cells and is a precursor of both testosterone and estradiol [39]. The first use of DHEA as adjuvant pretreatment in PORs in IVF was reported by Casson *et al.* [40].

It has been demonstrated that androgens increase the number of preantral follicles and protect follicles from atresia relating to the polycystic ovary syndrome (PCOS) model, and the different aspects of follicular development following androgen stimulation in various species have been investigated in both in vivo and in vitro studies [41;42].

Some data have been published promoting the efficacy of androgen use in IVF cycles as a pretreatment.

A Cochrane systematic review included 1496 POR patients in 17 RCTs. When DHEA or testosterone was compared with no treatment or placebo, the RCTs suggested that there will be a higher live birth rate and ongoing pregnancy rate in favor of DHEA or testosterone. However, no benefit was found when studies with bias were excluded [43].

In 2016, a systematic review reported an increase in clinical pregnancy, live birth, and implantation rate and a decrease in miscarriage rate [44]. More high-quality RCTs are required to determine the potential of routine use of DHEA with more precision of the dosage and the timing of administration [44;45].

Growth Hormone

Growth hormone is a peptide, synthesized and secreted by somatotroph cells in the anterior pituitary gland [46]. It appears that this hormone increases local production of insulin-like growth factor 1 (IGF-1). The IGF-1 stimulates follicular development, ovarian steroidogenesis, and oocyte maturation [47].

In a systematic review, including 169 PORs patients in six randomized trials, treated with GnRH agonist and gonadotropins, the addition of growth hormone resulted in a significant increase in clinical pregnancy and live birth rates, with a reduction in cycle cancellation [48]. This study included a heterogeneous population regarding the lack of definition, ovarian stimulation protocol employed, and the dose of growth hormone.

A Cochrane review reported that growth hormone addition to poor-responder patients in IVF protocols improved significantly the live birth and pregnancy rate. The authors recommended cautious interpretation of the results due to the limited number of trials included in the meta-analysis and the small sample size in the trials [46]. This finding has been recently confirmed in a systematic review with high evidence [49].

Estradiol Priming

Estradiol priming in the luteal phase in the GnRH antagonist protocol may induce FSH receptor formation in more resistant follicles and result in a more coordinated gonadotropin response [50]. The effectiveness of this approach to synchronize follicle growth and to optimize ovarian response to gonadotropin has been demonstrated [51].

In POR patients, estradiol priming to COH has been evaluated in a systematic review. An increase chance of CPR and a significant decrease of cycle cancellation were reported [52].

A Cochrane review concluded no clear evidence of a difference in live birth rate, ongoing pregnancy rate, or pregnancy loss, when estradiol was used as priming during COH with an antagonist protocol compared with either antagonist or agonist protocols without estradiol priming in a general IVF population [53].

Oral Contraceptive Pill (OCP)

Pretreatment with OCP in GnRH antagonist protocols is the most popular option for schedule cycles in IVF [54]. The OCP administration inhibits FSH and LH secretion and alters follicular growth [55].

Other negative impacts of OCP pretreatment are related to the low LH level which may impair oocyte competence and endometrial receptivity [56].

In 2010, a significantly lower pregnancy rate, -5 percent per patient with OCP pretreatment in GnRH antagonist protocol, was reported [56].

However, some studies reported no negative impact in GnRH antagonist OCP pretreatment on endometrial receptivity when stimulation was started after a washout period [54]. There is no modification in gene expression in the endometrium related to embryo implantation [57].

A Cochrane review including 1335 general population analyzed six RCTs and concluded live birth rate and ongoing pregnancy rate were lower in women with OCP pretreatment in GnRH antagonist cycles compared with cycles without OCP. There was no evidence of a difference in outcomes in low response patients [53].

Duo Stimulation

Duo stimulation, also known as double stimulation, was reported for the first time in a prospective study in 2014 by Kuang *et al.* [58]. A novel theory of follicular wave development has been reported recently, and based on this concept a new strategy of ovarian stimulation took place [59] (Figure 12.2).

The pilot study has successfully demonstrated that double stimulation is an effective strategy for providing more oocytes and more embryos, giving new hope for poor-responder patients [58].

This strategy combines a conventional ovarian stimulation in both follicular phase and luteal phase with embryo vitrification. More recently, studies showed that the oocytes collected from luteal phase stimulation are competent, as well as those collected from follicular phase stimulation in terms of blastocyst euploidy [60;61].

Dual Trigger for Final Oocyte Maturation

Introduction of a GnRH agonist trigger in GnRH antagonist protocols in IVF cycles provides the release of endogenous FSH and LH surge like in the natural cycle for maturation of follicles with the aim of a greater number of mature oocytes [62].

The dual trigger for final oocyte maturation – GnRH agonist combined with human chorionic gonadotropin – used in normal responder patients has showed an increase in clinical pregnancy, implantation, and live birth rate [63].

Unfortunately, this new concept of trigger, when tried for poor responder patients, has not yet proved to be efficient [64;65]. The lack of these studies was mostly the retrospective design with the small sample size. Further studies are required.

The Freeze-All and Embryo Banking Strategy

The recent advances in oocyte cryopreservation by the vitrification techniques allowed the development of new strategies for managing poor responder patients in IVF cycles.

High rate of dropout has been reported in conventional ovarian hyperstimulation in PORs [66]. Accumulation of oocytes or embryos from several COH cycles and replacement in subsequent thawed cycles appeared to be very promising with high live birth rate and cumulative live birth rate [66;67]. However, recent studies did not succeed in reproducing the same positive results [68].

Freeze-all in POR patients does not appear to be as efficient as it is in good-prognosis patients. Further studies are needed [69].

Summary

- ESHRE consensus on the definition of poor response to ovarian stimulation for IVF known as the Bologna criteria allowed better classification of POR patients and enhanced the quality studies. However, the management of PORs is still a challenge
- Different strategies were evaluated by many authors with conflicting results
- Downregulation regimens, maximizing dose of gonadotropins, and LH supplementation therapies do not appeared to improve the pregnancy outcomes. Androgens and growth hormones are not yet recommended in routine use; their efficacy has to be proven by well-designed studies
- Otherwise, mild ovarian stimulation protocol with or without oral agents is recommended by the practice committee of ASRM
- Dual stimulation seems to be a promising strategy for PORs
- At the moment, a new window of hope has been opened for POR patients by autologous stem cell ovarian transplant. Nevertheless, further works are needed to validate the preliminary findings

Acknowledgments

We would like to express our deepest appreciation to Professor Mohamed Aboulghar and Professor

113

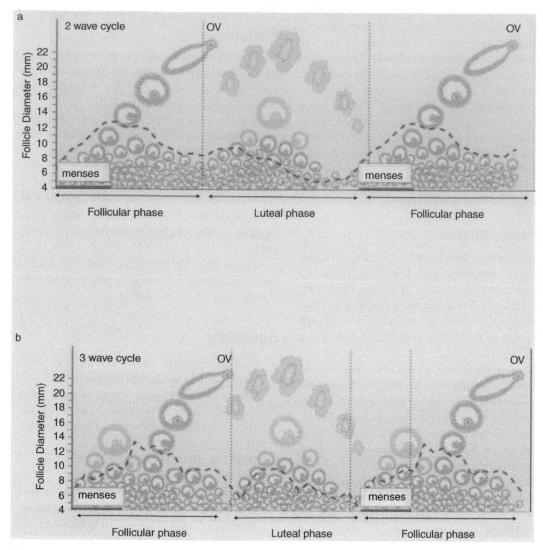

Figure 12.2 The wave theory of follicle recruitment suggests that two or more waves of antral follicles emerge during the ovarian cycle. In women with two follicular waves (a), an anovulatory wave emerged at the early luteal phase followed by emergence of the ovulatory wave during the early follicular phase. In women with three waves (b), an anovulatory wave emerged at the time of ovulation (ov), a second anovulatory wave emerged during the mid to late luteal phase and the ovulatory wave emerged in the early to mid-follicular phase. The dominant follicle develops in a minority of anovulatory waves. Follicle "cyclic recruitment" is the process by which a single "dominant" follicle is chosen from the recruited cohort or wave for preferential growth (modified with permission from Baerwald et al., 2012). From Sighinolfi G et al. [71], with permission.

Botros Rizk for giving us the opportunity to update the chapter of Ovarian hyperstimulation for poor responders from the first edition of *Ovarian Stimulation*.

We are thankful to Professor William B. Schoolcraft and Dr. Eric S. Surrey who gave us the permission to use the chapter as a basis for its revision.

Furthermore we would like to acknowledge with much appreciation Ms. Karima Djerroudib and Mrs. Fatima Nanouche for their crucial help and support.

References

1. Keay SD, Liversedge NH, Mathur RS, Jenkins JM. Assisted conception following poor ovarian response to gonadotrophin stimulation. *Br J Obstet Gynaecol* 1997;**104**(5):521–527.

2. Polyzos NP, Nwoye M, Corona R, *et al.* Live birth rates in Bologna poor responders treated with

ovarian stimulation for IVF/ICSI. *Reprod Biomed Online* 2014;**28**(4):469–474.

3. Ferraretti AP, La Marca A, Fauser BCJM, *et al.*; ESHRE working group on Poor Ovarian Response Definition. ESHRE consensus on the definition of 'poor response' to ovarian stimulation for in vitro fertilization: the Bologna criteria *Hum Reprod* 2011;**26**(7):1616–1624. https://doi.org/10.1093/humrep/der092.

4. Younis JS. The Bologna criteria for poor ovarian response; has the job been accomplished? *Hum Reprod* 2012;27(6): 1874–1875. https://doi.org/10.1093/humrep/des118.

5. Frydman R. Poor responders: still a problem *Fertil Steril* 2011;**96**(5):1057. https://doi.org/10.1016/j.fertnstert.2011.09.051.

6. Humaidan P, Alviggi C, Fischer R, Esteves SC. The novel POSEIDON stratification of 'Low prognosis patients in Assisted Reproductive Technology' and its proposed marker of successful outcome. *F1000Res* 2016;5:2911. doi:10.12688/f1000research.10382.1.

7. Younis JS. Ovarian aging and implications for fertility female health. *Minerva Endocrinol* 2012;**37**(1):41–57.

8. De Ziegler D, Borghese B, Chapron C. Endometriosis and infertility: pathophysiology and management. *Lancet* 2010;**376**(9742):730–738. doi:10.1016/S0140-6736(10)60490-4.

9. Coccia ME, Rizzello F, Mariani G, *et al.* Ovarian surgery for bilateral endometriomas influences age at menopause. *Hum Reprod* 2011;**26**(11):3000–3007. https://doi.org/10.1093/humrep/der286.

10. Wouter JK, Hehenkamp NA, Volkers FJM, *et al.* Loss of ovarian reserve after uterine artery embolization: a randomized comparison with hysterectomy. *Hum Reprod* 2007;**22**(7):1996–2005. https://doi.org/10.1093/humrep/dem105.

11. Almog B, Shehata F, Sheizaf B, Tan SL, Tulandi T. Effects of ovarian endometrioma on the number of oocytes retrieved for in vitro fertilization. *Fertil Steril* 2011;**95**(2):525–527.

12. Soto N, Iñiguez G, López P, *et al.* Anti-Müllerian hormone and inhibin B levels as markers of premature ovarian aging and transition to menopause in type 1 diabetes mellitus *Hum Reprod* 2009;**24**(11):2838–2844. https://doi.org/10.1093/humrep/dep276.

13. Chang H, Chen M, Lu M, *et al.* Iron overload is associated with low anti-müllerian hormone in women with transfusion-dependent β-thalassaemia. *BJOG* 2011;**118**: 825–831. doi:10.1111/j.1471-0528.2011.02927.x.

14. De Vos M, Devroey P, Fauser BC. Primary ovarian insufficiency. *Lancet* 2010;**376**(9744):911–921.

15. Fritz MA, Speroff L. *Clinical Gynecologic Endocrinology and Infertility*, 8th ed. Philadelphia: Wolters Kluwer Health/Lippincott Williams & Wilkins; 2011.

16. Persani L, Rossetti R, Cacciatore C. Genes involved in human premature ovarian failure. *J Mol Endocrinol* 2010;**45**(5):257–279. https://jme.bioscientifica.com/view/journals/jme/45/5/257.xml.

17. Broer SL, Dólleman M, van Disseldorp J, *et al.*; IPD-EXPORT Study Group. Prediction of an excessive response in in vitro fertilization from patient characteristics and ovarian reserve tests and comparison in subgroups: an individual patient data meta-analysis. *Fertil Steril* 2013;**100**(2):420.e7–429.e7.

18. La Marca A, Sunkara SK. Individualization of controlled ovarian stimulation in IVF using ovarian reserve markers: from theory to practice. *Hum Reprod Update* 2014;**20**(1):124–140. https://doi.org/10.1093/humupd/dmt037.

19. Surrey S, Schoolcraft WB. Evaluating strategies for improving ovarian response of the poor responder undergoing assisted reproductive techniques. *Fertil Steril* 2000;**73**(4):667–676.

20. Al-Inany H, Aboulghar M. GnRH antagonist in assisted reproduction: a Cochrane review. *Hum Reprod* 2002;**17**(4):874–885. https://doi.org/10.1093/humrep/17.4.874.

21. Land JA, Yarmolinskaya MI, Dumoulin JC, Evers JL. High-dose human menopausal gonadotropin stimulation in poor responders does not improve in vitro fertilization outcome. *Fertil Steril* 1996;**65**(5):961–965.

22. Tarlatzis BC, Zepiridis L, Grimbizis G, Bontis J. Clinical management of low ovarian response to stimulation for IVF: a systematic review. *Hum Reprod Update* 2003;**9**(1):61–76.

23. Pandian Z, McTavish AR, Aucott L, Hamilton MPR, Bhattacharya S. Interventions for 'poor responders' to controlled ovarian hyper stimulation (COH) in in-vitro fertilisation (IVF). *Cochrane Database Syst Rev* 2010;**1**:CD004379. doi: 10.1002/14651858.CD004379.pub3.

24. Pu D, Wu J, Liu J. Comparisons of GnRH antagonist versus GnRH agonist protocol in poor ovarian responders undergoing IVF. *Hum Reprod* 2011;**26**(10):2742–2749. https://doi.org/10.1093/humrep/der240.

25. Sunkara SK, Coomarasamy A, Faris R, Braude P, Khalaf Y. Long gonadotropin-releasing hormone agonist versus short agonist versus antagonist regimens in poor responders undergoing in vitro

fertilization: a randomized controlled trial. *Fertil Steril* 2014;**101**(1):147–153.

26. Lambalk CB, Banga FR, Huirne JA, *et al.* GnRH antagonist versus long agonist protocols in IVF: a systematic review and meta-analysis accounting for patient type. *Hum Reprod Update* 2017;**23** (5):560–579. https://doi.org/10.1093/humupd/dmx017.

27. Sunkara SK, Rittenberg V, Raine-Fenning N, *et al.* Association between the number of eggs and live birth in IVF treatment: an analysis of 400 135 treatment cycles. *Hum Reprod* 2011;**26**:1768–1774.

28. Drakopoulos P, Blockeel C, Stoop D, *et al.* Conventional ovarian stimulation and single embryo transfer for IVF/ICSI. How many oocytes do we need to maximize cumulative live birth rates after utilization of all fresh and frozen embryos? *Hum Reprod* 2016;**31**(2):370–376. https://doi.org/10.1093/humrep/dev316.

29. Youssef MA, van Wely M, Mochtar M, *et al.* Low dosing of gonadotropins in in vitro fertilization cycles for women with poor ovarian reserve: systematic review and meta-analysis. *Fertil Steril* 2017;**109**(2): 289–301.

30. Practice Committee of the American Society for Reproductive Medicine. Electronic address: ASRM@asrm.org. Comparison of pregnancy rates for poor responders using IVF with mild ovarian stimulation versus conventional IVF: a guideline *Fertil Steril* 2018;**109**(6):993–999.

31. Park J-Y, Su Y-Q, Ariga M, *et al.* EGF-like growth factors as mediators of LH action in the ovulatory follicle. *Science* 2004;**303**:682–684.

32. Lehert P, Kolibianakis EM, Venetis CA, *et al.* Recombinant human follicle-stimulating hormone (r-hFSH) plus recombinant luteinizing hormone versus r-hFSH alone for ovarian stimulation during assisted reproductive technology: systematic review and meta-analysis. *Reprod Biol Endocrinol* 2014;**12**:17. https://doi.org/10.1186/1477-7827-12-17.

33. Mochtar MH, Danhof NA, Ayeleke RO, Van der Veen F, van Wely M. Recombinant luteinizing hormone (rLH) and recombinant follicle stimulating hormone (rFSH) for ovarian stimulation in IVF/ICSI cycles. *Cochrane Database Syst Rev* 2017;**5**:CD005070. doi: 10.1002/14651858.CD005070.pub3.

34. Humaidan P, Chin W, Rogoff D, *et al.* Efficacy and safety of follitropin alfa/lutropin alfa in ART: a randomized controlled trial in poor ovarian responders. *Hum Reprod* 2017;**32**(7):1537–1538.

35. Alviggi C, Conforti A, Esteves SC, *et al.* Recombinant luteinizing hormone supplementation in assisted reproductive

technology: a systematic review. *Fertil Steril* 2018;**109**(4):644–664.

36. Fauser BC, Alper MM, Ledger W, *et al.* Pharmacokinetics and follicular dynamics of corifollitropin alfa versus recombinant FSH during ovarian stimulation for IVF. *Reprod Biomed Online* 2010;**21**(5):593–601.

37. Polyzos NP, Devos M, Humaidan P, *et al.* Corifollitropin alfa followed by rFSH in a GnRH antagonist protocol for poor ovarian responder patients: an observational pilot study. *Fertil Steril* 2013;**99**(2):422–426.

38. Kolibianakis EM, C.A. Venetis CA, J.K. Bosdou JK, *et al.* Corifollitropin alfa compared with follitropin beta in poor responders undergoing ICSI: a randomized controlled trial. *Hum Reprod* 2015;**30**(2):432–440. https://doi.org/10.1093/humrep/deu301.

39. Fabozzi G, Giannini A, Piscitelli VP, Colicchia A. Adjuvants therapies for women undergoing IVF: is there any evidence of their safety and efficacy? An updated mini-review. *Obstet Gynecol Int J* 2017;**7**(4):00254. doi: 10.15406/ogij.2017.07.00254.

40. Casson PR, Lindsay MS, Pisarska MD, Carson SA, Buster JE. Dehydroepiandrosterone supplementation augments ovarian stimulation in poor responders: a case series. *Hum Reprod* 2000;**15**(10):2129–2132.

41. Weil S, Vendola K, Zhou J, Bondy CA. Androgen and follicle-stimulating hormone interactions in primate ovarian follicle development. *J Clin Endocrinol Metab* 1999;**84** (8):2951–2956.

42. Prizant H, Gleicher N, Sen A. Androgen actions in the ovary: balance is key. *J Endocrinol* 2014;**222**(3): R141–R151. https://joe.bioscientifica.com/view/journals/joe/222/3/R141.xml.

43. Nagels HE, Rishworth JR, Siristatidis CS, Kroon B. Androgens (dehydroepiandrosterone or testosterone) for women undergoing assisted reproduction. *Cochrane Database Syst Rev* 2015;**11**:CD009749. doi:10.1002/14651858.CD009749.pub2.

44. Zhang M, Niu W, Wang Y, *et al.* Dehydroepiandrosterone treatment in women with poor ovarian response undergoing IVF or ICSI: a systematic review and meta-analysis. *J Assist Reprod Genet* 2016;**33**:981–991. doi 10.1007/s10815-016-0713-5.

45. Haahr T, Esteves SC, Humaidan P. Individualized controlled ovarian stimulation in expected poor-responders: an update. *Reprod Biol Endocrinol* 2018;**16**(1):20. doi:10.1186/s12958-018-0342-1.

46. Duffy JMN, Ahmad G, Mohiyiddeen L, Nardo LG, Watson A. Growth hormone for in vitro fertilization. *Cochrane Database Syst Rev* 2010;**1**: CD000099. doi: 10.1002/14651858.CD000099 .pub3.

47. Yoshimura Y, Ando M, Nagamatsu S, *et al.* Effects of insulin-like growth factor-I on follicle growth, oocyte maturation, and ovarian steroidogenesis and plasminogen activator activity in the rabbit. *Biol Reprod* 1996;**55**(1):152–160.

48. Kolibianakis E, Venetis C, Diedrich K, Tarlatzis B, Griessinger G. Addition of growth hormone to gonadotropins in ovarian stimulation of poor responders treated by in-vitro fertilization: a systemic review and meta-analysis. *Hum Reprod Update* 2009;**15**:613–622.

49. Jeve YB, Bhandari HM. Effective treatment protocol for poor ovarian response: a systematic review and meta-analysis. *J Hum Reprod Sci* 2016;**9**:70–81.

50. Fanchin R, Cunha-Filho JS, Schonäuer LM, *et al.* Coordination of early antral follicles by luteal estradiol administration provides a basis for alternative controlled ovarian hyperstimulation regimens. *Fertil Steril* 2003;**79**:316–321.

51. Fanchin R, Salomon L, Castelo-Branco A, *et al.* Luteal estradiol pre-treatment coordinates follicular growth during controlled ovarian hyperstimulation with GnRH antagonists. *Hum Reprod* 2003;**18**(12):2698–2703. https://doi.org/10 .1093/humrep/deg516.

52. Reynolds KA, Omurtag KR, Jimenez PT, *et al.* Cycle cancellation and pregnancy after luteal estradiol priming in women defined as poor responders: a systematic review and meta-analysis. *Hum Reprod* 2013;**28**(11):2981–2989.

53. Farquhar C, Rombauts L, Kremer JAM, Lethaby A, Ayeleke RO. Oral contraceptive pill, progestogen or oestrogen pretreatment for ovarian stimulation protocols for women undergoing assisted reproductive techniques. *Cochrane Database Syst Rev* 2017;**5**:CD006109. doi: 10.1002/14651858 .CD006109.pub3.

54. Garcia-Velasco JA, Fatemi HM. To pill or not to pill in GnRH antagonist cycles: that is the question! *Reprod Biomed Online* 2014;**30** (1):39–42.

55. Cédrin-Durnerin B, Bständig I, Parneix V, *et al.* Effects of oral contraceptive, synthetic progestogen or natural estrogen pre-treatments on the hormonal profile and the antral follicle cohort before GnRH antagonist protocol. *Hum Reprod* 2007;**22**(1):109–116. https://doi.org/10.1093/ humrep/del340.

56. Griesinger G, Kolibianakis EM, Venetis C, Diedrich K, Tarlatzis B. Oral contraceptive pretreatment significantly reduces ongoing pregnancy likelihood in gonadotropin-releasing hormone antagonist cycles: an updated meta-analysis. *Fertil Steril* 2010;**94**(6):2382–2384.

57. Bermejo A, Iglesias C, Ruiz-Alonso M, *et al.* The impact of using the combined oral contraceptive pill for cycle scheduling on gene expression related to endometrial receptivity. *Hum Reprod* 2014;**29** (6):1271–1278. https://doi.org/10.1093/humrep/ deu065.

58. Kuang Y, Chen Q, Hong Q, *et al.* Double stimulations during the follicular and luteal phases of poor responders in IVF/ICSI programmes (Shanghai protocol). *Reprod Biomed Online* 2014; **29**(6):684–691.

59. Baerwald AR, Adams GP, Pierson RA. Characterization of ovarian follicular wave dynamics in women. *Biol Reprod* 2003;**69** (3):1023–1031. https://doi.org/10.1095/biolreprod .103.017772.

60. Ubaldi FM, Capalbo A, Vaiarelli A, *et al.* Follicular versus luteal phase ovarian stimulation during the same menstrual cycle (DuoStim) in a reduced ovarian reserve population results in a similar euploid blastocyst formation rate: new insight in ovarian reserve exploitation. *Fertil Steril* 2016;**105**:1488.e1–1495.e1.

61. Cimadomo D, Vaiarelli A, Colamaria S, *et al.* Luteal phase anovulatory follicles result in the production of competent oocytes: intra-patient paired case-control study comparing follicular versus luteal phase stimulations in the same ovarian cycle. *Hum Reprod* 2018;**33**(8):1442–1448. https://doi.org/10.1093/humrep/dey217.

62. Humaidan P, Ejdrup Bredkjær H, Bungum L, *et al.* GnRH agonist (buserelin) or hCG for ovulation induction in GnRH antagonist IVF/ICSI cycles: a prospective randomized study. *Hum Reprod* 2005;**20**(5):1213–1220. https://doi.org/10.1093/ humrep/deh765.

63. Lin MH, Wu FS, Lee RK, *et al.* Dual trigger with combination of gonadotropin-releasing hormone agonist and human chorionic gonadotropin significantly improves the live-birth rate for normal responders in GnRH-antagonist cycles. *Fertil Steril* 2013;**100**(5):1296–1302.

64. Zhang J, Wang Y, Mao X, *et al.* Dual trigger of final oocyte maturation in poor ovarian responders undergoing IVF/ICSI cycles. *Reprod Biomed Online* 2017;**35**(6):701–707.

65. Eser A, Devranoğlu B, Bostanc Ergen E, Yayla Abide Ç. Dual trigger with gonadotropin-releasing hormone and human chorionic gonadotropin for

poor responders. *J Turk Ger Gynecol Assoc* 2018;**19**(2):98–103.

66. Cobo A, Garrido N, Crespo J, José R, Pellicer A. Accumulation of oocytes: a new strategy for managing low-responder patients. *Reprod Biomed Online* 2012;**24**(4):424–432.

67. Chatziparasidou A, Nijs M, Moisidou M, *et al.* Accumulation of oocytes and/or embryos by vitrification: a new strategy for managing poor responder patients undergoing pre implantation diagnosis. *F1000Res* 2014;**2**:240.

68. Çelik S, Turgut NE, Cengiz Çelik D, *et al.* The effect of the pooling method on the live birth rate in poor ovarian responders according to the Bologna criteria. *Turk J Obstet Gynecol* 2018;**15**(1):39–45.

69. Roque M, Valle M, Sampaio M, Geber S. Does freeze-all policy affect IVF outcomes in poor responders? *Ultrasound Obstet Gynecol* 2018;**52**(4):530–534. https://doi.org/10.1002/uog.19000.

70. Haahr T, Esteves SC, Humaidan P. Individualized controlled ovarian stimulation in expected poor-responders: an update. *Reprod Biol Endocrinol* 2018;**16**(1):20. doi:10.1186/s12958-018-0342-1.

71. Sighinolfi G, Sunkara SK, La Marca A. New strategies of ovarian stimulation based on the concept of ovarian follicular waves: from conventional to random and double stimulation. *Reprod Biomed Online* 2018;**37**(4):489–497.

Polycystic Ovary Syndrome: Ovulation Induction Strategies

13

Lina El-Taha, Botros Rizk, William Ledger, Raja Sayegh, and Johnny Awwad

Introduction

Polycystic ovarian syndrome (PCOS) is one of the most prevalent endocrinopathies affecting 5 to 10 percent of women of reproductive age [1;2]. Characteristic clinical features of PCOS include menstrual irregularity such as oligomenorrhea/amenorrhea and signs of hyperandrogenemia including hirsutism, acne, and/or obesity. The syndrome was first clearly described by Stein and Leventhal in 1935 [3]. While the primary etiology remains poorly defined [4], insulin resistance with compensatory hyperinsulinemia is a prominent feature of the condition and appears to be an underlying cause of hyperandrogenemia identified in both lean and obese women [5]. Hyperinsulinemia promotes increased ovarian androgen biosynthesis in vivo and in vitro [6;7]. It also decreases sex hormone-binding globulin production in the liver [8], which results in the increased bioavailability of free androgens and exacerbates the signs of androgen excess.

PCOS is a heterogeneous condition with concurrent symptoms, signs, and biochemical features. As such, a universal definition of this disorder integrating the various diagnostic features relative to each other has been the subject of much debate. In 1990, the National Institute of Health concluded that hyperandrogenism and menstrual dysfunction are the major criteria for diagnosing PCOS after excluding other known disorders [9]. In 2003, a joint meeting of the European Society of Human Reproduction and Embryology (ESHRE) and the American Society for Reproductive Medicine (ASRM) in Rotterdam revised the definition of PCOS and incorporated ultrasonographic features [10]. Accordingly, the diagnosis of PCOS requires two of the following three criteria:

1. Oligo- and/or anovulation
2. Hyperandrogenism (clinical and/or biochemical)
3. Polycystic ovaries, with the exclusion of other etiologies such as congenital adrenal hyperplasia due to 21-hydroxylase deficiency

The definition was later refined to encompass a description of the morphology of the polycystic ovary. The criteria required to diagnose a polycystic ovary on ultrasound scan include at least one of the following: either 12 or more follicles measuring 2–9 mm in diameter or increased ovarian volume (> 10 cm³). The distribution of the follicles and the description of the stroma are not required in this diagnosis.

While the debate on a universal definition of PCOS is far from settled, a characterization that incorporates a critical number of clinical and/or biochemical abnormalities has been suggested. This allows the appreciation of the complexity of PCOS as a spectrum of phenotypes with various severities, metabolic and reproductive implications [11].

1. Phenotype A: Frank PCOS (ovulatory dysfunction, hyperandrogenism, PCO morphology)
2. Phenotype B: Ovulatory PCOS (hyperandrogenism, PCO morphology, regular cycles)
3. Phenotype C: Non-PCO PCOS (hyperandrogenism, ovulatory dysfunction)
4. Phenotype D: Normoandrogenic PCOS (ovulatory dysfunction, PCO morphology)

Obesity and Lifestyle Interventions

Obesity is a condition characterized by excessive storage of triglycerides in adipose cells and is defined as a body mass index (BMI) higher than 30 kg/m² [12]. While the overall prevalence of obesity has increased dramatically over the past few decades, it is estimated that 40 to 60 percent of women with PCOS are overweight or obese depending on the population and ethnic group of interest [13–15]. Obese PCOS women have greater abdominal/visceral adiposity compared with weight-matched controls which further worsens insulin resistance and compensatory hyperinsulinemia [16].

Pathophysiology

This condition contributes to a large number of health problems, including type II diabetes, hypertension, coronary heart disease, dyslipidemia, respiratory dysfunction, sleep apnea, non-alcoholic steatohepatitis, reflux esophagitis, osteoarthritis, urinary incontinence, and increases in breast, endometrial, ovarian, and colon cancers [17]. In addition to medical complications, obesity has an adverse effect on fertility. In 2017, the National Institute for Health and Care Excellence (NICE) published guidelines regarding the assessment and treatment of infertility, and recommended that women with a BMI of more than 29 kg/m^2 should be informed that they are likely to take longer to conceive. If not ovulating, they should be informed that losing weight is likely to increase their chance of conception [18]. This is in concordance with findings of the Pregnancy in Polycystic Ovary Syndrome II (PPCOS II) trial of increased time to live birth with increased BMI [19;20].

To date, the etiology of the metabolic syndrome in PCOS women has not been entirely elucidated; nevertheless, obesity has been proposed as an underlying contributor in these patients [21]. In obese patients, adipose tissue secretes fatty acids and tumor necrosis factor-α (TNF-α) which play a role in the development and worsening of insulin resistance [22].

Clinical Correlates

Furthermore, obesity has a substantial influence on the manifestations of PCOS. Menstrual irregularity in obese women correlates with elevated BMI and increased truncal obesity, thereby contributing to decreased fertility [23–25]. Excess weight might promote a more severe phenotype of PCOS in susceptible women [26]. Even in ovulatory women, obesity appears to decrease fecundity [27]. Obesity is also associated with an increased risk of pregnancy loss [28], and when pregnant these women are at an increased risk of obstetrical complications such as pre-eclampsia, gestational diabetes, and cesarean delivery [29;30].

For those women who are obese and require medically assisted reproduction (MAR), the evidence regarding obesity and its effect on assisted conception is conflicting. A review article highlighted the controversy of evidence regarding effect of obesity on assisted reproductive treatments [31]. Several chart review studies reported adverse effects of obesity on assisted reproductive technology (ART) outcomes including lower implantation, pregnancy, and live birth rates, as well as higher spontaneous miscarriage rates [32;33]. A large retrospective study of 5019 in vitro fertilization (IVF) cycles revealed that obesity was associated with a longer duration of stimulation, increased amount of gonadotropin consumption, increased frequency of cycle cancellation, and lower oocyte yield [28]. This review did not identify an association between obesity and poor embryo quality, nonetheless. Conversely, other retrospective studies showed conflicting results suggesting comparable outcomes in women undergoing MAR irrespective of their obesity status. These studies showed no significant adverse effects of obesity on ovarian response during controlled ovarian stimulation in ART cycles [34–36]. Cycle characteristics, follicular response, and oocyte efficiency parameters were comparable between obese and non-obese women [35]. Similarly, there was no significant difference in the reproductive outcomes including implantation and pregnancy rates [34]. These findings were also recently confirmed by a large retrospective study of the Latin American registry of ART involving more than 100 000 women undergoing intracytoplasmic sperm injection over four years. Though obesity was found to be associated with increased odds of cycle cancellation and decreased number of oocytes retrieved; obesity was not associated with a change in odds for miscarriages and live births after adjusting for age, number of embryos transferred, and stage of embryo development at transfer [37].

On the other hand, the evidence regarding the effect of obesity on oocyte and embryo quality is no less controversial. While several studies suggest that obesity has an adverse effect on oocyte and embryo quality [38–43], other studies do not concur [44].

A recent review of the literature concluded that obesity is associated with a progressive worsening of pregnancy outcomes with increasing BMI in fresh ART and donor/recipient cycles

[45;46]. A systematic review of 33 IVF studies including more than 47 000 cycles emphasized the negative impact of obesity on reproductive outcomes [47]. However, this meta-analysis was limited by the heterogeneity of studies included and the bias of reporting outcomes per cycle rather than per woman. Despite the general consensus on the effects of obesity on outcomes of MAR, it is important to note that the majority of studies are retrospective in nature with no evidence derived from randomized trials to guide best practice management. This does not exclude, nonetheless, the need to counsel obese women planning ART about pregnancy outcomes and complications related to obesity before receiving fertility treatment.

Lifestyle Interventions

It follows that obese PCOS patients should also be advised that weight loss may potentially restore menstrual cyclicity, and improve hormonal profile, inflammatory markers, and fecundity.

Many inflammatory markers have been correlated to the severity of both PCOS and obesity and were suggested to be reflective of improvement after weight loss. C-reactive protein (CRP), secreted by the liver in response to circulating cytokines mainly TNF-α and interleukin 6, is commonly elevated with insulin resistance and metabolic syndrome [48]. Though not consistent, possibly due to individual genetic polymorphism, increased CRP level is also positively correlated to severity of obesity by virtue of increased adipose tissue and subsequent cytokine levels [49;50]. Adiponectin is yet another inflammatory marker with insulin-sensitizing properties and anti-inflammatory effects which is secreted by adipocytes [51]. An inverse relationship exists between adiponectin and CRP levels such as obese PCOS patients tend to have higher CRP levels and lower adiponectin levels [52;53]. Many studies have illustrated how weight loss decreases CRP and increases adiponectin levels in both obese PCOS patients and obese non-PCOS patients [54;55], which are paralleled by improved insulin sensitivity [56].

The first-line treatment for PCOS women is therefore weight loss with lifestyle modifications including calorie restriction and regular exercise. A multidisciplinary approach is required to achieve the optimal results incorporating the assistance of dieticians and counselors. It has been shown that women participating in structured weight loss programs involving a behavioral modification component are more successful than those who attempt weight loss on their own [57;58]. In addition to lifestyle changes pharmacotherapy may be beneficial to a subpopulation of patients. The majority of currently FDA approved pharmacological agents for weight loss promote satiety. These include phentermine, combination of phentermine and extended release topiramate, bupropion, combination of bupropion and naltrexone, and lorcaserin. Few medication classes are associated with weight loss without targeting appetite mechanisms: orlistat, liraglutide, and SGLT-2 inhibitors [59;60]. Extreme caution is to be practiced in the use of pharmacological agents as they may be associated with side effects. One such example is orlistat, a lipase inhibitor which decreases the absorption of fat from the intestine by 30 percent. However, it also decreases the absorption of fat-soluble vitamins, such as vitamin D [61]. The ASRM recommends supplementation with a multivitamin containing vitamin D at least 2 hours before or after orlistat treatment [17]. Patients should be advised about the gastrointestinal side effects of this medication and its contraindication in cholestasis and malabsorption syndromes.

However appealing, the magnitude of the weight loss usually attained after implementation of dietary modifications in combination with increased physical activity is usually 5 to 10 percent of the initial body weight, which has been shown to be sufficient to improve the chance of natural conception [62]. Maintenance of weight loss is challenging and usually short-lived. Under very specific circumstances and strict criteria, surgical management of obesity has shown to be an effective alternative therapeutic approach for ameliorating the metabolic dysfunction in PCOS patients when lifestyle modifications and pharmacological intervention have failed in attaining the goal.

Increasingly, bariatric surgery is being used in the treatment of morbid obesity to ameliorate obesity-related medical problems such as diabetes and hypertension. In addition, this surgery has been shown to improve menstrual regularity and fertility in women [63]. There is plenty of evidence supporting the efficacy of bariatric surgery not only in significantly reducing weight of obese PCOS women but also in decreasing hirsutism score, androstenedione, dehydroepiandrosterone sulfate, and testosterone levels, and in improving insulin resistance [64;65].

The success of the surgery is dependent on the careful selection of patients. In addition to BMI, adjunct selection criteria include failed dietary therapy, psychological stability, high motivation, knowledge of the operation and its sequelae, and most importantly the likelihood of surviving surgery [17]. The patients should be informed that pregnancy is not recommended in the first year following bariatric surgery as this is the time when the majority of weight loss occurs [17]. Studies have shown that previous bariatric surgery is not associated with an increased risk of adverse perinatal outcomes [66–68], but the incidence of anemia due to iron, folate, vitamin B12, and nutritional deficiencies may be increased [17].

The treatment of subfertility is one in which many patients may feel a loss of control, but lifestyle is a contributing factor which only the motivated patient can change. Although lifestyle alterations, including diet modification and regular exercise, are the essential steps in a weight loss program, inevitably weight will be regained when lifestyle changes are not maintained. Most expert opinions and guidelines indicate the necessity for weight loss in obese women before MAR on the basis of the documented impact of obesity on pregnancy outcomes and complications in natural conceptions. For example, the national guidelines in the UK for managing women with PCOS who are overweight primarily advise weight loss preferably to a BMI < 30 kg/m^2 prior to commencing ovulation induction medications. Public funding for MAR may be withheld by authorities before the imposed BMI threshold is attained. Despite epidemiological studies suggesting a clear link between obesity and the chances of fertility in women seeking natural conception, the findings of well-designed randomized clinical trials evaluating the effects of a lifestyle program before MAR on reproductive outcomes found no compelling evidence of the value of weight loss intervention on live birth rates [69–71].

In a randomized trial of 577 women with a BMI of ≥ 29 kg/m^2, the Dutch LIFESTYLE program evaluated a 6-month program with the goal of losing 5% to 10% of body weight [69]. Despite a statistically significant mean weight loss of 4.4 kg, less singleton live births were delivered vaginally at term in the intervention group

(27%) compared with controls (35%) (odds ratio [OR] 0.77, 95% confidence interval [CI] 0.60–0.99). It should be noted nonetheless that the intervention arm showed a higher spontaneous pregnancy rate prior to the start of ART and high cancellation rates. In a similar study design of 317 women with a BMI between 30 and 35 kg/m^2, a Swedish study evaluated the impact of an intensive 16-week weight reduction program on ART outcome [70]. Following a mean weight reduction of 9.44 kg in the intervention group and a mean weight gain of 1.19 kg in the control group, live birth rates were comparable (29.6% and 27.5%, respectively) with no statistically significant differences in miscarriage rates or obstetric outcomes between the two study arms. Subgroup analysis showed no statistical improvement in live birth rates in PCOS women who achieved a BMI of 25 kg/m^2 or less in the intervention group.

In the absence of compelling evidence of the value of lifestyle intervention for weight loss on live birth rates after MAR, and considering the biological and psychological adverse effects of time delay when ART is warranted, it may be neither medically nor ethically justified to deny reproductive care to obese women on the basis of their BMI [71].

Ovulation Induction: Oral Agents

If lifestyle changes and weight loss to attain a healthy BMI fail to achieve ovulatory cycles in PCOS women, or if the benefit of weight loss is outweighed by the risk of declining fertility potential with advancing age, the next step is the use of pharmacotherapy.

Clomiphene Citrate

Traditionally, clomiphene (clomifene) citrate has been the standard treatment for induction of ovulation in women with anovulatory infertility for many years [72]. Clomiphene citrate is a selective estrogen receptor modulator which acts by competitive inhibition of estrogen binding to estrogen receptors, resulting in mixed agonist and antagonist action depending on the target tissue. Clomiphene citrate affects ovulation induction mainly by binding to estrogen receptors of the hypothalamus, pituitary, and ovary blocking the negative feedback effect of endogenous estrogen, leading to increased stimulation by endogenous gonadotropins [73]. However, unlike endogenous estrogen, the prolonged binding of clomiphene citrate to nuclear estrogen receptors downregulates these receptors [74]. The effectiveness of clomiphene citrate for induction of ovulation in normally estrogenized women is well established. Studies have shown an ovulation rate of 60–85% and a pregnancy rate of 30–40% [75–77]. The discrepancy between ovulation and pregnancy rate has been attributed to the antiestrogenic effects of clomiphene on the uterus, cervix, and vagina, resulting in a thin endometrial lining [78–80] and poor cervical mucus [77;81]. Clomiphene citrate is conventionally commenced on day 2 to 6 of the cycle and prescribed for five days. If the patient is oligo/amenorrheic, it is necessary to exclude pregnancy and then induce a withdrawal bleed with a course of either medroxyprogesterone acetate or norethisterone. The starting dose of clomiphene citrate is 50 mg which may be increased by increments of 50 mg in subsequent cycles until ovulation is achieved, for a maximum dose of 150 mg/day. However, the maximum dose approved by the FDA for ovulation induction is 100 mg/day in accordance with ASRM suggestion that doses over 100 mg/day contributes minimally to increasing clinical pregnancy rate [74]. When couples with other factors contributing to subfertility are excluded, the cumulative conception rate continues to rise after six months of treatment with clomiphene citrate, reaches a plateau by treatment cycle 12, and approaches that of the normal population [82]. It has been accepted that a single midluteal serum progesterone measurement is adequate to assess ovulation [83;84].

The Royal College of Obstetricians and Gynaecologists (RCOG) published guidelines advise that patients should be informed of the risks of multiple pregnancy when prescribed clomiphene citrate. Centers are encouraged to adopt protocols which minimize the risk of ovarian hyperstimulation and multiple pregnancy rate which may be 10 times that of spontaneous pregnancy [85]. Expert groups, such as RCOG and NICE, advise that ovulation induction with clomiphene should be performed in circumstances which allow access to ovarian ultrasound monitoring. Serial pelvic ultrasonography provides accurate monitoring of follicular development which helps to reduce the risk of multiple pregnancy and provides information as to the endometrial thickness, which is the minimal distance between the echogenic interfaces of myometrium and endometrium, measured in the plane through the central longitudinal axis of the uterine body [86]. Studies suggest a minimal endometrial thickness of 7–8 mm to be a prerequisite for successful embryo implantation during IVF cycles [87–90]. Some women may respond to treatment in terms of follicle development but have a thin endometrium which is believed to decrease their chance of success. These women may benefit from hysteroscopic assessment of their uterine cavity to investigate any potential underlying cause of poor endometrial development such as uterine adhesions. Suboptimal endometrial development is not a condition synonymous with PCOS. PCOS patients tend to be well estrogenized and as a result of prolonged periods of oligo/amenorrhea are at risk of endometrial hyperplasia which if untreated may result in endometrial cancer. Hence the importance of inducing artificial cycles in amenorrheic PCOS patients. In addition, pelvic ultrasonography enables the time of ovulation to be identified accurately, ensuring correct timing of intercourse, which is particularly helpful in women with a variable cycle length. It is also possible to identify either those patients who do not develop a dominant follicle in response to clomiphene (clomiphene resistant) or those with multiple follicles who are at risk of multiple pregnancy, and to adjust the dose or medication used in a subsequent cycle.

The factors influencing response to clomiphene citrate and treatment outcome are unclear but there is evidence to suggest that increased BMI adversely affects response to clomiphene [91;92]. It is estimated that 15 to 25 percent of women may fail to ovulate in response to clomiphene treatment. Predictors of clomiphene resistance have been shown to be advancing age, menstrual history, insulin resistance, ovarian volume, and androgen index [93]. In normogonadotropic PCOS, about 47 percent of women are expected to conceive during the first three months of clomiphene citrate treatment, and 73 percent following nine months of treatment. Predictive modeling found age and menstrual history to be the most powerful predictors of pregnancy outcome after clomiphene therapy. Primarily, female age may represent an important factor influencing ovulatory response, pregnancy outcome, and risk of multiple pregnancy after clomiphene treatment, as the age-dependent decline in female fertility is well documented [94]. The NICE published guidelines in 2016 concurred with the RCOG recommendations in terms of patient education regarding the risk of multiple pregnancy associated with clomiphene treatment. It has also been suggested that administration of clomiphene for more than 12 months may be associated with an increased risk of ovarian cancer [95] although several subsequent studies have failed to confirm this suggestion. Nonetheless, the Policy and Practice Subcommittee of the British Fertility Society (BFS) has recommended limiting the use of clomiphene to 6 months [96].

Aromatase Inhibitors

Recently, an aromatase inhibitor namely letrozole has been suggested as a first-line agent for ovulation induction in PCOS patients as an alternative to clomiphene citrate for the purpose of avoiding antiestrogenic effects and/or as a second-line agent in cases of clomiphene resistance [97]. Letrozole is a non-steroidal, reversible aromatase inhibitor which was initially used in the treatment of postmenopausal breast cancer. Letrozole inhibits the conversion of androgens to estrogen, resulting in an increase of follicle-stimulating hormone (FSH) following release of the hypothalamus–pituitary axis from the negative feedback of excessive estradiol. Evidence suggests that aromatase inhibitors are effective in the induction of ovulation in WHO type II anovulation [98;99]. In comparison to clomiphene citrate, treatment with letrozole does not require the same intensity of serial ultrasound monitoring of follicular development as the risk of multifollicular development is relatively low. In contrast to clomiphene, letrozole does not deplete estrogen receptors. Therefore, as the dominant follicle develops, increasing estradiol level suppresses FSH resulting mainly in monofollicular development [100]. This is particularly advantageous in PCOS patients who are at risk of hyperstimulation. A second advantage is the avoidance of the antiestrogenic effects seen with clomiphene. A cohort study reviewed the clinical outcome of pregnancies following the administration of aromatase inhibitors for ovulation induction or controlled ovarian stimulation for intrauterine insemination and compared the outcomes with pregnancies achieved

following other ovarian stimulation techniques and those occurring spontaneously [101]. Pregnancies conceived after aromatase inhibitor treatments were associated with comparable miscarriage and ectopic pregnancy rates to all other groups, including the spontaneous conceptions. Letrozole use was found to be associated with a significantly lower rate of multiple gestation compared with clomiphene citrate (4.3% vs. 22%, respectively). These results were reaffirmed in the PPCOS II randomized trial which showed significantly higher cumulative live birth rates after letrozole (27.5% vs. 19.1%, respectively; $p = 0.007$), and higher cumulative ovulation rates (61.7% vs. 48.3%, respectively; $p < 0.001$). Miscarriage rates were comparable in women who received letrozole and women who received clomiphene (31.8% vs. 29.1%, respectively) [20]. BMI tertile was a significant factor in the primary outcome of live birth, as women with elevated BMI showed more improvement in outcomes with letrozole treatment. Although this study was underpowered for detection of significant difference in multiple gestation rate, letrozole was found to be associated with lower twin pregnancy rate compared with clomiphene.

The 2018 Cochrane review which included 42 randomized controlled trials (RCTs) and over 7000 women concluded that letrozole is superior to clomiphene in terms of live birth rate (OR 1.64, 95% CI 1.32–2.04) and increased clinical pregnancy rate (OR 1.40, 95% CI 1.18–1.65) with comparable miscarriage rates [102].

In an abstract presentation at the 2005 annual ASRM meeting, letrozole use was suggested to increase the risk of fetal cardiac and skeletal malformations following ovulation induction [103]. Though the presented evidence was of poor quality and the study was never published in a peer-reviewed journal, this prompted the manufacturer to add a label warning for use of letrozole in premenopausal women. A subsequent multicenter study did not find any increase in the rates of major and minor malformations in newborns conceived after letrozole treatment [104]. The study included 911 babies, 514 born after letrozole treatment and 397 after clomiphene treatment. Reassuringly, the incidence of cardiac anomalies in the letrozole group was slightly lower than the rate of congenital cardiac anomalies reported among all births (0.4–1.2%).

Based on current evidence, the American College of Obstetrics and Gynecology (ACOG) revised its recommendations to consider letrozole as first-line agent for ovulation induction in women with PCOS regardless of BMI [105]. It is important to note however that when prescribing letrozole, patients should be counseled that it is not FDA approved for ovulation induction and is used off label. As such, RCOG continues to recommend clomiphene as first-line agent.

Ovulation Induction: Adjunctive Therapy

Insulin-Sensitizing Agents

Metformin, a biguanide and insulin-sensitizing drug used in the treatment of type 2 diabetes mellitus, has been introduced in the treatment of anovulation in PCOS women since 1994 [106]. Metformin gained popularity due to the prevalence of insulin resistance in PCOS, and also due to a lower risk of multiple pregnancy and ovarian cyst formation when compared with clomiphene treatment. Although not proven to decrease weight in obese PCOS women [107–109], metformin treatment can decrease the risk of progression to diabetes by 31 percent in prediabetics [110]. Prior to commencing metformin, a baseline investigation is recommended, including an oral glucose tolerance test, full blood count, urea and electrolytes, and liver function tests. Side effects of this medication are predominantly gastrointestinal and may be reduced by a gradual increase in dose and by taking the medication preprandially. The most serious side effect of this treatment is lactic acidosis, but the risk is minimal in non-diabetic women with normal renal and liver function. Metformin is contraindicated in the presence of renal impairment for this reason and it is important to discontinue treatment with metformin for three days following the administration of iodine-containing contrast media. While it is not known to be teratogenic, the current practice is to discontinue its use when pregnancy is confirmed as evidence regarding its safety in pregnancy is not complete.

Metformin and Obstetrical Outcomes

A case–control study aimed to evaluate pregnancy outcomes in women with PCOS who conceived while on metformin treatment and continued the medication for variable lengths of time in pregnancy [111]. Of the 137 subfertile women with a diagnosis of PCOS according to the Rotterdam criteria, 105 conceived while taking metformin and the remaining 32 women conceived spontaneously without metformin (controls). Cases were divided into three groups: group A, 40 women who discontinued metformin between 4 and 16 weeks of pregnancy; group B, 20 women who received metformin to 32 weeks' gestation; group C, 45 women who continued metformin throughout pregnancy. All the groups were matched by age, height, and weight. Comparisons were made in terms of early and late pregnancy complications, intrauterine growth restriction, and live birth rates. The authors concluded that in women with PCOS, continuous use of metformin during pregnancy significantly reduced the rate of miscarriage, gestational diabetes requiring insulin treatment, and fetal growth restriction. No congenital anomaly, intrauterine death, or stillbirth were reported in this study. However, encouraging the results of this study, there is a need for large prospective randomized controlled studies to provide definitive evidence to recommend the use of metformin in pregnancy in PCOS women who conceive while taking this treatment.

Metformin and Pregnancy Outcomes

The role of metformin in the management of anovulation in PCOS patients has been controversial. Early data suggested that metformin use was effective in inducing ovulation in anovulatory PCOS women [112]. The pregnancy in polycystic ovarian syndrome trial I (PPCOS I) evaluated the use of extended release metformin alone or in combination with clomiphene for ovulation induction. This study concluded that clomiphene was three times more effective than metformin alone in attaining live birth [20;113].

The evidence regarding the superiority of metformin alone or in combination with clomiphene citrate as a first-step approach in treating anovulatory infertility in women with PCOS is somewhat conflicting. A meta-analysis evaluated the effectiveness of metformin in subfertile women with PCOS [114]. Only RCTs were included in this meta-analysis and the definition of PCOS was consistent with the Rotterdam consensus criteria. The primary outcome was live birth rate and 27 trials were identified in the literature search. This meta-analysis concluded that there was no evidence of a difference in live birth rate when metformin was compared with clomiphene citrate and when comparing metformin and clomiphene citrate in combination with clomiphene citrate. However, this study identified a benefit in terms of a higher live birth rate when clomiphene citrate-resistant women received both clomiphene and metformin treatment in combination. The authors concluded that clomiphene is the first-choice therapy for women with PCOS and that in clomiphene-resistant women, the combination of clomiphene and metformin is the preferred treatment option prior to proceeding with gonadotropin administration or laparoscopic ovarian diathermy. However, there are some weaknesses in this meta-analysis as only 17 of 27 trials used an appropriate method of randomization and employed adequate concealment. Trial sizes varied from 17 to 626 women and a power calculation was only reported in eight trials. Eight studies excluded women over the age of 35 and most studies did not have restrictions concerning BMI.

A systematic review aimed to define the best evidence-based recommendations regarding the use of clomiphene citrate and/or metformin as the initial treatment of PCOS women with anovulatory infertility [115]. The primary endpoint was the live birth rate and secondary endpoints were the rates of ovulation, pregnancy, abortion, and discontinuation for adverse events. Four head-to-head RCTs were identified and qualified for inclusion in the analysis. The meta-analysis revealed that metformin and clomiphene citrate did not differ with respect to rates of cumulative ovulation, pregnancy, live birth, and abortion. As significant heterogeneity existed among studies these findings cannot be regarded as conclusive. Analysis of homogeneous data indicated that both medications were safe and rates of discontinuation for adverse events were low. This study concluded that in PCOS women with anovulatory infertility and not previously treated, the administration of metformin plus clomiphene is not better than monotherapy (metformin or clomiphene citrate alone). The aim of this study was not achieved, in that no specific recommendation could be given regarding the use of clomiphene citrate or metformin as a first-line therapy in anovulatory PCOS women seeking pregnancy.

The latest Cochrane review investigating the role of insulin-sensitizing agents included 40 studies that examined metformin use. It concluded that clinical pregnancy rate was improved when adding metformin to clomiphene citrate in clomiphene-resistant women regardless of BMI (OR 1.59, 95% CI 1.25–2.02), with no improvement in live birth rate (OR 1.21, 95% CI 0.91–1.61) [116].

Recently published ASRM guidelines advised against the use of metformin monotherapy for ovulation induction especially that letrozole or clomiphene alone have proven more effective first-line agents [117]. However, the use of metformin in combination with clomiphene citrate may be beneficial in clomiphene-resistant PCOS women. Although metformin was not shown to increase live birth rate, individualizing its use to specific PCOS phenotypes to improve ovulation rates and insulin resistance may prove beneficial in enhancing pregnancy rates on the long term. The concluding remarks of this document were the need for more sufficiently powered randomized trials to delineate the PCOS patients' phenotypes that would benefit most from metformin therapy [117].

Dexamethasone

Other adjunctive treatments evaluated in ovulation induction of PCOS women include dexamethasone. Evidence regarding use of combination therapy including dexamethasone in clomiphene-resistant patients has been conflicting. A 2006 randomized trial involving 80 patients had promising results. It concluded that the addition of 2 mg dexamethasone daily divided in two doses to clomiphene increases ovulation and pregnancy rates in clomiphene citrate-resistant PCOS women [118]. A subsequent trial including 60 patients using the same protocol showed a significant increase in the number of mature follicles but no significant difference in ovulation and pregnancy rate [119]. Recently a randomized trial compared the combination of clomiphene and dexamethasone to letrozole and dexamethasone for ovulation induction in PCOS patients. It showed a significantly higher ovulation rate (62.5% vs. 37.5%, respectively; $p < 0.05$) and pregnancy rate (68.8% vs. 31.2%, respectively; $p = 0.05$) in the combination of letrozole and dexamethasone group [120].

There is scarce data evaluating the use of *N*-acetyl cysteine (NAC) in inducing ovulation in PCOS patients. A 2007 cross-over study suggested that NAC may enhance the effect of clomiphene citrate in inducing ovulation [121]. However, a recent randomized trial showed it to be ineffective in inducing or enhancing ovulation in non-clomiphene-resistant PCOS women candidates for intrauterine insemination [122]. A major limitation of these studies is the small sample size involved which calls for larger, adequately powered randomized trials before strong evidence-based recommendations can be drawn.

References

1. Frank S. Polycystic ovarian syndrome. *N Engl J Med* 1995;**333**:853–861.

2. Homburg R. Polycystic ovary syndrome–from gynaecological curiosity to multisystem endocrinopathy. *Hum Reprod* 1996;**11**:29–39.

3. Stein IF, Leventhal ML. Amenorrhea associated with bilateral polycystic ovaries. *Am J Obstet Gynecol* 1935;**29**:181–191.

4. Balen A. The pathophysiology of polycystic ovary syndrome: trying to understand PCOS and its endocrinology. *Best Pract Res Clin Obstet Gynaecol* 2004;**18**:685–706.

5. Dunaif A, Segal KR, Futterweit W, Dobrjansky A. Profound peripheral insulin resistance, independent of obesity, in polycystic ovary syndrome. *Diabetes* 1989;**38**:1165–1174.

6. Adashi EY, Resnick CE, D'Ercole AJ, Svoboda ME, Van Wyk JJ. Insulin-like growth factors as intraovarian regulators of granulosa cell growth and function. *Endocr Rev* 1985;**6**:400–420.

7. Barbieri RL, Makris A, Randall RW, *et al.* Insulin stimulates androgen accumulation in incubations of ovarian stroma obtained from women with hyperandrogenism. *J Clin Endocrinol Metab* 1986;**62**:904–910.

8. Nestler JE, Powers LP, Matt DW, *et al.* A direct effect of hyperinsulinemia on serum sex hormone-binding globulin levels in obese women with the polycystic ovary syndrome. *J Clin Endocrinol Metab* 1991;**72**:83–89.

9. Zawadzki JK, Dunaif A. Diagnostic criteria for polycystic syndrome: towards a rational approach. In: Dunaif A, Givens JR, Haseltine FP, *et al.*, eds. Polycystic ovary syndrome. Boston: Blackwell Scientific; 1992:337–384.

10. Rotterdam ESHRE/ASRM-Sponsored PCOS Consensus Workshop Group. Revised 2003 consensus on diagnostic criteria and long-term

11. Lizneva D, Suturina L, Walker W, *et al.* Criteria, prevalence, and phenotypes of polycystic ovary syndrome. *Fertil Steril* 2016;**106**(1):6–15.

12. Erel CT, Senturk LM. The impact of body mass index on assisted reproduction. *Curr Opin Obstet Gynecol* 2009;**21**:228–235.

13. Balen AH, Conway GS, Kaltsas G, *et al.* Polycystic ovary syndrome: the spectrum of the disorder in 1741 patients. *Hum Reprod* 1995;**10**:2107–2111.

14. Kiddy DS, Sharp PS, White DM, *et al.* Differences in clinical and endocrine features between obese and non-obese subjects with polycystic ovary syndrome: an analysis of 263 consecutive cases. *Clin Endocrinol (Oxf)* 1990;**32**:213–220.

15. Goldzieher JW, Axelrod LR. Clinical and biochemical features of polycystic ovarian disease. *Fertil Steril* 1963;**14**:631–653.

16. Moran LJ, Pasquali R, Teede HJ, Hoeger KM, Norman RJ. Treatment of obesity in polycystic ovary syndrome: a position statement of the Androgen Excess and Polycystic Ovary Syndrome Society. *Fertil Steril* 2009;**92**(6):1966–1982.

17. Practice Committee of the American Society for Reproductive Medicine. Obesity and reproduction: a committee opinion. *Fertil Steril* 2015;**104**(5):1116–1126.

18. National Institute for Clinical Excellence. Fertility: assessment and treatment for people with fertility problems. Clinical Guideline; London: RCOG Press; 2004.

19. Legro RS, Kunselman AR, Brzyski RG, *et al.* The Pregnancy in Polycystic Ovary Syndrome II (PPCOS II) trial: rationale and design of a double-blind randomized trial of clomiphene citrate and letrozole for the treatment of infertility in women with polycystic ovary syndrome. *Contemp Clin Trials* 2012;**33**(3):470–481.

20. Legro RS, Brzyski RG, Diamond MP, *et al.* Letrozole versus clomiphene for infertility in the polycystic ovary syndrome. *N Engl J Med* 2014;**371**:119–129.

21. Caserta D, Adducchio G, Picchia S, *et al.* Metabolic syndrome and polycystic ovary syndrome: an intriguing overlapping. *Gynecol Endocrinol* 2014;**30**(6):397–402.

22. Salehi M, Bravo-Vera R, Sheikh A, Gouller A, Poretsky L. Pathogenesis of polycystic ovary syndrome: what is the role of obesity? *Metabolism* 2004;**53**(3):358–376.

23. Douchi T, Kuwahata R, Yamamoto S, *et al.* Relationship of upper body obesity to menstrual

disorders. *Acta Obstet Gynecol Scand* 2002;**81**:147–150.

24. Hartz AJ, Rupley DC, Rimm AA. The association of girth measurements with disease in 32,856 women. *Am J Epidemiol* 1984;**119**:71–80.

25. Pasquali R, Pelusi C, Genghini S, Cacciari M, Gambineri A. Obesity and reproductive disorders in women. *Hum Reprod Update* 2003;**9**:359–372.

26. Norman RJ, Masters SC, Hague W, *et al*. Metabolic approaches to the subclassification of polycystic ovary syndrome. *Fertil Steril* 1995;**63**(2):329–335.

27. Gesink Law DC, Maclehose RF, Longnecker MP. Obesity and time to pregnancy. *Hum Reprod* 2007;**22**:414–420.

28. Fedorcsak P, Dale PO, Storeng R, *et al*. Impact of overweight and underweight on assisted reproduction treatment. *Hum Reprod* 2004;**19**:2523–2528.

29. Cedergren MI. Maternal morbid obesity and the risk of adverse pregnancy outcome. *Obstet Gynecol* 2004;**103**:219–224.

30. Weiss JL, Malone FD, Emig D, *et al*. FASTER Research Consortium. Obesity, obstetric complications and cesarean delivery rate: a population-based screening study. *Am J Obstet Gynecol* 2004;**190**:1091–1097.

31. Metwally M, Ledger WL, Li TC. Reproductive endocrinology and clinical aspects of obesity in women. *Ann N Y Acad Sci* 2008;**1127**:140–146.

32. Lintsen AM, Pasker-de Jong PC, De Boer EJ, *et al*. Effects of subfertility cause, smoking and body weight on the success rate of IVF. *Hum Reprod* 2005;**20**(7):1867–1875.

33. Loveland JB, McClamrock HD, Malinow AM, Sharara FI. Clinical assisted reproduction: increased body mass index has a deleterious effect on in vitro fertilization outcome. *J Assist Reprod Genet* 2001;**18**(7):382–386.

34. Dechaud H, Anahory T, Reyftmann L, *et al*. Obesity does not adversely affect results in patients who are undergoing in vitro fertilization and embryo transfer. *Eur J Obstet Gynecol Reprod Biol* 2006;**127**:88–93.

35. Lashen H, Ledger W, Bernal AL, Barlow D. Extremes of body mass do not adversely affect the outcome of superovulation and in-vitro fertilization. *Hum Reprod* 1999;**14**:712–715.

36. Martinuzzi K, Ryan S, Luna M, Copperman AB. Elevated body mass index (BMI) does not adversely affect in vitro fertilization outcome in young women. *J Assist Reprod Genet* 2008;**25**:169–175.

37. MacKenna A, Schwarze JE, Crosby JA, Zegers-Hochschild F. Outcome of assisted reproductive technology in overweight and obese women. *JBRA Assist Reprod* 2017;**21**(2):79–83.

38. Balaban B, Urman B. Effect of oocyte morphology on embryo development and implantation. *Reprod Biomed Online* 2006;**12**:608–615.

39. Carrell DT, Jones KP, Peterson CM, *et al*. Body mass index is inversely related to intrafollicular HCG concentrations, embryo quality and IVF outcome. *Reprod Biomed Online* 2001;**3**:109–111.

40. Esinler I, Bozdag G, Yarali H. Impact of isolated obesity on ICSI outcome. *Reprod Biomed Online* 2008;**17**:583–587.

41. Wittemer C, Ohl J, Bailly M, *et al*. Does body mass index of infertile women have an impact on IVF procedure and outcome? *J Assist Reprod Genet* 2000;**17**:547–552.

42. Jungheim ES, Moley KH. Current knowledge of obesity's effects in the pre- and periconceptional periods and avenues for future research. *Am J Obstet Gynecol* 2010;**203**(6):525–530.

43. Pandey S, Pandey S, Maheshwari A, Bhattacharya S. The impact of female obesity on the outcome of fertility treatment. *J Hum Reprod Sci* 2010;**3**(2):62–67.

44. Metwally M, Cutting R, Tipton A, *et al*. Effect of increased body mass index on oocyte and embryo quality in IVF patients. *Reprod Biomed Online* 2007;**15**:532–538.

45. Provost MP, Acharya KS, Acharya CR, *et al*. Pregnancy outcomes decline with increasing body mass index: analysis of 239,127 fresh autologous in vitro fertilization cycles from the 2008–2010 Society for Assisted Reproductive Technology registry. *Fertil Steril* 2016;**105**(3):663–669.

46. Provost MP, Acharya KS, Acharya CR, *et al*. Pregnancy outcomes decline with increasing recipient body mass index: an analysis of 22,317 fresh donor/recipient cycles from the 2008–2010 Society for Assisted Reproductive Technology Clinic Outcome Reporting System registry. *Fertil Steril* 2016;**105**(2):364–368.

47. Rittenberg V, Seshadri S, Sunkara SK, *et al*. Effect of body mass index on IVF treatment outcome: an updated systematic review and meta-analysis. *Reprod Biomed Online* 2011;**23**(4):421–439.

48. Escobar-Morreale HF, Luque-Ramírez M, González F. Circulating inflammatory markers in polycystic ovary syndrome: a systematic review and meta analysis. *Fertil Steril* 2011;**95**(3):1048–1058.

49. Paepegaey AC, Genser L, Bouillot JL, *et al*. High levels of CRP in morbid obesity: the central role of adipose tissue and lessons for clinical practice

before and after bariatric surgery. *Surg Obes Relat Dis* 2015;**11**(1):148–154.

50. Faucher G, Guénard F, Bouchard L, *et al.* Genetic contribution to C-reactive protein levels in severe obesity. *Mol Genet Metab* 2012;**105**(3):494–501.

51. Kadowaki T. Yamauchi T. Adiponectin and adiponectin receptors. *Endocr Rev* 2005;**26**:439–451.

52. Yuan G, Zhou L, Tang J, *et al.* Serum CRP levels are equally elevated in newly diagnosed type 2 diabetes and impaired glucose tolerance and related to adiponectin levels and insulin sensitivity. *Diabetes Res clin Pract* 2006;**72** (3):244–250.

53. Sieminska L, Marek B, Kos-Kudla B, *et al.* Serum adiponectin in women with polycystic ovarian syndrome and its relation to clinical, metabolic and endocrine parameters. *J Endocrinol Investig* 2004;**27**(6):528–534.

54. Kopp HP, Krzyzanowska K, Möhlig M, *et al.* Effects of marked weight loss on plasma levels of adiponectin, markers of chronic subclinical inflammation and insulin resistance in morbidly obese women. *Int J Obes* 2005;**29**(7):766–771.

55. Esposito K, Pontillo A, Di Palo C, *et al.* Effect of weight loss and lifestyle changes on vascular inflammatory markers in obese women: a randomized trial. *JAMA* 2003;**289** (14):1799–1804.

56. Woelnerhanssen B, Peterli R, Steinert RE, *et al.* Effects of postbariatric surgery weight loss on adipokines and metabolic parameters: comparison of laparoscopic Roux-en-Y gastric bypass and laparoscopic sleeve gastrectomy – a prospective randomized trial. *Surg Obes Relat Dis* 2011;**7** (5):561–568.

57. Wadden TA, Foster GD. Behavioral treatment of obesity. *Med Clin N Am* 2000;**84**(2):441–461.

58. Wadden TA, Webb VL, Moran CH, Bailer BA. Lifestyle modification for obesity: new developments in diet, physical activity, and behavior therapy. *Circulation* 2012;**125** (9):1157–1170.

59. Pucci A, Finer N. New medications for treatment of obesity: metabolic and cardiovascular effects. *Can J Cardiol* 2015;**31**(2):142–152.

60. Apovian CM, Aronne LJ, Bessesen DH, et al. Pharmacological management of obesity: an Endocrine Society clinical practice guideline. *J Clin Endocrinol Metab* 2015;**100**(2):342–362.

61. Keating GM, Jarvis B. Orlistat: in the prevention and treatment of type 2 diabetes mellitus. *Drugs* 2001;**61**:2107–2119.

62. Inge TH, Jenkins TM, Zeller M, *et al.* Baseline BMI is a strong predictor of nadir BMI after adolescent gastric bypass. *J Pediatr* 2010;**156**(1):103–108.

63. Deitel M, Stone E, Kassam HA, Wilk EJ, Sutherland DJ. Gynecologic-obstetric changes after loss of massive excess weight following bariatric surgery. *J Am Coll Nutr* 1988;**7**:147–153.

64. Abiad F, Abbas HA, Hamadi C, Ghazeeri G. Bariatric surgery in the management of adolescent and adult obese patients with polycystic ovarian syndrome. *J Obes Weight Loss Ther* 2016;**6**:303.

65. Abiad F, Khalife D, Safadi B, *et al.* The effect of bariatric surgery on inflammatory markers in women with polycystic ovarian syndrome. *Diabetes Metab Syndr* 2018;**12**(6):999–1005.

66. Sheiner E, Levy A, Silverberg D, *et al.* Pregnancy after bariatric surgery is not associated with adverse perinatal outcome. *Am J Obstet Gynecol* 2004;**190**:1335–1340.

67. Printen KJ, Scott D. Pregnancy following gastric bypass for the treatment of morbid obesity. *Am Surg* 1982;**48**:363–365.

68. Marceau P, Kaufman D, Biron S, *et al.* Outcome of pregnancies after biliopancreatic diversion. *Obes Surg* 2004;**14**:318–324.

69. Mutsaerts MA, van Oers AM, Groen H, *et al.* Randomized trial of a lifestyle program in obese infertile women. *N Engl J Med* 2016;**374**:1942–1953.

70. Einarsson S, Bergh C, Friberg B, *et al.* Weight reduction intervention for obese infertile women prior to IVF: a randomized controlled trial. *Hum Reprod* 2017;**32**:1621–1630.

71. Norman RJ, Mol BWJ. Successful weight loss interventions before in vitro fertilization: fat chance? *Fertil Steril* 2018;**110**:581–586.

72. Greenblatt RB, Barfield WE, Jungck EC, Ray AW. Induction of ovulation with MRL/41. Preliminary report. *J Am Med Assoc* 1961;**178**:101–104.

73. Ecklund LC, Usadi RS. Endocrine and reproductive effects of polycystic ovarian syndrome. *Obstet Gynecol Clin North Am* 2015;**42** (1):55–65.

74. Practice Committee of the American Society for Reproductive Medicine. Use of clomiphene citrate in infertile women: a committee opinion. *Fertil Steril* 2013;**100**(2):341–348.

75. Hammond MG. Monitoring techniques for improved pregnancy rates during clomifene ovulation induction. *Fertil Steril* 1984;**42**:499–508.

76. Dickey RP, Taylor SN, Curole DN, *et al.* Incidence of spontaneous abortion in clomifene pregnancies. *Hum Reprod* 1996;**11**:2623–2628.

77. Gysler M, March CM, Mishell DR Jr., Bailey EJ. A decade's experience with an individualized clomiphene treatment regimen including its effect on the postcoital test. *Fertil Steril* 1982;37:161–167.

78. Eden JA, Place J, Carter GD, et al. The effect of clomiphene citrate on follicular phase increase in endometrial thickness and uterine volume. *Fertil Steril* 1989;73:187–190.

79. Bonhoff AJ, Naether OG, Johannisson E. Effects of clomiphene citrate stimulation on endometrial structure in infertile women. *Hum Reprod* 1996;11 (4):844–849.

80. Dehbashi S, Parsanezhad ME, Alborzi S, Zarei A. Effect of clomiphene citrate on endometrium thickness and echogenic patterns. *Int J Gynaecol Obstet* 2003;80(1):49–53.

81. Thompson LA, Barratt CL, Thornton SJ, Bolton AE, Cooke ID. The effects of clomiphene citrate and cyclofenil on cervical mucus volume and receptivity over the periovulatory period. *Fertil Steril* 1993;59(1):125–129.

82. Kousta E, White DM, Franks S. Modern use of clomiphene citrate in induction of ovulation. *Hum Reprod Update* 1997;3(4):359–365.

83. Hull MG, Savage PE, Bromham DR, Ismail AA, Morris AF. The value of a single serum progesterone measurement in the midluteal phase as a criterion of a potentially fertile cycle ('ovulation') derived from treated and untreated conception cycles. *Fertil Steril* 1982;37(3):355–360.

84. Talbert LM. Clomiphene citrate induction of ovulation. *Fertil Steril* 1983;39(6):742–743.

85. Chaabane S, Sheehy O, Monnier P, et al. Ovarian stimulation, intrauterine insemination, multiple pregnancy and major congenital malformations: a systematic review and meta-analysis-The ART_Rev Study. *Curr Drug Saf* 2016;11 (3):222–261.

86. Senturk LM, Erel CT. Thin endometrium in assisted reproductive technology. *Curr Opin Obstet Gynecol* 2008;20:221–228.

87. Oliveira JB, Baruffi RL, Mauri AL, et al. Endometrial ultrasonography as a predictor of pregnancy in an in-vitro fertilization programme after ovarian stimulation and gonadotrophin-releasing hormone and gonadotrophins. *Hum Reprod* 1997;12 (11):2515–2518.

88. Schild RL, Knobloch C, Dorn C, et al. Endometrial receptivity in an in vitro fertilization program as assessed by spiral artery blood flow, endometrial thickness, endometrial volume, and uterine artery blood flow. *Fertil Steril* 2001;75:361–366.

89. Wu Y, Gao X, Lu X, et al. Endometrial thickness affects the outcome of in vitro fertilization and embryo transfer in normal responders after GnRH antagonist administration. *Reprod Biol Endocrinol* 2014;12(1):96.

90. Wang Y, Zhu Y, Sun Y, et al. Ideal embryo transfer position and endometrial thickness in IVF embryo transfer treatment. *Int J Gynecol Obstet* 2018;143(3):282–288.

91. Lobo RA, Gysler M, March CM, Goebelsmann U, Mishell DR Jr. Clinical and laboratory predictors of clomiphene response. *Fertil Steril* 1982;37 (2):168–174.

92. Douchi T, Oki T, Yamasaki H, et al. Body fat patterning in polycystic ovary syndrome women as a predictor of the response to clomiphene. *Acta Obstet Gynecol Scand* 2004;83:838–841.

93. Imani B, Eijkemans MJ, te Velde ER, Habbema JD, Fauser BC. Predictors of chances to conceive in ovulatory patients during clomiphene citrate induction of ovulation in normogonadotropic oligoamenorrheic infertility. *J Clin Endocrinol Metab* 1999;84(5):1617–1622.

94. Gindoff PR, Jewelewicz R. Reproductive potential in the older woman. *Fertil Steril* 1986;46 (6):989–1001.

95. Rossing MA, Daling JR, Weiss NS, et al. Ovarian tumors in a cohort of infertile women. *N Engl J Med* 1994;331:771–776.

96. Balen A. Anovulatory infertility and ovulation induction. Policy and Practice subcommittee of the British Fertility Society. *Hum Reprod* 1997;12 (11 Suppl):83–87.

97. Balen AH, Morley LC, Misso M, et al. The management of anovulatory infertility in women with polycystic ovary syndrome: an analysis of the evidence to support the development of global WHO guidance. *Hum Reprod Update* 2016;22(6):687–708.

98. Palomba S. Aromatase inhibitors for ovulation induction. *J Clin Endocrinol Metab* 2015;100 (5):1742–1747.

99. Holzer H, Casper R, Tulandi T. A new era in ovulation induction. *Fertil Steril* 2006;85 (2):277–284.

100. Kar S. Current evidence supporting "letrozole" for ovulation induction. *J Hum Reprod Sci* 2013;6 (2):93–98.

101. Mitwally MF, Biljan MM, Casper RF. Pregnancy outcome after the use of an aromatase inhibitor for ovarian stimulation. *Am J Obstet Gynecol* 2005;192(2):381–386.

102. Franik S, Eltrop SM, Kremer JA, Kiesel L, Farquhar C. Aromatase inhibitors (letrozole) for

subfertile women with polycystic ovary syndrome. *Cochrane Database Syst Rev* 2018;5: CD010287.

103. Biljan MM, Hemmings R, Brassard N. The outcome of 150 babies following the treatment with letrozole or letrozole and gonadotropins. *Fertil Steril* 2005;**84**:S95.

104. Tulandi T, Martin J, Al-Fadhli R, *et al.* Congenital malformations among 911 newborns conceived after infertility treatment with letrozole or clomiphene citrate. *Fertil Steril* 2006;**85**(6):1761–1765.

105. American College of Obstetricians and Gynecologists. Polycystic ovary syndrome. ACOG practice bulletin no. 194. *Obstet Gynecol* 2018;**11**:131.

106. Velazquez EM, Mendoza S, Hamer T, Sosa F, Glueck CJ. Metformin therapy in polycystic ovary syndrome reduces hyperinsulinemia, insulin resistance, hyperandrogenemia, and systolic blood pressure, while facilitating normal menses and pregnancy. *Metabolism* 1994;**43**:647–654.

107. Williamson DF, Pamuk E, Thun M, *et al.* Prospective study of intentional weight loss and mortality in never-smoking overweight US white women aged 40–64 years. *Am J Epidemiol* 1995;**141**:1128–1141.

108. Kiddy DS, Hamilton-Fairley D, Bush A, *et al.* Improvement in endocrine and ovarian function during dietary treatment of obese women with polycystic ovary syndrome. *Clin Endocrinol* 1992;**36**:105–111.

109. Crosignani PG, Colombo M, Vegetti W, *et al.* Overweight and obese anovulatory patients with polycystic ovaries: parallel improvements in anthropometric indices, ovarian physiology and fertility rate induced by diet. *Hum Reprod* 2003;**18**:1928–1932.

110. Harborne L, Fleming R, Lyall H, Norman J, Sattar N. Descriptive review of the evidence for the use of metformin in polycystic ovary syndrome. *Lancet* 2003;**361**:1894–1901.

111. Nawaz FH, Khalid R, Naru T, Rizvi J. Does continuous use of metformin throughout pregnancy improve pregnancy outcomes in women with polycystic ovarian syndrome? *J Obstet Gynaecol Res* 2008;**34**(5):832–837.

112. Morley LC, Tang TM, Balen AH. Metformin therapy for the management of infertility in women with polycystic ovary syndrome: Scientific Impact Paper No. 13. *BJOG* 2017;**124**(12):E306–E313.

113. Legro RS, Barnhart HX, Schlaff WD, *et al.* Clomiphene, metformin, or both for infertility in the polycystic ovary syndrome. *N Engl J Med* 2007;**356**(6):551–566.

114. Moll E, van der Veen F, van Wely M. The role of metformin in polycystic ovary syndrome: a systematic review. *Hum Reprod Update* 2007;**13**(6):527–537.

115. Palomba S, Pasquali R, Orio JF, Nestler JE. Clomiphene citrate, metformin or both as first-step approach in treating anovulatory infertility in patients with polycystic ovary syndrome (PCOS): a systematic review of head-to-head randomized controlled studies and meta-analysis. *Clin Endocrinol* 2009;**70**:311–321.

116. Morley LC, Tang T, Yasmin E, Norman RJ, Balen AH. Insulin-sensitising drugs (metformin, rosiglitazone, pioglitazone, D-chiro-inositol) for women with polycystic ovary syndrome, oligo amenorrhoea and subfertility. *Cochrane Database Syst Rev* 2017;**11**:CD003053.

117. Practice Committee of the American Society for Reproductive Medicine. Role of metformin for ovulation induction in infertile patients with polycystic ovary syndrome (PCOS): a guideline. *Fertil Steril* 2017;**108**(3):426–441.

118. Elnashar A, Abdelmageed E, Fayed M, Sharaf M. Clomiphene citrate and dexamethazone in treatment of clomiphene citrate-resistant polycystic ovary syndrome: a prospective placebo-controlled study. *Hum Reprod* 2006;**21**(7):1805–1808.

119. Esmaeilzadeh S, Amiri MG, Basirat Z, Shirazi M. Does adding dexamethasone to clomiphene citrate improve ovulation in PCOS patients? A triple-blind randomized clinical trial study. *Int J Fertil Steril* 2011;**5**(1):9–12.

120. Shabana AA, Al-Halby AE, Abd Hamid ES, El-Naggar AM. Letrozole with dexamethasone versus clomiphene citrate with dexamethasone for induction of ovulation in polycystic ovary. *Menoufia Med J* 2018;**31**(1):38–45.

121. Badawy A, State O, Abdelgawad S. N-acetyl cysteine and clomiphene citrate for induction of ovulation in polycystic ovary syndrome: a cross-over trial. *Acta Obstet Gynecol Scand* 2007;**86**(2):218–222.

122. Lak TB, Hajshafiha M, Nanbakhsh F, Oshnouei S. N-acetyl cysteine in ovulation induction of PCOS women underwent intrauterine insemination: An RCT. *Int J Reprod Biomed* 2017;**15**(4):203–206.

Chapter

14

Polycystic Ovary Syndrome: Controlled Ovarian Stimulation

Lina El-Taha, Botros Rizk, William Ledger, Raja Sayegh, and Johnny Awwad

Laparoscopic Ovarian Diathermy

Surgical methods of ovulation induction for women with clomiphene (clomifene) citrate-resistant polycystic ovary syndrome (PCOS) include laparoscopic ovarian drilling with diathermy. This technique has replaced the more invasive and damaging technique of ovarian wedge resection first introduced by Gjønnaess in the early 1980s [1]. Laparoscopic ovarian surgery is free from the risks of multiple pregnancy and ovarian hyperstimulation, which makes it an attractive procedure for PCOS women, but surgery is not without risks. The techniques of laparoscopic ovarian diathermy have been described previously [2;3]. Studies suggest that four punctures per ovary with application of diathermy current via needle cautery set at 30 watts for 5 seconds per puncture (i.e., no more than 600 J per ovary) should produce an optimal response. The greater the damage to the surface of the ovary the greater the risk of peri-ovarian adhesions estimated at 60 percent (ranging from 0 to 100 percent) in treated women. An additional concern is the risk of premature ovarian failure should the procedure be aggressively performed and therefore, a minimal amount of ovarian destruction is advised. Unilateral ovarian diathermy has been shown to result in bilateral ovarian activity indicating that ovarian diathermy achieves its effect by potentially altering ovarian-pituitary feedback [4]. A recently published Cochrane review evaluated available evidence on the effects of diathermy on live births and miscarriages as poor quality and insufficient to justify conclusions due to increased bias, heterogeneity, and small sample size [5].

Early studies investigating the efficacy of laparoscopic ovarian diathermy in PCOS women are encouraging with 70–94% chance of successful ovulation and 60–70% chance of spontaneous conception [6]. Cycle-by-cycle analysis demonstrated that the clinical response to diathermy may be immediate, with a remarkable ovulation rate per cycle of 60% during the first three cycles. With restoration of ovarian activity following ovarian diathermy it has been shown that serum concentrations of luteinizing hormone (LH) and testosterone fall. The reduction in serum LH concentrations appears to increase the chance of conception and reduce the risk of miscarriage. A randomized controlled trial comparing PCOS women receiving clomiphene citrate treatment and those undergoing ovarian diathermy concluded that medical intervention is more effective in terms of cumulative live birth over a 12-month period at lower treatment costs and hazards [7].

A 2002 study has investigated the long-term effects of laparoscopic ovarian drilling in 116 anovulatory women with PCOS [8]. PCOS women were requested to attend for a transvaginal ultrasound scan and blood sampling to measure serum concentrations of LH, follicle-stimulating hormone (FSH), testosterone, androstenedione, and sex hormone-binding globulin prior to the procedure and at different intervals following their surgery, short (< 1 year), medium (1–3 years), and long term (4–9 years). This study found that the LH:FSH ratio, mean serum concentrations of LH and testosterone, and free androgen index decreased significantly after laparoscopic ovarian diathermy and remained low during the medium- and long- term follow-up periods. The mean ovarian volume decreased significantly ($p < 0.05$) from 11 ml before surgery to 8.5 ml at medium-term and remained low (8.4 ml) at long-term follow-up. The authors concluded that the beneficial endocrinological and morphological effects of laparoscopic ovarian diathermy appear to be sustained for up to nine years in most patients with PCOS. On the contrary, patterns of anti-Müllerian hormone (AMH) did not seem to mirror those of the endocrinological profile. A recently published meta-analysis showed significant decline in AMH levels six months following laparoscopic ovarian diathermy in PCOS women. Yet, these findings call for more studies to address the ambiguity in whether they reflect damage to the ovaries or normalization of the preoperative endocrine dysfunction [9].

It should be noted however that about one-third of patients may not manifest any significant clinical benefit following laparoscopic ovarian diathermy. Accurate identification of poor prognostic indicators would have economic benefits in terms of reduced theater costs and avoidance of potential risks associated with surgery. A retrospective study was carried out to identify factors that may help to predict the outcome of laparoscopic ovarian diathermy in 200 patients with anovulatory infertility secondary to PCOS [10]. This study concluded that marked obesity (body mass index [BMI] $\geq$ 35 kg/m^2), marked hyperandrogenism (free androgen index $\geq$ 15 and/or testosterone $\geq$ 4.5 nmol/L), and/or long duration of infertility (> 3 years) in women with PCOS seem to predict resistance to laparoscopic ovarian diathermy. Elevated AMH serum levels ($\geq$ 7.7 ng/ml) have also been associated with treatment failures.

Laparoscopic ovarian diathermy has been studied as a measure to prevent ovarian hyperstimulation syndrome (OHSS) in women with PCOS undergoing in vitro fertilization (IVF), but to date the evidence is unconvincing. While acknowledging moderate quality evidence, laparoscopic ovarian diathermy was recommended as first line in infertile PCOS women if laparoscopy was indicated for another reason and as second line in clomiphene-resistant, anovulatory PCOS women [11]. However, these recommendations are debatable given a 2020 Cochrane review highlighting the poor- quality evidence for the majority of available data. This is particularly revealed considering a sensitivity analysis limited only to four randomized trials with low risk of selection bias, which highlights the uncertainty of whether a difference exists between medical induction of ovulation and laparoscopic ovarian diathermy in terms of live birth rate (odds ratio [OR] 0.90, 95% confidence interval [CI] 0.59–1.36) [6]. At present it does not seem justifiable to perform this procedure with the sole aim of preventing OHSS in the IVF treatment cycle. Although previous recommendations were in favor of this procedure as an

appropriate treatment in the management of clomiphene-resistant PCOS women, we expect new updates reflecting findings of recently published reviews.

Ovulation Induction: Gonadotropins

Patients who fail to conceive following the use of first-line ovulatory induction medications and/or laparoscopic ovarian diathermy may then progress to gonadotropin ovulation induction in conjunction with either timed sexual intercourse or intrauterine insemination. To this end, the step-up stimulation protocol is advised and commences with the lowest dose of FSH followed by incremental increases until follicular development is identified, the time at which the dose is then maintained. The aim of ovulation induction in PCOS patients is to achieve monofollicular development and avoid the complication of OHSS. Studies have shown that the risk of overstimulation is lower with the step-up protocol and it is the protocol of choice for patients at risk of multifollicular development particularly PCOS women. For PCOS women who prove to be resistant to clomiphene, a low-dose step-up protocol using recombinant FSH at a starting dose of 50 IU is appropriate. Increments in dose (50 IU) every five to seven days may be made according to follicular response as determined by transvaginal ultrasound monitoring. Evidence is available to suggest that this regimen is efficient, safe, and well tolerated despite a particularly protracted duration of stimulation in some cases. In a randomized controlled trial, the use of gonadotropins resulted in more miscarriages (relative risk [RR] 2.23, 95% CI 1.11–4.47), significantly higher live births (RR 1.24, 95% CI 1.05–1.46), and higher clinical pregnancies (RR 1.31, 95% CI 1.13–1.52) compared with clomiphene citrate [12;13].

It is imperative that patients are carefully monitored during the treatment cycle to detect multifollicular development with the associated risks of multiple pregnancy and ovarian hyperstimulation. Careful monitoring of patients requires serial pelvic ultrasound scans to monitor follicle growth and endometrial thickness. Serial monitoring of serum estradiol is of benefit as plasma estradiol is an index of follicular maturity. When the mean diameter of the leading follicle is 17 mm, human chorionic gonadotropin (hCG) is administered to promote follicular maturation and rupture. The patient will then be advised as to the optimum time for sexual intercourse or intrauterine insemination. The insemination is timed to ensure that viable spermatozoa are present in the female reproductive tract at the time of ovulation. In a stimulated cycle, rupture of the follicle is expected to occur on average 36–40 hours from the time of hCG administration [14]. Because gonadotropin follicle stimulation is associated with luteal phase defect, progesterone luteal supplementation was found to improve the pregnancy outcome in these patients.

In Vitro Fertilization

Favorable IVF outcomes have been reported in cases of PCOS [15]. A meta-analysis comparing outcomes of conventional IVF in PCOS women as per Rotterdam consensus and a matched control group of ovulatory patients was performed [16]. Nine out of 290 identified studies reporting data on 458 PCOS patients (793 cycles) and 694 matched controls (1116 cycles) fulfilled the inclusion criteria. This meta-analysis demonstrated an increased cycle cancellation rate, higher number of oocytes retrieved, and lower fertilization rate in PCOS patients undergoing IVF. Overall, PCOS and control patients achieved similar pregnancy and live birth rates per cycle. A subsequent meta-analysis emphasized the higher risk of adverse pregnancy-related outcomes in PCOS women undergoing IVF, namely miscarriages (OR 1.41, 95% CI 1.04–1.91), OHSS (OR 4.96, 95% CI 3.73–6.60), gestational diabetes mellitus (OR 2.67, 95% CI 1.43–4.98), hypertensive disorders of pregnancy (OR 2.06, 95% CI 1.45–2.91), preterm birth (OR 1.60, 95% CI 1.25–2.04), and large for gestational age (OR 2.10, 95% CI 1.01–4.37) [17].

It follows that while IVF is considered an appropriate treatment option for PCOS patients, the risk of ovarian hyperstimulation should not be underestimated. OHSS is an iatrogenic and potentially life-threatening complication of superovulation. The severe form of OHSS occurs in 0.5 to 2 percent of IVF cycles and PCOS patients are at increased risk. The underlying pathophysiology of OHSS is an increased capillary permeability leading to third-space fluid accumulation with resultant intravascular dehydration. The severe form of OHSS is a condition of massive ovarian enlargement with ascites and pleural effusions and hemoconcentration; in the critical form, it may be complicated by arterial and venous thromboembolism, respiratory distress syndrome, and myocardial infarction.

Clinics that provide ovarian stimulation should have protocols in place for the prevention, diagnosis, and management of OHSS. The primary aim in the management of OHSS should be prediction and prevention. Risk factors for this condition include young age, high basal antral follicular count, high baseline AMH level, ovarian hyper-responsiveness, (large number of stimulated follicles especially intermediate size follicles 11–14 mm in size, and/or large number of retrieved oocytes), high serum estradiol, and the presence of polycystic ovaries. Anti-Müllerian hormone produced in the granulosa cells of ovarian follicles and secreted into the circulation is a good indicator of ovarian reserve. In contrast to FSH, serum levels may be taken at any time in the cycle and levels do not fluctuate. AMH may serve as a marker of risk of OHSS in an IVF treatment cycle. Women with polycystic ovaries tend to have higher serum levels of AMH ($\geq$ 3.5 ng/dl). If polycystic ovaries are identified by transvaginal ultrasound prior to commencing assisted conception treatment it is reasonable to adopt measures which may reduce the risk of OHSS. These should include use of a gonadotropin-releasing hormone (GnRH) antagonist to prevent premature LH rises during stimulation, use of low doses of FSH, use of a GnRH agonist (GnRHa) rather than hCG to trigger final oocyte maturation along with a policy of "freeze-all" embryos to avoid a fresh embryo transfer [18].

In Vitro Maturation

In vitro maturation (IVM) involves the collection of immature oocytes from unstimulated or minimally stimulated ovaries, and then maturing them in vitro in distinct media. IVM protocols are proposed as a potential alternative to conventional ovarian stimulation during IVF as a strategy to prevent OHSS. Conventional IVF entails significant expenses due to medication cost, and increased requirement for biochemical and ultrasound monitoring. It also has potential side effects for the patient, the most serious of which is OHSS. For these reasons, IVM has attracted considerable attention as a potential alternative particularly for patients at risk for OHSS. This approach has been hampered in the past with limitations including failed oocyte retrieval, poor in vitro oocyte maturation, poor embryo development, and high likelihood of no embryos for transfer. Polycystic ovaries by definition have 12 or more follicles measuring 2–9 mm in diameter and immature oocytes from these follicles retain their maturational and developmental competence [19] and pregnancies have been reported [20]. In 2009, a study evaluated the value of IVM in 350 cycles from 262 unstimulated patients diagnosed with PCOS [21]. These patients were primed with hCG before oocyte retrieval. In order to improve nuclear and cytoplasmic maturation, growth hormone was added to the maturation medium. Oocytes were recovered in 94.8 percent of the cycles, with a mean number of nine cumulus-oocyte complexes retrieved. An ongoing pregnancy rate of 15.2 percent was obtained with an elevated miscarriage rate of 28 percent. High miscarriages could not be attributed to oocyte quality as cytogenetic and DNA fragmentation analyses of the embryos were not fundamentally different from what is classically observed in routine IVF. The authors suggested that endometrial receptivity should be considered as a possible cause especially in IVM cycles where the follicular phase was considerably shortened.

A Cochrane review of available published trials concluded that though the data seem promising, the evidence is insufficient to base best practice recommendations regarding IVM versus IVF/intracytoplasmic sperm injection (ICSI) in women with PCOS [22].

The Use of GnRH Antagonists for Pituitary Suppression

GnRH antagonists induce a prompt inhibition of LH and FSH secretion without inducing the transient "flare" known to be associated with GnRHa. When administered in the follicular phase of the cycle, GnRH antagonists can either prevent or interrupt LH surges. GnRH antagonist IVF cycles are patient friendly in that the protocol is simple and has less side effects in comparison to GnRHa cycles. In one of the earliest landmark studies, Albano and colleagues published the results of an open randomized trial comparing antagonist multiple-dose protocol (0.25 mg/day of either cetrorelix or ganirelix) with GnRHa suppression in IVF cycles [23]. In total, 188 patients were treated with cetrorelix, and 85 with the long

(buserelin) agonist protocol. While the clinical pregnancy rates were comparable, the duration of gonadotropin treatment, serum estradiol levels on the day of hCG, and the incidence of OHSS were lower in the antagonist (cetrorelix) group. In another controlled, multicenter, randomized trial, the differences in clinical pregnancy rates per attempt were likewise not statistically significant, but the incidence of OHSS was lower in the multiple-dose GnRH antagonist group [24]. A recent meta-analysis including PCOS women randomized either to GnRH antagonist or GnRHa protocol showed no significant differences in live birth rate (RR 0.90, 95% CI: 0.69–1.19). However, the use of the GnRH antagonist significantly reduced the risk of OHSS compared with GnRHa long protocol (RR 0.53, 95% CI 0.30–0.95) [25;26].

On the basis of available evidence, it is reasonable to conclude that the GnRH antagonist protocol is an effective and more appropriate alternative to the standard long suppression protocol for PCOS patients at risk of OHSS.

GnRH Agonist Triggering of Final Oocyte Maturation

Administration of a single bolus of GnRHa in cycles co-treated with a GnRH antagonist for pituitary suppression induces an endogenous LH rise which results in successful induction of nuclear oocyte maturation [27]. Because of the short duration of the endogenous GnRHa-induced LH surge, agonist triggering of final oocyte maturation is associated with significant reduction in the risk of severe OHSS compared with conventional hCG.

By the same token, the main limitation of the GnRHa trigger is the induction of an inadequate luteal phase and impaired ovarian steroid production [28]. An earlier systematic review confirmed associations between the use of standard luteal support in GnRHa-triggered cycles and lower clinical pregnancy rates (OR 0.22, 95% CI 0.05–0.85) and higher miscarriages (OR 11.5, 95% CI 0.95–138.98) compared with hCG [29]. These findings clearly indicate the need to modify luteal phase support when a GnRHa is used to trigger ovulation. Different strategies have been published for this purpose, including the use of intensive estrogen and progesterone luteal supplementation.

A prospective randomized controlled trial evaluated the incidence of OHSS and implantation rates in high-risk patients undergoing IVF using either exogenous hCG trigger after luteal pituitary suppression or GnRHa trigger after co-treatment with a GnRH antagonist [30]. The study findings indicated that the use of a GnRHa trigger after GnRH antagonist co-treatment combined with intensive luteal phase supplementation, consisting of a daily dose of 50 mg of progesterone intramuscularly in combination with 0.3 mg of transdermal estradiol patches every other day until 10 weeks of gestation, reduces the risk of OHSS in high-risk patients undergoing IVF without affecting implantation rates (36.0% vs. 31.0%; $p > 0.05$) and ongoing pregnancy rates (53.3% vs. 48.3%; $p > 0.05$). Close monitoring of luteal estradiol and progesterone levels was also performed with dose adjustment of luteal support in order to maintain serum progesterone levels above 20 ng/ml and estradiol levels above 200 pg/ml. It should be noted that 31 percent of women in the hCG group developed some form of OHSS while none in the GnRHa group had similar manifestations. Cycle predictors for successful embryo implantation after GnRHa triggering have been evaluated and positive associations found between pregnancy and peak serum estradiol levels > 4000 pg/ml and LH levels >3.5 IU/L on the day of trigger [31].

Another alternative to support the luteal phase after GnRHa triggering of final oocyte maturation consists of preventing the demise of the corpus luteum by administering a low hCG dose concurrently at the time of ovulation trigger or oocyte collection. In order to assess the risk of OHSS after dual trigger, Griffin *et al.* conducted a retrospective cohort study in high responders in which they compared GnRHa alone and GnRHa/hCG for triggering of ovulation [32]. The dual trigger group showed significantly higher live birth (52.9% vs. 30.9%) and embryo implantation (41.9% vs. 22.1%) compared with the GnRHa alone group without an increased risk of OHSS. Using a prospective controlled design, Humaidan *et al.* randomized normogonadotropic women to receive either hCG trigger or GnRHa trigger followed by 1500 IU hCG at 35 hours [33]. They found no statistically significant differences in live births. It should be noted however that the safety of this protocol in high-responder women, particularly PCOS women, has not yet been fully

established. Two retrospective studies of women at high risk for OHSS showed that this protocol was associated with severe early OHSS in 8 to 26 percent of cases [34;35].

In order to circumvent the risk of late-onset OHSS, several investigators introduced the concept of cycle segmentation with cryopreservation of all embryos for replacement in a subsequent cycle as the safest approach to high-risk women undergoing ovarian stimulation [18;36;37].

Metformin Co-administration

Insulin stimulates serum vascular endothelial growth factor (VEGF) expression and secretion [38]. Investigators have studied the use of metformin (insulin-sensitizer) co-treatment during ovarian stimulation to improve follicular response and reduce the risk of OHSS. Although metformin pretreatment does not appear to improve pregnancy outcomes, some evidence is available to suggest that its co-administration during gonadotropin ovarian stimulation in women with PCOS undergoing IVF reduces the risk of OHSS. In 2013, a systematic review including 10 randomized trials with a total of 845 PCOS women showed that metformin therapy in IVF/ICSI cycles significantly reduced the risk for OHSS (OR 0.27, 95% CI 0.16–0.46), but had no effects on clinical pregnancy (OR 1.20, 95% CI 0.90–1.61) and live birth rates (OR 1.69, 95% CI 0.85–3.34) [39]. Furthermore, a recent double-blinded placebo-controlled randomized trial confirmed the lack of beneficial effect of metformin on live birth (25.5% vs. 17.6%, $p = 0.34$), implantation (15.7% vs. 11.8%, $p = 0.32$), multiple pregnancies (13.4% vs. 3.9%, $p = 0.08$), and miscarriages (23.5% vs. 35.7%, $p = 0.46$) in PCOS women with a BMI > 24 kg/m^2 [40]. The reported reduction in OHSS with metformin administration compared with placebo was found in a published randomized trial [41]. A subsequent Cochrane review including nine randomized trials confirmed the favorable effect of metformin pretreatment in IVF/ICSI cycles on risk reduction for OHSS [42].

Although metformin was shown to reduce the risk for OHSS in stimulated cycles, the size of the protective effect is by no means comparable to that derived from the use of GnRHa triggering of final oocyte maturation in cycles with GnRH antagonist suppression.

Alternative Pretreatment Strategies: Myo-inositol

Given the complexity of PCOS, it is no surprise that over past decades it has been one of the most studied and researched medical conditions. Recently, there has been growing interest in the use of myo-inositol to improve the safety, quality, and outcome of fertility management of PCOS women. Myo-inositol has been traditionally classified as a non-essential nutrient, a component of vitamin B complex, that can be synthesized from glucose in the human body. However, it is mainly derived from dietary sources and converted to D-chiro-inositol in the presence of insulin [43]. There is evidence to support the use of myo-inositol to ameliorate the metabolic and hormonal profiles associated with PCOS. Myo-inositol supplementation was found to significantly reduce LH, prolactin, LH/FSH ratio, testosterone, and insulin levels and to remarkably improve insulin sensitivity, menstrual cyclicity, and lipid profile [44–47] in treated women. In a meta-analysis of six randomized trials, including 355 PCOS patients, myo-inositol was found to be superior to metformin in terms of adverse side effects, while inducing comparable improvement in the hormonal profile [48].

In addition, myo-inositol participates in FSH signaling, including FSH-induced production of AMH which is critical for modulating the sensitivity of follicles to FSH [49]. As such myo-inositol is proposed to play a crucial role in enhancing oocyte health (oocyte development and maturation), fertilization, and subsequent embryo development and quality [50–52]. Unfortunately, published studies investigating the effects of myo-inositol on oocyte quality are limited by their small sample size. In 2009, a randomized trial randomized 60 PCOS women to receive either 2 g myo-inositol combined with folic acid twice a day or folic acid alone [53]. The total dose of gonadotropins used and days of stimulation were significantly reduced in the myo-inositol treatment group. The average number of oocytes retrieved did not differ in the two groups, although the mean numbers of germinal vesicles and degenerated oocytes were significantly reduced with myo-inositol co-treatment, with a trend for more mature oocytes [53].

Ciotta *et al.* published a double-blinded study comparing oocyte quality in 34 PCOS women receiving a similar protocol: 2 g of myo-inositol with 200 µg of folic acid twice daily versus 200 µg of folic acid alone twice daily for three months [50]. The investigators reported significantly higher numbers of follicles > 15 mm, oocytes recovered, and embryos available for transfer in the group treated with myo-inositol. Given the paucity of high-quality evidence supporting the use of myo-inositol in infertile PCOS women planning IVF, these preliminary findings paved the way for larger more powered ongoing trials.

Two recent systematic reviews advocated the benefits of myo-inositol in infertile PCOS women undergoing IVF on the basis of a more significant reduction in recombinant FSH requirements, shortening in the duration of stimulation [54], as well as increase in clinical pregnancies (95% CI 1.04–1.96, $p = 0.03$) and decrease in miscarriages (95% CI 0.08–0.50, $p = 0.0006$) [55].

Conclusion

The missing pieces of the PCOS puzzle are yet to be unraveled. As the prevalence of obesity rises, PCOS genes appear to be unmasked and reproductive medicine centers will be increasingly challenged by patients with the "double whammy" of PCOS and obesity. The results of ovarian stimulation in women with PCOS are less predictable and more prone to over-response than in women without the condition. The skill is in anticipation and prevention of ovarian hyperstimulation. Extra vigilance is necessary to ensure patient safety and optimum outcome in this group of patients, but with proper knowledge and diligent care, outcomes should be comparable with those seen for other groups of infertile women.

References

1. Gjønnaess H. Ovarian electrocautery in the treatment of women with polycystic ovary syndrome (PCOS): factors affecting the results. *Acta Obstet Gynecol Scand* 1994;**73**(5):407–412.

2. Li TC, Saravelos H, Chow MS, Chisabingo R, Cooke ID. Factors affecting the outcome of laparoscopic ovarian drilling for polycystic ovary syndrome in women with anovulatory infertility. *Br J Obstet Gynaecol* 1998;**105**:338–344.

3. Armar NA, McGarrigle HHG, Honour J, *et al.* Laparoscopic ovarian diathermy in the

management of anovulatory infertility in women with polycystic ovaries: endocrine changes and clinical outcome. *Fertil Steril* 1990;**53**:45–49.

4. Balen AH, Jacobs HS. A prospective study comparing unilateral and bilateral laparoscopic ovarian diathermy in women with the polycystic ovary syndrome. *Fertil Steril* 1994;**62**:921–925.

5. Bordewijk EM, Ng KY, Rakic L, *et al*. Laparoscopic ovarian drilling for ovulation induction in women with anovulatory polycystic ovary syndrome. *Cochrane Database Syst Rev* 2020;**2**:CD001122.

6. Api M, Gorgen H, Cetin A. Laparoscopic ovarian drilling in polycystic ovary syndrome. *Eur J Obstet Gynecol Reprod Biol* 2005;**119**:76–81.

7. Amer SA, Li TC, Metwally M, Emarh M, Ledger WL. Randomized controlled trial comparing laparoscopic ovarian diathermy with clomiphene citrate as a first-line method of ovulation induction in women with polycystic ovary syndrome. *Hum Reprod* 2009;**24**:219–225.

8. Amer S, Banu Z, Li TC, Cooke ID. Long-term follow-up of patients with polycystic ovary syndrome after laparoscopic ovarian drilling: endocrine and ultrasonographic outcomes. *Hum Reprod* 2002;**17**(11):2851–2857.

9. Amer SA, El Shamy TT, James C, Yosef AH, Mohamed AA. The impact of laparoscopic ovarian drilling on AMH and ovarian reserve: a meta-analysis. *Reproduction* 2017;**154**(1):R13–R21.

10. Amer S, Li TC, Ledger WL. Ovulation induction using laparoscopic ovarian drilling in women with polycystic ovarian syndrome: predictors of success. *Hum Reprod* 2004;**19**(8):1719–1724.

11. Balen AH, Morley LC, Misso M, *et al*. The management of anovulatory infertility in women with polycystic ovary syndrome: an analysis of the evidence to support the development of global WHO guidance. *Hum Reprod Update* 2016;**22**(6):687–708.

12. Weiss NS, Nahuis MJ, Bordewijk E, *et al*. Gonadotrophins versus clomifene citrate with or without intrauterine insemination in women with normogonadotropic anovulation and clomifene failure (M-OVIN): a randomised, two-by-two factorial trial. *Lancet* 2018;**391**(10122):758–765.

13. Weiss NS, Kostova E, Nahuis M, *et al*. Gonadotrophins for ovulation induction in women with polycystic ovary syndrome. *Cochrane Database Syst Rev* 2019;**1**:CD010290.

14. Pardo M, Bancells N. Artificial insemination with husband's sperm (AIH). Techniques for sperm selection. *Arch Androl* 1989;**22**:15–27.

15. Tan SL, Child TJ. In-vitro maturation of oocytes from unstimulated polycystic ovaries. *Reprod Biomed Online* 2002;**4**:18–23.

16. Heijnen E, Eijkemans M, Hughes E, *et al*. A meta-analysis of outcomes of conventional IVF in women with polycystic ovary syndrome. *Hum Reprod Update* 2006;**12**(1):13–21.

17. Sha T, Wang X, Cheng W, Yan Y. A meta-analysis of pregnancy-related outcomes and complications in women with polycystic ovary syndrome undergoing in vitro fertilization. *Reprod Biomed Online* 2019;**39**(2):281–293.

18. Devroey P, Polyzos NP, Blockeel C. An OHSS-free clinic by segmentation of IVF treatment. *Hum Reprod* 2011;**26**(10):2593–2597.

19. Trounson A, Wood C, Kausche A. In vitro maturation and the fertilization and developmental competence of oocytes recovered from untreated polycystic ovarian patients. *Fertil Steril* 1994;**62**(2):353–362.

20. Barnes FL, Crombie A, Gardner DK, *et al*. Blastocyst development and birth after in-vitro maturation of human primary oocytes, intracytoplasmic sperm injection and assisted hatching. *Hum Reprod* 1995;**10**(12):3243–3247.

21. Benkhalifa M, Demirol A, Ménézo Y, *et al*. Natural cycle IVF and oocyte in-vitro maturation in polycystic ovary syndrome: a collaborative prospective study. *Reprod Biomed Online* 2009;**18**(1):29–36.

22. Siristatidis CS, Maheshwari A, Vaidakis D, Bhattacharya S. In vitro maturation in subfertile women with polycystic ovarian syndrome undergoing assisted reproduction. *Cochrane Database Syst Rev* 2018;**11**:CD006606.

23. Albano C, Felberbaum RE, Smitz J, *et al*. Ovarian stimulation with HMG: results of a prospective randomized phase III European study comparing the luteinizing hormone-releasing hormone (LHRH)-antagonist cetrorelix and the LHRH-agonist buserelin. *Hum Reprod* 2000;**15**(3):526–531.

24. Borm G, Mannaerts B. Treatment with the gonadotrophin-releasing hormone antagonist ganirelix in women undergoing ovarian stimulation with recombinant follicle stimulating hormone is effective, safe and convenient: results of a controlled, randomized, multicentre trial. The European Orgalutran Study Group. *Hum Reprod* 2000;**15**(7):1490–1498.

25. Lambalk CB, Banga FR, Huirne JA, *et al*. GnRH antagonist versus long agonist protocols in IVF: a systematic review and meta-analysis accounting for patient type. *Hum Reprod Update* 2017;**23**(5):560–579.

26. Shin JJ, Park KE, Choi YM, *et al.* Early gonadotropin-releasing hormone antagonist protocol in women with polycystic ovary syndrome: a preliminary randomized trial. *Clin Exp Reprod Med* 2018;**45**(3):135–142.

27. Olivennes F, Fanchin R, Bouchard P, *et al.* Triggering of ovulation by a gonadotropin-releasing hormone (GnRH) agonist in patients pretreated with a GnRH antagonist. *Fertil Steril* 1996;**66**:151–153.

28. Fauser BC, de Jong D, Olivennes F, *et al.* Endocrine profiles after triggering of final oocyte maturation with GnRH agonist after cotreatment with the GnRH antagonist ganirelix during ovarian hyperstimulation for in vitro fertilization. *J Clin Endocrinol Metab* 2002;**87**:709–715.

29. Griesinger G, Diedrich K, Devroey P, Kolibianakis EM. GnRH agonist for triggering final oocyte maturation in the GnRH antagonist ovarian hyperstimulation protocol: a systematic review and meta-analysis. *Hum Reprod Update* 2006;**12**:159–168.

30. Engmann L, DiLuigi A, Schmidt D, *et al.* The use of gonadotropin-releasing hormone (GnRH) agonist to induce oocyte maturation after cotreatment with GnRH antagonist in high-risk patients undergoing in vitro fertilization prevents the risk of ovarian hyperstimulation syndrome: a prospective randomized controlled study. *Fertil Steril* 2008;**89**(1):84–91.

31. Kummer N, Benadiva C, Feinn R, *et al.* Factors that predict the probability of a successful clinical outcome after induction of oocyte maturation with a gonadotropin-releasing hormone agonist. *Fertil Steril* 2011;**96**(1):63–68.

32. Griffin D, Benadiva C, Kummer N, *et al.* Dual trigger of oocyte maturation with gonadotropin-releasing hormone agonist and low-dose human chorionic gonadotropin to optimize live birth rates in high responders. *Fertil Steril* 2012;**97**(6):1316–1320.

33. Humaidan P, Bredkjær HE, Westergaard LG, *et al.* 1,500 IU human chorionic gonadotropin administered at oocyte retrieval rescues the luteal phase when gonadotropin-releasing hormone agonist is used for ovulation induction: a prospective, randomized, controlled study. *Fertil Steril* 2010;**93**(3):847–854.

34. Seyhan A, Ata B, Polat M, *et al.* Severe early ovarian hyperstimulation syndrome following GnRH agonist trigger with the addition of 1500 IU hCG. *Hum Reprod* 2013;**28**(9):2522–2528.

35. O'Neill KE, Senapati S, Maina I, *et al.* GnRH agonist with low-dose hCG (dual trigger) is associated with higher risk of severe ovarian hyperstimulation syndrome compared to GnRH agonist alone. *J Assist Reprod Genet* 2016;**33**(9):1175–1184.

36. Fatemi HM, Popovic-Todorovic B. Implantation in assisted reproduction: a look at endometrial receptivity. *Reprod Biomed Online* 2013;**27**(5):530–538.

37. Garcia-Velasco JA. Agonist trigger: what is the best approach? Agonist trigger with vitrification of oocytes or embryos. *Fertil Steril* 2012;**97**(3):527–528.

38. Doronzo G, Russo I, Mattiello L, *et al.* Insulin activates vascular endothelial growth factor in vascular smooth muscle cells: influence of nitric oxide and of insulin resistance. *Eur J Clin Invest* 2004;**34**:664–673.

39. Palomba S, Falbo A, La Sala GB. Effects of metformin in women with polycystic ovary syndrome treated with gonadotrophins for in vitro fertilisation and intracytoplasmic sperm injection cycles: a systematic review and meta-analysis of randomised controlled trials. *BJOG* 2013;**120**(3):267–276.

40. Palomba S, Falbo A, Carrillo L, *et al.* Metformin reduces risk of ovarian hyperstimulation syndrome in patients with polycystic ovary syndrome during gonadotropin-stimulated in vitro fertilization cycles: a randomized, controlled trial. *Fertil Steril* 2011;**96**(6):1384–1390.

41. Abdalmageed OS, Farghaly TA, Abdalaleem AA, *et al.* Impact of metformin on IVF outcomes in overweight and obese women with polycystic ovary syndrome: a randomized double-blind controlled trial. *Reprod Sci* 2019;**26**(10):1336–1342.

42. Tso LO, Costello MF, Albuquerque LE, Andriolo RB, Macedo CR. Metformin treatment before and during IVF or ICSI in women with polycystic ovary syndrome. *Cochrane Database Syst Rev* 2014;**11**:CD006105.

43. Bevilacqua A, Bizzarri M. Inositols in insulin signaling and glucose metabolism. *Int J Endocrinol* 2018;**2018**:1968450.

44. Genazzani AD, Lanzoni C, Ricchieri F, Jasonni VM. Myo-inositol administration positively affects hyperinsulinemia and hormonal parameters in overweight patients with polycystic ovary syndrome. *Gynecol Endocrinol* 2008;**24**(3):139–144.

45. Costantino D, Minozzi G, Minozzi E, Guaraldi C. Metabolic and hormonal effects of myo-inositol in women with polycystic ovary syndrome: a double-blind trial. *Eur Rev Med Pharmacol Sci* 2009;**13**(2):105–110.

46. Minozzi M, Nordio M, Pajalich R. The combined therapy myo-inositol plus D-chiro-inositol, in a physiological ratio, reduces the cardiovascular risk by improving the lipid profile in PCOS patients. *Eur Rev Med Pharmacol Sci* 2013;**17**(4):537–540.

47. Gateva A, Unfer V, Kamenov Z. The use of inositol (s) isomers in the management of polycystic ovary syndrome: a comprehensive review. *Gynecol Endocrinol* 2018;**34**(7):545–550.

48. Facchinetti F, Orrù B, Grandi G, Unfer V. Short-term effects of metformin and myo-inositol in women with polycystic ovarian syndrome (PCOS): a meta-analysis of randomized clinical trials. *Gynecol Endocrinol* 2019;**35**(3):198–206.

49. Taieb J, Grynberg M, Pierre A, *et al.* FSH and its second messenger cAMP stimulate the transcription of human anti-Müllerian hormone in cultured granulosa cells. *Mol Endocrinol* 2011;**25**(4):645–655.

50. Ciotta L, Stracquadanio M, Pagano I, *et al.* Effects of myo-inositol supplementation on oocyte's quality in PCOS patients: a double blind trial. *Eur Rev Med Pharmacol Sci* 2011;**15**(5):509–514.

51. Unfer V, Porcaro G. Updates on the myo-inositol plus D-chiro-inositol combined therapy in polycystic ovary syndrome. *Expert Rev Clin Pharmacol* 2014;**7**(5):623–631.

52. Colazingari S, Fiorenza MT, Carlomagno G, Najjar R, Bevilacqua A. Improvement of mouse embryo quality by myo-inositol supplementation of IVF media. *J Assist Reprod Genet* 2014;**31** (4):463–469.

53. Papaleo E, Unfer V, Baillargeon JP, *et al.* Myo-inositol may improve oocyte quality in intracytoplasmic sperm injection cycles. A prospective, controlled, randomized trial. *Fertil Steril* 2009;**91**(5):1750–1754.

54. Laganà AS, Vitagliano A, Noventa M, Ambrosini G, D'Anna R. Myo-inositol supplementation reduces the amount of gonadotropins and length of ovarian stimulation in women undergoing IVF: a systematic review and meta-analysis of randomized controlled trials. *Arch Gynecol Obstet* 2018;**298**(4):675–684.

55. Zheng X, Lin D, Zhang Y, *et al.* Inositol supplement improves clinical pregnancy rate in infertile women undergoing ovulation induction for ICSI or IVF-ET. *Medicine (Baltimore)* 2017;**96** (49):e8842.

Chapter

15

Prevention of Ovarian Hyperstimulation Syndrome

Mohamed Youssef, Abdel-Maguid Ramzy, and Botros Rizk

Introduction

Ovarian hyperstimulation syndrome (OHSS) is the most serious iatrogenic complication of excessive response to ovulation induction or ovarian stimulation during in vitro fertilization/intracytoplasmic sperm injection (IVF/ICSI) treatment cycles [1–5] The incidence of OHSS has been estimated at 20–33% for mild cases, 3–6% for moderate cases, and 0.1% and 2% for severe cases [6–8]. OHSS is characterized by bilateral, multiple follicular and theca-lutein ovarian cysts (Figure 15.1) and an acute shift in body fluid distribution resulting in ascites (Figure 15.2) and pleural effusion. Rizk and Smitz [9], in an analytical study of the factors that influence the incidence of OHSS, found a wide variation among different centers. This is partly because of different definitions for the grades of severity and partly because of the adoption of different criteria for prevention.

OHSS Classifications

OHSS may be mild, moderate, severe, or critical in severity; early (< 9 days) or late in onset; spontaneous or iatrogenic in etiology. Early OHSS presented 3 to 7 days after the ovulatory dose of human chorionic gonadotropin (hCG) whereas late OHSS presented 12 to 17 days after hCG. Early OHSS relates to "excessive" preovulatory response to stimulation, whereas late OHSS depends on the occurrence of pregnancy, is more likely to be severe, and is only poorly related to preovulatory events. Most cases of OHSS are iatrogenic following excessive ovarian stimulation with gonadotropins. Rarely, OHSS may be spontaneous occurring as a result of mutations in the follicle-stimulating hormone (FSH) receptor resulting in stimulation of the FSH receptor by chorionic gonadotropin that is abundant in early pregnancy.

Although OHSS classification helps us to predict and prevent OHSS by comparing the

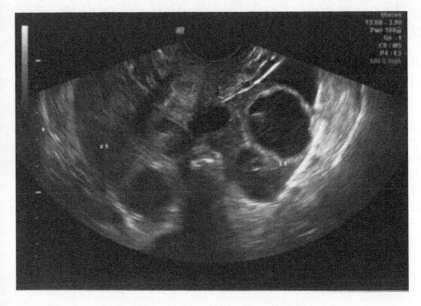

Figure 15.1 Bilateral enlarged cystic ovaries. Reproduced with permission from Rizk *et al.* [110].

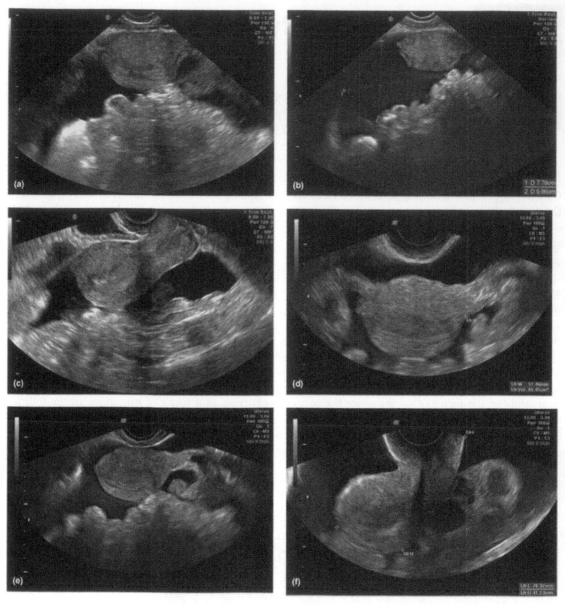

Figure 15.2 Ascites in severe ovarian hyperstimulation syndrome. Reproduced with permission from Rizk *et al.* [110].

incidence of different severity grades and to individualize the treatment options, there has been no unanimity in classifying OHSS and divergent classifications have made comparisons between studies difficult [10]. Aboulghar and Mansour reviewed the classifications used for OHSS (Table 15.1) [2]. A classification was introduced in 1999 by Rizk and Aboulghar [11]. They classified the syndrome into only two categories, moderate and severe with the purpose of categorizing patients into more

defined clinical groups that correlate with the prognosis of the syndrome. The mild degree of OHSS used by most previous authors was omitted from the classification, as this degree occurs in the majority of cases of ovarian stimulation and does not require special treatment. The great majority of cases of OHSS present with symptoms belong to category of moderate OHSS. In addition to the presence of ascites on ultrasound, the patient's complaints are usually limited to mild abdominal pain and distension

Table 15.1 Classification of OHSS

- Moderate OHSS
  - Discomfort, pain, nausea, abdominal distension, no clinical evidence of ascites, but ultrasonic evidence of ascites and enlarged ovaries, normal hematological and biological profiles; can be treated on an outpatient basis with extreme vigilance
- Severe OHSS
  - Grade A: Dyspnea, oliguria, nausea, vomiting, diarrhea, abdominal pain; clinical evidence of ascites plus marked distension of abdomen or hydrothorax; ultrasound scan showing large ovaries and marked ascites; normal biochemical profiles; can be treated as inpatient or outpatient depending on the physician's comfort, the patient's compliance, and medical facility
  - Grade B: All symptoms of grade A, plus massive tension ascites, markedly enlarged ovaries, severe dyspnea, and marked oliguria; Biochemical changes in the form of increased hematocrit, elevated serum creatinine, and liver dysfunction; would be treated in an inpatient hospital setting with expert supervision
  - Grade C: OHSS complicated by respiratory distress syndrome, renal shut-down, or venous thrombosis; which is critical and would be treated in an intensive care setting.

and their hematological and biochemical are normal.

In 2009, the Golan classification considered life-threatening OHSS including complications such as renal failure, thromboembolism, and adult respiratory syndrome as a "Grade 6 OHSS" [12]. In 2010, Humaidan *et al.* provided a classification scheme for grading OHSS that incorporates vaginal sonography and laboratory parameters to objectively relate symptoms to severity [13]. In this system, mild, moderate, and severe forms of OHSS are distinguished by the extent of fluid shift into body cavities, with moderate disease defined by shifts of 500 ml, and severe disease characterized by laboratory signs of hepatorenal dysfunction due to hemoconcentration and hypovolemia.

Pathophysiology of OHSS

The exact pathophysiology and etiology of OHSS remains unknown, but increased capillary permeability with the resulting loss of fluid into the third space is common to the syndrome [14]. Administration of hCG for final follicle maturation and triggering of ovulation appears to be the pivotal stimulus in a susceptible patient, by releasing vasoactive–angiogenic substances such as vascular endothelial growth factor (VEGF) from the ovaries hyperstimulated with gonadotropins (Figure 15.3) [15]. VEGF has been found to be expressed in human ovaries and it has been observed that VEGF mRNA levels increase after hCG administration in granulosa cells and elevated levels of the secreted proteins have been detected in serum, plasma, and peritoneal fluids in women at risk or with OHSS. Other mediators

such as angiotensin II, insulin-like growth factor 1, pro-inflammatory interleukin-6, and tumor necrosis factor have been implicated in the pathogenesis of OHSS [16–18]. OHSS is characterized by bilateral ovarian cystic enlargement and third-space fluid shift. The ovaries are noted to have a significant degree of stromal edema, interspersed with multiple hemorrhagic follicular and thecalutein cysts, areas of cortical necrosis, and neovascularization. The second pathological phenomenon is that of acute body fluid shifts, which in turn causes hemoconcentration with reduced organ perfusion, alterations in blood coagulation and the resulting risk of thromboembolism, and leakage of fluids into the peritoneal cavity and lungs [2].

Prediction of OHSS

There are several pretreatment characteristics such as young age, black race, ovulation disorder, and polycystic ovarian syndrome (PCOS), which have been introduced as predictive markers of OHSS [2;19–21]. Furthermore, biomarkers of the ovarian reserve such as an elevated anti-Müllerian hormone (> 3.4 ng/ml) or elevated antral follicle count (> 24) have been proven to be significantly more specific and sensitive and are now routinely recommended for the pretreatment identification of patients at risk and for planning of ovarian stimulation cycles [22]. Once patients have commenced treatment, additional characteristics related to the extent of multifollicular growth such as visualization of ≥ 25 follicles, estradiol on the day of trigger > 3500 pg/ml, or ≥ 24 oocytes retrieved may aid in the prediction of patients who will develop OHSS (Table 15.2) [8;23].

Pathophysiology:

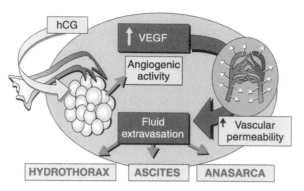

Figure 15.3 Pathophysiology of hCG in ovarian hyperstimulation syndrome. Reproduced with permission from Rizk et al. [110].

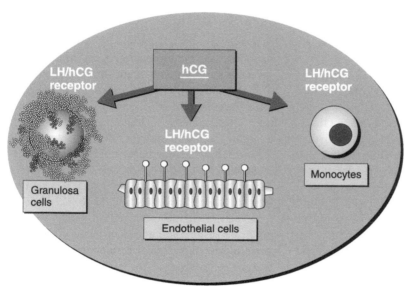

Transvaginal ultrasonography (TVUS) plus/or serum estradiol levels has been suggested to be an effective intervention in reducing the incidence and severity of OHSS. A Cochrane systematic review evaluated the effect of monitoring controlled ovarian stimulation in IVF/ICSI cycles with TVUS only versus TVUS plus serum estradiol concentration, with respect to rates of live birth, pregnancy, and OHSS [24;25]. Six randomized controlled trials (RCTs) with 781 women were included in the analysis. The combined monitoring by TVUS and serum estradiol was not superior to the monitoring by ultrasound alone with regard to pregnancy rate and OHSS incidence.

Prevention of OHSS

As the treatment of OHSS involves supportive management such as antiemetics, analgesics, fluid intake, and paracentesis, in severe cases, while the condition slowly improves, the mainstay of management of women at risk of OHSS resolves around the prevention of this complication in the first instance [26]. By identifying women at risk, several preventive approaches have been suggested to reduce the risk of OHSS; these approaches could be divided into primary and secondary [27]. Primary prevention includes mild doses of gonadotropins [28–31], use of gonadotropin-releasing hormone (GnRH) antagonists [3;32–34], and in vitro maturation (IVM) [35–37]. Secondary prevention includes all strategies directed to counteract an excessive ovarian response, cycle cancellation [38], coasting [39–41], ovulation triggering by low doses of hCG [42;43] or by a GnRH agonist [44–46], dopamine agonist administration around the time of follicle aspiration [47–50]; intravenous

Table 15.2 Prediction of OHSS

Predictors	Cut-off value	Statistical significance
Before initiation of ovarian stimulation		
Age	< 33 years	
BMI/weight	Does not currently appear to be a useful marker for increased risk of *OHSS*	
AFC	• 14 may predict hyper-response • 24 follicles in both ovaries	
AMH [111;112]	• 3.36 ng/ml • 6.85 ng/ml for PCOS patients • 4.85 ng/ml in non-PCOS patients • 1.5 ng/ml in serum with 80% detection rate of OHSS	Sensitivity: 90.5% Specificity: 80% Sensitivity: 66.7% Specificity: 68.7% Sensitivity: 85.7 % Specificity: 89.7%
Previous OHSS	Moderate or severe cases especially when hospitalization required	
PCOS	≥ 12 antral follicles 2–8 mm in diameter	10–12% incidence of moderate/severe OHSS in PCOS
During controlled ovarian stimulation and before hCG trigger		
Total dose of gonadotropins	1700 IU or less threshold 85% of the cases of severe OHSS were identified	PPV: 0.85% NPV: 99.92%
High number of growing follicles on the day of hCG	• ≥ 15 follicles of diameters > 10 mm for identification of severe OHSS • ≥ 12 follicles ≥ 10 mm for identification of moderate OHSS • Combination of 25 follicles at aspiration, 19 large/medium-sized follicles before hCG and 24 oocytes	AUC = 0.904, 95% CI 0.895–0.912 Sensitivity: 82% Specificity: 99% for requiring hospitalization
High serum estradiol level on the day of hCG	• ≥ 2201 pg/ml, this cut-off value identified 85% of cases of severe OHSS by 13 times • Combination of ≥ 18 follicles and/or estradiol of 5000 pg/ml	OR 13.2, 95% CI: 3.9–44.8 Predicts 83% of severe OHSS
Number of oocytes retrieved [113]	> 15 oocytes	
Non-applicable markers	VEGF, follicular fluid IL-6 and IL-8 levels	

BMI = body mass index; AFC = antral follicle count; AMH = anti-Müllerian hormone; PCOS = polycystic ovary syndrome; PPV = positive predictive value; NPV = negative predictive value; AUC = area under curve; CI = confidence interval; OR = odds ratio; VEGF = vascular endothelial growth factor; IL = interleukin.

volume expanders administration at the time of follicle aspiration [51;52], or calcium gluconate infusion [53], cryopreservation of oocytes or embryos [54;55] and suppression of luteal phase steroids after oocyte retrieval, together with embryo cryopreservation, using letrozole, mifepristone, GnRH antagonist, or three-drug combinations [56–58]. Moreover, incorporating two or more of the previous strategies has been suggested as an alternative approach. So, OHSS is a great challenge, and although there are a huge number of interventions available, the evidence to support one over the other was limited. Thus, in this chapter we set out to identify and evaluate the most widely used interventions for predicting and preventing OHSS.

GnRH Antagonists for Pituitary Desensitization

GnRH antagonists can be used to prevent a luteinizing hormone (LH) surge during controlled ovarian hyperstimulation without the hypoestrogenic side effects, flare-up, or long downregulation period associated with agonists [59]. The antagonists directly and rapidly inhibit gonadotropin release within several hours through competitive binding to pituitary GnRH receptors. This property allows their use at any time during the follicular phase. Several different regimens have been described including multiple-dose fixed (0.25 mg daily from day 6 to 7 of stimulation), multiple-dose flexible (0.25 mg daily when leading follicle is 14 to 15 mm), and single-dose (single administration of 3 mg on day 7 to 8 of stimulation) protocols, with or without the addition of an oral contraceptive pill.

A Cochrane systematic review was published on the effectiveness and safety of GnRH antagonists compared with the standard long protocol of GnRH agonists for controlled ovarian hyperstimulation in assisted conception cycles. The review included 73 RCTs, totaling 12 212 women. Primary outcome measure of effectiveness was live birth rate and primary outcome measure of safety was OHSS incidence. Secondary outcome measures were ongoing pregnancy rate, clinical pregnancy rate, miscarriage rate, and cycle cancellation rate [3]. Forty-five RCTs (n = 7511) comparing the antagonist to the long agonist protocols fulfilled the inclusion criteria. There was no evidence of a statistically significant difference in rates of live births (odds ratio [OR] 0.86, 95% confidence interval [CI] 0.69–1.08). There was a statistically significant lower incidence of OHSS in the GnRH antagonist group (OR 0.43, 95% CI 0.33–0.57) [3]. Based on this, finding the short GnRH antagonist protocol should be the protocol of choice for women undergoing IVF/ICSI cycles and at an increased risk of severe OHSS [60].

Another systematic review and meta-analysis accounted for various patient populations, such as ovulatory women, women with polycystic ovary syndrome (PCOS), or women with poor ovarian response [61]. Antagonist treatment in the general population resulted in a significantly lower OHSS rate than agonist (relative risk [RR] 0.63, 95% CI 0.50–0.81). Compared to a control OHSS rate of 6.2 percent following the agonist protocol, the development of OHSS following the antagonist protocol would be at a rate of 3.7 percent, with an absolute risk difference of 2.5 percent. In women with PCOS, the OHSS rate was significantly lower when antagonist was used instead of agonist (RR 0.53, 95% CI 0.30–0.95). Assuming comparable clinical outcomes for the antagonist and agonist protocols, these benefits would justify a change from the standard long agonist protocol to antagonist regimens.

Mild Ovarian Stimulation

Mild stimulation IVF is defined as a protocol in which ovaries are stimulated with gonadotropins and/or oral compounds such as clomiphene (clomifene) citrate or letrozole to limit the number of oocytes and to avoid OHSS [62;63]. Mild stimulation has benefits of less stress [64] and lower cost [28]. In hyper-responder women, mild stimulation IVF has not achieved wide acceptance in practice because of concerns about its clinical effectiveness and currently the availability of GnRH antagonist–GnRH agonist trigger and freeze-all policy [65;66].

In Vitro Maturation

IVM has been proposed to reduce the risk of OHSS in women with PCOS. IVM involves earlier retrieval of immature oocytes, from the germinal vesicle stage, that may or may not have been exposed to gonadotropins, followed by their maturation in the laboratory until the metaphase II stage and ready to undergo fertilization [67]. IVM treatment is still considered to be experimental and currently there is no evidence to base any practice recommendation regarding IVM before IVF/ICSI [68].

Coasting

Coasting means omission of gonadotropins and continued administration of GnRH agonist or antagonist (Figure 15.4). A recent Cochrane systematic review, including eight RCTs, found that the rates of OHSS were lower in the coasting group (OR 0.11, 95% CI 0.05–0.24) (Figure 15.4), suggesting that if 45 percent of women developed moderate or severe OHSS without coasting, between 4 and 17 percent of women would develop it with coasting [69]. However, the evidence to suggest that coasting reduced rates of moderate or severe OHSS more than no coasting was of low quality.

GnRH Agonist Trigger for Final Oocyte Maturation in GnRH Antagonist Cycles

Traditionally a bolus of hCG has been the gold standard for ovulation induction and final oocyte maturation in assisted reproductive technology (ART) cycles as a surrogate for the natural mid-cycle luteinizing hormone (LH) surge. When

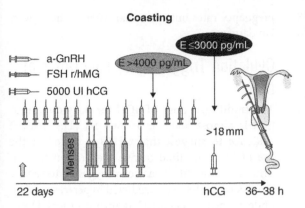

Coasting

⊨— a-GnRH
⊨— FSH r/hMG
⊨— 5000 UI hCG

E >4000 pg/mL
E ≤3000 pg/mL

Menses

>18 mm

22 days

hCG   36–38 h

Figure 15.4 Coasting versus no coasting for prevention of ovarian hyperstimulation syndrome. Reproduced with permission from Rizk *et al.* [110].

GnRH antagonist protocols were introduced for the prevention of a premature LH surge it became possible to trigger final oocyte maturation and ovulation with a GnRH agonist as an alternative to hCG. A midcycle single bolus of GnRH agonist may be injected subcutaneously (0.2 to 0.5 mg of triptorelin, leuprorelin, or buserelin) [70] or administered intranasally (200 µg buserelin) [71;72].

Consequently, oocyte maturation triggering with GnRH agonists may provide several advantages over that achieved with hCG. First, GnRH agonists reduce the risk of OHSS due to quick and irreversible luteolysis [72]. Second, a more physiological LH and FSH surge is induced by the agonists, which may result in better oocyte and embryo quality [70]. Third, GnRH agonists may improve endometrial quality as a result of the lower luteal phase steroid levels [72;73].

A Cochrane review on the effectiveness and safety of GnRH agonists in comparison with hCG for triggering final oocyte maturation in IVF and ICSI for women undergoing controlled ovarian hyperstimulation in a GnRH antagonist protocol has been performed [46]. Primary outcome measure of effectiveness was live birth rate and primary outcome measure of safety was OHSS. Secondary outcome measures were ongoing pregnancy rates, clinical pregnancy rates, and miscarriage rate. It included 17 RCTs (*n* = 1847), of which 13 studies assessed fresh autologous cycles and 4 studies assessed donor-recipient cycles. Final oocyte maturation triggering with GnRH agonist instead of hCG in fresh autologous GnRH antagonist IVF/ICSI treatment cycles prevents OHSS (OR 0.15, 95% CI 0.05–0.47) to the detriment of the live birth rate due to the short duration of the induced LH/FSH peak. Thus,

GnRH agonist as an oocyte maturation trigger could be useful for women who choose to avoid fresh transfers, women who donate oocytes to recipients, or women who wish to freeze their eggs for later use in the context of fertility preservation.

Different modified luteal phase support strategies have been provided to overcome the luteal phase deficiency, in terms of small boluses of hCG [13], or daily recombinant LH or GnRH agonist [74]. In the OHSS risk patient, GnRH agonist trigger can be safely performed, followed by a "freeze-all" policy with a minimal risk of OHSS development and high live birth rates in the subsequent frozen embryo transfer cycle [74;75]. Furthermore, converting OHSS risk patients during stimulation from a long GnRH agonist protocol to a GnRH antagonist protocol and subsequent GnRH agonist trigger is a plausible rescue option in patients at high risk of OHSS development [76].

Metformin

The use of insulin sensitizers, such as metformin, an oral biguanide, is recognized to reduce OHSS in women with PCOS who are undergoing GnRH agonist IVF cycles (OR 0.27, 95% CI 0.16–0.47) [77]. Meanwhile, its role in a GnRH antagonist protocol is controversial. A recent Cochrane overview concluded that clinicians should consider metformin treatment before and during IVF/ICSI cycles for women with PCOS (moderate-quality evidence) [78]. A RCT evaluated the use of a short course of metformin for the prevention of OHSS in 153 women with PCOS undergoing GnRH antagonist IVF cycles and concluded that metformin does not reduce the incidence of OHSS [79]. Furthermore the fact that treatment with metformin during ovarian stimulation was still associated with an overall occurrence of moderate to severe OHSS of 14.1 percent in cycles triggered with hCG is no longer acceptable given that a substantive reduction in OHSS may be achieved by simply replacing hCG with a GnRH agonist trigger.

Ovarian Drilling in PCOS Patients

Laparoscopic ovarian drilling has been used for prevention of OHSS in patients with polycystic ovaries undergoing ovulation induction [80]. A RCT evaluated the effect of laparoscopic ovarian drilling in 120 women with clomiphene citrate-resistant polycystic ovary compared with GnRH antagonist plus dopamine agonist a day before hCG and for eight days in 130 women [81]. None of the women in the ovarian drilling group developed severe OHSS.

Ultrasound-guided transvaginal ovarian needle drilling (UTND) and ovarian stroma hydrocoagulation for ovarian stimulation has also been reported in patients with clomiphene-resistant PCOS [82]. The mechanism of UTND is not well understood but it might be similar to ovarian wedge resection and laparoscopic ovarian drilling. Ovary puncture and aspiration of follicular fluid through UTND reduces intraovarian androgen and other steroids rapidly and directly [83]. Serum androgen and LH levels also decrease remarkably after UTND [84]. It has been suggested that transvaginal ovarian drilling has been effective in improving IVF results in difficult cases and is less invasive and expensive when compared with laparoscopic ovarian drilling. A recent meta-analysis included five RCTs involving 639 clomiphene-resistant women with PCOS to evaluate UTND compared with laparoscopic ovarian drilling or with gonadotropins; there were no studies reported on the incidence of OHSS [85]. The technique is relatively straightforward: a triple puncture laparoscopy is usually performed and the ovary is grasped by the ovarian ligament. A variety of instruments have been used for many years with tremendous variation in the literature regarding the three variables involved, which are the number of ovarian punctures, the duration of diathermy, and the wattage used. Generally no fewer than 4 and no more than 10 punctures to a depth of 4–10 mm on each ovary should be made. Fewer than four punctures on each ovary results in lower

pregnancy rates but more than 10 may cause ovarian damage.

Ovulation Triggering by Low Doses of hCG

The traditional dose of hCG for oocyte maturation is almost 5000 or 10 000 IU [1]. There is evidence to suggest that OHSS is linked to the use of hCG for final oocyte maturation trigger. Thus, low-dose hCG has been suggested to reduce the risk of OHSS in unpredicted hyper-responders undergoing a long GnRH agonist protocol. Doses of either 2500 IU [86] or 2000 IU of hCG [87] were given. The low dose of hCG was feasible to prevent OHSS without compromising IVF outcomes. On the other hand, the use of a very low dose of hCG, 2000 IU, would definitely impact the number of mature oocytes that can be retrieved; however, there seems to be no difference in the incidence of severe OHSS when patients are given 5000 IU of hCG or 10 000 IU hCG [88].

Several studies suggested that lower dose of hCG plus FSH supplementation –mimicking the naturally occurring FSH surge during the LH surge – may be associated with decreased OHSS compared with conventional triggers without compromising IVF outcomes [89;90]. A retrospective cohort study, comparing 1500 IU hCG plus 450 IU FSH with 3300 IU hCG, GnRH agonist alone, or GnRH agonist plus 1500 IU hCG, concluded that this modified trigger seems to be an alternative option for GnRH agonist-IVF cycles at high risk for OHSS [5].

Cycle Cancellation (hCG Withholding)

Although cycle cancellation is a valid and safe option that prevents both early- and late-onset OHSS, it results in financial and emotional disturbances for both woman and physician especially of cycles that would not have progressed to clinical OHSS [38;91]. Because of the availability of other more safe interventions such as GnRH antagonist–GnRH agonist trigger and freeze-all policy [46], termination of the cycle should only be considered as a last option for severe OHSS cases.

Dopamine Agonist Administration around the Time of Follicle Aspiration

A potential strategy to prevent OHSS and reduce the severity is the use of a dopamine agonist around the time of hCG administration or ovum pickup [92]. It was observed that the administration of a dopamine agonist in immature rats at low doses simultaneously with hCG prevented an increase in vascular permeability and did not affect angiogenesis [4]; the effect was due to the availability of dopamine type 2 receptors (Figures 15.5 and 15.6).

Two systematic reviews and meta-analyses of randomized trials comparing the prophylactic effect of the dopamine agonist cabergoline versus no treatment in IVF/ICSI cycles have been conducted. Primary outcome was OHSS incidence per randomized woman. Secondary outcomes were live birth rate, ongoing pregnancy rate, clinical pregnancy rate, and miscarriage rate. In Youssef *et al.* [47], four randomized trials entailing 570 women were included. There was evidence of a statistically significant reduction in the incidence of OHSS in the cabergoline group (OR 0.41, 95% CI 0.25–0.66) with an absolute risk reduction of 12 percent (95% CI 6.1–18.2%), but there was no statistically significant evidence of a reduction in severe OHSS (OR 0.50, 95% CI 0.20–1.26) [47].

In Tang *et al.*, 16 RCTs were included involving 2091 high-risk women. They evaluated three types of dopamine agonist: cabergoline, quinagolide, and bromocriptine. When compared with placebo or no intervention, the dopamine agonists seemed effective in the prevention of moderate or severe OHSS (OR 0.27, 95% CI 0.19–0.39). This suggests that if 29 percent of women undergoing ART experience moderate or severe OHSS, the use of dopamine agonists will lower this to 7 to 14 percent of women. There was no evidence of a difference in live birth rate, clinical pregnancy rate, multiple pregnancy rate, or miscarriage rate. However, taking dopamine agonists (especially quinagolide) may increase the incidence of adverse events such as gastrointestinal adverse effects (OR 4.54, 95% CI 1.49–13.84) [93].

Intravenous Volume Expanders' Administration at the Time of Follicle Aspiration

A number of clinical studies with conflicting results have reported on the use of plasma expanders such as albumin, hydroxyethyl starch (HES), mannitol, polygeline (Haemaccel), and dextran as a possible intervention for the prevention of OHSS [94]. Women who are considered at high risk are those with specific estradiol threshold levels, a threshold number of follicles or oocytes retrieved, or women with PCOS.

A Cochrane review evaluated the effectiveness and safety of the administration of intravenous fluids such as albumin, HES, Haemaccel, and

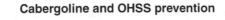

Cabergoline and OHSS prevention

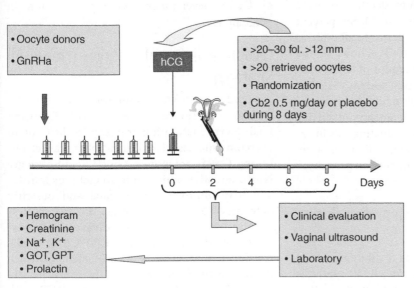

Figure 15.5 Cabergoline versus placebo/no treatment for prevention of ovarian hyperstimulation syndrome Cabergoline and prevention of ovarian hyperstimulation syndrome. Reproduced with permission from Rizk *et al.* [110].

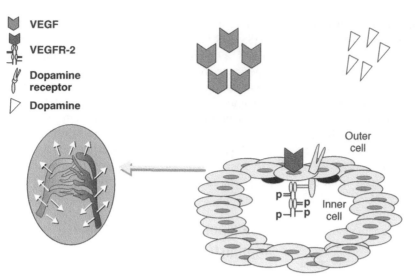

VEGF

VEGFR-2

Dopamine receptor

Dopamine

Outer cell

Inner cell

Figure 15.6 Molecular mechanism of dopamine agonist on vascular permeability. Reproduced with permission from Rizk *et al.* [110].

dextran in the prevention of severe OHSS in IVF or ICSI treatment cycles. Nine RCTs, totaling 2147 women, were included. Primary outcome measure was the incidence of severe OHSS and secondary outcomes were pregnancy rates and adverse events. The authors concluded that there was no evidence that intravenous albumin administration has any effect on the incidence of severe OHSS, but albumin possibly reduces the incidence of moderate OHSS in high-risk women undergoing controlled ovarian hyperstimulation (OR 0.71, 95% CI 0.47–1.07). There was moderate-quality evidence suggesting that HES might reduce the incidence of both moderate and severe OHSS (OR 0.13, 95% CI 0.02–0.75). Six percent HES has been proven to be superior to albumin as a volume expander in many studies; however, the evidence was inconclusive because of small sample size and observational study designs [95]. The administration of mannitol might also reduce both moderate and severe incidence of OHSS, but there was only one RCT evaluating this intervention. There was no evidence that albumin, HES, or mannitol had any influence on pregnancy rates [52].

Calcium Gluconate Infusion after Oocyte Retrieval

Low intracellular calcium has a stimulatory role on adenylyl cyclase resulting in cAMP synthesis and thus renin release. By increasing circulating calcium concentrations by infusion of 10 ml of 10% calcium gluconate solution in 200 ml physiological saline within 30 minutes of ovum pickup and continued thereafter on day 1, day 2, and day 3, it was speculated that this would inhibit cAMP-stimulated renin release, and decrease angiotensin II synthesis and VEGF production [53]. Four studies evaluated the infusion of calcium gluconate alone [53;96;97] or in combination with cabergoline, albumin infusion, GnRH antagonist in luteal phase in addition to elective cryopreservations of embryos [98]. It was concluded that intravenous calcium infusion effectively reduced the incidence of OHSS development without reduction in pregnancy.

Cryopreservation of Embryos (Freeze-All Strategy)

Currently, embryo cryopreservation for the avoidance of severe late-onset OHSS following final oocyte maturation trigger with hCG or to overcome the associated luteal phase defect following GnRH antagonist–GnRH agonist trigger is an alternative option to fresh embryos transfer and may improve the neonatal and obstetric outcomes [99–101]. In contrast, a Cochrane systematic overview evaluating different interventions for the prevention of OHSS in ART concluded that there was insufficient evidence to show benefit for routine embryo cryopreservation [78;102]. A large multicenter RCT, with

1508 infertile women with PCOS who were undergoing their first IVF cycle to undergo either fresh embryo transfer or embryo cryopreservation followed by frozen embryo transfer, reported that in infertile women with PCOS, frozen embryo transfer was associated with a lower risk of OHSS (RR 0.19, 95% CI 0.10–0.37) and higher live birth rate (RR 1.17, 95% CI 1.05–1.31) [103].

Suppression of Luteal Phase Steroids

Suppression of luteal phase steroids after oocyte retrieval, together with embryo cryopreservation, was suggested for preventing severe OHSS in high-risk women. Several trials evaluated letrozole (7.5 mg daily for 3 days), mifepristone, GnRH antagonist (0.25 mg SC daily for 3 days) and three-drug combinations during the luteal phase in 294 women. There were no evidence of a statistically significant difference in incidence of severe OHSS, the paracentesis rate, and the duration of hospitalization between study and control groups [56–58].

Letrozole Administration for the Prevention of OHSS

It has been proposed that administration of 2.5 mg of letrozole – for 1–3 days – either before the final oocyte maturation trigger with hCG [104] or during the luteal phase [58;105] in women with PCOS who underwent IVF is associated with lower risk of OHSS as a result of luteolysis rather than the effect of VEGF [106]. Letrozole is an aromatase inhibitor that prevents aromatase from producing estrogens, and lowers the level of estradiol; as letrozole does not affect the central nervous system, the process of follicular growth and ovulation continues normally.

Luteal GnRH Antagonist for the Prevention of OHSS

There are limited data regarding the ability of luteal GnRH antagonist to reduce the risk of severe OHSS and the mechanism is unclear. A prospective cohort study compared subcutaneous luteal GnRH antagonist administration – from day 3 to day 5 after oocyte retrieval – in 65 women with high risk of developing OHSS undergoing cryopreservation of all embryos with no drug in the control group [107]. The risk of moderate and severe OHSS was markedly lower in the luteal GnRH antagonist group (18.03% and 37.14%, $p = 0.037$). Another cohort study evaluated the impact of administration of low-dose GnRH antagonist from day 5 to day 7 after oocyte retrieval in 192 women who developed severe early OHSS after fresh embryo transfer compared to no drug [108]. There was no significant difference between both groups in either the live birth rate or risk of OHSS. A small pilot study investigated the kinetics of serum VEGF following GnRH antagonist administration in the luteal phase in 12 women with severe OHSS [109]. The levels of VEGF were higher five days after oocyte retrieval and there was a marked decline of VEGF after luteal GnRH antagonist administration and regression of severe OHSS.

Key Points

- OHSS is a broad spectrum of signs and symptoms that include abdominal distension and discomfort, enlarged ovaries, ascites, and other complications of enhanced vascular permeability
- The exact pathophysiology of OHSS remains unknown, but increased capillary permeability with the resulting loss of fluid into the third space is common to the syndrome
- There is evidence to suggest that OHSS is linked to the use of hCG for final oocyte maturation trigger by releasing VEGF from the ovary
- Identifying women at risk is the cornerstone of successful prevention of OHSS
- The combined monitoring by TVUS and serum estradiol was not superior to the monitoring by ultrasound alone with regard to pregnancy rate and OHSS incidence
- Effective prevention includes individualized ovarian stimulation protocols with mild doses of gonadotropins and/or the use of GnRH antagonists for pituitary downregulation, ovulation triggering by a GnRH agonist instead of hCG, and cryopreservation of all embryos
- Dopamine agonist and calcium infusion administration around the time of follicle aspiration seems to be a promising intervention
- Alternative preventive strategies such as luteal phase estradiol administration and GnRH antagonist are promising and further RCTs are required

References

1. Abdalla HI, Ah-Moye M, Brinsden P, *et al.* The effect of the dose of human chorionic gonadotropin and the type of gonadotropin stimulation on oocyte recovery rates in an in vitro fertilization program. *Fertil Steril* 1987;**48** (6):958–963.

2. Aboulghar MA, Mansour RT. Ovarian hyperstimulation syndrome: classifications and critical analysis of preventive measures. *Hum Reprod Update* 2003;**9**:275–289.

3. Al-Inany HG, Youssef MA, Ayeleke RO, *et al.* Gonadotrophin-releasing hormone antagonists for assisted reproductive technology. *Cochrane Database Syst Rev* 2016;**4**:CD001750.

4. Alvarez C, Martí-Bonmatí L, Novella-Maestre E, *et al.* Dopamine agonist cabergoline reduces hemoconcentration and ascites in hyperstimulated women undergoing assisted reproduction. *J Clin Endocrinol Metab* 2007;**92**(8):2931–2937.

5. Anaya Y, Mata DA, Letourneau J, *et al.* A novel oocyte maturation trigger using 1500 IU of human chorionic gonadotropin plus 450 IU of follicle-stimulating hormone may decrease ovarian hyperstimulation syndrome across all in vitro fertilization stimulation protocols [published correction appears in *J Assist Reprod Genet* 2017;35(2):309]. *J Assist Reprod Genet* 2018;**35**(2):297–307.

6. Serour GI, Aboulghar MA, Mansour R, *et al.* Complications of medically assisted conception in 3,500 cycles. *Fertil Steril* 1998;**70**:638–642.

7. Mathur RS, Akande AV, Keay SD, *et al.* Distinction between early and late ovarian hyperstimulation syndrome. *Fertil Steril* 2000;**73**:901–907.

8. Papanikolaou EG, Pozzobon C, Kolibianakis EM, *et al.* Incidence and prediction of ovarian hyperstimulation syndrome in women undergoing gonadotropin-releasing hormone antagonist in vitro fertilization cycles. *Fertil Steril* 2006;**85**:112–120.

9. Rizk B, Smitz J. Ovarian hyperstimulation syndrome after superovulation for IVF and related procedures. *Hum Reprod* 1992;**7**:320–327.

10. Rizk B. Ovarian hyperstimulation syndrome. In: Studd J, ed. *Progress in Obstetrics and Gynecology*, Vol. 11. Edinburgh: Churchill Livingstone; 1993:311–349.

11. Rizk B, Aboulghar MA. Classification, pathophysiology and management of ovarian hyperstimulation syndrome. In: Brinsden P, ed. *A Textbook of In-vitro Fertilization and Assisted Reproduction*, 2nd ed. Carnforth-Lancs, UK: The Parthenon Publishing Group; 1999:131–155.

12. Golan A, Weissman A. Symposium: update on prediction and management of OHSS. A modern classification of OHSS. *Reprod Biomed Online* 2009;**19**(1):28–32. doi: 10.1016/s1472-6483(10)60042-9.

13. Humaidan P, Quartarolo J, Papanikolaou EG. Preventing ovarian hyperstimulation syndrome: guidance for the clinician. *Fertil Steril* 2010;**94** (2):389–400.

14. Ferrero H, García-Pascual CM, Gómez R, *et al.* Dopamine receptor 2 activation inhibits ovarian vascular endothelial growth factor secretion in vitro: implications for treatment of ovarian hyperstimulation syndrome with dopamine receptor 2 agonists. *Fertil Steril* 2014;**101** (5):1411–1418.

15. Nastri CO, Ferriani RA, Rocha IA, Martins WP. Ovarian hyperstimulation syndrome: pathophysiology and prevention. *J Assist Reprod Genet* 2010;**27**:121–128.

16. Geva E, Jaffe RB. Role of vascular endothelial growth factor in ovarian physiology and pathology. *Fertil Steril* 2000;**74**(3):429–438. doi: 10.1016/s0015-0282(00)00670-1.

17. Naredi N, Talwar P, Sandeep K. VEGF antagonist for the prevention of ovarian hyperstimulation syndrome: current status. *Med J Armed Forces India* 2014;**70**(1):58–63. doi: 10.1016/j.mjafi.2012.03.005.

18. Kaiser UB. The pathogenesis of the ovarian hyperstimulation syndrome. *N Engl J Med* 2003;**349**:729–732.

19. Aboulghar MA, Mansour RT, Serour GI, El Helw BA, Shaarawy M. Elevated levels of interleukin-2, soluble interleukin-2 receptor alpha, interleukin-6, soluble interleukin-6 receptor and vascular endothelial growth factor in serum and ascitic fluid of patients with severe ovarian hyperstimulation syndrome. *Eur J Obstet Gynecol Reprod Biol* 1999;**87**(1):81–85. doi: 10.1016/s0301-2115(99)00082-2.

20. Luke B, Brown MB, Morbeck DE, *et al.* Factors associated with ovarian hyperstimulation syndrome (OHSS) and its effect on assisted reproductive technology (ART) treatment and outcome. *Fertil Steril* 2010;**94**(4):1399–1404. doi: 10.1016/j.fertnstert.2009.05.092.

21. Tarlatzi TB, Venetis CA, Devreker F, Englert Y, Delbaere A. What is the best predictor of severe ovarian hyperstimulation syndrome in IVF? A cohort study. *J Assist Reprod Genet* 2017;**34** (10):1341–1351.

22. Iliodromiti S, Anderson RA, Nelson SM. Technical and performance characteristics of anti-Müllerian hormone and antral follicle count as biomarkers of ovarian response. *Hum Reprod Update* 2015;**21**(6):698–710.

23. Lee TH, Liu CH, Huang CC, et al. Serum anti-mullerian hormone and estradiol levels as predictors of ovarian hyperstimulation syndrome in assisted reproduction technology cycles. *Hum Reprod* 2008;**23**:160–167.

24. Kwan I, Bhattacharya S, McNeil A, van Rumste MM. Monitoring of stimulated cycles in assisted reproduction (IVF and ICSI). *Cochrane Database Syst Rev* 2008;**2**:CD005289. doi: 10.1002/14651858.CD005289.pub2.

25. Kwan I, Bhattacharya S, Kang A, Woolner A. Monitoring of stimulated cycles in assisted reproduction (IVF and ICSI). *Cochrane Database Syst Rev* 2014;**2014**(8):CD005289.

26. Nelson SM. Prevention and management of ovarian hyperstimulation syndrome. *Thromb Res* 2017;**151** Suppl 1:S61–S64.

27. Papanikolaou EG, Humaidan P, Polyzos NP, Tarlatzis B. Identification of the high-risk patient for ovarian hyperstimulation syndrome. *Semin Reprod Med* 2010;**28**(6):458–462.

28. Heijnen EM, Eijkemans MJ, De Klerk C, et al. A mild treatment strategy for in-vitro fertilisation: a randomised non-inferiority trial. *Lancet* 2007;**369**(9563):743–749.

29. Karimzadeh MA, Ahmadi S, Oskouian H, Rahmani E. Comparison of mild stimulation and conventional stimulation in ART outcome. *Arch Gynecol Obstet* 2010;**281**(4):741–746.

30. Casano S, Guidetti D, Patriarca A, et al. MILD ovarian stimulation with GnRH-antagonist vs. long protocol with low dose FSH for non-PCO high responders undergoing IVF: a prospective, randomized study including thawing cycles. *J Assist Reprod Genet* 2012;**29**(12):1343–1351.

31. Rinaldi L, Lisi F, Selman H. Mild/minimal stimulation protocol for ovarian stimulation of patients at high risk of developing ovarian hyperstimulation syndrome. *J Endocrinol Invest* 2014;**37**(1):65–70.

32. Onofriescu A, Bors A, Luca A, et al. GnRH antagonist IVF protocol in PCOS. *Curr Health Sci J* 2013;**39**(1):20–25.

33. Ozmen B, Sükür YE, Seval MM, et al. Dual suppression with oral contraceptive pills in GnRH antagonist cycles for patients with polycystic ovary syndrome undergoing intracytoplasmic sperm injection. *Eur J Obstet Gynecol Reprod Biol* 2014;**183**:137–140.

34. Xing W, Lin H, Li Y, et al. Is the GnRH antagonist protocol effective at preventing OHSS for potentially high responders undergoing IVF/ICSI? *PLoS One* 2015; **10**(10):e0140286.

35. Yu R, Lin J, Zhao JZ, et al. Study on clinical effect on infertility women with polycystic ovary syndrome treated by in vitro maturation and in vitro fertilization-embryo transfer. *Zhonghua Fu Chan Ke Za Zhi* 2012;**47**(4):250–254.

36. Das M, Son WY, Buckett W, Tulandi T, Holzer H. In-vitro maturation versus IVF with GnRH antagonist for women with polycystic ovary syndrome: treatment outcome and rates of ovarian hyperstimulation syndrome. *Reprod Biomed Online* 2014;**29**(5):545–551.

37. Walls ML, Hunter T, Ryan JP, et al. In vitro maturation as an alternative to standard in vitro fertilization for patients diagnosed with polycystic ovaries: a comparative analysis of fresh, frozen and cumulative cycle outcomes. *Hum Reprod* 2015;**30**(1):88–96.

38. Rizk B, Aboulghar M. Modern management of ovarian hyperstimulation syndrome. *Hum Reprod* 1991;**6**(8):1082–1087.

39. Sher G, Zouves C, Feinman M, Maassarani G. 'Prolonged coasting': an effective method for preventing severe ovarian hyperstimulation syndrome in patients undergoing in-vitro fertilization. *Hum Reprod* 1995;**10**(12):3107–3109.

40. Kovács P, Mátyás S, Kaali SG. Effect of coasting on cycle outcome during in vitro fertilization/intracytoplasmic sperm injection cycles in hyper-responders. *Fertil Steril* 2006;**85**(4):913–917.

41. D'Angelo A, Brown J, Amso NN. Coasting (withholding gonadotrophins) for preventing ovarian hyperstimulation syndrome. *Cochrane Database Syst Rev* 2011;**6**:CD002811.

42. Kosmas IP, Zikopoulos K, Georgiou I, et al. Low-dose HCG may improve pregnancy rates and lower OHSS in antagonist cycles: a meta-analysis. *Reprod Biomed Online* 2009; 19(5):619–630.

43. Tiboni GM, Colangelo EC, Ponzano A. Reducing the trigger dose of recombinant hCG in high-responder patients attending an assisted reproductive technology program: an observational study. *Drug Des Devel Ther* 2016;**10**:1691–1694.

44. Gülekli B, Göde F, Sertkaya Z, Işık AZ. Gonadotropin-releasing hormone agonist triggering is effective, even at a low dose, for final oocyte maturation in ART cycles: case series. *J Turk Ger Gynecol Assoc* 2015;**16**(1):35–40.

45. Casper RF. Introduction: gonadotropin-releasing hormone agonist triggering of final follicular

maturation for in vitro fertilization. *Fertil Steril* 2015;**103**(4):865–866.

46. Youssef MA, Van der Veen F, Al-Inany HG, *et al.* Gonadotropin-releasing hormone agonist versus HCG for oocyte triggering in antagonist-assisted reproductive technology. *Cochrane Database Syst Rev* 2014;**10**:CD008046.

47. Youssef MA, van Wely M, Hassan MA, *et al.* Can dopamine agonists reduce the incidence and severity of OHSS in IVF/ICSI treatment cycles? A systematic review and meta-analysis. *Hum Reprod Update* 2010;**16**(5):459–466.

48. Baumgarten M, Polanski L, Campbell B, Raine-Fenning N. Do dopamine agonists prevent or reduce the severity of ovarian hyperstimulation syndrome in women undergoing assisted reproduction? A systematic review and meta-analysis. *Hum Fertil* 2013;**16**(3):168–174.

49. Kasum M, Vrčić H, Stanić P, *et al.* Dopamine agonists in prevention of ovarian hyperstimulation syndrome. *Gynecol Endocrinol* 2014;**30**(12):845–849.

50. Leitao VM, Moroni RM, Seko LM, Nastri CO, Martins WP. Cabergoline for the prevention of ovarian hyperstimulation syndrome: systematic review and meta-analysis of randomized controlled trials. *Fertil Steril* 2014;**101**(3):664–675.

51. Gokmen O, Ugur M, Ekin M, *et al.* Intravenous albumin versus hydroxyethyl starch for the prevention of ovarian hyperstimulation in an in vitro fertilization programme: a prospective randomized placebo controlled study. *Eur J Obstet Gynecol Reprod Biol* 2001;**96**(2):187–192.

52. Youssef MA, Mourad S. Volume expanders for the prevention of ovarian hyperstimulation syndrome. *Cochrane Database Syst Rev* 2016;**8**:CD001302.

53. Naredi N, Karunakaran S. Calcium gluconate infusion is as effective as the vascular endothelial growth factor antagonist cabergoline for the prevention of ovarian hyperstimulation syndrome. *J Hum Reprod Sci* 2013;**6**(4):248–252. doi: 10.4103/0974-1208.126293.

54. Boothroyd C, Karia S, Andreadis N, *et al.*; Australasian CREI Consensus Expert Panel on Trial evidence (ACCEPT) group. Consensus statement on prevention and detection of ovarian hyperstimulation syndrome. *Aust N Z J Obstet Gynaecol* 2015;**55**(6):523–534.

55. Borges E Jr., Braga DP, Setti AS, *et al.* Strategies for the management of OHSS: results from freezing-all cycles. *JBRA Assist Reprod* 2016;**20**(1):8–12.

56. He Q, Xu J, Cui S, Li H, Zhang C. Relationship between letrozole administration during the luteal phase after oocyte retrieval and the early-stage ovarian hyperstimulation syndrome occurrence. *Zhonghua Fu Chan Ke Za Zhi* 2014;**49**(12):909–913.

57. Wang YQ, Luo J, Xu WM, *et al.* Can steroidal ovarian suppression during the luteal phase after oocyte retrieval reduce the risk of severe OHSS? *J Ovarian Res* 2015;**8**:63.

58. Cheng ZX, Kong G, Zhang CL, Zhao YN. Letrozole versus gonadotropin-releasing hormone antagonist during luteal phase in the prevention of ovarian hyperstimulation syndrome: a randomized controlled trial. *Zhonghua Fu Chan Ke Za Zhi* 2020;**55**(1):9–14.

59. Kol S, Homburg R, Alsbjerg B, Humaidan P. The gonadotropin-releasing hormone antagonist protocol–the protocol of choice for the polycystic ovary syndrome patient undergoing controlled ovarian stimulation. *Acta Obstet Gynecol Scand* 2012;**91**(6):643–647.

60. Toftager M, Bogstad J, Bryndorf T, *et al.* Risk of severe ovarian hyperstimulation syndrome in GnRH antagonist versus GnRH agonist protocol: RCT including 1050 first IVF/ICSI cycles. *Hum Reprod* 2016;**31**(6):1253–1264.

61. Lambalk CB, Banga FR, Huirne JA, *et al.* GnRH antagonist versus long agonist protocols in IVF: a systematic review and meta-analysis accounting for patient type *Hum Reprod Update* 2017;**23**(5):560–579.

62. Verberg MF, Macklon NS, Nargund G, *et al.* Mild ovarian stimulation for IVF. *Hum Reprod Update* 2009;**15**(1):13–29.

63. Zegers-Hochschild F, Adamson GD, de Mouzon J, *et al.* The International Committee for Monitoring Assisted Reproductive Technology (ICMART) and the World Health Organization (WHO) Revised Glossary on ART Terminology, 2009. *Hum Reprod* 2009;**24**(11):2683–2687.

64. Baart EB, Martini E, Eijkemans MJ, *et al.* Milder ovarian stimulation for in-vitro fertilization reduces aneuploidy in the human preimplantation embryo: a randomized controlled trial. *Hum Reprod* 2007;**22**(4):980–988.

65. Nargund G, Datta AK, Fauser B. Mild stimulation for in vitro fertilization. *Fertil Steril* 2017;**108**:558–567.

66. Roque M, Haahr T, Geber S, Esteves SC, Humaidan P. Fresh versus elective frozen embryo transfer in IVF/ICSI cycles: a systematic review and meta-analysis of reproductive outcomes. *Hum Reprod Update* 2019;**25**(1):2–14.

67. Yang ZY, Chian RC. Development of in vitro maturation techniques for clinical applications. *Fertil Steril* 2017;**108**(4):577–584.

68. Siristatidis CS, Maheshwari A, Vaidakis D, Bhattacharya S. In vitro maturation in subfertile women with polycystic ovarian syndrome undergoing assisted reproduction. *Cochrane Database Syst Rev* 2018;**11**(11):CD006606.

69. D'Angelo A, Amso NN, Hassan R. Coasting (withholding gonadotrophins) for preventing ovarian hyperstimulation syndrome. *Cochrane Database Syst Rev* 2017;**5**:CD002811. doi: 10.1002/14651858.CD002811.pub4.

70. Humaidan P, Bredkjær HE, Bungum L, *et al.* GnRH agonist (buserelin) or hCG for ovulation induction in GnRH antagonist IVF/ICSI cycles: a prospective randomized study. *Huan Reprod* 2005;**20**(5):1213–1220.

71. Pirard C, Donnez J, Loumaye E. GnRH agonist as luteal phase support in assisted reproduction technique cycles: results of a pilot study. *Hum Reprod* 2006;**21**(7):1894–1900.

72. Kol S. Luteolysis induced by a gonadotropin-releasing hormone agonist is the key to prevention of ovarian hyperstimulation syndrome. *Fertil Steril* 2004;**81**(1):1–5.

73. Simon C, Cano F, Valbuena D, Remohi J, Pellicer A. Clinical evidence for a detrimental effect on uterine receptivity of high serum estradiol concentrations in high and normal responders. *Hum Reprod* 1995;**10**:2432–2437.

74. Haahr T, Roque M, Esteves SC, Humaidan P. GnRH agonist trigger and LH activity luteal phase support versus hCG trigger and conventional luteal phase support in fresh embryo transfer IVF/ICSI cycles-a systematic PRISMA review and meta-analysis. *Front Endocrinol (Lausanne)* 2017;**8**:116.

75. Castillo JC, Haahr T, Martínez-Moya M, Humaidan P. Gonadotropin-releasing hormone agonist for ovulation trigger – OHSS prevention and use of modified luteal phase support for fresh embryo transfer. *Ups J Med Sci* 2020;**125**(2):131–137.

76. Martínez F, Mancini F, Solé M, *et al.* Antagonist rescue of agonist IVF cycle at risk of OHSS: a case series. *Gynecol Endocrinol* 2014;**30**:145–148.

77. Tso LO, Costello MF, Albuquerque LE, Andriolo RB, Macedo CR. Metformin treatment before and during IVF or ICSI in women with polycystic ovary syndrome. *Cochrane Database Syst Rev* 2014;**11**:CD006105.

78. Mourad S, Brown J, Farquhar C. Interventions for the prevention of OHSS in ART cycles: an overview of Cochrane reviews. *Cochrane Database Syst Rev* 2017;**1**: CD012103. doi: 10.1002/14651858.CD012103.pub2.

79. Jacob SL, Brewer C, Tang T, *et al.* A short course of metformin does not reduce OHSS in a GnRH antagonist cycle for women with PCOS undergoing IVF: a randomised placebo-controlled trial. *Hum Reprod* 2016;**31**(12):2756–2764.

80. Eftekhar M, Deghani Firoozabadi R, Khani P, Ziaei Bideh E, Forghani H. Effect of laparoscopic ovarian drilling on outcomes of in vitro fertilization in clomiphene-resistant women with polycystic ovary syndrome. *Int J Fertil Steril* 2016;**10**(1):42–47. doi: 10.22074/ijfs.2016.4767.

81. Seyam E, Hefzy E. Laparoscopic ovarian drilling versus GnRH antagonist combined with cabergoline as a prophylaxis against the re-development of ovarian hyperstimulation syndrome. *Gynecol Endocrinol* 2018;**34**(7):616–622. doi: 10.1080/09513590.2018.1425989.

82. Ramzy A, Al-Inany H, Aboulfoutouh I. Ultrasonographic guided ovarian stroma hydrocoagulation for ovarian stimulation in polycystic ovary syndrome. *Acta Obstet Gynecol Scand* 2001;**80**:1046–1050.

83. McNatty KP, Smith DM, Makris A, *et al.* The intraovarian sites of androgen and estrogen formation in women with normal and hyperandrogenic ovaries as judged by in vitro experiments. *J Clin Endocrinol Metab* 1980;**50**(4):755–763.

84. Badawy A, Khiary M, Ragab A, Hassan M, Sherief L. Ultrasound-guided transvaginal ovarian needle drilling (UTND) for treatment of polycystic ovary syndrome: a randomized controlled trial. *Fertil Steril* 2009;**91**(4):1164–1167.

85. Zhang J, Tang L, Kong L, *et al.* Ultrasound-guided transvaginal ovarian needle drilling for clomiphene-resistant polycystic ovarian syndrome in subfertile women [published online ahead of print, 2019 Jul 31]. *Cochrane Database Syst Rev* 2019;**7**(7):CD008583.

86. Nargund G, Hutchison L, Scaramuzzi R, Campbell S. Low-dose HCG is useful in preventing OHSS in high-risk women without adversely affecting the outcome of IVF cycles. *Reprod Biomed Online* 2007;**14**(6):682–685. doi: 10.1016/s1472-6483(10)60668-2.

87. Chen X, Chen S, He Y, *et al.* Minimum dose of hCG to trigger final oocyte maturation and prevent OHSS in a long GnRHa protocol. *J Huazhong Univ Sci Technol* 2013;**33**:133–136.

88. Tsoumpou I, Muglu J, Gelbaya TA, Nardo LG. Symposium: update on prediction and management of OHSS. Optimal dose of HCG for final oocyte maturation in IVF cycles: absence of

evidence? *Reprod Biomed Online* 2009;**19**
(1):52–58.

89. Tapanainen JS, Lapolt PS, Perlas E, Hsueh AJ.
Induction of ovarian follicle luteinization by
recombinant follicle-stimulating hormone.
Endocrinology 1993;**133**(6):2875–2880.

90. Zelinski-Wooten MB, Hutchison JS, Hess DL,
Wolf DP, Stouffer RL. A bolus of recombinant
human follicle stimulating hormone at midcycle
induces periovulatory events following multiple
follicular development in macaques. *Hum Reprod*
1998;**13**(3):554–560.

91. Busso CE, Garcia-Velasco JA, Simon C, Pellicer A.
Prevention of OHSS: current strategies and new
insights. *Middle East Fertil Soc J* 2010;**15**
(4):223–230.

92. Knoepfelmacher M, Danilovic DL, Rosa
Nasser RH, Mendonca BB. Effectiveness of
treating ovarian hyperstimulation syndrome with
cabergoline in two patients with gonadotropin-
producing pituitary adenomas. *Fertil Steril*
2006;**86**(3):719.e15–719.e18.

93. Tang H, Mourad S, Zhai SD, Hart RJ. Dopamine
agonists for preventing ovarian hyperstimulation
syndrome. *Cochrane Database Syst Rev* 2016;**11**:
CD008605. doi: 10.1002/14651858.CD008605.
pub3.

94. Kissler S, Neidhardt B, Siebzehnrübl E, *et al.* The
detrimental role of colloidal volume substitutes in
severe ovarian hyperstimulation syndrome: a case
report. *Eur J Obstet Gynecol Reprod Biol* 2001;**99**
(1):131–134.

95. Morris RS, Wong IL, Kirkman E, Gentschein E,
Paulson RJ. Inhibition of ovarian-derived
prorenin to angiotensin cascade in the treatment of
ovarian hyperstimulation syndrome. *Hum Reprod*
1995;**10**:1355–1358.

96. Gurgan T, Demirol A, Guven S, *et al.* Intravenous
calcium infusion as a novel preventive therapy of
ovarian hyperstimulation syndrome for patients
with polycystic ovarian syndrome. *Fertil Steril*
2011;**96**(1):53–57.

97. El-Khayat W, Elsadek M. Calcium infusion for the
prevention of ovarian hyperstimulation
syndrome: a double-blind randomized controlled
trial. *Fertil Steril* 2015;**103**(1):101–105. doi:
10.1016/j.fertnstert.2014.09.046.

98. Naredi N, Singh SK, Lele P, Nagraj N. Severe
ovarian hyperstimulation syndrome: can we
eliminate it through a multipronged approach?
Med J Armed Forces India 2018;**74**(1):44–50. doi:
10.1016/j.mjafi.2017.04.006.

99. Davenport MJ, Vollenhoven B, Talmor AJ.
Gonadotropin-releasing hormone-agonist
triggering and a freeze-all approach: the final step

in eliminating ovarian hyperstimulation
syndrome? *Obstet Gynecol Surv* 2017;**72**
(5):296–308.

100. Atkinson P, Koch J, Ledger WL. GnRH agonist
trigger and a freeze-all strategy to prevent ovarian
hyperstimulation syndrome: a retrospective
study of OHSS risk and pregnancy rates. *Aust
N Z J Obstet Gynaecol* 2014;**54**(6):581–585.

101. Shin JJ, Jeong Y, Nho E, Jee BC. Clinical
outcomes of frozen embryo transfer cycles after
freeze-all policy to prevent ovarian
hyperstimulation syndrome. *Obstet Gynecol Sci*
2018;**61**(4):497–504.

102. D'Angelo A, Amso NN. Embryo freezing for
preventing ovarian hyperstimulation syndrome.
Cochrane Database Syst Rev 2007;**3**:CD002806.
doi: 10.1002/14651858.CD002806.pub2.

103. Chen ZJ, Shi Y, Sun Y, *et al.* Fresh versus frozen
embryos for infertility in the polycystic ovary
syndrome. *N Engl J Med* 2016;**375**(6):523–533.

104. Chen Y, Yang T, Hao C, Zhao J.
A retrospective study of letrozole treatment
prior to human chorionic gonadotropin in
women with polycystic ovary syndrome
undergoing in vitro fertilization at risk of
ovarian hyperstimulation syndrome. *Med Sci
Monit* 2018;**24**:4248–4253.

105. Tshzmachyan R, Hambartsoumian E. The role of
letrozole (LE) in controlled ovarian stimulation
(COS) in patients at high risk to develop ovarian
hyper stimulation syndrome (OHSS).
A prospective randomized controlled pilot study.
J Gynecol Obstet Hum Reprod 2020;**49**(2):101643.
doi: 10.1016/j.jogoh.2019.101643.

106. Mai Q, Hu X, Yang G, *et al.* Effect of letrozole on
moderate and severe early-onset ovarian
hyperstimulation syndrome in high-risk women:
a prospective randomized trial. *Am J Obstet
Gynecol* 2017;**216**(1):42.e1–42.e10.

107. Zeng C, Shang J, Jin AM, *et al.* The effect of luteal
GnRH antagonist on moderate and severe early
ovarian hyperstimulation syndrome during
in vitro fertilization treatment: a prospective
cohort study. *Arch Gynecol Obstet* 2019;**300**
(1):223–233.

108. Lainas GT, Kolibianakis EM, Sfontouris IA, *et al.*
Pregnancy and neonatal outcomes following
luteal GnRH antagonist administration in
patients with severe early OHSS. *Hum Reprod*
2013;**28**(7):1929–1942. doi: 10.1093/humrep/
det114.

109. Lainas GT, Kolibianakis EM, Sfontouris IA, *et al.*
Serum vascular endothelial growth factor levels
following luteal gonadotrophin-releasing
hormone antagonist administration in women

with severe early ovarian hyperstimulation syndrome. *BJOG* 2014;**121**(7):848–855.

110. Rizk B, Rizk CB, Nawar MG, Garcia-Velasco JA, Sallam HN. Ultrasonography in the prediction and management of ovarian hyperstimulation syndrome In: Rizk B, ed. *Ultrasonography in Reproductive Medicine and Infertility.* Cambridge, UK : Cambridge University Press; 2010:299–312.

111. Salmassi A, Mettler L, Hedderich J, *et al.* Cut-off levels of anti-Mullerian hormone for the prediction of ovarian response, in vitro fertilization outcome and ovarian

hyperstimulation syndrome. *Int J Fertil Steril* 2015;**9**(2):157–167.

112. Vembu R, Reddy NS. Serum AMH level to predict the hyper response in women with PCOS and non-PCOS undergoing controlled ovarian stimulation in ART. *J Hum Reprod Sci* 2017;**10**(2):91–94. doi: 10.4103/jhrs. JHRS_15_16.

113. Steward RG, Lan L, Shah AA, *et al.* Oocyte number as a predictor for ovarian hyperstimulation syndrome and live birth: an analysis of 256,381 in vitro fertilization cycles. *Fertil Steril* 2014;**101**(4):967–973.

Chapter 16

Treatment of Ovarian Hyperstimulation Syndrome

Mohamed Youssef, Abdel-Maguid Ramzy, and Botros Rizk

Although, ovarian hyperstimulation syndrome (OHSS) is the most serious iatrogenic complication of ovarian stimulation, the condition usually resolves within 14 days in women who are subjected to freeze-all embryos policy; meanwhile symptoms may extend through the first trimester in women who do become pregnant as endogenous human chorionic gonadotropin (hCG) levels continue to stimulate the ovaries. The exact pathophysiology and etiology of OHSS remains unknown, but increased capillary permeability with the resulting loss of fluid into the third space is common to the syndrome [1]. Administration of hCG for final follicle maturation and triggering of ovulation appears to be the pivotal stimulus in a susceptible patient, by releasing vasoactive–angiogenic substances such as vascular endothelial growth factor from the ovaries hyperstimulated with gonadotropins [2].

OHSS is characterized by bilateral ovarian cystic enlargement and third-space fluid shift. The ovaries are noted to have a significant degree of stromal edema, interspersed with multiple hemorrhagic follicular and theca-lutein cysts, areas of cortical necrosis and neovascularization. The other pathological phenomenon is that of acute body fluid shifts, which in turn causes hemoconcentration with reduced organ perfusion, alterations in blood coagulation and the resulting risk of thromboembolism, and leakage of fluids into the peritoneal cavity and lungs [3]. OHSS presents either early (< 10 days after hCG administration) or late (≥ 10 days after oocyte retrieval) [4].

Outpatient Management of Moderate and Severe OHSS

The clinical diagnosis and management is based on severity of the disease (Table 16.1), it involves preventive strategies coupled with supportive management such as antiemetic, analgesics, fluid intake to maintain intravascular volume, correction of electrolyte imbalance, and prophylactic anticoagulation

in cases of severe OHSS and multiple paracentesis while the condition slowly improves [5].

Several studies evaluated the value of aggressive outpatient treatment of ascites with paracentesis under ultrasound guidance and proper hydration with IV crystalloids and albumin until resolution of symptoms, or hospitalization in addition to anticoagulation [5]. Following this regimen, the majority of patients either avoided hospitalization or had significantly fewer days of hospitalization [6]. A systematic review included 12 studies evaluating outpatient management of severe OHSS, in 356 patients. Only 16 out of 356 women required hospital admission because of intolerable pain, vomiting or development of critical OHSS with pleural effusion. A total of 95 percent of patients included were successfully treated on an outpatient basis without subsequent hospital admission [5]. Outpatient treatment involved administration of gonadotropin-releasing hormone (GnRH) antagonist in the luteal phase and early therapeutic paracentesis combined with rehydration and thromboprophylaxis.

Outpatient Monitoring

Based on the classification of Rizk and Aboulghar [7], moderate OHSS will be followed up by regular telephone calls (daily at least) and twice weekly office visits. The assessment at the office includes pelvic ultrasound, complete blood count, liver function tests, and coagulation profile. The patient should be instructed to report to the hospital if she develops dyspnea, if the volume of urine is diminished, or upon development of any unusual symptoms such as leg swelling, dizziness, numbness, and neurological problems.

Administration of GnRH Antagonist in the Luteal Phase

Administration of GnRH antagonist (0.25 mg) daily from days 5 to 8 after oocyte retrieval, combined

Table 16.1 Classification of OHSS [36;37]

	Clinical feature	Laboratory features
Mild	Abdominal distension/discomfort Mild nausea/vomiting Mild dyspnea Diarrhea Enlarged ovaries	No important alterations
Moderate	Mild features Ultrasonographic evidence of ascites	Hct > 41% WBC > 15 000/ml
Severe	Mild and moderate features Clinical evidence of ascites Hydrothorax Severe dyspnea Oliguria/anuria Intractable nausea/vomiting	Hct > 55% WBC > 25 000/ml CrCl < 50 ml/min Cr > 1.6 mg/dl Na+ < 135 mEq/L K+ > 5 mEq/L Elevated liver enzymes
Critical	Low blood/central venous pressure Pleural effusion Rapid weight gain (> 1 kg in 24 h) Syncope Severe abdominal pain venous thrombosis Anuria/acute renal failure Arrhythmia Thromboembolism Pericardial effusion Massive hydrothorax Arterial thrombosis Adult respiratory distress syndrome Sepsis	Worsening of findings

Hct: hematocrit; WBC: white blood cell; CrCl: creatinine clearance; Cr: creatinine; Na+: sodium; K+: potassium
From Practice Committee of the American Society for Reproductive Medicine 2016 [26].

with cryopreservation of all embryos, has been evaluated in a cohort study where 40 patients out of 353 were diagnosed with severe OHSS [8]. Severe OHSS was diagnosed in the presence of moderate or marked ascites with large ovaries, hematocrit > 45%, white blood cell (WBC) count > 15 000/mm^3, hydrothorax, oliguria, or abnormal liver function tests. None of the patients required hospitalization following luteal GnRH antagonist administration and embryo cryopreservation. Moreover, ovarian volume, ascites, hematocrit, serum estradiol, progesterone, and WBC decreased markedly indicating rapid resolution of severe OHSS without jeopardizing the live birth rate [9].

An observational study evaluated administration of a second dose of GnRH agonist 12 hours after the first GnRH agonist trigger combined with 0.25 mg of GnRH antagonist administrated for three days from the day of oocyte retrieval onwards in 21 women diagnosed with severe early OHSS [10]. None of the included patients developed moderate to severe OHSS. Moreover, patients'

symptoms, reproductive hormone levels, and ultrasound findings were improved significantly.

Fluid Balance

There is insufficient evidence in the literature to determine the optimum method of achieving fluid balance in women with severe OHSS. Intravenous fluid therapy in the presence of increased capillary permeability carries a risk of increasing ascites and effusions. Oral fluid intake, guided by the patient's thirst, allows a more physiological approach to fluid replacement and is the preferred method of fluid management. Patients should be encouraged to drink to thirst rather than to an arbitrary volume. Pain relief and antiemetic therapy may be required to help the patient achieve oral hydration. Intravenous fluid has a role where the patient is unable to drink, or for initial rehydration when the patient presents with severe hemoconcentration. Initial replacement is with crystalloids such as normal saline. If elevated hematocrit and poor urine output persist despite crystalloid infusion, colloids such as human albumin or hydroxyethyl starch (HES) have a role. Strict input/output recording, and daily weight and abdominal girth recording are important parts of the inpatient management of OHSS. Increasing weight and girth with output lagging behind intake are signs of worsening fluid retention. Conversely, an increased urine output and negative fluid balance is an early sign of recovery from OHSS. Electrolyte imbalances affect around 50 percent of patients with severe OHSS. Characteristic problems include hyponatremia and hyperkalemia, which usually respond to correction of dehydration. Diuretics should generally be avoided as they may worsen hypovolemia; although there may be a role for diuretic use if urine output remains poor despite adequate fluid replacement (as judged by invasive hemodynamic monitoring). Low-dose dopamine infusion has been used in such situations. Often these patients will be seriously ill and input should be sought from intensive care and/or renal colleagues.

Measures against Thromboembolism

The reported incidence of thrombosis with OHSS ranges from 0.7 to 10 percent. Women with OHSS are at an increased risk of thrombosis, probably secondary to high estrogen levels, dehydration, specific cytokine effect, and the effects of ascites and enlarged ovaries on venous return. Thromboembolism is a life-threatening complication of severe OHSS and prophylactic measures are warranted despite the lack of clinical studies on the value of thromboprophylaxis. Signs and symptoms of thromboembolism demand prompt additional diagnostic measures (arterial blood gas measurements, ventilation/perfusion scan) and therapeutic anticoagulation when the diagnosis is confirmed or strongly suspected. Thrombosis in women with OHSS frequently affects upper body sites and the arterial system.

Thromboprophylaxis in the form of venous support stockings and prophylactic low molecular weight heparin should be used in all women admitted with OHSS, cases of severe OHSS, and in individuals with preexisting risk factors for thrombosis. It is unclear on how long to continue thromboprophylaxis. In women who conceive, there are several reports of thrombosis following apparent improvement of OHSS up to the 13th week of pregnancy. Current Royal College of Obstetricians and Gynaecologists guidelines recommend continuing prophylactic measures until the end of the first trimester of pregnancy. However, patients should be individualized and counseled depending on their risk factors, and in some cases it may be reasonable to continue thromboprophylaxis for the duration of pregnancy. In women who do not conceive, thromboprophylaxis is discontinued at the time of the withdrawal bleed.

Analgesia

Analgesia is provided by paracetamol and codeine. Injectable opiates may be used for more severe pain. However, the occurrence of severe pain should prompt a search for a complication or coincident problem such as ovarian torsion, cyst rupture, or ectopic pregnancy. Non-steroidal anti-inflammatory medications should be avoided as they may compromise renal function.

Circulatory Volume Correction

The main line of treatment is correction of the circulatory volume and the electrolyte imbalance. Every effort should be directed toward restoring a normal intravascular volume and preserving adequate renal function. Volume replacement should begin with intravenous crystalloid fluids at 125–150 ml/h. Normal saline and lactated Ringer have been successfully used. Plasma colloid expanders may be used if necessary. One concern with using plasma expanders is that the beneficial effect is transitory before their redistribution into the extravascular space, further exacerbating ascites formation. Albumin, dextran, mannitol, fresh frozen plasma, and HES have also been used. HES has the advantage of a non-biological origin and high molecular weight (200–1000 kD vs. 69 kD for albumin). Abramov et al. compared the efficacy of HES and human albumin for the treatment of 16 patients with severe OHSS [11]. They observed a higher urine output, fewer paracenteses, and shorter hospital stays with HES solution. Gamzu et al. compared HES 10% and polygeline (Haemaccel) and found no clinical advantage for HES [12]. In another retrospective cohort study 293 women with severe OHSS received either intravenous artificial colloids or human albumin [13]. There was no significant difference between both groups in terms of the length of hospital stay or development of thromboembolism.

Electrolyte Replacement

Appropriate solutions will correct electrolyte imbalances. If hypokalemia is significant, a cation exchange resin may be needed. Sodium and water restriction has been used but others found no change in the patient's weight, abdominal circumference, or peripheral edema when sodium and water were restricted. Therefore, salt and water restriction are not widely advocated [14].

Anticoagulant Therapy

Anticoagulant therapy is indicated if there is clinical evidence of thromboembolic complications or laboratory evidence of hypercoagulability [15]. Venous thrombosis is the most common serious complication of OHSS. Preventative treatment with heparin should be used whenever there is a thromboembolic risk. In cases of severe OHSS, the following situations are recognized as indicating an increased risk of thromboembolism: immobilization, compression of pelvic vessels by large ovaries or ascites, pregnancy coagulation abnormalities, and hyperestrogenemia. Prevention using mobilization and antithrombosis stockings is insufficient as thrombosis may occur at all localizations and may be systemic in nature. Prophylaxis with heparin remains debatable for the reason that there are no randomized studies proving its efficacy in preventing thromboembolic complications during severe OHSS; in some clinical scenarios, thromboembolism still occurs despite giving heparin [14]. Despite these reservations Rizk recommend giving heparin or enoxaparin (Lovenox) for patients with severe OHSS [14]. The incidence of deep vein thrombosis is markedly increased in patients with Leiden factor V mutation one of the thrombophilias [16]. Others are: protein C and protein S deficiency, and antithrombin III deficiency. Leiden factor V mutation occurs in 4 percent of Northern European women. Patients should be questioned about a history of personal or familial thrombosis, and if positive should be tested for Leiden factor V mutation. If OHSS occurs in patients with Leiden factor V mutation, they should be placed on prophylactic heparin. The duration of anticoagulant administration is debatable. Some

investigators have reported late thrombosis up to 20 weeks after transfer and many investigators are in favor of maintaining heparin therapy for many weeks [17]. Severity of OHSS must be separated from risk of thromboembolism because intrinsic coagulopathy may trigger the problem even in moderate cases. However, those who have followed a more liberal policy for prophylaxis have had to deal with operating on ruptured ectopic pregnancies in anticoagulated patients. Therefore, thromboembolism will remain a more difficult complication to prevent and may complicate the outcome.

Antibiotic Treatment

Infections are not uncommon in the setting of treatment of OHSS because of frequent catheterizations, venipuncture, transvaginal aspiration of ascitic fluid, and pleural drainage. Furthermore, hypoglobulinemia is present in severe cases. Preoperative antibiotic prophylaxis is highly recommended. Some authors suggested the administration of immunoglobulins for the treatment of infections associated with severe OHSS. However, this intervention still awaits further evaluation.

Diuretics

Diuretic therapy without prior volume expansion may prove detrimental, by further contracting the intravascular volume, thereby worsening hypotension and its sequelae. Diuretics will increase blood viscosity and increase the risk of venous thrombosis. Diuretics use should be restricted to the management of pulmonary edema.

Aspiration of Ascitic Fluid and Pleural Effusion in Severe OHSS

The presence of ascites is the hallmark of OHSS. Symptoms resulting from ascites are the most common reason for hospitalization. Aspiration is not indicated in every patient. Paracentesis by the transabdominal or transvaginal route is indicated for severe abdominal pain, pulmonary compromise as demonstrated by pulse oximetry, and tachypnea and renal compromise as demonstrated by oliguria and increased creatinine concentration [18;19].

Paracentesis is followed by increased urinary output shortly after the procedure, with a concomitant decrease in the patient's weight, leg edema, and abdominal circumference. Also creatinine clearance rate is increased following the procedure. Paracentesis offers temporary relief of respiratory and abdominal distress, but, since the fluid tends to recur, some patients need repeated paracentesis and drainage of effusions before spontaneous improvement occurs. Placement of pigtail catheter has been proposed to be safe and effective outpatient management for drainage of ascites in patients with OHSS [20], an alternative to multiple vaginal or abdominal paracentesis [14]. In a retrospective analysis of 33 patients who underwent in vitro fertilization (IVF) and developed severe/critical OHSS, pigtail catheter placement was performed. In nine of the patients OHSS started early, requiring placement of a pigtail catheter almost four days after retrieval. In 30 patients OHSS started late. The mean amount of ascitic fluid drained immediately after placement of the catheter was 2085 ± 1018 cc. The pigtail catheter was removed after 7.8 ± 5.3 days. Of the 31 patients who had embryo transfer, 84 percent conceived. Twenty-nine patients were managed on outpatient basis without any complications. Four patients required hospital admission for one to seven days. One patient with severe OHSS was admitted for workup for chest pain. Three patients with critical OHSS with severe pleural effusion requiring thoracentesis were admitted for supportive measures [21]. Removal of fluid up to 7.5 liters on one occasion and 45 liters in total has been reported in cases with severe OHSS [22;23].

The risk of injury to ovaries is minimized by ultrasonographic guidance. Monitoring of plasma proteins is essential and human albumin should be infused whenever necessary. Percutaneous placement of a pigtail catheter is a safe and effective treatment modality for severe OHSS that may represent an alternative to multiple vaginal or abdominal paracentesis. On the other hand, transvaginal ultrasound-guided aspiration is an effective and safe procedure. Injury to the ovary is easily avoided by puncture under ultrasonic visualization. No anesthesia is required for the procedure, and better drainage of the ascetic fluid is accomplished because the pouch of Douglas is the most dependent part [24].

Evaluation and treatment of patients with severe OHSS complaining of dyspnea includes physical examination, chest ultrasound and X-ray, and arterial blood gases. It is essential to evaluate accurately any pulmonary complications that may result in hypoxia. If a pulmonary embolus is suspected, a CT scan or ventilation/perfusion scan should be performed. Pulmonary compromise should be treated with oxygen supplementation. Thoracocentesis may be necessary for patients with significant hydrothorax. However, a dramatic improvement in the clinical status may occur after paracentesis. Pericardial effusion rarely occurs, but if it does, drainage by specialists may be necessary [25].

Acute respiratory distress syndrome (ARDS) is encountered after fluid overload. The importance of a strict fluid input/output balance in patients with moderate complications of OHSS is stressed. Optimum management may require admission to an intensive care unit. ARDS subsides after three to six days with fluid restriction, forced diuresis, and dopamine therapy.

In-Hospital Management of Severe OHSS

According to the American Society of Reproductive Medicine (ASRM) clinical and laboratory criteria of OHSS severity (Table 16.1) patients with severe/critical OHSS grades are admitted to hospital for treatment [26]. The British Fertility Society guidelines recommended outpatient management for cases with mild OHSS with regular follow-up, while inpatient management was recommended for those with severe OHSS [27].

Surgical Treatment

Anesthesia Considerations in OHSS Patients

Surgery is infrequently needed, but if required there are several aspects important for the anesthesiologist (Table 16.2). Careful positioning of patients during surgery is important as the Trendelenburg position may further compromise the residual pulmonary functional capacity. Establishment of access lines may be necessary in patients with contracted vascular volume. Drainage of pleural effusions may assist in improving pulmonary status.

Ruptured Cysts

Laparotomy, in general, should be avoided in OHSS. If deemed necessary, in cases of hemorrhagic ovarian cysts, it should be performed by an experienced gynecologist and only hemostatic measures undertaken so as to preserve the ovaries.

Table 16.2 Challenges to the anesthesiologist in OHSS

- Pulmonary compromise
- Severe hemoconcentration
- Pleural effusions
- Restricted IV access
- Infections and febrile morbidity
- Difficult positioning in surgery
- Thrombophlebitis
- Pelvic masses
- Ascites
- Electrolytic disturbances

Ovarian Torsion

Ovarian stimulation during IVF-embryo transfer treatment is a risk factor for ovarian torsion [28–30]. Presenting symptoms are severe unilateral adnexal pain, in a patient with enlarged ovaries due to ovulation stimulation, or with multiple pregnancy. Sonography with Doppler flow analysis can be diagnostic but a finding of apparently normal blood flow does not rule out ovarian torsion [31]. In a review of 77 cases of ovarian torsion at a single hospital, Doppler flow sonography was performed preoperatively in 90 percent of cases but demonstrated compromised blood flow in only 29 percent of those scanned [32]. Of these, 39 (51%) required oophorectomy. Ovarian torsion followed ovulation induction in 21 of the 77 cases, and of these only one required oophorectomy, possibly because of earlier diagnosis. Twenty-four patients were pregnant, two-thirds as a result of ovulation induction. The mean gestational age was 10.4 weeks at the time of ovarian torsion. Although the adnexa usually appear dark, hemorrhagic and ischemic, they can be saved, if the diagnosis is made soon enough, by simply unwinding often as a laparoscopy procedure [32].

Ectopic Pregnancy

IVF and OHSS are a known risk factor for ectopic pregnancy with an incidence of 2 to 3 percent [33;34]. Excessive ovarian response, IVF as opposed to intracytoplasmic sperm injection, and GnRH agonist trigger were found to be independent risk factors for ectopic pregnancy [34;35].

Other Surgery

Mesenteric resection after massive arterial infarction has been reported. Rarely vascular surgery is required to treat thromboses that are complicated by recurrent emboli or resistant to medical intervention. Posterolateral thoracotomy and subclavian arteriotomy and thromboarterectomy by the Fogarthy technique have been reported. Inferior vena cava interruption to prevent massive thromboembolism has also been used [14].

Pregnancy Termination

Pregnancy termination is performed in extreme cases and has been reported to improve the clinical picture of neurological, hematological, and vascular complications. [14].

References

1. Ferrero H, García-Pascual CM, Gómez R, *et al.* Dopamine receptor 2 activation inhibits ovarian vascular endothelial growth factor secretion in vitro: implications for treatment of ovarian hyperstimulation syndrome with dopamine receptor 2 agonists. *Fertil Steril* 2014;**101** (5):1411–1418.

2. Nastri CO, Ferriani RA, Rocha IA, Martins WP. Ovarian hyperstimulation syndrome: pathophysiology and prevention. *J Assist Reprod Genet* 2010;**27**:121–128.

3. Aboulghar MA, Mansour RT. Ovarian hyperstimulation syndrome: classifications and critical analysis of preventive measures. *Hum Reprod Update* 2003;**9**:275–289.

4. Mathur RS, Akande AV, Keay SD, Hunt LP, Jenkins JM. Distinction between early and late ovarian hyperstimulation syndrome. *Fertil Steril* 2000;**73**(5):901–907.

5. Gebril A, Hamoda H, Mathur R. Outpatient management of severe ovarian hyperstimulation syndrome: a systematic review and a review of existing guidelines. *Hum Fertil (Camb)* 2018;**21** (2):98–105.

6. Smith LP, Hacker MR, Alper MM. Patients with severe ovarian hyperstimulation syndrome can be managed safely with aggressive outpatient transvaginal paracentesis. *Fertil Steril* 2009;**92** (6):1953–1959.

7. Rizk B, Aboulghar MA. Classification, pathophysiology and management of ovarian hyperstimulation syndrome. In: Brinsden P, ed. *A Textbook of In-vitro Fertilization and Assisted Reproduction*, 2nd ed. Carnforth-Lancs, UK. The Parthenon Publishing Group; 1999:131–155.

8. Lainas GT, Kolibianakis EM, Sfontouris IA, *et al.* Outpatient management of severe early OHSS by administration of GnRH antagonist in the luteal

phase: an observational cohort study. *Reprod Biol Endocrinol* 2012;**10**:69.

9. Lainas GT, Kolibianakis EM, Sfontouris IA, *et al.* Pregnancy and neonatal outcomes following luteal GnRH antagonist administration in patients with severe early OHSS. *Hum Reprod* 2013;**28**(7):1929–1942.

10. Deng L, Li XL, Ye DS, *et al.* A second dose of GnRHa in combination with luteal GnRH antagonist may eliminate ovarian hyperstimulation syndrome in women with ≥30 follicles measuring ≥11 mm in diameter on trigger day and/or pre-trigger peak estradiol exceeding 10 000 pg/mL. *Curr Med Sci* 2019;**39**(2):278–284.

11. Abramov Y, Fatum M, Abrahomov D, *et al.* Hydroxyethyl starch versus human albumin for the treatment of severe ovarian hyperstimulation syndrome: a preliminary report. *Fertil Steril* 2001;**75**:1228–1230.

12. Gamzu R, Almog B, Levin Y, *et al.* Efficacy of hydroxyethyl starch and Haemaccel for the treatment of severe ovarian hyperstimulation syndrome. *Fertil Steril* 2002;**77**:1302–1303.

13. Minami T, Mph, Yamana H, *et al.* Artificial colloids versus human albumin for the treatment of ovarian hyperstimulation syndrome: a retrospective cohort study. *Int J Reprod Biomed* 2019;**17**(10):709–716.

14. Rizk B. *Ovarian Hyperstimulation Syndrome: Epidemiology, Pathophysiology, Prevention and Management.* Cambridge, UK: Cambridge University Press; 2006.

15. Fabregues Tassies D, Reverter JC, Reverter JC, *et al.* Prevalence of thrombophilia in women with severe ovarian hyperstimulation syndrome and cost-effectiveness of screening. *Fertil Steril* 2004;**81**:989–995.

16. Mikhail S, Rizk RMB, Nawar MG, Rizk CB. Thrombophilia and implantation failure. In: Rizk B, Garcia-Velasco JA, Sallam HN, Makrigiannakis A, eds. *Infertility and Assisted Reproduction.* Cambridge, UK: Cambridge University Press; 2008:407–415.

17. Serour GI, Aboulghar MA, Mansour R, *et al.* Complications of medically assisted conception in 3,500 cycles. *Fertil Steril* 1998;**70**:638–642.

18. Lee TH, Liu CH, Huang CC, *et al.* Serum anti-mullerian hormone and estradiol levels as predictors of ovarian hyperstimulation syndrome in assisted reproduction technology cycles. *Hum Reprod* 2008;**23**:160–167.

19. Lambalk CB, Banga FR, Huirne JA, *et al.* GnRH antagonist versus long agonist protocols in IVF: a systematic review and meta-analysis accounting

for patient type. *Hum Reprod Update* 2017;**23**(5):560–579.

20. Çağlar Aytaç P, Kalaycı H, Yetkinel S, *et al.* Effect of pigtail catheter application on obstetric outcomes in in vitro fertilization/intracytoplasmic sperm injection pregnancies following hyperstimulation syndrome. *Turk J Obstet Gynecol* 2017;**14**(2):94–99.

21. Abuzeid M, Warda H, Joseph S, *et al.* Outpatient management of severe ovarian hyperstimulation syndrome (OHSS) with placement of pigtail catheter. *Facts Views Vis Obgyn* 2014;**6**(1):31–37.

22. Ozgun MT, Batukan C, Oner G, *et al.* Removal of ascites up to 7.5 liters on one occasion and 45 liters in total may be safe in patients with severe ovarian hyperstimulation syndrome. *Gynecol Endocrinol* 2008;**24**(11):656–658.

23. Agarwal N, Ghosh S, Bathwal S, Chakravarty B. Large-volume paracentesis, up to 27 L, with adjuvant vaginal cabergoline in the case of severe ovarian hyperstimulation syndrome with successful pregnancy outcome: a case report. *J Hum Reprod Sci* 2017;**10**(3):235–237.

24. Raziel A, Friedler S, Schachter M, *et al.* Transvaginal drainage of ascites as an alternative to abdominal paracentesis in patients with severe ovarian hyperstimulation syndrome, obesity, and generalized edema. *Fertil Steril* 1998;**69**(4):780–783.

25. Brinsden PR, Wada I, Tan SL, *et al.* Diagnosis, prevention and management of ovarian hyperstimulation syndrome. *Br J Obstet Gynecol* 1995;**102**:767–772.

26. Practice Committee of the American Society for Reproductive Medicine. Electronic address: ASRM@asrm.org; Practice Committee of the American Society for Reproductive Medicine. Prevention and treatment of moderate and severe ovarian hyperstimulation syndrome: a guideline. *Fertil Steril* 2016;**106**(7):1634–1647.

27. Tan BK, Mathur R. Management of ovarian hyperstimulation syndrome. Produced on behalf of the BFS Policy and Practice Committee. *Hum Fertil (Camb)* 2013;**16**(3):151–159.

28. Busso CE. Prevention of OHSS – dopamine agonists. *Reprod Biomed Online* 2009;**19**(1):43–51.

29. Spitzer D, Wirleitner B, Steiner H, Zech NH. Adnexal torsion in pregnancy after assisted reproduction – case study and review of the literature. *Geburtshilfe Frauenheilkd* 2012;**72**(8):716–720.

30. Tsai HC, Kuo TN, Chung MT, *et al.* Acute abdomen in early pregnancy due to ovarian torsion following successful in vitro fertilization

treatment. *Taiwan J Obstet Gynecol* 2015;**54**(4):438–441.

31. Busso C, Fernandez-Sanchez M, Garcia-Velasco JA, *et al.* The non-ergot derived dopamine agonist quinagolide in prevention of early ovarian hyperstimulation syndrome in IVF patients: a randomized, double-blind, placebo-controlled trial. *Hum Reprod* 2010;**25**(4):995–1004. doi: 10.1093/humrep/deq005.

32. Kanayama S, Kaniwa H, Tomimoto M, *et al.* Laparoscopic detorsion of the ovary in ovarian hyperstimulation syndrome during the sixth week of gestation: a case report and review. *Int J Surg Case Rep* 2019;**59**:50–53.

33. Orvieto R, Vanni VS. Ovarian hyperstimulation syndrome following GnRH agonist trigger-think ectopic. *J Assist Reprod Genet* 2017;**34**(9):1161–1165. doi: 10.1007/s10815-017-0960-0.

34. Weiss A, Beck-Fruchter R, Golan J, *et al.* Ectopic pregnancy risk factors for ART patients undergoing the GnRH antagonist protocol: a retrospective study. *Reprod Biol Endocrinol* 2016;**14**:12.

35. Chang HJ, Suh CS. Ectopic pregnancy after assisted reproductive technology: what are the risk factors? *Curr Opin Obstet Gynecol* 2010;**22**(3):202–207.

36. Navot D, Bergh PA, Laufer N. Ovarian hyperstimulation syndrome in novel reproductive technologies: prevention and treatment. *Fertil Steril* 1992;**58**:249–261.

37. Fiedler K, Ezcurra D. Predicting and preventing ovarian hyperstimulation syndrome (OHSS): the need for individualized not standardized treatment. *Reprod Biol Endocrinol* 2012;**10**:32.

How to Individualize Ovarian Stimulation Protocols to Avoid Difficulties and Complications

Suleiman Ghunaim, Raja Sayegh, and Johnny Awwad

Introduction

Traditionally, controlled ovarian stimulation in women undergoing assisted reproductive technology (ART) treatment was designed in a standardized fashion taking into account the age and body weight of the patient. A standardized treatment protocol has been described as a "one-size-fits-all" approach that does not take into account inter-individual differences.

Because of our improved understanding of genomic and proteomic functions, individualized medicine has made its way with measurable progress into some aspects of medicine, namely oncology and chemotherapy. The case of reproductive medicine is nonetheless different, in that the development of individually tailored ovarian stimulation protocols has been sluggish over the past decade. It should be noted that the range of available treatment options for ovarian stimulation is very limited while the dose–response relationship remains poorly defined. In addition, the success of fertility treatment depends on a wide range of intertwined factors beyond the ovarian response per se.

Ovarian Physiology

It is believed that an estimated 20 to 30 antral follicles are recruited every menstrual cycle with only a single one allowed to reach dominance and ovulation. Numerous endocrine events contribute to this selection process. The initial follicle-stimulating hormone (FSH) rise in the early follicular phase stimulates the growth of multiple antral follicles. The resulting expansion of the granulosa cell mass and associated rise in serum estradiol and inhibin B levels subsequently down-regulate FSH production leading to a midfollicular decline in serum levels. The time-restricted nature of the "FSH window" appears to favor the selection of a single dominant follicle while forcing other less privileged antral follicles into atresia. By extending the "FSH window," more follicles may be recruited, which constitutes the principle of controlled ovarian stimulation, the cornerstone of modern in vitro fertilization (IVF) treatment.

Prolonged supraphysiological FSH exposure associated with the administration of exogenous gonadotropins is associated with an exaggerated ovarian response of variable intensity. Individual response variability has been attributed to antral follicle count, differential FSH sensitivity, body weight, and genetic variants. This explains why dosing of exogenous gonadotropin administration has not always been successful in generating a predictable and reproducible follicular response.

What Is the Optimal Number of Oocytes Required for a Successful ART Treatment Cycle?

The spectrum of optimal ovarian response has been arbitrarily defined on the basis of risk benefit equations. Ovarian stimulation leading to a "normal range" follicular response is estimated to yield 5 to 15 oocytes at the time of transvaginal retrieval. Outside this range, a "low" ovarian response is likely to be associated with a low reproductive outcome and a high risk for cycle cancellation, while a "high" response predisposes to the hazards of ovarian hyperstimulation syndrome (OHSS). It should be noted however that the most reliable predictor of a live birth remains the age of the woman, which determines the likelihood of obtaining implantable euploid embryos.

The most widely used predictors of ovarian response currently include the serum anti-Müllerian hormone (AMH) and the antral follicle count (AFC). AMH assays have been the subject of much scrutiny over the past decade due to wide inter-assay variations and poor reproducibility of results. The introduction of on-site automated systems has largely patched the shortcomings associated with earlier assays [1;2]. On the other hand, limitations associated with the use of the AFC include interobserver variation and dependence on the technical performance of the ultrasound equipment [3;4]. The limited sensitivity of 60 to 70 percent for detecting "out of the normal range" responders has rendered the reliability of these tests of ovarian response imprecise in guiding the process of gonadotropin dosing.

Because of a positive association between the number of oocytes collected and cumulative live births, a high ovarian response has been suggested as a positive predictor of ART success [5–10]. A large UK registry analysis evaluating live births following 400 135 fresh IVF/intracytoplasmic sperm injection (ICSI) treatment cycles showed a strong association between the number of oocytes collected and live birth rate (LBR) [7]. More specifically, LBR was shown to rise with an increasing number of oocytes up to 15, achieve a plateau between 15 and 20 oocytes, and finally steadily decline beyond 20 oocytes. A SART registry analysis of 256 381 IVF/ICSI cycles showed a similar increase in live births up to 15 oocytes, followed by a plateau [8]. Most of these studies however reported on the outcome of fresh IVF cycles in a heterogeneous group of women with variable ovarian stimulation protocols and different numbers of embryos transferred. Furthermore, reporting of results was made as per patient cycle irrespective of cycle rank. Cumulative pregnancy outcome following the transfer of fresh and cryopreserved embryos was evaluated in a large cohort study of 1099 women undergoing their first IVF cycle and planning for elective single embryo transfer in their fresh cycle [6]. High responders with more than 15 oocytes collected at the time of retrieval demonstrated a significantly higher LBR in fresh cycles. Multivariate logistic regression analysis showed that ovarian response remained an independent predictive factor for cumulative LBR ($p < 0.0001$) irrespective of the number of oocytes obtained.

It should be noted however that the older dictum of "more is better" has been challenged by studies suggesting that high ovarian response may be associated with inferior oocyte quality,

high oocyte wastage, and less favorable endometrial receptivity in fresh autologous embryo transfers [11].

Individualization in Ovarian Stimulation

Pituitary Suppression

Earlier on, phase III studies reporting on pituitary suppression during ART showed significantly lower pregnancy outcomes in gonadotropin-releasing hormone (GnRH) antagonist cycles compared with conventional long suppression GnRH agonist cycles [12]. These preliminary findings were initially believed to be the outcome of limited experience in the manipulation of newly introduced medications. Recently, however, a published overview suggested the cause to be due to a higher incidence of premature luteinizing hormone (LH) surges (8%) in antagonist cycles as a result of insufficient suppression of endogenous pituitary gonadotropin secretion and advanced follicular development compared with long agonist cycles (less than 1%) [13]. With the widespread use of GnRH antagonists lately, the previously observed reproductive performance gap between both analogues has been reportedly bridged [14–16].

In a Cochrane review, Al-Inany et al. found no evidence of a difference in LBR between GnRH antagonist and long suppression GnRH agonist cycles (odds ratio [OR] 1.02, 95% confidence interval [CI] 0.85–1.23; 12 randomized controlled trials [RCTs], $n = 2303$, $I^2 = 27\%$, moderate-quality evidence). GnRH antagonist cycles were associated with a lower incidence of OHSS nonetheless compared with agonist cycles (OR 0.61, 95% CI 0.51–0.72; 36 RCTs, $n = 7944$, $I^2 = 31\%$, moderate-quality evidence). In women who received the antagonist, cycle cancellations due to high risk for OHSS were significantly lower, and those cancellations due to poor ovarian response were significantly higher [14].

In another meta-analysis, Lambalk et al. found the ongoing pregnancy rate (OPR) to be significantly lower in the antagonist group in the general ART population compared with the agonist group (relative risk [RR] 0.89, 95% CI 0.82–0.96). In women with polycystic ovary syndrome (PCOS) and in those with poor ovarian response, no significant differences in OPR between both groups were observed. Subgroup analyses for various antagonist treatment schedules showed a significantly lower OPR when oral contraceptive pill pretreatment was combined with a flexible protocol, but not with a fixed one [16]. This meta-analysis however has been criticized for methodological flaws including misclassification of one study of poor responders in the general ART population [13]. After correcting for study flaws, the probability of ongoing pregnancy in the general ART population was no more dependent on the type of GnRH analogue used (RR 0.920, 95% CI 0.836–1.013).

Overall, in all reported meta-analyses, antagonists resulted in significantly lower OHSS rates both in the general ART population and in women at risk for OHSS [14–16]. Moreover, the GnRH antagonist protocol was shown to perform well in patients with expected normal or high ovarian response, with no sufficient data against its use in women with expected poor response [17]. As a general consensus, the use of the GnRH antagonist for pituitary suppression is preferred during standardized stimulation protocols and/or for women with predicted high response because of the option of using a GnRH agonist trigger to increase safety without compromising efficacy.

Quantification of the Gonadotropin Dose

The optimal starting gonadotropin dose during the first treatment cycle in women undergoing IVF/ICSI remains controversial. Earlier research suggested the standardization of the gonadotropin dose on the basis of general patient characteristics [18–21]. The "optimal standard dose" was reported to vary between 100 and 250 IU/day depending on what reproductive physicians estimated as desired oocyte yield. A wide range of oocyte numbers were obtained nonetheless when the same dose of gonadotropins was administered on the basis of standardization characteristics [21].

Studies evaluating the dose response relationship of exogenous gonadotropins suggest that a 150–225 IU daily dose is appropriate in most instances to obtain a reasonable number of 8 to 15 oocytes [11;22;23].

Multiple regression analyses of reproductive data collected from 145 women treated with 150 IU/day of recombinant FSH (rFSH) on their first stimulation cycle showed that the total number of antral follicles, total Doppler score, smoking status and serum testosterone level were independent predictors of the number of oocytes retrieved [24]. Backwards stepwise regression modeling of a population of 2280 normo-ovulatory women undergoing IVF/ICSI from 11 randomized clinical trials indicated that predictive factors for ovarian response included basal FSH, body mass index (BMI), age, and number of follicles < 11 mm at baseline screening [25].

Using a combination of these predictive factors, various rFSH starting dose calculators were developed for use in clinical practice with the aim of optimizing ovarian response. The relevance of these developed algorithms was evaluated in prospective clinical trials [26;27]. Using a prospective randomized study design, Popovic-Todorovic *et al.* found that individualized dosage algorithms increased the proportion of appropriate ovarian response and decreased the need for dose adjustments during controlled ovarian stimulation compared with standard dosing [26]. In a randomized, controlled, open-label, phase IV study, Olivennes *et al.* evaluated ovarian response using the CONSORT calculator to determine the rFSH starting dose in women undergoing IVF/ICSI treatment [27]. The primary efficacy analysis found the CONSORT calculator to be inferior to standard dosing (150 IU) for the number of oocytes retrieved, and comparable for the rates of poor and excessive ovarian response, as well as clinical pregnancy rates per fresh embryo transfer.

Subsequent studies focused on exploring the value of various tests of ovarian response in tailoring the dose of gonadotropins to individual patients. Compared with basal FSH, estradiol, and inhibin B, AFC and AMH have shown to perform better in predicting low response and hyper-response following ovarian stimulation [28]. Ovarian response test (ORT) thresholds predicting low response were an AFC < 7 and an AMH < 1.1 ng/ml, while those predicting hyper-response were an AFC > 14 and an AMH > 3.5 ng/ml [29;30]. Both ORTs nonetheless did not appear to add relevant information when applied simultaneously and were weaker predictors of live birth compared with women's age [29].

Although tests of ovarian reserve have been demonstrated to predict follicle response in normal and high responders, a well-defined dose–response relationship in poor responders is still lacking.

Individualized Gonadotropin Dosing in the General ART Population

Using a prospective controlled single-center study design, Magnusson et al. randomly assigned 308 patients starting their first IVF/ICSI cycle to one of two dosage algorithms, one including AMH, AFC, age, and BMI (intervention group), or another including only AFC, age, and BMI (control group) [31]. Cycles with poor response (< 5 oocytes) were more frequent in the intervention group (25.7% vs. 11.0%; $p < 0.01$), while the rates of over-response and live births were no different between groups. The addition of AMH to an individualized dosage regimen including AFC in an unselected patient group did not appear to alter the number of women achieving the targeted number of oocytes nor improve reproductive outcomes.

In a dual-center open-label RCT, Friis Petersen et al. randomized 490 women in a 2:1 ratio between an individualized and a standard dosing approach. Participants were divided into expected low (AMH < 12 pmol/L), medium (AMH 12–24 pmol/L), and high (AMH > 24 pmol/L) response groups. Compared with the standard dosing group (150 IU/day), individualized FSH dosing increased unintended low response in the high pretreatment AMH stratum, and reduced the proportion of unintended low responders in the low pretreatment AMH stratum [32].

The ESTHER-1 study, a randomized, multi-center, assessor-blinded, non-inferiority trial, randomized 1329 women on the basis of AMH and body weight to an individualized follitropin delta dosing protocol and a standard follitropin alfa (150 IU/day) regimen [33]. While ongoing pregnancy, implantation, and LBRs were similar between groups, the individualized protocol was associated with more women with target response, fewer poor responses, fewer excessive responses, and fewer measures taken to prevent OHSS.

A meta-analysis of five randomized controlled studies which evaluated the merits of ORT-based individualized gonadotropin dosing in the general ART population over standard management (150 IU daily) found moderate-quality evidence

for the absence of a difference in live births (OR 1.04, 95% CI 0.88–1.23) and low-quality evidence for a reduced incidence of moderate to severe OHSS (OR 0.58, 95% CI 0.34–1.00) [34]. For predicted normal responders, the same study demonstrated a higher oocyte yield following 200–225 IU FSH daily doses compared with 100–150 IU. No significant differences were observed between 225 IU and 300 IU daily doses.

Studies comparing the use of AMH versus AFC for gonadotropin dosing in the same population have not shown any significant differences in clinical or safety outcomes [35].

Individualized Gonadotropin Dosing in Predicted Poor Responders

Clinical research suggests that ORT-based gonadotropin dosing does not seem to improve the clinical outcome of "predicted low responders." In this group of responders, a daily gonadotropin dose of 300 IU or more was found to be associated with more oocytes collected and less cycle cancellations due to insufficient ovarian response compared with 150 IU, with no significant improvements in live births [34]. The OPTIMIST study, an open-label multicenter randomized clinical trial in women with predicted poor responders (AFC < 11), demonstrated higher oocyte yield and reduced cycle cancellation in individualized high FSH dosing (225–450 IU) compared with standard FSH dosing (150 IU) [36]. Increased FSH dosing did not improve LBRs, while it increased significantly treatment costs compared to the standard dose protocol.

A randomized controlled non-inferiority trial demonstrated that mild ovarian stimulation consisting of low-dose gonadotropins (150 IU rFSH) and pituitary downregulation with a GnRH antagonist did not reduce ongoing pregnancies despite a reduction in the number of oocytes and embryos available for transfer, compared with high-dose gonadotropins (450 IU hMG) and pituitary downregulation with a long midluteal GnRH agonist [37]. The interpretation of these findings however should be done with caution considering the heterogeneity in gonadotropin formulations and GnRH analogue suppression protocols between comparison arms.

It should be noted that actual prognosis for a live birth appears to be highly dependent on age in this particular group of women [38;39]. Hence, the combination of ORT and women's age may be more valuable in counseling patients on the prognosis of further fertility management considering the higher incidence of aneuploidy oocytes in women of advanced age [40].

Individualized Gonadotropin Dosing in Predicted High Responders

The use of ORT-based individualization of the gonadotropin dose in "predicted high responders" has been shown to be associated with improved safety of IVF/ICSI treatment with a significant reduction in the incidence of OHSS [33;37]. It follows therefore that ovarian reserve testing could be an effective tool for the primary prevention of OHSS in women undergoing IVF treatment.

In the OPTIMIST study, an open-label multicenter RCT in non-PCOS women with regular menstrual cycles and an AFC > 15, a reduced FSH dose (100 IU/day) resulted in similar cumulative LBRs (RR 0.95, 95% CI 0.85–1.07, $p = 0.423$), higher first cycle cancellation rate for insufficient follicle response (20.9% vs. 3.4%, $p < 0.001$), lower mild to moderate OHSS (RR 0.44, 95% CI 0.28–0.71, $p = 0.001$), and similar severe OHSS rate (RR 1.25, 95% CI 0.38–4.07, $p = 0.728$) compared with a standard dose (150 IU/day) [36]. It should be noted that the study did not include the strategy of GnRH agonist triggering of final oocyte maturation for hyper-responders; and that cycle cancellation for low response occurred twice as often in the first cycle in the reduced-dose group.

On the basis of the best available evidence, one may therefore argue that the use of a standard gonadotropin 150 IU daily dose with GnRH antagonist co-treatment offers an equally effective and safe stimulation approach in this particular category of high responders. Excessive ovarian response may be managed by the use of GnRH agonist triggering of final oocyte maturation with freeze-all policy to enhance patient safety.

Qualification of Gonadotropins

Several gonadotropin preparations are available in the market today. The major breakthrough has been the development of recombinant FSH and LH preparations with less reliance on urinary-derived products [41]. The question whether LH supplementation is required at all or in a subset of patients such as poor responders and advanced age remains inconclusive after more than three decades of heated debate [42–44]. The only group of women who were shown to benefit from FSH and LH combination remains patients with hypothalamic amenorrhea (WHO group I).

Future Perspectives

The aim of ovarian stimulation is to obtain a number of oocytes deemed optimal for the successful and safe achievement of a live birth. In the era of gamete/embryo vitrification, the debate on whether more oocytes is better for improving the cumulative prospect of pregnancy remains inconclusive. The use of markers of ovarian reserve to generate the most optimal follicular response associated with the best prognosis for a live birth is complicated by the presence of other contributing confounders such as the woman's age, body weight, and previous ovarian response. Studies using ovarian reserve testing for gonadotropin dosing did not demonstrate an improvement in IVF success, albeit a significant reduction in treatment-associated complications. More specifically, dosage individualization, while not resulting in a demonstrative improvement in pregnancy outcome, appears to be associated with elevated treatment cost in predicted low responders and a reduction in the risk of OHSS in predicted high responders. Tailoring of gonadotropin dosing nonetheless reduces cycle cancellation in unexpected low responders. Finally, it should be noted that the recent introduction of GnRH agonist triggering of final oocyte maturation in GnRH antagonist-suppressed cycles have rendered the management of high responders much safer and the reliance on gonadotropin dose individualization less relevant.

References

1. Nelson SM, Pastuszek E, Kloss G, *et al.* Two new automated, compared with two enzyme-linked immunosorbent, antimüllerian hormone assays. *Fertil Steril* 2015;**104**(4):1016–1021.

2. Iliodromiti S, Salje B, Dewailly D, *et al.* Non-equivalence of anti-Müllerian hormone automated assays – clinical implications for use as a companion diagnostic for individualised gonadotrophin dosing. *Hum Reprod* 2017;**32**(8):1710–1715.

3. Broekmans FJ, de Ziegler D, Howles CM, *et al.* The antral follicle count: practical recommendations for

better standardization. *Fert Steril* 2010;**94** (3):1044–1051.

4. Haadsma ML, Bukman A, Groen H, *et al.* The number of small antral follicles (2–6 mm) determines the outcome of endocrine ovarian reserve tests in a subfertile population. *Hum Reprod* 2007;**22**(7):1925–1931.

5. Bosch E, Labarta E, Pellicer A. Does cumulative live birth plateau beyond a certain ovarian response? *Fertil Steril* 2017;**108**(6):943.

6. Drakopoulos P, Blockeel C, Stoop D, *et al.* Conventional ovarian stimulation and single embryo transfer for IVF/ICSI. How many oocytes do we need to maximize cumulative live birth rates after utilization of all fresh and frozen embryos? *Hum Reprod* 2016;**31**(2):370–376.

7. Sunkara SK, Rittenberg V, Raine-Fenning N, *et al.* Association between the number of eggs and live birth in IVF treatment: an analysis of 400 135 treatment cycles. *Hum Reprod* 2011;**26** (7):1768–1774.

8. Steward RG, Lan L, Shah AA, *et al.* Oocyte number as a predictor for ovarian hyperstimulation syndrome and live birth: an analysis of 256,381 in vitro fertilization cycles. *Fertil Steril* 2014;**101** (4):967–973.

9. Baker VL, Brown MB, Luke B, Conrad KP. Association of number of retrieved oocytes with live birth rate and birth weight: an analysis of 231,815 cycles of in vitro fertilization. *Fertil Steril* 2015;**103**(4):931–938.

10. Briggs R, Kovacs G, MacLachlan V, Motteram C, Baker HG. Can you ever collect too many oocytes? *Hum Reprod* 2014;**30**(1):81–87.

11. Arce JC, Andersen AN, Fernández-Sánchez M, *et al.* Ovarian response to recombinant human follicle-stimulating hormone: a randomized, antimüllerian hormone–stratified, dose–response trial in women undergoing in vitro fertilization/ intracytoplasmic sperm injection. *Fertil Steril* 2014;**102**(6):1633–1640.

12. Kolibianakis EM, Griesinger G, Venetis CA. GnRH antagonists vs. long GnRH agonists in IVF: significant flaws in a meta-analysis lead to invalid conclusions. *Hum Reprod Update* 2017;**24** (2):242–243.

13. Kolibianakis EM, Venetis CA, Kalogeropoulou L, Papanikolaou E, Tarlatzis BC. Fixed versus flexible gonadotropin-releasing hormone antagonist administration in in vitro fertilization: a randomized controlled trial. *Fertil Steril* 2011;**95**:558–562.

14. Al-Inany HG, Youssef MA, Ayeleke RO, *et al.* Gonadotrophin-releasing hormone antagonists for assisted reproductive technology. *Cochrane Database Syst Rev* 2016;**4**:CD001750.

15. Xiao JS, Su CM, Zeng XT. Comparisons of GnRH antagonist versus GnRH agonist protocol in supposed normal ovarian responders undergoing IVF: a systematic review and meta-analysis. *PLoS One* 2014;**9**:e106854.

16. Lambalk CB, Banga FR, Huirne JA, *et al.* GnRH antagonist versus long agonist protocols in IVF: a systematic review and meta-analysis accounting for patient type. *Hum Reprod Update* 2017;**23**:560–579.

17. Mol BW, Bossuyt PM, Sunkara SK, *et al.* Personalized ovarian stimulation for assisted reproductive technology: study design considerations to move from hype to added value for patients. *Fertil Steril* 2018;**109**(6):968–979.

18. Devroey P, Tournaye H, Van Steirteghem A, Hendrix P, Out HJ. The use of a 100 IU starting dose of recombinant follicle stimulating hormone (Puregon) in in-vitro fertilization. *Hum Reprod* 1998;**13**:565–566.

19. Out HJ, Lindenberg S, Mikkelsen AL, *et al.* A prospective, randomized, double-blind clinical trial to study the efficacy and efficiency of a fixed dose of recombinant follicle stimulating hormone (Puregon) in women undergoing ovarian stimulation. *Hum Reprod* 1999;**14**:622–627.

20. Out HJ, Braat DD, Lintsen BM, *et al.* Increasing the daily dose of recombinant follicle stimulating hormone (Puregon) does not compensate for the age-related decline in retrievable oocytes after ovarian stimulation. *Hum Reprod* 2000;**15**:29–35.

21. Out HJ, David I, Ron-El R, *et al.* A randomized, double blind clinical trial using fixed daily doses of 100 or 200 IU of recombinant FSH in ICSI cycles. *Hum Reprod* 2001;**16**:1104–1109.

22. Sterrenburg MD, Veltman-Verhulst SM, Eijkemans MJ, *et al.* Clinical outcomes in relation to the daily dose of recombinant follicle-stimulating hormone for ovarian stimulation in in vitro fertilization in presumed normal responders younger than 39 years: a meta-analysis. *Hum Reprod Update* 2011;**17**:184–196.

23. Van der Meer M, Hompes PG, Scheele F, *et al.* Follicle stimulating hormone (FSH) dynamics of low dose step-up ovulation induction with FSH in patients with polycystic ovary syndrome. *Hum Reprod* 1994;**9**:1612–1617.

24. Popovic-Todorovic B, Loft A, Lindhard A, *et al.* A prospective study of predictive factors of ovarian response in 'standard' IVF/ICSI patients treated with recombinant FSH. A suggestion for

a recombinant FSH dosage normogram. *Hum Reprod* 2003;**18**:781–787.

25. Howles CM, Saunders H, Alam V, Engrand P; FSH Treatment Guidelines Clinical Panel. Predictive factors and a corresponding treatment algorithm for controlled ovarian stimulation in patients treated with recombinant human follicle stimulating hormone (follitropin alfa) during assisted reproduction technology (ART) procedures. An analysis of 1378 patients. *Curr Med Res Opin* 2006;**22**:907–918.

26. Popovic-Todorovic B, Loft A, Ejdrup Bredkjær H, *et al.* A prospective randomized clinical trial comparing an individual dose of recombinant FSH based on predictive factors versus a 'standard' dose of 150 IU/day in 'standard' patients undergoing IVF/ICSI treatment. *Hum Reprod* 2003;**18**:2275–2282.

27. Olivennes F, Howles CM, Borini A, *et al.* Individualizing FSH dose for assisted reproduction using a novel algorithm: the CONSORT study. *Reprod Biomed Online* 2009;**18**:195–204.

28. Broekmans FJ, Kwee J, Hendriks DJ, Mol BW, Lambalk CB. A systematic review of tests predicting ovarian reserve and IVF outcome. *Hum Reprod Update* 2006;**12**:685–718.

29. Broer SL, van Disseldorp J, Broeze KA, *et al.* Added value of ovarian reserve testing on patient characteristics in the prediction of ovarian response and ongoing pregnancy: an individual patient data approach. *Hum Reprod Update* 2013;**19**:26–36.

30. Aflatoonian A, Oskouian H, Ahmadi S, Oskouian L. Prediction of high ovarian response to controlled ovarian hyperstimulation: anti-Mullerian hormone versus small antral follicle count (2-6 mm). *J Assist Reprod Genet* 2009;**26**:319–325.

31. Magnusson A, Kallen K, Thurin-Kjellberg A, Bergh C. The number of oocytes retrieved during IVF: a balance between efficacy and safety. *Hum Reprod* 2018;**33**:58–64.

32. Friis Petersen J, Løkkegaard E, Andersen LF, *et al.* A randomized controlled trial of AMH-based individualized FSH dosing in a GnRH antagonist protocol for IVF. *Hum Reprod Open* 2019;**2019**(1): hoz003.

33. Nyboe Andersen A, Nelson SM, Fauser BC, *et al.* Individualized versus conventional ovarian stimulation for in vitro fertilization: a multicenter, randomized, controlled, assessor blinded, phase three non-inferiority trial. *Fertil Steril* 2017;**107**:396.e4.

34. Lensen SF, Wilkinson J, Leijdekkers JA, *et al.* Individualised gonadotropin dose selection using markers of ovarian reserve for women undergoing in vitro fertilization plus intracytoplasmic sperm injection (IVF/ICSI). *Cochrane Database Syst Rev* 2018;**2**:CD012693.

35. Lan VT, Linh NK, Tuong HM, Wong PC, Howles CM. Anti-mullerian hormone versus antral follicle count for defining the starting dose of FSH. *Reprod Biomed Online* 2013;**27**:390–399.

36. Van Tilborg TC, Torrance HL, Oudshoorn SC, *et al.* Individualized versus standard FSH dosing in women starting IVF/ICSI: an RCT. Part 1: The predicted poor responder. *Hum Reprod* 2017;**32**:2496–2505.

37. Youssef MA, Van Wely M, Al-Inany H, *et al.* A mild ovarian stimulation strategy in women with poor ovarian reserve undergoing IVF: a multicenter randomized non-inferiority trial. *Hum Reprod* 2016;**32**(1):112–118.

38. Oudendijk JF, Yarde F, Eijkemans MJ, Broekmans FJ, Broer SL. The poor responder in IVF: is the prognosis always poor? A systematic review. *Hum Reprod Update* 2012;**18**:1–11.

39. Hamdine O, Eijkemans MJC, Lentjes EGW, *et al.* Antimullerian hormone: prediction of cumulative live birth in gonadotropin-releasing hormone antagonist treatment for in vitro fertilization. *Fertil Steril* 2015;**104**:898.e2.

40. Esteves SC, Roque M, Bedoschi GM, *et al.* Defining low prognosis patients undergoing assisted reproductive technology: POSEIDON criteria–the why. *Front Endocrinol (Lausanne)* 2018;**9**:461.

41. Mochtar MH, Van der Veen F, Ziech M, van Wely M, Musters A. Recombinant luteinizing hormone (rLH) for controlled ovarian hyperstimulation in assisted reproductive cycles. *Cochrane Database Syst Rev* 2007;**2**:CD005070.

42. Lahoud R, Ryan J, Illingworth P, Quinn F, Costello M. Recombinant LH supplementation in patients with a relative reduction in LH levels during IVF/ICSI cycles: a prospective randomized controlled trial. *Eur J Obstet Gynecol Reprod Biol* 2017;**210**:300–305.

43. Humaidan P, Chin W, Rogoff D, *et al.* Efficacy and safety of follitropin alfa/lutropin alfa in ART: a randomized controlled trial in poor ovarian responders. *Hum Reprod* 2017;**32**:544–555.

44. Griesinger G, Boostanfar R, Gordon K, *et al.* Corifollitropin alfa versus recombinant follicle-stimulating hormone: an individual patient data meta-analysis. *Reprod Biomed Online* 2016;**33**:56–60.

Endometrial Receptivity

Eva Gómez, Jose Miravet-Valenciano, Diana Valbuena,
and Carlos Simón

Introduction

Human reproduction is highly inefficient, and that is why it has been widely observed and documented since the ancient civilizations. Fertility has been a main concern along the history. Greeks already described "the best time for fruitful intercourse" [1] understanding that women are not fertile all days of the menstrual cycle. The poor effectiveness of the human species continuity is due to a fair number of factors involved to achieve a successful pregnancy: quality and quantity of sperm, ovum and embryo quality, chromosomal abnormalities, and the capability of the endometrium to harbor the embryo among others. The synchrony between the embryo development and the endometrium maturation must work as perfectly as the gear of a watch.

The endometrium is an extremely plastic organ: every month it suffers morphological changes in response to the influence of hormones and when there is no pregnancy, tissue breakdown and regeneration occurs. During almost all the menstrual cycle, the endometrium is refractory to the embryo and only for a few hours acquires the ability to be adhesive. This short period of time is known as "endometrial receptivity" and it has been widely studied in the last century from different points of view to try to understand what actually happens and how it is achieved. The aim of this chapter is to introduce a complete and summarized review about the current knowledge of this outstanding process.

Window of Implantation

The term "window of implantation" (WOI) is referred to as the period of time in which the endometrium is receptive to harbor the embryo. It occurs during the mid-secretory phase and was suggested for the first time in 1956 by Herting *et al.* [2], but it was not confirmed until the 1990s when Navot demonstrated through human conception in vitro that successful embryo implantation only occurred when the embryos were transferred between days 17 and 19 of the cycle [3]. In 1992, Michael J. K. Harper finally coined this term and defined the implantation window as the "period when the uterus is receptive for implantation of the free-lying blastocyst" as a consequence of the action exerted by estrogen and progesterone on the endometrium, and suggested that apposition occurs between 6 and 10 days after the luteinizing hormone (LH) surge [4]. In 1999 Wilcox *et al.* reported the idea that implantation happens between days 8 and 10 after ovulation and this assertion has been universally accepted by the clinical community [5].

Nowadays, with the extraordinary development of the assisted reproductive techniques, this window of opportunity has been located around day 7 after the LH surge. Despite the timing and length of the WOI varying, in most women it lasts between 12 and 48 hours and starts 6 days after ovulation as a response to the exposure of the endometrium to progesterone, which is secreted by the corpus luteum. The endometrium is a strongly hormone-regulated organ. The acquisition of receptivity is not possible without the stimuli of estrogen and progesterone, which involve deep changes at the molecular level resulting in phenotypic modifications in the endometrium. Luminal epithelium suffers flattening of the apical surface, gradual loss of cellular polarity, and the appearance of ectoplasmic projections on the luminal surface called pinopodes or uterodomes. In the glandular epithelium, the secretory glands increase in size and become sinuous. They will be responsible for the main uterine secretions needed for the embryo implantation process and subsequent survival of the blastocyst. When the cells surrounding spiral arteries acquire a rounded aspect at the stromal compartment, store lipids and glycogen, and a vascular reorganization occurs, the receptive period ends. This phenomenon is known as "decidualization" and it is essential to coordinate trophoblast invasion and posterior placentation [6;7].

Even though the receptivity has been correctly achieved, implantation may fail if it is not coordinated with the required stage of embryonic development. Timing between the two partners is the key (Figure 18.1). Thanks to the molecular approaches that have emerged in recent years, nowadays it is possible to detect alterations of the normal acquisition of the WOI related to its duration or to its location inside the menstrual cycle. In 2013, Ruiz-Alonso *et al.* estimated that around 25 percent of patients with repeat implantations failure (RIF) have a displaced WOI [8].

Searching for a Unique Receptivity Marker

The endometrium suffers a fair number of events at the molecular level as well as morphological changes to reach receptivity. Some of them have been widely studied looking for the best marker to identify this moment but none has turned out to be the only one so far. In fact, all of them intervene

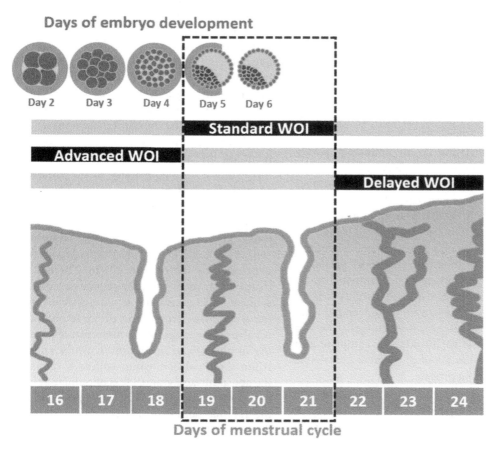

Figure 18.1 The synchrony between the embryo development and the endometrium maturation is critical for a successful implantation process. An advanced WOI matches with a premature embryo stage unready to implant. A delayed WOI does not match with blastocyst stage, leading to implantation failure.

in a complex network of events that should be studied together. The main markers involved in endometrial receptivity and their function are summarized below.

Cellular Anti-adhesion Molecules: MUC-1

Mucins act as a physical and chemical barrier being protectors against bacterial and proteolytic attacks, and they also often play an inhibitory role. MUC-1 is the most widely studied mucin in comparison with MUC-4 and MUC-16 that are also present in the endometrial epithelium. It is a glycoprotein located in the surface of the luminal epithelium and its abundance increases, due to the presence of progesterone, two to three days after the LH surge in fertile women. In contrast, patients with RIF and recurrent miscarriage present lower levels. It has been demonstrated that the blastocyst induces a break or specific cleavage of MUC-1 in the area of the epithelium where it is going to adhere. Therefore, in the human species the expression of MUC-1 is regulated during appositional and adhesion phases [7;9].

Cellular Adhesion Molecules (CAMs)

CAMs are cell surface glycoproteins that mediate cell–cell adhesion, as well as cell adhesion with the extracellular matrix. The main families are: cadherins, selectins, immunoglobulin superfamily, and integrins, with L-selectin and integrins being the most studied. L-selectin is used by the embryo to initiate adhesion with the ligands of the endometrium. On their side, integrins have been considered for decades as the best biochemical receptivity markers. They are a family of transmembrane glycoproteins. Some of them are constitutively expressed in the endometrium but others, such as $\alpha_1\beta_1$, $\alpha_4\beta_1$, and $\alpha_v\beta_3$, are regulated by hormones and cytokines and their expression is periodic, reaching the maximum during the mid-secretory phase. Some authors support the relationship between an abnormal expression of these three integrins and unexplained infertility although this is not universally accepted. The most studied integrin is $\alpha_v\beta_3$, whose expression is limited by β_3 subunit production which in turn is regulated by HOXA10, a transcriptional factor present in the uterus and necessary for decidualization. Deficiencies in the expression of HOXA10

and absence of β_3 subunit has been associated with endometriosis. On the other hand, osteopontin (OPN) acts as a ligand for β_3 and is differentially expressed through the menstrual cycle, reaching its maximum when the implantation window is open. Expression of OPN-$\alpha_v\beta_3$ complex occurs in the apical surface of the luminal epithelium and it is suggested that it could promote the embryo adhesion [6;7;9].

Cytokines

Cytokines are low molecular weight soluble proteins essential not only for the communication between endometrial cells but also for the communication between endometrial cells and the embryo. Once joined with their specific receptors, they cause the activation of several processes such as cell differentiation, cell maturation, and inflammation among many others. Oocytes and embryos also produce cytokines, so it seems quite clear that they are involved in embryo implantation. The interleukin (IL)-6 family includes four important cytokines: IL-1, IL-6, IL-11, and leukemia inhibitory factor (LIF), which are activators of STAT3. In mice, uterine deletion of STAT3 and GP130 were demonstrated to be critical for uterine receptivity and implantation [7].

LIF is a pro-inflammatory cytokine that is highly expressed during the mid to late secretory phase in the luminal and glandular epithelium. Decreased levels of LIF have been found in endometrial fluid of patients with implantation failure, although a multicentric study injecting subcutaneous recombinant LIF to this type of patient did not demonstrate any improvement. Despite this, some functions related to endometrial receptivity have been attributed to LIF, such as behaving as a mediator between trophoblast and decidual leukocytes and being an immune-cell regulator controlling their number and proportions during implantation. LIF also participates in pinopode formation [9].

IL-1 stimulates the production of LIF by the endometrium and plays an important role in decidualization, mediating the production of leptin and its receptor by increasing the expression of integrin β_3 subunit. IL-11 defects seem to be related to infertility. Its cyclic expression during the menstrual cycle has been described, with it achieving a maximum level in stromal cells during decidualization. However, its receptor does not present these cyclical variations. IL-6 may play a role in the preimplantation period and its abnormal expression during the mid-secretory phase has been related to recurrent abortion [7].

Growth Factors

Growth factors regulate many aspects of cellular function, including survival, proliferation, migration, and differentiation. Usually they are proteins or steroid hormones. Heparin binding-epidermal growth factor (HB-EGF) is anchored to the membrane of the luminal epithelium. It shows a low expression during the proliferative phase, but its expression is maximal just before the WOI. It is hypothesized that this growth factor plays a role as a mediator in the adhesion of the blastocyst to the endometrium [6].

Prostaglandins

Prostaglandins (PGs) are autocrine and paracrine lipid mediators synthesized from arachidonic acid that are implicated in several processes related to menstruation, ovulation, decidualization, fertilization, embryo transport, trophoblast invasion, and blastocyst growth and development among others. Four PGs are known to be directly related to implantation: PGD_2, PGE_2, $PGF_{2\alpha}$, and PGI_2. PGD_2 causes vasoconstriction; PGE_2 has been detected in all stages of the menstrual cycle and induces proliferation of glandular epithelial cells; $PGF_{2\alpha}$ and PGI_2 induce epithelial cell proliferation; PGE_2 and $PGF_{2\alpha}$ concentrations are significantly increased during the WOI [7].

Endometrial Immune Cells (uNK)

Among the different leukocyte subpopulations present in the human endometrium, it is worth mentioning uterine natural killer cells (uNK). Although they are found throughout the menstrual cycle, during the WOI and late secretory phase they are the most abundant immune cells in the endometrium.

The number of CD16+ macrophage cells and NLp46 receptors seems to be significantly higher in women with unexplained pregnancy loss and unexplained infertility than in fertile patients [7].

miRNAs

Regarding implantation, microRNAs (miRNAs) are small highly conserved non-coding RNA sequences (19–22 nucleotides) that have been proposed as key mediators of receptivity. They are secreted by the endometrial cells and by the embryo. Different miRNAs have been isolated in the mid-secretory phase. It has been suggested that they are involved in the regulation of the proliferation and differentiation of epithelial cells during cyclic changes of the endometrium. Differentially expressed miRNAs have been identified in pre-receptive and receptive endometrium. Besides, differences have been found in expression between the genes in which these miRNAs act, suggesting that miRNAs also play an important role in the acquisition of receptivity and early gestation. Nevertheless, the exact role is still unknown [10].

Endometrial Receptivity Assessment

Several tools of receptivity assessment have been released since the mid-twentieth century based on morphological endometrial changes, identification of molecular receptivity markers, or using expression arrays to study the transcriptomic endometrial profile among others. In the current decade, the use of next-generation sequencing (NGS) techniques is leading to the development of more accurate diagnostic methods. The most used methods are described below.

Noyes Criteria

In 1950 Noyes, Herting, and Rock described the histological changes suffered by the different compartments of the endometrium during the menstrual cycle in endometrial biopsies and developed a classification criteria method that has been considered for a long time as the "gold standard" method for endometrial status assessment. However, randomized clinical trials, prospective and retrospective studies, revealed that Noyes dating criteria are an inaccurate diagnostic tool because of the subjectivity of the observer and the influence of other variables such as the state of the biopsy, intercycle variations, and tissue fixation techniques [10].

Pinopodes

Identified in 1958 in mouse, these ectoplasmic projections have been considered for a long time as an unequivocal receptivity marker but in recent years this idea has been debated. Pinopodes appear around the 20th day of the menstrual cycle. They absorb part of the endometrial fluid and macromolecules present in the uterine cavity by pinocytosis and endocytosis respectively, allowing the blastocyst to approach the endometrium and favoring the contact between both. Several molecules, also suggested as receptivity markers, are related to their presence including integrins, LIF, L-selectin, HOXA10, HB-EGF, and mucins. Moreover, it has been demonstrated that miRNAs, whose role in implantation has already been discussed, could affect the expression of pinopodes. However, some studies show that the presence of pinopodes persists in the post-receptive phase suggesting that they would not be useful as indicators of receptivity. In contrast, it is not fully clear whether implantation is possible in the absence of pinopodes [7;11].

Menstrual Cycle and LH Surge

One of the first methods used to identify the fertile period was based on the observation of the changes that occurred across the menstrual cycle. Changes in basal temperature or in the appearance of cervical mucus have traditionally been used as indicators of ovulation. Based on these parameters, some tools were developed, such as LH surge detection strips in urine that try to recognize the WOI between five and seven days after this peak. Nowadays it is known that receptivity is not always reached in the expected days, so these methods have become obsolete [10].

Ultrasonography

The application of ultrasonographic techniques revealed certain characteristics that were supposed to be related to a receptive endometrium, such as a trilaminar pattern and a thickness between 6 and 12 mm. Most recently, the development of three-dimensional ultrasound and power Doppler angiography has allowed the study of the volume, the vascularization, and the endometrial blood flow. Although echography is very useful in identifying reproductive disorders, its utility to predict endometrial receptivity was less than expected because the achievement of this status is due to other events apart from the morphological changes that are visually distinguishable [10].

E-tegrity Test and Endometrial Function Test

The E-tegrity test and the Endometrial Function Test (EFT) combine histological staining and molecular markers.

The E-tegrity test to evaluate endometrial receptivity was developed based on the expression of β_3 integrin. This test combines classical histological dating using the Noyes criteria with the presence/absence of β_3 integrin in endometrial biopsies taken between days LH+7 and LH+11. The main weakness of this test lies mainly in two aspects: on the one hand the subjectivity and imprecision of the Noyes criteria and on the other hand the diagnosis based on a single protein. However, this test seems to be useful for the diagnosis of defects during the luteal phase, unexplained infertility, hydrosalpinx, and endometriosis [10;12;13].

The development of the EFT is based on the presence or absence of cyclin E and cyclin-dependent kinase inhibitor p27 in a subcellular localization of the endometrial cells during the acquisition of receptivity. These two cyclins are involved in the endometrial cell's mitotic cycle and have been used to determine the endometrial receptivity in donor ovum recipients [14;15].

Natural Killer Cells

The assessment of the degree of activation of NK cells in endometrial biopsies and peripheral blood has been suggested as a method for evaluating endometrial receptivity and embryo implantation. Different studies have linked an increase in uNK and pNK (peripheral natural killer) cells with reproductive disorders such as unexplained infertility, RIF, and endometriosis. However, some studies have shown no association between the pNK/uNK and RIF [10].

-Omics Sciences

The emergence of the "-omics sciences" in the 2000s has led to numerous studies regarding genomics, secretomics, proteomics, lipidomics, transcriptomics, and interactomics analysis, extending the knowledge of the complex process of receptivity acquisition and opening the possibilities to new receptivity assessment approaches.

In the proteomic field, the latest advances in mass spectrometry have increased the number of studies related to protein profiles expressed in endometrial tissue and in endometrial fluid and have improved the understanding about the underlying biological processes. Different levels of protein can be detected, demonstrating the upregulation or downregulation of the expression of certain proteins related to the acquisition of receptivity. As an example, it has been published that annexin A2 and stathmin 1 (proteins involved in the regulation of the assembly of microtubules) are differently expressed between the pre-receptive (LH+2) and receptive phases (LH+7). This fact is consistent with the changes that occur in the epithelial cells in the course of pre-receptivity to receptivity [16].

The study of lipidomics has allowed the determination of important lipids related to receptivity and implantation phenomena. PGs are essential lipids presents in the endometrial fluid. A mass spectrometry assay showed a significant increase in the level of expression of PGE_2 and $PGF_{2\alpha}$ during the implantation window in fertile women and exhibited a specific lipidomic signature. This finding was thought to be useful to predict a successful pregnancy outcome by quantifying PGE_2 and $PGF_{2\alpha}$ concentrations in endometrial fluids of patients undergoing IVF 24 hours before the embryo transfer [17].

Advances in the development of molecular tools led to the search of the transcriptomic signature of endometrial receptivity. Several groups have described long lists of genes whose expression is regulated during the mid-secretory phase and that are involved in the achievement of the receptivity status. Due to the identification of the transcriptomic signature, a receptivity commercial test with successful clinical application was released in 2011: the Endometrial Receptivity Analysis (ERA) test [18]. The ERA test can predict the moment in which the WOI is opened. This publication analyzed the gene expression profile of endometrial biopsies by hybridization of the extracted mRNA with a customized microarray coupled to a computational predictor specially designed for such use. The main advantage of the ERA test over other tests is that it does not only identify whether the endometrium is receptive or not, but also identifies advanced or delayed displacements of the WOI, according to the standard day. This ability to locate the WOI of each patient (pWOI) makes feasible a personalized embryo transfer (pET) on the day when the

endometrium is really receptive and thus achieves a significant increase in the implantation rate, converting it into a good therapeutic option [8;19]. The ERA outcomes are accurate, reproducible, and consistent over time and support the existence of specific patterns of the secretory phase [20;21]. After analyzing over 35 000 transcriptomic profiles, in 2017 a new algorithm was developed to provide a new computational predictor based on NGS technology. The new ERA predictor defines the WOI with higher precision, indicating the optimal moment for the pET with a margin of only 6 hours [15]. The ERA test has also been applied to obtain information about the influence of certain factors on endometrial receptivity, such as obesity, ethnicity, endometrial thickness, or diseases such as endometriosis, thus providing new clinical data [10].

Factors Affecting Endometrial Receptivity

Sundry factors could affect the endometrial receptivity acquisition and the use of the newest molecular tools may be a good option to identify them. The ERA test has been used to evaluate whether obesity, ethnicity, endometrial thickness, and endometriosis are related to disorders in receptivity achievement.

Obesity

Obesity is an excessive fat accumulation condition traditionally linked with infertility and several other pathologies. Maternal obesity may affect both oocyte and embryo quality as well as endometrial functionality. The endometrial factor has been analyzed from the transcriptomic point of view. The results of the ERA test in five groups of infertile patients were compared. The groups were stratified by body mass index (BMI) as: normal weight (18.5–24.9 kg/m^2), overweight (25.0–29.9 kg/m^2), obesity class I (30.0–34.9 kg/m^2), obesity class II (35.0–39.9 kg/m^2), and obesity class III (over 40.0 kg/m^2) and nine genes were founded significantly dysregulated during the WOI in the receptive endometrium of obese patients. The proportion of non-receptive patients was higher as the BMI increased resulting in the conclusion that obesity may cause displacement of the WOI that results in RIF due to the endometrial factor [22;23].

Ethnicity

Whether ethnicity has an influence on the endometrial receptivity acquisition remains uncertain. Comparing the ERA results of patients from six different ethnicities, a lower number of receptive patients was observed in only one group. No significance differences were found between Arabian, Caucasian, East Asian, Hispanic, and South Asian patients but the African women showed more pre-receptive transcriptomic profiles than the other groups. However, this group presented a significantly higher BMI than the others making it difficult to know if the cause of the higher proportion in WOI displacements was either the ethnicity or the higher weight of the patients [23].

Endometrial Thickness

An insufficient endometrial growth may be directly related to defects in receptivity. It is widely accepted that an endometrial thickness between 6 and 12 mm before progesterone administration is an indicator of receptivity. To verify this assertion, a retrospective analysis of samples stratified in three ranges of thickness, measured by ultrasound, was performed. All samples were taken after five days of progesterone administration because it is the expected receptivity day. ERA test results showed a significant increase in the percentage of pre-receptive endometrial profile in the group of patients with atrophic endometrium (less than 6 mm) compared with the other two groups, while the percentage between the normal patient group (6–12 mm) and hypertrophic endometrium patient group (greater than 12 mm) presented a normal ratio of receptive versus non-receptive profiles. These results suggest a relation between a delay in the achievement of the WOI and an insufficient endometrial growth [23].

Endometriosis

Endometriosis affects around 10 percent of women and is directly related to infertility, though it does not seem to be associated with infertility due to the endometrial factor and nothing indicates that the origin of the endometriosis is related with a disruption of endometrial genes. Endometriosis is the growth of endometrial tissue outside the uterine cavity causing fallopian tube obstruction, chronic pain, dysmenorrhea, painful intercourse, and many other symptoms. The origin of this disorder is the study objective of many research groups. Seventeen infertile patients diagnosed with endometriosis (stages I–IV) were compared to five fertile patients using the ERA test. Biopsies were taken between days 18 and 20 of the natural cycle. The results showed that samples were only clustered according to the day when biopsy is performed, regardless of whether they were from healthy or affected patients [23;24].

Microbiome: The Unexpected Endometrial Factor

The endometrium has been traditionally considered a sterile organ, considering the cervix as an important barrier which avoided uterine cavity colonization. At the end of the 1990s and earlier 2000s, some publications described the existence of microbiota in the cervix by culture of the tips of endometrial catheters used to perform embryo transfers. The presence of some of these isolated bacterial species did not seem to affect implantation and pregnancy rates while others were associated with a decrease in implantation rate and poor pregnancy outcome. Recently, the use of NGS techniques has allowed a better insight of microbiota because some bacterial species are difficult to culture and remained undetected with classical methods. Using molecular methodologies, in 2015 the presence of endometrial microbiota in hysterectomized wombs for benign indications was demonstrated. In 2016, two independent groups used the 16S rRNA sequencing to study the endometrial microbiome: Franasiak et al., analyzing the transfer catheter tips, reported the identification of Lactobacillus as the most represented bacteria [25], while Moreno et al. analyzed endometrial fluid and vaginal aspirates, demonstrating the existence of specific endometrial microbiota, and a relationship between this microbiome population and reproductive clinical outcomes, concluding that a non-Lactobacillus-dominated flora in the receptive endometrium is associated with decreases in implantation, pregnancy, ongoing pregnancy, and live birth rates. So, microorganisms can cause implantation failure and pregnancy loss. These interesting new findings highlight the necessity of a more complete endometrial evaluation including the microbiological assessment (Figure 18.2) [26].

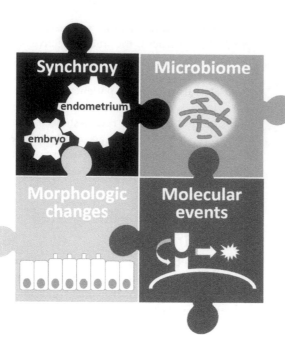

Figure 18.2 The complex network of events that compose the puzzle of the endometrial factor should be studied together.

Conclusions

The assessment of endometrial receptivity is an essential component in IVF and assisted reproductive techniques to avoid implantation failure and improve pregnancy outcomes since the implantation of a healthy embryo depends not only on the embryo itself and on an effective endometrium–embryo dialogue, but also on diseases or disorders in the endometrium and an imbalance of the endometrial microbiome.

In this trip to find a unique marker to be translated to the clinic and develop a diagnosing tool to find the WOI, the endometrial receptivity has been extensively investigated from diverse points of view. All the molecules, hormones, miRNAs, lipids, proteins, transcripts, and other known markers are ensembled participating in the complex building of receptivity. The uprising of molecular techniques has led to the substitution of other classic biochemical and morphological markers, whose effectiveness has been frequently questioned. Nowadays, the use of NGS techniques allows us to find the personal receptive transcriptomic profile and the endometrial microbiome balance of every single patient to synchronize embryo transfer during the optimal receptive period.

Technological advances in genetics should be used to expand our knowledge and improve the current assessment tools allowing their clinical application and helping to achieve an actual personalized reproductive medicine. Since the association of single-nucleotide polymorphisms or genetic variants with several traits and diseases have been studied, genome-wide association studies would be helpful to identify genetic variants in non-receptive patients that are causative of a displacement of the WOI.

References

1. Temkin O. *Soranus' Gynaecology*. Baltimore: John Hopkins University Press; 1956:xlix, 258 pp.

2. Herting AT, Rock J, Adams EC. A description of 34 human ova within the first 17 days of development. *Dev Dyn* 1956;**98**:435–493.

3. Navot D, Scott RT, Droesch K, *et al.* The window of embryo transfer and the efficiency of human conception in vitro. *Fertil Steril* 1991;**55**(1):114–118. doi:10.1016/s0015-0282(16)54069-2.

4. Harper MJ. The implantation window. *Baillieres Clin Obstet Gynaecol* 1992;**6**(2):351–371.

5. Wilcox AJ, Baird DD, Weinberg CR. Time of implantation of the conceptus and loss of pregnancy. *N Engl J Med* 1999;**340**(23):1796–1799. doi:10.1056/nejm199906103402304.

6. Grasso A, Balaguer N, Vilella F. Receptividad endometrial: expresión génica y otros biomarcadores. In:García-Velasco JA, ed. *Cuadernos de Medicina Reproductiva*, Vol. 23, No. 3. Edita Anarr. Nuevo Siglo,S.L.; 2017:45–57.

7. Miravet-Valenciano JA, Balaguer N, Vilella F, Simon C. Molecular diagnosis of endometrial receptivity. In: Simón C, Giudice L, eds. *The Endometrial Factor, A Reproductive Precision Medicine Approach*. Boca Raton: Taylor & Francis Group; 2017:36–49.

8. Ruiz-Alonso M, Blesa D, Díaz-Gimeno P, *et al.* The endometrial receptivity array for diagnosis and personalized embryo transfer as a treatment for patients with repeated implantation failure. *Fertil Steril* 2013;**100**(3):818–24.

9. Domínguez F, Loro F, Simón C. Funcionalidad del endometrio. In: *El Endometrio Humano: Desde la investigación a la clínica*. Madrid: Editorial Panamericana; 2009:19–37.

10. Gómez E, Marín C, Ruiz-Alonso M, Miravet-Valenciano JA, Simón C. Papel del test ERA en el fallo repetido de la implantación. In: Nadal J, ed. *Banco de óvulos*. Madrid: Editorial Panamericana; 2017:67–77.

11. Rarani FZ, Borhani F, Rashidi B. Endometrial pinopode biomarkers: molecules and microRNAs. *Cell Physiol* 2018;**233**(12):9145–9158.

12. Lessey BA, Castlebaum AJ, Sawin SW, *et al.* Abberant integrin expression in the endometrium of women with endometriosis. *J Clin Endocrinol Metab* 1994;**79**:643–649.

13. Lessey BA, Castlebaum AJ, Sawin SW, Sun JJF. Integrins as markers of uterine receptivity in women with primary unexplained infertility. *Fertil Steril* 1995;**63**(3):535–542.

14. Kliman H, Honig S, Walls D, *et al.* Optimization of endometrial preparation results in a normal endometrial function test (EFT) and good reproductive outcome in donor ovum recipients. *J Assist Reprod Genet* 2006;**23**(7–8):299–303.

15. Miravet-Valenciano J, Ruiz-Alonso M, Simón C. Modern evaluation of endometrial receptivity. In: Stadtmauer A, Tur-Kaspa I, eds. *Ultrasound Imaging in Reproductive Medicine: Advances in Infertility Work-up, Treatment and ART*, 2nd ed. Cham: Springer; 2019:357–368.

16. Domınguez F, Garrido-Gómez T, Lopez JA, *et al.* Proteomic analysis of the human receptive versus non-receptive endometrium using differential in-gel electrophoresis and MALDI-MS unveils stathmin 1 and annexin A2 as differentially regulated. *Hum Reprod* 2009;**24**:2607–2617.

17. Vilella F, Ramirez L, Berlanga O, *et al.* PGE2 and PGF2 concentrations in human endometrial fluid as biomarkers for embryonic implantation. *J Clin Endocrinol Metab* 2013;**98**(10):4123–4132.

18. Díaz-Gimeno P, Horcajadas JA, Martínez-Conejero JA, *et al.* A genomic diagnostic tool for human endometrial receptivity based on the transcriptomic signature. *Fertil Steril* 2011;**95**(1):50–60, 60.e1–60.e15.

19. Blesa D, Ruiz-Alonso M, Simón C. Clinical management of endometrial receptivity. *Semin Reprod Med* 2014;**32**(5):410–413.

20. Garrido-Gómez T, Ruiz-Alonso M, Blesa D, *et al.* Profiling the gene signature of endometrial receptivity: clinical results. *Fertil Steril* 2010;**99**(4):1078–1085.

21. Díaz-Gimeno P, Ruíz-Alonso M, Blesa D, *et al.* The accuracy and reproducibility of the endometrial receptivity array is superior to histology as a diagnostic method for endometrial receptivity. *Fertil Steril* 2013;**99**:508–517.

22. Comstock IA, Diaz-Gimeno P, Cabanillas S, *et al.* Does an increased body mass index affect endometrial gene expression patterns in infertile patients? A functional genomic analysis. *Fertil Steril* 2017;**107**(3):740–748.

23. Miravet-Valenciano J, Ruiz-Alonso M, Simón C. The transcriptomics of the human endometrium and embryo implantation. In: Leung PCK, Qiao J, eds. *Human Reproductive and Prenatal Genetics*. London: Academic Press; 2018:271–291.

24. Garcia-Velasco JA, Fassbender A, Ruiz-Alonso M, *et al.* Is endometrial receptivity transcriptomics affected in women with endometriosis? A pilot study. *Reprod Biomed Online* 2015;**31**(5):647–654.

25. Franasiak JM, Werner MD, Juneau CR, *et al.* Endometrial microbiome at the time of embryo transfer: next-generation sequencing of the 16S ribosomal subunit. *J Assist Reprod Genet* 2016;**33**:129–136.

26. Moreno I, Codoñer FM, Vilella F, *et al.* Evidence that the endometrial microbiota has an effect on implantation success or failure. *Am J Obstet Gynecol* 2016;**215**(6):684–703.

Chapter 19

Folliculogenesis and Implantation Failure

Antonis Makrigiannakis and Panagiotis Drakopoulos

Normal Implantation

Following fertilization in the fallopian tube approximately 24 to 48 hours after ovulation, the zygote migrates through the fallopian tube to the uterine cavity at the stage of morula on day 18 of an ideal 28-day cycle [1]. On day 19, a 32- to 256-cell blastocyst forms, sheds its zona pellucida (known as hatching), superficially apposes, and adheres to the endometrium [2]. This is followed by trophoblast invasion through the endometrial epithelium and underlying stroma, the inner third of the myometrium, and the uterine vasculature, all of which finally result in placentation [3]. The success of each step is crucial in order to advance toward the next stage.

Implantation occurs only during the "window of implantation," which corresponds to days 8 to 10 after ovulation [4]. The concept of endometrial receptivity and the presence of a "window of implantation" was first introduced by Hertig *et al.* in the 1950s [5] and was further developed by others using the luteinizing hormone (LH) peak as reference for the detection of the optimal period of endometrial receptivity [6]. Nonetheless, despite the well-known limitations of the use of LH measurements to detect ovulation, it is still believed by many that all patients become receptive during these three days, irrespective of individual variations or hormonal treatment received (natural cycle, conventional ovarian stimulation [COS] cycles, artificially prepared cycles). The "window of implantation" is transient in humans, and implantation after this period results in spontaneous miscarriages.

In natural cycles, implantation rate (IR) is difficult to estimate, given that although ovulation can be confirmed, fertilization and migration of the embryo to the uterus cannot be directly assessed. In this regard, implantation failure may occur very early, during the attachment or migration of the embryo and in that case there is no objective evidence of pregnancy (i.e., negative human chorionic gonadotropin [hCG] test), or later on, following successful migration and production of hCG by the embryo. The estimated IR in natural cycles is poor, approximately 15 to 30 percent, and seems to decrease with maternal age, especially after the age of 35 [7;8]. On the other hand, in assisted reproduction and more specifically in COS cycles, implantation is considered to be successful if an intrauterine gestational sac is detectable by ultrasound, usually about three weeks following oocyte retrieval. The IR in in vitro fertilization (IVF) treatment is defined as the number of gestational sacs divided by the total number of embryos transferred, and ranges between 25 and 40 percent [9].

From the clinical point of view, the term "implantation failure" may refer to two distinct conditions: (1) those that have never had evidence of implantation (no detectable hCG production) and (2) those that have evidence of implantation (detectable hCG) but the embryo did not advance and therefore no gestational sac was visible on ultrasound. It is well established that both embryo and endometrial factors can result in implantation failure.

Hormones and Implantation

Steroid Hormones and the Endometrium during Implantation

Implantation is a dynamic and strictly regulated process occurring between a good-quality developing embryo and a synchronized endometrium. To achieve successful implantation, the uterus should undergo structural and functional remodeling, which is mainly regulated by hormones secreted by the ovary (estrogen [E] and progesterone [P]), whose role is to make the endometrium receptive to the embryo that will implant during the so-called "window of implantation."

At the moment of implantation, the endometrium has morphologically differentiated into two layers: the basal layer (which represents the lower one-third of the endometrium and is most adjacent to the myometrium, a layer which remains relatively unchanged throughout the menstrual cycle and is critical for endometrial regeneration following menstruation) and the functional layer (which represents the upper two-thirds of the endometrium and is the site of proliferation, secretion, and degeneration) [10].

In particular, during the proliferative (follicular) phase of the menstrual cycle, under the effect of E produced by the growing ovarian follicles, the functionalis layer regenerates, ciliogenesis occurs (appearance of ciliated cells around gland openings), and the uterine epithelial cells proliferate and differentiate [11]. E levels rise prior to the receptive phase, although whether this E elevation is required for implantation in humans is currently unknown [12]. Furthermore, although E can induce uterine receptivity, the "window of implantation" remains open for an extended period at lower E levels and precipitously closes at higher levels in mice [13].

Serum P levels remain low throughout the follicular phase until ovulation (median of 0.30 ng/ml and 95% confidence interval of 0.19–0.51 ng/ml) [14]. At midcycle, there is a pick of gonadotropins, namely LH, resulting in ovulation. The LH surge causes a slight late-follicular phase P rise, which seems to be essential for ovulation timing and follicular development [15]. Following ovulation, P impairs the proliferation of the endometrium by directly inhibiting the function of E and the expression of E-binding receptors and in the meantime stimulates the development of vascular and glandular structures [16]. Peak secretory activity is reached approximately seven days after the LH surge and is characterized by an extremely edematous endometrial stroma, though decidualization (the differentiation of endometrial stromal cells to decidual cells) occurs later in the luteal phase and involves augmented mitosis and differentiation of stromal cells [17]. In the absence of implantation, the corpus luteum undergoes regression, which is followed by a sharp decline in E and P, and tissue breakdown and regeneration.

The successive morphological changes induced by P follow a day-by-day sequence of development and were the basis of the histological endometrial dating classification system developed by Noyes *et al.* [18]. This classic endometrial classification system was, until recently, the gold standard for the evaluation of luteal phase, where endometrial tissue samples with a greater than two to three days' lag in endometrial maturation were considered to be "out of phase." However, the results of a large prospective multicenter randomized controlled trial, showing no significant difference in abnormal endometrial biopsies between fertile and infertile women, led to the conclusion that endometrial dating should probably be eliminated as part of the infertility workup [19].

Conclusively, the "window of implantation" opens due to the effects of P on an E-primed endometrium. The necessity of ovarian steroids in implantation can also be noticed from clinical experience in IVF practice, given that E and P supplementation alone is sufficient to induce endometrial receptivity in frozen/thawed embryo transfer cycles [20].

Mechanisms of Steroids' Action during Implantation

E and P have a key role in the dynamic process of implantation by mobilizing several molecular modulators in a spatiotemporal manner; albeit transcription factors whose expressions are not altered by these hormones and are also related to implantation have recently been identified [21]. The molecular crosstalk that originates locally from the mother/embryo and results in the orderly chronological transitions for successful implantation is not completely understood. Ethical issues have delayed and even precluded the conduction of studies on human implantation and evidence is mainly derived by transgenic mouse models (Table 19.1) [21]. These models have allowed the discovery of new regulators that mimic human pregnancy events and have provided conceptual advances in the understanding of the complex phenomenon of implantation.

The effect of E and P is mediated through their intracellular receptors: E and P have two receptors subtypes, α and β and A and B, respectively [22]. Estrogen receptor (ER)-α is expressed by endometrial epithelial and stromal cells during the follicular

Table 19.1 Reproductive function in animals with targeted disruption of genes important in the Implantation process

Gene	Reproductive (uterine, implantation) function
Alk3	Implantation failure
Bmp2	Incapable of undergoing the decidual reaction
Cdh1	Implantation failure
CSF-1/M-CSF	op/op and op/op crosses are infertile, op/op females and op/+ males are subfertile
E-cadherin	Implantation failure; failed to artificially induce decidualization
ERα	Infertile owing to complete ovarian inefficiency; able to induce and support decidualization
ERβ	Subfertile (fewer and smaller litters) owing to reduced ovarian efficiency
Egfr	Implantation site demise due to a failure in the maintenance and progression of decidualization
Fkbp52	Compromised P4 activity; impaired implantation and decidualization
HOXA10	Oviductal transformation of the proximal third of the uterus, defective implantation and embryonic reabsorption in the early postimplantation period
HOXA11	Diminished uterine glands; partial homeotic transformation of uterus to oviduct, defective implantation
Hand2	Impaired progesterone receptor's function
IHH	Implantation failure
IL-6	Subfertile, viable implantation sites are decreased by 50 percent
IL-11Rα	Infertile owing to defective decidualization
IL-1β	Fertile, no major reproductive defects
IL-1 Rt1	Fertile, slightly smaller litters
IL-15	Fertile, lack of uterine natural killer (uNK) cells at the implantation, impaired decidual integrity, unmodified spiral arteries
LIF	Infertile owing to complete implantation failure, unable to induce and support decidualization
LIFR	Intrauterine lethality
PRA	Infertile, subovulatory, unable to induce and support decidualization
PRB	Fertile, normal ovarian and uterine response to progesterone
Stat3	Implantation failure
TGF-β1	Intrauterine and early postnatal lethality
Wnt4	Implantation defect failed to undergo the artificially induced decidual response
Wnt7a	Implantation failure

Alk3 = activin-like kinase 3; Bmp2 = bone morphogenetic protein 2; Cdh1 = E-cadherin; Egfr = epidermal growth factor receptor; Fkbp52 = FK506-binding protein-4; CSF-1 = colony stimulating factor-1; IHH = Indian hedgehog homolog; IL = interleukin; IL-11Rα = type α IL-11 receptor; IL-1Rt1 = interleukin-1 receptor type 1; M-CSF = macrophage-colony stimulating factor; TGF-β1 = transforming growth factor-β1, ER = estrogen receptor; PR = progesterone receptor; LIF = leukemia inhibitory factor; LIFR = LIF receptor; HOXA10 and HOXA11 = Hox genes; Hand2 = heart and neural crest derivatives expressed transcript 2; Stat3 = signal transducer and activator of transcription 3; Wnt4 = wingless-related MMTV integration site 4; Wnt7a = wingless-related MMTV integration site 7a.

phase, and decreases during the secretory phase, while the expression of ERβ is low and limited to glandular epithelial cells only [22]. ERα is the primary driver of E action, as ERα$^{-/-}$ mice have a hypoplastic uterus and are infertile [23]. One major mediator of E action is leukemia inhibitory factor (LIF), a member of the interleukin-6 family of cytokines. LIF binds to its receptor (LIFR) and further activates the downstream signaling via signal transducer and activator of transcription 3 [24]. LIF is essential for uterine receptivity and implantation and its deletion results in implantation failure in mice, though its role in humans remains unclear. LIF administration in infertile patients does not seem to improve reproductive outcomes [25].

Progesterone receptor (PR)-A is expressed in the epithelium and stroma during the proliferative and secretory phase of the menstrual cycle, whereas PRB is present only in the proliferative phase [26]. PRA is crucial for implantation, based on the fact that mice lacking both PRA and PRB are infertile, while mice lacking only PRB have normal fertility [27]. P_4, which is considered the "hormone of pregnancy," stimulates the induction of several genes in the uterus that are involved in peri-implantation events. For instance, FKBP52, a P_4-inducible co-chaperone, is required for optimizing PR activity. Fkbp52$^{-/-}$ female mice are infertile with decreased uterine P_4 responsiveness and are more susceptible to oxidative stress [28;29]. P_4 also induces Indian hedgehog (Ihh) in the uterus, which acts as a paracrine signal for epithelial–stromal interaction, and its uterine deletion results in implantation failure and impaired endometrial receptivity [30;31]. In the same vein, Hand2, a P_4-induced transcription factor in the endometrial stroma, has also been reported to be involved in implantation in mice [32].

Although the most important molecular mediators of E and P have been outlined above, studies have identified several other E- and P-regulated factors taking part in the cascade of implantation, including, among others, cytokines, matrix metalloproteinases, growth factors, adhesion molecules, extracellular matrix components, and homeobox element-containing genes [33].

Finally, it should be mentioned that unlike the embryo, the transition from anatomical to molecular medicine in the evaluation of endometrial receptivity happened only a decade ago. Since, several studies have evaluated potential markers of endometrial receptivity as predictors of successful implantation and, by doing so, have contributed to a better understanding of the physiological pathway of implantation. These markers include pinopodes, cell adhesion molecules, growth factors, cytokines, homeobox (HOX) genes, prostaglandins, peptide hormones, matrix metalloproteinases, and their inhibitors [10]. Besides, transcriptomic profiling of the endometrium throughout the menstrual cycle, as well as during the "window of implantation" [34], gave rise to the identification of the transcriptomic signature of endometrial receptivity and the development of tests evaluating endometrial receptivity on an individual basis [35]. In the same context, the advent of advanced omics technologies has provided new insights for the understanding of embryo implantation by identifying endometrial epithelial cellular and secreted protein changes in response to ovarian steroid hormones [36]. Nonetheless, findings regarding the role of all these markers as predictors of successful implantation remain controversial and further studies are warranted in the era of endometrial receptivity.

The Effect of Supraphysiological Circulating Hormone Levels on Endometrial Receptivity

Although the duration of the follicular phase of the human menstrual cycle may be subject to both intercycle and inter-patient variability, endogenous sexual hormones remain within relatively low levels prior to ovulation, specifically a median (5th and 95th percentiles) of 182.80 pg/ml (131.30–388.28 pg/ml) for estradiol (E_2) and 0.80 ng/ml (0.39–1.30 ng/ml) for P [14]. On the other hand, the same hormones reach significantly higher levels in controlled ovarian stimulation. These supraphysiological hormone concentrations have been shown to have a negative impact on endometrial receptivity, given that endometrial biopsies performed on the day of oocyte retrieval were found to have histological and gene expression patterns suggestive of endometrial advancement [37]. If we further take into consideration that high E levels may render the endometrium non-receptive as discussed previously, it becomes evident that one reason for implantation failure in IVF programs may be related to the increased E levels associated with controlled ovarian stimulation [38]. Furthermore, there is accumulated evidence demonstrating a direct relationship between late-follicular elevated P and endometrial receptivity in IVF cycles. Specifically values of P above 1.50 ng/ml have been associated with histological endometrial advancement, abnormal expression of implantation regulating proteins, and dysregulation of key endometrial genes [37]. The results of a recent meta-analysis including more than 60 000 IVF cycles clearly showed that high P has a negative impact on reproductive outcomes of patients undergoing fresh embryo transfer [39]. These findings have led many reproductive medicine centers to change their policy, so as to measure serum P levels on the day of ovulation triggering and to implement a "freeze-all" strategy when the threshold of 1.50 ng/ml is surpassed [40]. Nonetheless, the mechanism by which the rise of

P during the follicular phase affects pregnancy rates is still not completely elucidated and further studies are warranted, especially if we consider that emerging evidence associates high P not only with endometrium–embryo asynchrony, but also with poor embryo quality [41].

References

1. Croxatto HB, Diaz S, Fuentealba B, *et al.* Studies on the duration of egg transport in the human oviduct. I. The time interval between ovulation and egg recovery from the uterus in normal women. *Fertil Steril* 1972;**23**(7):447–458. doi: 10.1016/s0015-0282(16)39069-0.

2. Enders AC, Schlafke S. Cytological aspects of trophoblast-uterine interaction in early implantation. *Am J Anat* 1969;**125**(1):1–29. doi: 10.1002/aja.1001250102.

3. Cross JC, Werb Z, Fisher SJ. Implantation and the placenta: key pieces of the development puzzle. *Science* 1994;**266**(5190):1508–1518. doi: 10.1126/science.7985020.

4. Wilcox AJ, Baird DD, Weinberg CR. Time of implantation of the conceptus and loss of pregnancy. *N Engl J Med* 1999;**340**(23):1796–1799. doi: 10.1056/NEJM199906103402304.

5. Hertig AT, Rock J, Adams EC. A description of 34 human ova within the first 17 days of development. *Am J Anat* 1956;**98**(3):435–493. doi: 10.1002/aja.1000980306.

6. Acosta AA, Elberger L, Borghi M, *et al.* Endometrial dating and determination of the window of implantation in healthy fertile women. *Fertil Steril* 2000;**73**(4):788–798. doi: 10.1016/s0015-0282(99)00605-6.

7. Miller JF, Williamson E, Glue J, *et al.* Fetal loss after implantation. A prospective study. *Lancet* 1980;**2**(8194):554–556. doi: 10.1016/s0140-6736(80)91991-1.

8. Spandorfer SD, Chung PH, Kligman I, *et al.* An analysis of the effect of age on implantation rates. *J Assist Reprod Genet* 2000;**17**(6):303–306. doi: 10.1023/a:1009422725434.

9. Coughlan C, Ledger W, Wang Q, *et al.* Recurrent implantation failure: definition and management. *Reprod Biomed Online* 2014;**28**(1):14–38. doi: 10.1016/j.rbmo.2013.08.011.

10. Kodaman PH, Taylor HS. Hormonal regulation of implantation. *Obstet Gynecol Clin North Am* 2004;**31**(4):745–766, ix. doi: 10.1016/j.ogc.2004.08.008.

11. Ludwig H, Spornitz UM. Microarchitecture of the human endometrium by scanning electron microscopy: menstrual desquamation and remodeling. *Ann N Y Acad Sci* 1991;**622**:28–46. doi: 10.1111/j.1749-6632.1991.tb37848.x.

12. Rao AJ, Ramachandra SG, Ramesh V, *et al.* Establishment of the need for oestrogen during implantation in non-human primates. *Reprod Biomed Online* 2007;**14**(5):563–571. doi: 10.1016/s1472-6483(10)61047-4.

13. Ma WG, Song H, Das SK, *et al.* Estrogen is a critical determinant that specifies the duration of the window of uterine receptivity for implantation. *Proc Natl Acad Sci U S A* 2003;**100**(5):2963–2968. doi: 10.1073/pnas.0530162100.

14. Stricker R, Eberhart R, Chevailler MC, *et al.* Establishment of detailed reference values for luteinizing hormone, follicle stimulating hormone, estradiol, and progesterone during different phases of the menstrual cycle on the Abbott ARCHITECT analyzer. *Clin Chem Lab Med* 2006;**44**(7):883–887. doi: 10.1515/CCLM.2006.160.

15. Hild-Petito S, Stouffer RL, Brenner RM. Immunocytochemical localization of estradiol and progesterone receptors in the monkey ovary throughout the menstrual cycle. *Endocrinology* 1988;**123**(6):2896–2905. doi: 10.1210/endo-123-6-2896.

16. Scublinsky A, Marin C, Gurpide E. Localization of estradiol 17beta dehydrogenase in human endometrium. *J Steroid Biochem* 1976;**7**(10):745–7. doi: 10.1016/0022-4731(76)90174-6.

17. Bulmer JN, Morrison L, Longfellow M, *et al.* Granulated lymphocytes in human endometrium: histochemical and immunohistochemical studies. *Hum Reprod* 1991;**6**(6):791–798. doi: 10.1093/oxfordjournals.humrep.a137430.

18. Noyes RW, Hertig AT, Rock J. Dating the endometrial biopsy. *Am J Obstet Gynecol* 1975;**122**(2):262–263. doi: 10.1016/s0002-9378(16)33500-1.

19. McGovern PG, Myers ER, Silva S, *et al.* Absence of secretory endometrium after false-positive home urine luteinizing hormone testing. *Fertil Steril* 2004;**82**(5):1273–7. doi: 10.1016/j.fertnstert.2004.03.070.

20. Racca A, Drakopoulos P, Van Landuyt L, *et al.* Single and double embryo transfer provide similar live birth rates in frozen cycles. *Gynecol Endocrinol* 2020;**36**(9):824–828. doi: 10.1080/09513590.2020.1712697.

21. Cha J, Sun X, Dey SK. Mechanisms of implantation: strategies for successful pregnancy. *Nat Med* 2012;**18**(12):1754–1767. doi: 10.1038/nm.3012.

22. Lessey BA, Killam AP, Metzger DA, *et al.* Immunohistochemical analysis of human uterine estrogen and progesterone receptors throughout the menstrual cycle. *J Clin Endocrinol Metab* 1988;**67**(2):334–340. doi: 10.1210/jcem-67-2-334.

23. Lubahn DB, Moyer JS, Golding TS, *et al.* Alteration of reproductive function but not prenatal sexual development after insertional disruption of the mouse estrogen receptor gene. *Proc Natl Acad Sci U S A* 1993;**90** (23):11162–11166. doi: 10.1073/pnas.90.23.11162.

24. Niwa H, Burdon T, Chambers I, *et al.* Self-renewal of pluripotent embryonic stem cells is mediated via activation of STAT3. *Genes Dev* 1998;**12** (13):2048–2060. doi: 10.1101/gad.12.13.2048.

25. Brinsden PR, Alam V, de Moustier B, *et al.* Recombinant human leukemia inhibitory factor does not improve implantation and pregnancy outcomes after assisted reproductive techniques in women with recurrent unexplained implantation failure. *Fertil Steril* 2009;**91**(4Suppl): 1445–1447. doi: 10.1016/j.fertnstert.2008.06.047.

26. Stavreus-Evers A, Nikas G, Sahlin L, *et al.* Formation of pinopodes in human endometrium is associated with the concentrations of progesterone and progesterone receptors. *Fertil Steril* 2001;**76**(4):782–791. doi: 10.1016/s0015-0282(01)01993-8.

27. Mulac-Jericevic B, Mullinax RA, DeMayo FJ, *et al.* Subgroup of reproductive functions of progesterone mediated by progesterone receptor-B isoform. *Science* 2000;**289** (5485):1751–1754. doi: 10.1126/science.289.5485.1751.

28. Tranguch S, Wang H, Daikoku T, *et al.* FKBP52 deficiency-conferred uterine progesterone resistance is genetic background and pregnancy stage specific. *J Clin Invest* 2007;**117**(7):1824–1834. doi: 10.1172/JCI31622.

29. Hirota Y, Acar N, Tranguch S, *et al.* Uterine FK506-binding protein 52 (FKBP52)-peroxiredoxin-6 (PRDX6) signaling protects pregnancy from overt oxidative stress. *Proc Natl Acad Sci U S A* 2010;**107** (35):15577–15582. doi: 10.1073/pnas.1009324107.

30. Lee K, Jeong J, Kwak I, *et al.* Indian hedgehog is a major mediator of progesterone signaling in the mouse uterus. *Nat Genet* 2006;**38**(10):1204–1209. doi: 10.1038/ng1874.

31. Franco HL, Rubel CA, Large MJ, *et al.* Epithelial progesterone receptor exhibits pleiotropic roles in uterine development and function. *FASEB J* 2012;**26**(3):1218–1227. doi: 10.1096/fj.11-193334.

32. Huyen DV, Bany BM. Evidence for a conserved function of heart and neural crest derivatives expressed transcript 2 in mouse and human decidualization. *Reproduction* 2011;**142** (2):353–368. doi: 10.1530/REP-11-0060.

33. Dey SK, Lim H, Das SK, *et al.* Molecular cues to implantation. *Endocr Rev* 2004;**25**(3):341–373. doi: 10.1210/er.2003-0020.

34. Riesewijk A, Martin J, van Os R, *et al.* Gene expression profiling of human endometrial receptivity on days LH+2 versus LH+7 by microarray technology. *Mol Hum Reprod* 2003;**9** (5):253–264. doi: 10.1093/molehr/gag037.

35. Diaz-Gimeno P, Horcajadas JA, Martinez-Conejero JA, *et al.* A genomic diagnostic tool for human endometrial receptivity based on the transcriptomic signature. *Fertil Steril* 2011; **95**(1):50–60, 60.e1–60.e15. doi: 10.1016/j.fertnstert.2010.04.063.

36. Greening DW, Nguyen HP, Evans J, *et al.* Modulating the endometrial epithelial proteome and secretome in preparation for pregnancy: the role of ovarian steroid and pregnancy hormones. *J Proteomics* 2016;**144**:99–112. doi: 10.1016/j.jprot.2016.05.026.

37. Labarta E, Martinez-Conejero JA, Alama P, *et al.* Endometrial receptivity is affected in women with high circulating progesterone levels at the end of the follicular phase: a functional genomics analysis. *Hum Reprod* 2011;**26**(7):1813–1825. doi: 10.1093/humrep/der126.

38. Simon C, Garcia Velasco JJ, Valbuena D, *et al.* Increasing uterine receptivity by decreasing estradiol levels during the preimplantation period in high responders with the use of a follicle-stimulating hormone step-down regimen. *Fertil Steril* 1998;**70**(2):234–239. doi: 10.1016/s0015-0282(98)00140-x.

39. Venetis CA, Kolibianakis EM, Bosdou JK, *et al.* Progesterone elevation and probability of pregnancy after IVF: a systematic review and meta-analysis of over 60 000 cycles. *Hum Reprod Update* 2013;**19**(5):433–457. doi: 10.1093/humupd/dmt014.

40. Drakopoulos P, Racca A, Errazuriz J, *et al.* The role of progesterone elevation in IVF. *Reprod Biol* 2019;**19**(1):1–5. doi: 10.1016/j.repbio.2019.02.003.

41. Racca A, Santos-Ribeiro S, De Munck N, *et al.* Impact of late-follicular phase elevated serum progesterone on cumulative live birth rates: is there a deleterious effect on embryo quality? *Hum Reprod* 2018;**33**(5):860–868. doi: 10.1093/humrep/dey031.

Adjuncts for Ovarian Stimulation

Alexander M. Quaas and David R. Meldrum

Introduction

Clomiphene (clomifene) citrate (CC) and follicle-stimulating hormone (FSH) have traditionally been considered the two main modalities used for ovarian stimulation (OS). However, many adjuncts have been used to maximize the convenience and effectiveness of these two agents, often specifically targeted to subsets of women undergoing stimulation. Most of these adjuncts are not officially approved for these indications. Therefore, educators and practitioners must take it upon themselves to assess the evidence supporting their use, and make treatment recommendations and decisions accordingly. We have outlined in an editorial in *Fertility and Sterility* a process to aid in this endeavor [1]. Decisions are based not only on randomized clinical trials (RCT), but also on other basic science and clinical evidence supporting their use.

Leuprolide Acetate and Other Gonadotropin-Releasing Hormone Agonists

Primarily developed for treatment of prostate cancer, the usefulness of gonadotropin-releasing hormone (GnRH) agonists in preventing premature luteinizing hormone (LH) release became immediately apparent, leading to the suggestion for routine use in all in vitro fertilization (IVF) cycles [2]. Despite a reduction of premature ovulation from over 20 percent to almost zero and a subsequent meta-analysis showing a twofold increase of the pregnancy rate [3], the principle GnRH agonist used in the USA, leuprolide acetate, is still "off-label" for this indication. Further benefits have been increased numbers of retrieved oocytes and embryos for fresh transfer and for cryopreservation, as well as the ability to schedule procedures for patients' or programs' convenience. Disadvantages have been an increased rate

of ovarian hyperstimulation syndrome (OHSS), ovarian cyst development due to the agonist phase of treatment, and symptoms due to low estrogen levels prior to the ovarian response to stimulation, which sometimes can be severe.

In "poor responders," a "microdose flare" protocol using leuprolide acetate may be used for stimulation, taking advantage of the initial "flare" effect of GnRH agonists in the early follicular phase to stimulate follicular recruitment through endogenous gonadotropins.

Gonadotropin-Releasing Hormone Antagonists

Gonadotropin-releasing hormone antagonists competitively block pituitary GnRH receptors, producing a fast and reversible suppression of gonadotropin secretion.

They have been increasingly used as part of IVF stimulation protocols to replace the role of pre-stimulation GnRH agonists in preventing premature LH release [4]. Because of their ability to rapidly suppress gonadotropin release at the level of the pituitary gland, GnRH antagonists can be started after initiation of gonadotropin stimulation, with no impact on early follicular recruitment. In practice, GnRH antagonists are typically started when the lead follicle during OS reaches a size of 14 mm.

Given that the suppressive effect of GnRH agonist downregulation is removed, protocols using GnRH antagonists represent an attractive option for "poor responders." Another advantage of GnRH antagonist protocols is the fact that GnRH agonists may be used to trigger ovulation instead of human chorionic gonadotropin (hCG), which is associated with a lower risk of OHSS. Therefore, protocols involving GnRH antagonists are also frequently used for patients with polycystic ovary syndrome (PCOS) and egg donors. In addition, GnRH antagonist use to prevent premature ovulation simplifies stimulation regimens and may be more convenient to patients. A systematic review of published trials comparing GnRH antagonist versus long agonist protocols in IVF found lower rates of OHSS in "general IVF patients" and in women with PCOS [5], and no difference in ongoing clinical pregnancy rates in patients with PCOS and poor responders. In "general IVF patients," the ongoing pregnancy was lower in the antagonist group than in the agonist group, specifically when oral contraceptive (OC) pretreatment was combined with the flexible antagonist protocol [5]. However, with the many additional modifications to contemporary IVF protocols (including "freeze-only" approaches and the use of other adjuvants), and because of many other advantages outlined above, more and more practices are now exclusively using GnRH antagonist protocols for OS in all patients.

Oral Contraceptive Pretreatment

Pretreatment with OC was found to markedly reduce the occurrence of ovarian cysts with GnRH agonist treatment, and allows programming of cycles with a reduced interval of low estrogen levels prior to the ovarian response to stimulation. Overlap of OC and agonist has most commonly been five days, but the regimen appears to be equally effective with as little as one day [6]. Less gonadotropin is needed to achieve the same level of stimulation [6], provided stimulation is not begun prior to the fifth day off OC, when endogenous levels of gonadotropins have increased toward normal [7].

Estrogen Pretreatment

Oral estrogen was first used to schedule OS cycles using 4 mg daily of estradiol valerate beginning in the midluteal phase of the prior menstrual cycle, with the onset of stimulation on the day following discontinuation [8]. With this pretreatment, the resting follicles have less variation in size and the response to stimulation is increased [9], suggesting that both OC and estrogen increase ovarian response by improving synchrony of the cohort of follicles capable of responding to FSH. This approach has also been used to improve OS in poor responders [10].

Dexamethasone

Dexamethasone (DEX) was first shown to improve response to OS when combined with CC in a RCT showing a higher rate of ovulation with CC when

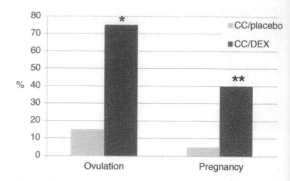

Figure 20.1 Ovulation and pregnancy rates were increased five- and eightfold with DEX compared with placebo (* $p < 0.001$, ** $p < 0.05$) [13].

0.5 mg of DEX was given continuously [11]. More recently, two RCTs in women failing to ovulate with up to 150–250 mg of CC have shown increases of ovulation of 4- to 5-fold and pregnancy of 8- to 10-fold with adjunctive use of DEX. In those studies, a higher dose of 2 mg was given, but only during the five days of CC and for the following five days [12;13]. Ovulation was routinely triggered with hCG. The mean body mass index in these two studies was 29–30 kg/m^2. The more recent study had a superior design [13], with ovulation in both groups triggered when at least one follicle reached 18 mm (Figure 20.1). In a further randomized trial of 1 mg of DEX during stimulation for IVF, a dramatic decrease of canceled cycles from 12.4 to 2.8 percent was noted, and the implantation and pregnancy rates were higher in spite of inclusion of those poor-prognosis women going to egg retrieval [14]. The ratio of cortisol to cortisone in follicular fluid correlates with IVF success [15;16], and higher follicular fluid cortisol levels are associated with a higher number of total and mature oocytes retrieved during IVF [17]. These findings suggest that glucocorticoids improve both the response of follicles to stimulation and the health of their developing oocytes. Because DEX is simpler than metformin (Met) therapy, it appears to be the initial adjunct of choice for women failing to ovulate with CC, particularly in women who are not markedly obese. It also appears to be an excellent adjunct for poor responders undergoing IVF.

Metformin

Meta-analysis of 10 RCTs with adjunctive use of Met in women with PCOS having OS for IVF has shown a dramatic reduction of OHSS (odds ratio [OR] 0.27, 95% confidence interval (CI) 0.16–0.46, $p < 0.00001$, Figure 20.2) [18]. Insulin, which is elevated in PCOS and markedly reduced by Met, is one of the factors that stimulate luteinized granulosa cells to produce vascular endothelial growth factor (VEGF) [19], the principle cause of the increased vascular permeability responsible for the major manifestations of OHSS. Because OHSS can be associated with severe complications and even death, this finding alone makes the use of Met essential whenever OS in PCOS patients is expected to be accompanied by a significant risk of OHSS.

Metformin also appears to improve the odds of pregnancy with OS in women with PCOS. Meta-analysis of 17 RCTs in PCOS women has shown both increased ovulation (OR 4.39, 95% CI 1.94–9.96) and pregnancy (OR 2.67, 95% CI 1.54–4.94) when Met was added to CC [20]. This effect was found to be statistically significant in obese women with PCOS (OR 10.9), whereas it failed to reach significance in non-obese women with this condition (Figure 20.2). It therefore seems logical to routinely use Met with CC in obese women with PCOS, and to use DEX as the first adjunct of choice for non-obese PCOS women failing to respond to CC. Met has also been associated with an improved pregnancy rate in PCOS women having IVF [21;22], but when all 10 RCTs were combined, the 69 percent higher pregnancy rate was not statistically significant [18]. The implantation rate was significantly increased (OR 1.42, 95% CI 1.24–2.75) and miscarriage was significantly reduced

(OR 0.50, 95% CI 0.30–0.83). Because individual trials have achieved statistical significance, it is assumed that Met also improves the odds of pregnancy in PCOS women having IVF.

The increased chance of implantation in PCOS women having OS is supported by studies showing decreased glycodelin, uterine blood flow, and HOXA-10 in women with PCOS, with significant improvement of these parameters with Met [23;24]. These findings also may explain the increased rate of miscarriage in these women and the reduced fetal loss reported with Met [25]. However, there are no RCTs in women continuing Met during early pregnancy to verify this latter benefit.

Intraovarian androgen increases ovarian response by increasing FSH receptors on granulosa cells. Therefore, Met may produce a more controlled ovarian response in PCOS women by reducing insulin stimulation of ovarian androgen production. In women who were CC resistant, who also tend to be hyperinsulinemic, Met did reduce OS response for IVF [21]. Also, in PCOS women receiving low-dose FSH, Met reduced the number of mature follicles [26]. Recent studies have confirmed a relatively low incidence of ovulation and pregnancy with Met as a single agent, leading many to conclude that CC alone should be used in preference to a trial of Met alone. This approach may not take into account potential long-term benefits in reducing the sensitivity of the PCO to stimulation.

It is important to note that almost all OS studies in PCOS women have been based on

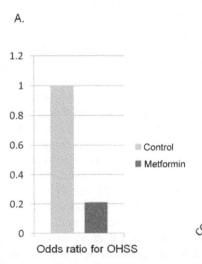

A.

Odds ratio for OHSS

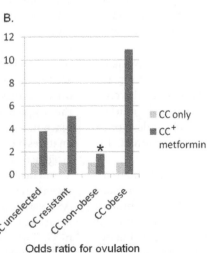

B.

Odds ratio for ovulation

Figure 20.2 A. OHSS was highly significantly decreased by almost 80% in women with PCOS having OS for IVF [18]. B. In women with PCOS having ovulation induction, the odds ratio for ovulation was 10.9 with Met versus placebo in obese women, but was not significantly improved (*) in women who were not obese. The favorable effect of Met was somewhat greater in CC-resistant PCOS [20].

a clinical diagnosis and not on the presence of decreased insulin sensitivity, with the exception of studies done in CC-resistant women, who are more often insulin resistant. Although the clinical criteria for the diagnosis of PCOS have varied in these studies, tests of insulin sensitivity are not required for the decision of whether to use Met as an adjunct to OS.

Mini-Dose Human Chorionic Gonadotropin

With some specific regimens for OS, use of FSH alone results in low levels of endogenous LH. This appears to be clearly the case when OC pretreatment is used for GnRH antagonist cycles, and results in a subset of patients with increased biochemical pregnancy loss [27]. In OC/antagonist cycles in egg donation recipients, recombinant LH reduced the rate of very early pregnancy loss and also increased implantation, showing that the impact of these very low LH levels was on the oocytes rather than on the endometrium [28]. In contrast to OC/antagonist cycles, there is no indication that supplementary LH activity is helpful when a GnRH antagonist is used without OC pretreatment, and there are indications that it may be detrimental. In a dose-finding study using ganirelix, when the dose of ganirelix was reduced below the optimum level, LH levels rose and the implantation rate fell [29]. In antagonist cycles not pretreated by OC, it has been published that very low LH levels benefited the pregnancy rate [30]. That study did show the benefit of lower LH levels, which is most likely also one reason why GnRH agonists improve implantation, but the numbers were too limited to make any statistically valid conclusion that very low levels were helpful and not detrimental.

Low levels of LH have also been associated with lower outcomes and increased early pregnancy loss with some potent GnRH agonist regimens [31]. It does appear that with marked agonist suppression, which would include agonist cycles overlapping with OC, supplementing LH is helpful.

With OS regimens in which supplementary LH improves pregnancy outcomes, the primary method has been to simply substitute human menopausal gonadotropin (hMG) for some of the pure FSH being used. However, the LH activity of hMG varies among suppliers and among batches of hMG. The most consistent way to supply this LH activity is to use very small doses of hCG, particularly because the major contributor to LH activity in hMG is the approximately 10 units of hCG contained in each 75 IU vial. This does require these small doses to be in a reasonable volume of diluent so that the amount delivered with injection is accurate. We have shown that a single dose of 50 IU of hCG raised the level of bioactive LH/hCG to normal in the mid to late follicular phase in women suppressed with a potent GnRH antagonist [32]. We suggested, based on the long half-life of hCG, that 20–30 units per day would replenish LH activity when exogenous LH is very low. Doses of 10–20 IU of hCG have been very successfully used in OC/antagonist cycles. A dose of 50 IU of hCG has been used successfully in a patient with hypogonadotropic hypogonadism treated with pure FSH.

Low-Dose Aspirin

Low-dose aspirin (ASA) was initially reported to improve ovarian and uterine blood flow and increase the pregnancy rate from IVF in a large, well-designed trial using 100 mg daily starting with midluteal agonist and continuing uninterrupted into early pregnancy [33]. ASA increases blood flow by increasing the amount of vasodilating prostacycline relative to thromboxane. Because stress has been associated with reduced IVF outcomes [34], it was hypothesized that the benefit of ASA was to counter the effect of stress in reducing pelvic blood flow. Thus, it may be necessary to begin ASA well before OS is begun and to continue it without interruption until oocyte retrieval to have a maximal effect on ovarian blood flow, ovarian response, and health of the oocyte, and the period between hCG and retrieval may be particularly important when chromosome segregation is taking place. Unfortunately, subsequent studies did not reproduce the parameters of the original study, including the fact that it took place in a busy and stressful environment. Meta-analyses have been published collating highly heterogeneous study designs, all resulting in a conclusion that ASA is of no benefit, the most recent one published in 2016 [35]. In two trials the ASA was begun on the day that OS was begun, and in another trial the ASA was stopped at the time of hCG. Two studies were in frozen embryo cycles and one was in oocyte donation recipients where an effect on ovarian response and oocyte quality would not be seen. One trial was in poor responders and one was in women refractory to usual doses of estrogen. The patient populations varied from a small town in Scandinavia to environments closer to that of the original trial. In a 2010 Hungarian RCT including 2425 IVF cycles using a GnRH agonist protocol, ASA resulted in a highly significant reduction of the incidence of severe OHSS, which would itself be a sufficient reason to continue use of this simple adjunct [36]. In addition, ASA may reduce the chance of a thromboembolic episode. A possible concern has been whether its use could increase the chance of bleeding following oocyte retrieval, but there have been no indications of such an effect.

Growth Hormone

Growth hormone (GH) and its intermediary insulin-like growth factor 1 (IGF-1) are extremely well characterized in promoting the health and proliferation of granulosa cells (GCs), which are in turn critical to the nourishment and health of the oocyte [37]. In a meta-analysis of RCTs in poor responders, adjunctive use of GH was found to be associated with three and fourfold increases of pregnancy and birth rates, although there was no impact on ovarian response, which was the original intent of those trials. The authors proposed that further evaluation of this potential benefit should be carried out [38]. Subsequently, a RCT was done in poor responders over age 40 and very similar results were obtained,

with four and fivefold increases of pregnancy and delivery with GH (Figure 20.3) [39]. Follicular fluid and circulating estradiol levels were significantly higher, consistent with improved proliferation of GCs. There was a significant increase of GH levels in follicular fluid. There was also a trend toward improved embryo quality (Figure 20.3). The GH was given at the dose of 8 IU daily from day 7 of stimulation until oocyte retrieval. This latter trial was done in a very poor-prognosis group of women having a mean age of 42 and three failed cycles. The peak estradiol level was 912 pg/ml in spite of stimulation with 600 IU of gonadotropins daily. The delivery rate of 22 percent in the treatment group was extremely good for such a difficult cohort of women. A meta-analysis from 2005 confirmed this benefit for poor responders, with an absolute difference of delivery rate of 17 percent [39]. That meta-analysis missed reference [40] in their search, but the absolute difference (22 – 4 = 18%) in that study was similar. A more recent systematic review and meta-analysis from 2017 on the influence of different GH addition protocols to poor ovarian responders demonstrated a lower canceled cycle rate, improvements in intermediate stimulation parameters, and increased clinical pregnancy rate and live birth rate in the GH group [41]. The exact treatment effect remains to be accurately defined; however, even a small increase of success for these couples would warrant the associated cost of the GH, a valuable adjunct to stimulation which is underutilized in poor responders [42].

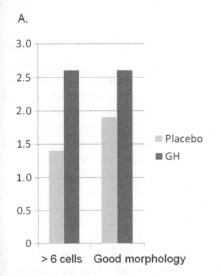

A.

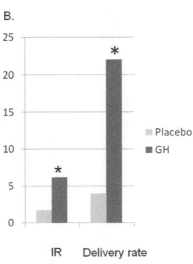

B.

Figure 20.3 A. Strong trends were observed for embryos with greater than six cells and with even cell division and minimal or no fragmentation with GH compared with placebo in poor-responding women over age 40. B. Significant increases of the implantation rate (IR) and delivery rate were also observed with GH (* $p < 0.05$) [39].

Dopamine Agonists

In an elegant RCT of oocyte donors at high risk for OHSS, cabergoline at the daily dose of 0.5 mg for eight days starting on the day of hCG was associated with less hemoconcentration, ascites (Figure 20.4), and increased vascular permeability compared with placebo [43]. The effect of follicular fluid from high responders on vascular permeability is almost completely abolished by an antibody to VEGF, showing that this GC product is sufficient to explain almost all of the vascular effects of OHSS [44]. Dopamine agonists like cabergoline decrease expression of the VEGF receptor and therefore the actions of VEGF. Dopamine itself is a highly effective treatment modality for established severe OHSS [45]. Concern over any adverse effect of cabergoline on implantation has been allayed by a pilot study in women having embryo transfer [46], and this agent is approved for women with hyperprolactinemia who are infertile and attempting conception. Side effects of headache, nausea, and dizziness can be generally avoided by administration at bedtime. The long-term effects of dopamine agonists on valvular heart disease occur at much higher doses and with more than six months of use. Considering the potential catastrophic complications of OHSS, the risk/benefit ratio of prophylactic use of cabergoline is very favorable. It should be started on the evening of hCG administration because GC VEGF production peaks at 48 hours following hCG.

Androgens and Androgenic Drugs

Testosterone (T) increases both antral follicles and GC proliferation and reduces GC apoptosis in subhuman primates [47], and androgen receptor

mRNA correlates positively with GC proliferation and negatively with GC apoptosis. This same dose of T has been shown to cause a marked increase of ovarian response in women who had a consistently poor response to repeated OS for IVF [48]. In a further randomized study this same group of investigators compared adjunctive T with a reduced agonist dose and an increased dose of gonadotropins. The days of stimulation, FSH dose, and percentage of poor responders were significantly decreased, but the mean number of oocytes increased only by 0.5, which was not significant. It was of considerable interest that the circulating levels of IGF-1 increased not only during the T therapy, but also during the 10 days of OS and in follicular fluid, and that the implantation rates following adjunctive T were also increased [48]. IGF-1 is presumed to be the intermediary of the GH effect on improving GC health and therefore on embryo implantation [38;39]. In those studies the T dose was the same as had produced a response in the monkey [47]. The dose per kilogram was adjusted by varying the number of hours per day the T patch was worn. The apparent benefit of adjunctive T remains to be shown by comparison with other poor-responder protocols.

In a 2011 Korean study, the effectiveness of transdermal testosterone gel (TTG) prior to controlled OS was studied in a cohort of 110 poor responders randomized to TTG or no pretreatment. Study participants in the TTG pretreatment group applied 12.5 mg TTG daily to both arms for 21 days, after a pilot study had determined that this was the minimum treatment length shown to be effective at this dose [49]. The total dose and days of FSH used were significantly fewer in the TTG pretreatment group than in the control group. The numbers of oocytes retrieved, mature oocytes, fertilized oocytes, and good-quality embryos were statistically significantly higher in the TTG pretreatment group. Embryo implantation rate (14.3% vs. 7.2%, $p = 0.019$) and clinical pregnancy rate (30.9% vs. 14.5%, $p = 0.041$) were also were significantly higher in the women pretreated with TTG, suggesting that TTG pretreatment can improve ovarian response to controlled ovarian stimulation and IVF outcome in low responders undergoing IVF/ICSI (intracytoplasmic sperm injection). In clinical practice, combination pretreatment of T patch and gel may be ideal, taking advantage of higher serum T levels during transdermal patch use, while maintaining

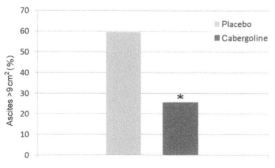

Figure 20.4 In high responders having OS for IVF, ascites > 9 cm^2 was observed significantly less often with cabergoline compared with placebo (* p < 0.005) [43].

the minimum T pretreatment duration needed to improve response.

Another approach used to increase local ovarian androgens more directly has been the use of letrozole. In a case–control study of poor responders given letrozole and gonadotropins following OC pretreatment, the mean number of oocytes was increased by two, and the embryo implantation rate was markedly increased from 9% to 25% ($p < 0.009$). In this study, T levels in follicular fluid were also increased, suggesting an action of letrozole throughout oocyte maturation and therefore a mechanism through which oocyte and embryo quality might be improved in addition to ovarian response [50]. Although not a RCT, this study's strength is that letrozole was the only difference in the OS protocol compared with control patients, whereas in other studies differences in OS protocols, such as the use or non-use of OC pretreatment, make firm conclusions difficult [51]. A 2014 meta-analysis of three trials including a total of 688 poor responders examined the efficacy of a GnRH antagonist/letrozole (A/L) protocol for OS compared with the GnRH agonist micro-dose flare (MF) protocol. The clinical pregnancy rate was significantly decreased in the A/L arm compared with the MF protocol (relative risk 0.70; 95% CI: 0.57–0.86; $p = 0.001$), possibly secondary to stimulation of intraovarian androgen production by GnRH agonist-induced LH secretion in the MF treatment group [52].

A third approach used to increase ovarian androgens and response in poor responders has been oral dehydroepiandrosterone (DHEA). Circulating DHEA levels decrease by about 50 percent between ages 25 and 45, and 50 percent of follicular fluid T is derived from circulating DHEA. Both serum T levels and number of oocytes retrieved decrease with age, and using multivariate analysis, baseline T levels independently correlate positively with the number of oocytes retrieved [53]. In a study using the patients' prior cycles as their own controls, a study design known to be influenced by regression to the mean, the number of oocytes increased significantly from 3.4 to 4.4 after an average of four months of 25 mg three times daily of oral DHEA [54]. A further case–control study by the same authors suggested that DHEA was associated with an increased chance of pregnancy with and without the use of IVF.

A fourth approach has been to increase LH activity during the week preceding OS using recombinant LH [55]. In that study a significant, though modest, increase in response was noted, with an increase in the number of embryos from normally fertilized oocytes, but the subjects were not poor responders.

Cumulatively these studies strongly suggest that increasing androgen concentrations around the resting follicles may increase ovarian response in poor responders. Also because the effect of androgens on the follicle is to reduce GC apoptosis and enhance GC proliferation, and because androgen increases IGF-1, an enhancer of GC health, androgens also have the potential of improving oocyte and embryo quality. The studies described have suggested that embryo implantation may be enhanced [50;54]. A Cochrane meta-analysis on the use of androgens in IVF based on available RCT evidence concluded that pretreatment with both T and DHEA was associated with increased live birth rates [56]. Use of more than one approach simultaneously is also an attractive possibility worthy of investigation.

Future Directions

Research into novel compounds to serve as adjuncts to stimulate ovarian function is ongoing. One area of investigation are compounds targeting the hypothalamic KISS1 system. Kisspeptins, a family of peptides encoded by the *Kiss1* gene, have been identified as upstream regulators of GnRH secretion. The use of kisspeptins holds promise for the treatment of reproductive disorders such as PCOS and idiopathic hypogonadotropic hypogonadism. In addition, kisspeptins could be used instead of hCG or GnRH agonists for ovulation induction.

Novel oral GnRH antagonists, developed for the treatment of endometriosis and uterine fibroids [57], could potentially be used instead of injectable GnRH antagonists as part of future OS.

In the future, advances in pharmacogenomics may assist providers in individualizing assisted reproductive technology protocols and the choice of adjunct medications based on unique patient characteristics, as potential genomic predictors of ovarian response are being identified.

Summary

Numerous adjuncts have been shown to be effective in enhancing outcomes in women having OS for IVF. Most of these adjuncts are medications approved for other uses but not specifically as adjuncts for OS. Because the risk/benefit ratio in their use is quite favorable, physicians should strongly consider incorporating them into IVF protocols.

References

1. Meldrum DR, Chang RJ, de Ziegler D, *et al*. Adjuncts for ovarian stimulation: when do we adopt "orphan indications" for approved drugs? *Fertil Steril* 2009;**92**:13–18.

2. Meldrum DR, Wisot A, Hamilton F, *et al*. Routine pituitary suppression with leuprolide before ovarian stimulation for oocyte retrieval. *Fertil Steril* 1989;**51**:455–459.

3. Hughes EG, Fedorkow DM, Daya S, *et al*. The routine use of gonadotropin-releasing hormone agonists prior to in vitro fertilization and gamete intrafallopian transfer: a meta-analysis of randomized controlled trials. *Fertil Steril* 1992;**58**:888–896.

4. Tarlatzis BC, Fauser BC, Kolibianakis EM, *et al*. GnRH antagonists in ovarian stimulation for IVF. *Hum Reprod Update* 2006;**12**:333–340.

5. Lambalk CB, Banga FR, Huirne JA, *et al*. GnRH antagonist versus long agonist protocols in IVF: a systematic review and meta-analysis accounting for patient type. *Hum Reprod Update* 2017;**23**:560–579.

6. Biljan MM, Mahutte NG, Dean N, *et al*. Effects of pretreatment with an oral contraceptive on the time required to achieve pituitary suppression with gonadotropin-releasing hormone analogues and on subsequent implantation and pregnancy rates. *Fertil Steril* 1998;**70**:1063–1069.

7. van Heusden AM, Fauser BC. Activity of the pituitary-ovarian axis in the pill-free interval during use of low-dose combined oral contraceptives. *Contraception* 1999;**59**:237–243.

8. de Ziegler D, Jaaskelainen AS, Brioschi PA, Fanchin R, Bulletti C. Synchronization of endogenous and exogenous FSH stimuli in controlled ovarian hyperstimulation (COH). *Hum Reprod* 1998;**13**:561–564.

9. Fanchin R, Salomon L, Castelo-Branco A, *et al*. Luteal estradiol pre-treatment coordinates follicular growth during controlled ovarian hyperstimulation with GnRH antagonists. *Hum Reprod* 2003;**18**:2698–2703.

10. Frattarelli JL, Hill MJ, McWilliams GD, *et al*. A luteal estradiol protocol for expected poor-responders improves embryo number and quality. *Fertil Steril* 2008;**89**:1118–1122.

11. Daly DC, Walters CA, Soto-Albors CE, Tohan N, Riddick DH. A randomized study of dexamethasone in ovulation induction with clomiphene citrate. *Fertil Steril* 1984;**41**:844–848.

12. Parsanezhad ME, Alborzi S, Motazedian S, Omrani G. Use of dexamethasone and clomiphene citrate in the treatment of clomiphene citrate-resistant patients with polycystic ovary syndrome and normal dehydroepiandrosterone sulfate levels: a prospective, double-blind, placebo-controlled trial. *Fertil Steril* 2002;**78**:1001–1004.

13. Elnashar A, Abdelmageed E, Fayed M, Sharaf M. Clomiphene citrate and dexamethazone in treatment of clomiphene citrate-resistant polycystic ovary syndrome: a prospective placebo-controlled study. *Hum Reprod* 2006;**21**:1805–1808.

14. Keay SD, Lenton EA, Cooke ID, Hull MG, Jenkins JM. Low-dose dexamethasone augments the ovarian response to exogenous gonadotrophins leading to a reduction in cycle cancellation rate in a standard IVF programme. *Hum Reprod* 2001;**16**:1861–1865.

15. Thurston LM, Norgate DP, Jonas KC, *et al*. Ovarian modulators of type 1 11beta-hydroxysteroid dehydrogenase (11betaHSD) activity and intra-follicular cortisol: cortisone ratios correlate with the clinical outcome of IVF. *Hum Reprod* 2003;**18**:1603–1612.

16. Lewicka S, von Hagens C, Hettinger U, *et al*. Cortisol and cortisone in human follicular fluid and serum and the outcome of IVF treatment. *Hum Reprod* 2003;**18**:1613–1617.

17. Simerman AA, Hill DL, Grogan TR, *et al*. Intrafollicular cortisol levels inversely correlate with cumulus cell lipid content as a possible energy source during oocyte meiotic resumption in women undergoing ovarian stimulation for in vitro fertilization. *Fertil Steril* 2015;**103**:249–257.

18. Palomba S, Falbo A, La Sala GB. Effects of metformin in women with polycystic ovary syndrome treated with gonadotrophins for in vitro fertilisation and intracytoplasmic sperm injection cycles: a systematic review and meta-analysis of randomised controlled trials. *BJOG* 2013;**120**:267–276.

19. Agrawal R, Jacobs H, Payne N, Conway G. Concentration of vascular endothelial growth factor released by cultured human luteinized

granulosa cells is higher in women with polycystic ovaries than in women with normal ovaries. *Fertil Steril* 2002;**78**:1164–1169.

20. Creanga AA, Bradley HM, McCormick C, Witkop CT. Use of metformin in polycystic ovary syndrome: a meta-analysis. *Obstet Gynecol* 2008;**111**:959–968.

21. Stadtmauer LA, Toma SK, Riehl RM, Talbert LM. Metformin treatment of patients with polycystic ovary syndrome undergoing in vitro fertilization improves outcomes and is associated with modulation of the insulin-like growth factors. *Fertil Steril* 2001;**75**:505–509.

22. Tang T, Glanville J, Orsi N, Barth JH, Balen AH. The use of metformin for women with PCOS undergoing IVF treatment. *Hum Reprod* 2006;**21**:1416–1425.

23. Jakubowicz DJ, Seppala M, Jakubowicz S, *et al.* Insulin reduction with metformin increases luteal phase serum glycodelin and insulin-like growth factor-binding protein 1 concentrations and enhances uterine vascularity and blood flow in the polycystic ovary syndrome. *J Clin Endocrinol Metab* 2001;**86**:1126–1133.

24. Cermik D, Selam B, Taylor HS. Regulation of HOXA-10 expression by testosterone in vitro and in the endometrium of patients with polycystic ovary syndrome. *J Clin Endocrinol Metab* 2003;**88**:238–243.

25. Jakubowicz DJ, Iuorno MJ, Jakubowicz S, Roberts KA, Nestler JE. Effects of metformin on early pregnancy loss in the polycystic ovary syndrome. *J Clin Endocrinol Metab* 2002;**87**:524–529.

26. De Leo V, la Marca A, Ditto A, Morgante G, Cianci A. Effects of metformin on gonadotropin-induced ovulation in women with polycystic ovary syndrome. *Fertil Steril* 1999;**72**:282–285.

27. Meldrum DR, Scott RT, Jr., Levy MJ, Alper MM, Noyes N. Oral contraceptive pretreatment in women undergoing controlled ovarian stimulation in ganirelix acetate cycles may, for a subset of patients, be associated with low serum luteinizing hormone levels, reduced ovarian response to gonadotropins, and early pregnancy loss. *Fertil Steril* 2009;**91**:1963–1965.

28. Acevedo B, Sanchez M, Gomez JL, *et al.* Luteinizing hormone supplementation increases pregnancy rates in gonadotropin-releasing hormone antagonist donor cycles. *Fertil Steril* 2004;**82**:343–347.

29. The ganirelix dose-finding group. A double-blind, randomized, dose-finding study to assess the efficacy of the gonadotrophin-releasing hormone antagonist ganirelix (Org 37462) to prevent premature luteinizing hormone surges in women undergoing ovarian stimulation with recombinant follicle stimulating hormone (Puregon). *Hum Reprod* 1998;**13**:3023–3031.

30. Kolibianakis EM, Zikopoulos K, Schiettecatte J, *et al.* Profound LH suppression after GnRH antagonist administration is associated with a significantly higher ongoing pregnancy rate in IVF. *Hum Reprod* 2004;**19**:24902496.

31. Coomarasamy A, Afnan M, Cheema D, *et al.* Urinary hMG versus recombinant FSH for controlled ovarian hyperstimulation following an agonist long down-regulation protocol in IVF or ICSI treatment: a systematic review and meta-analysis. *Hum Reprod* 2008;**23**:310–315.

32. Thompson KA, LaPolt PS, River J, *et al.* Gonadotropin requirements of the developing follicle. *Fertil Steril* 1995;**63**:273–276.

33. Rubinstein M, Marazzi A, Polak de Fried E. Low-dose aspirin treatment improves ovarian responsiveness, uterine and ovarian blood flow velocity, implantation, and pregnancy rates in patients undergoing in vitro fertilization: a prospective, randomized, double-blind placebo-controlled assay. *Fertil Steril* 1999;**71**:825–829.

34. Ebbesen SM, Zachariae R, Mehlsen MY, *et al.* Stressful life events are associated with a poor in-vitro fertilization (IVF) outcome: a prospective study. *Hum Reprod* 2009;**24**:2173–2182.

35. Siristatidis CS, Basios G, Pergialiotis V, Vogiatzi P. Aspirin for in vitro fertilisation. *Cochrane Database Syst Rev* 2016;**11**:CD004832.

36. Varnagy A, Bodis J, Manfai Z, et al. Low-dose aspirin therapy to prevent ovarian hyperstimulation syndrome. *Fertil Steril* 2010;**93**:2281–2284.

37. Bencomo E, Perez R, Arteaga MF, *et al.* Apoptosis of cultured granulosa-lutein cells is reduced by insulin-like growth factor I and may correlate with embryo fragmentation and pregnancy rate. *Fertil Steril* 2006;**85**:474–480.

38. Harper K, Proctor M, Hughes E. Growth hormone for in vitro fertilization. *Cochrane Database Syst Rev* 2003;**3**:CD000099.

39. Tesarik J, Hazout A, Mendoza C. Improvement of delivery and live birth rates after ICSI in women aged >40 years by ovarian co-stimulation with growth hormone. *Hum Reprod* 2005;**20**:2536–2541.

40. Kolibianakis EM, Venetis CA, Diedrich K, Tarlatzis BC, Griesinger G. Addition of growth hormone to gonadotrophins in ovarian stimulation of poor responders treated by in-vitro

fertilization: a systematic review and meta-analysis. *Hum Reprod Update* 2009;**15**:613–622.

41. Li XL, Wang L, Lv F, *et al.* The influence of different growth hormone addition protocols to poor ovarian responders on clinical outcomes in controlled ovary stimulation cycles: a systematic review and meta-analysis. *Medicine (Baltimore)* 2017;**96**:e6443.

42. Meldrum DR, Quaas AM, Su HI. Why is growth hormone underutilized for our most difficult IVF couples? *Fertil Steril* 2018;**110**:1261–1262.

43. Alvarez C, Marti-Bonmati L, Novella-Maestre E, *et al.* Dopamine agonist cabergoline reduces hemoconcentration and ascites in hyperstimulated women undergoing assisted reproduction. *J Clin Endocrinol Metab* 2007;**92**:2931–2937.

44. Levin ER, Rosen GF, Cassidenti DL, *et al.* Role of vascular endothelial cell growth factor in ovarian hyperstimulation syndrome. *J Clin Invest* 1998;**102**:1978–1985.

45. Ferraretti AP, Gianaroli L, Diotallevi L, Festi C, Trounson A. Dopamine treatment for severe ovarian hyperstimulation syndrome. *Hum Reprod* 1992;**7**:180–183.

46. Alvarez C, Alonso-Muriel I, Garcia G, *et al.* Implantation is apparently unaffected by the dopamine agonist cabergoline when administered to prevent ovarian hyperstimulation syndrome in women undergoing assisted reproduction treatment: a pilot study. *Hum Reprod* 2007;**22**:3210–3214.

47. Vendola KA, Zhou J, Adesanya OO, Weil SJ, Bondy CA. Androgens stimulate early stages of follicular growth in the primate ovary. *J Clin Invest* 1998;**101**:2622–2629.

48. Balasch J, Fabregues F, Penarrubia J, *et al.* Pretreatment with transdermal testosterone may improve ovarian response to gonadotrophins in poor-responder IVF patients with normal basal concentrations of FSH. *Hum Reprod* 2006;**21**:1884–1893.

49. Kim CH, Howles CM, Lee HA. The effect of transdermal testosterone gel pretreatment on controlled ovarian stimulation and IVF outcome in low responders. *Fertil Steril* 2011;**95**:679–683.

50. Garcia-Velasco JA, Moreno L, Pacheco A, *et al.* The aromatase inhibitor letrozole increases the concentration of intraovarian androgens and improves in vitro fertilization outcome in low responder patients: a pilot study. *Fertil Steril* 2005;**84**:82–87.

51. Schoolcraft WB, Surrey ES, Minjarez DA, Stevens JM, Gardner DK. Management of poor responders: can outcomes be improved with a novel gonadotropin-releasing hormone antagonist/letrozole protocol? *Fertil Steril* 2008;**89**:151–156.

52. Song Y, Li Z, Wu X, *et al.* Effectiveness of the antagonist/letrozole protocol for treating poor responders undergoing in vitro fertilization/intracytoplasmic sperm injection: a systematic review and meta-analysis. *Gynecol Endocrinol* 2014;**30**:330–334.

53. Frattarelli JL, Gerber MD. Basal and cycle androgen levels correlate with in vitro fertilization stimulation parameters but do not predict pregnancy outcome. *Fertil Steril* 2006;**86**:51–57.

54. Barad D, Gleicher N. Effect of dehydroepiandrosterone on oocyte and embryo yields, embryo grade and cell number in IVF. *Hum Reprod* 2006;**21**:2845–2849.

55. Barad D, Brill H, Gleicher N. Update on the use of dehydroepiandrosterone supplementation among women with diminished ovarian function. *J Assist Reprod Genet* 2007;**24**:629–634.

56. Nagels HE, Rishworth JR, Siristatidis CS, Kroon B. Androgens (dehydroepiandrosterone or testosterone) for women undergoing assisted reproduction. *Cochrane Database Syst Rev* 2015;**11**:CD009749.

57. Paulson RJ. At last, an orally active gonadotropin-releasing hormone antagonist. *Fertil Steril* 2019;**111**:30–31.

Luteinizing Hormone Supplementation during Ovarian Stimulation

Ioannis E. Messinis, Christina I. Messini, George Anifandis, and Alexandros Daponte

Introduction

Folliculogenesis in humans is a long process. It has become clear that there are two main time points in follicular development, the "initial recruitment" that takes place at the stage of primordial follicles and the "cyclic recruitment" at the stage of small antral follicles [1]. In humans, the initial recruitment is gonadotropin independent, while cyclic recruitment is entirely dependent on the action of both follicle-stimulating hormone (FSH) and luteinizing hormone (LH) [2]. Locally produced substances affect the action of gonadotrophins on follicle maturation. The balanced effect of FSH and LH in the normal menstrual cycle ensures the selection of a single follicle.

Physiology of Folliculogenesis

The Role of FSH and LH

During the luteal-follicular transition, the "intercycle rise" of FSH or "FSH window" is responsible for the recruitment of several follicles and the selection of a single dominant follicle [3]. The main action of FSH is the production of aromatase in the granulosa cells, while that of LH is the production of androgens in the theca cells. The two main androgens produced, androstenedione and testosterone, are converted by aromatase to estrone and estradiol respectively in the granulosa cells. The interaction between the theca and the granulosa cells in the presence of FSH and LH occurs in the context of the so-called "two-cell two-gonadotropin" theory (Figure 21.1). Of all the small antral follicles that are recruited, one, with the highest receptivity, will develop an estrogenic environment and will be selected for further maturation [3]. The increased amount of estradiol and inhibin B released in the circulation

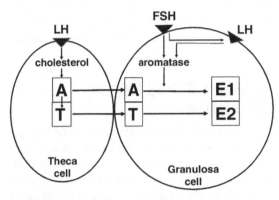

Figure 21.1 Two-cell two-gonadotropin theory. LH acts on the theca cells for the production of androgens, while FSH acts on the granulosa cells to stimulate the production of aromatase. This enzyme converts the androgens to estrogen in the granulosa cells. LH receptors appear on the granulosa cells for the first time in the dominant follicle after selection. A = androstenedione; T = testosterone; E1 = estrone; E2 = estradiol.

from the selected follicle suppresses FSH levels via the negative feedback mechanism and the intercycle rise of FSH is terminated. The closure, in this way, of the FSH window does not allow other follicles to be selected [4]. The selected dominant follicle is able to grow further to the preovulatory stage despite the declining concentrations of FSH, as it becomes gradually sensitive to LH due to the appearance of LH receptors in the granulosa cells [5]. From the midfollicular phase, LH takes over by increasing the expression of aromatase and stimulating proliferation of the granulosa cells. This action of LH is beyond its action in the theca cells where it stimulates the production of androgens. It is evident that for normal follicle maturation the two gonadotropins act synergistically, with FSH playing the key role in the first and LH in the second half of the follicular phase.

The Role of Local Regulators

Many local factors produced inside the ovaries can modify the action of gonadotropins and facilitate folliculogenesis [6]. Key roles are played by the system of inhibin and activin, the insulin-like growth factors and their binding proteins, androgens in low amounts and estrogen. Additionally, anti-Müllerian hormone produced by preantral and small antral follicles, by inhibiting the action of FSH on follicle maturation, is an important local regulator of folliculogenesis [7]. Finally, factors produced by the oocyte contribute to follicle maturation. Such factors include growth differentiation factor-9 and bone morphogenetic protein-15 [8].

LH Levels during Ovarian Stimulation

Ovarian stimulation is achieved by widening the FSH window with the exogenous administration of this hormone or following its hypersecretion from the pituitary during the administration of specific drugs, such as clomiphene (clomifene) citrate or letrozole. The widening of the FSH window leads to the rescue of many follicles, which otherwise would become atretic. Multiple follicular development affects endogenous hormone secretion and predisposes to the risk of ovarian hyperstimulation syndrome (OHSS). In cycles superovulated with FSH alone, there is a rapid increase in serum estradiol concentrations, which suppresses the secretion of LH and FSH from the pituitary and reduces markedly serum LH concentrations (Figure 21.2) [9;10]. The suppression is due to the potentiation of the ovarian negative feedback mechanism by the supraphysiological concentrations of estradiol and inhibin (Figure 21.3). On the other hand, the positive feedback mechanism is markedly attenuated due to overproduction of gonadotropin surge-attenuating factor from the ovaries (Figure 21.3) [11]. This may either block or markedly attenuate the endogenous LH surge. An attenuated LH surge can be premature in many cases, as the estradiol threshold for the positive feedback is exceeded early in the cycle, that is, before full follicle maturation to the preovulatory stage is achieved [10].

However, LH secretion is not suppressed in all treated cycles. For example, when clomiphene is included in the treatment regimen, LH levels

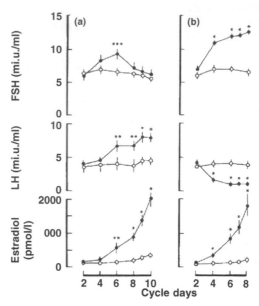

Figure 21.2 Serum concentrations of FSH, LH, and estradiol during the follicular phase of treated cycles (closed circles) with (a) clomiphene and (b) FSH in nine normally ovulating women. Comparison with untreated spontaneous cycles of the same women (open circles). Values are mean ± SEM for nine women in (a) and eight in (b) except for day 8 in the FSH cycles for which the number = 5. ***$p < 0.005$, **$p < 0.001$, *$p < 0.0001$ (compared to corresponding spontaneous cycles). Adapted from Messinis and Templeton (1989) [9] and reproduced with permission of the authors.

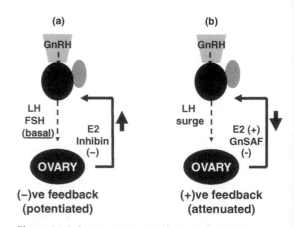

Figure 21.3 During ovarian stimulation with FSH, (a): secretion of LH from the pituitary is markedly suppressed, while during treatment with clomiphene citrate LH levels increase significantly due to overproduction of estradiol from the ovaries (potentiated negative feedback), (b): secretion of LH during the endogenous LH surge is markedly reduced due to an increase in the activity of gonadotropin surge-attenuating factor (GnSAF) (attenuated positive feedback).

increase (Figure 21.2) [9]. This is due to the fact that clomiphene, as an antiestrogen, blocks the negative feedback mechanism. Additionally, in the short gonadotropin-releasing hormone (GnRH) agonist protocol, due to the flare-up effect, LH levels fluctuate around the baseline level [12]. Therefore, in the current clinical practice, serum LH is expected to be markedly suppressed in three types of protocols, first when exogenous FSH is injected alone, that is, without a GnRH analogue, second when the long GnRH agonist protocol is used, and third in GnRH antagonist cycles. Especially, in the long agonist protocol, LH levels become very low before the onset of FSH administration, as a result of the pituitary downregulation [13]. On the other hand, in an antagonist protocol, LH is decreased, but this happens before starting the administration of the antagonist, that is, before day 7 of the cycle, due to the early increase in serum estradiol levels, while there is no further reduction in LH levels during treatment with the antagonist [14].

So far, there is no consensus on the LH level below which follicle maturation can be affected in superovulated cycles. It has been shown that LH levels below a threshold of 0.5 IU/L are associated with an adverse clinical outcome [15], although residual LH may be adequate for normal folliculogenesis and oocyte maturation [16]. There is no doubt that during ovarian stimulation, FSH, given exogenously, is the driving force throughout the whole follicular phase, while LH is needed mainly for steroidogenesis. However, the minimum LH value for optimal follicle maturation in such cycles still remains to be found.

Supplementation with Exogenous LH

Many studies have investigated the impact of supplementation of FSH treatment with exogenous LH during ovarian stimulation. It is likely that with milder ovarian stimulation, the decrease in LH is expected to be lower and therefore the need for LH supplementation is minimized. Alternatively, by reducing the dose of the GnRH agonist in a long protocol, LH might be suppressed less. Nevertheless, mild ovarian stimulation is not widely used, while in the long protocol, markedly lowered LH is an indication of attained pituitary downregulation and a prerequisite for initiating stimulation with FSH, while usually a fixed dose of the agonist is used. Furthermore, the tendency nowadays is to hyperstimulate the ovaries in order to obtain many oocytes that will create several embryos for cryopreservation and multiple embryo transfers in future cycles. Therefore, with the currently used protocols, endogenous LH is expected to decrease in most cases leading to the need to add exogenous hormone. Exogenous LH can be administered in the form of a recombinant preparation containing only LH activity. However, urinary products containing LH activity are also available. LH activity is also contained in human chorionic gonadotropin (hCG) preparations. In clinical practice, there is no clinical guideline that ovarian stimulation should begin with one or the other preparation, that is, with or without LH activity. Additionally, clinical studies have not shown differences in the outcome between protocols involving recombinant or urinary gonadotropins [17;18]. There are three main categories of patients where supplementation with LH has been attempted, that is, unselected population, poor ovarian responders and patients with hypogonadotropic hypogonadism, with equivocal results in most of them.

Unselected Population

Unselected or general population in infertility refers to all individuals without explicit selection criteria undergoing specific treatment, such as ovarian stimulation for in vitro fertilization (IVF). Many studies have tried to identify a beneficial effect of LH supplementation. One double-blind randomized controlled trial (RCT) using recombinant FSH (rFSH) has demonstrated no differences in pregnancy, miscarriage, and live birth rates when recombinant LH (rLH) was added from the time the follicle became 14 mm in diameter in a long GnRH agonist protocol [19]. A subsequent RCT, using a long GnRH agonist protocol with rLH from the midfollicular phase, has demonstrated no significant increase in the ongoing live gestation at 10–12 weeks, although in women older than 35 years there was a tendency for a significant difference [20]. Similarly, in an age-matched case–control study using a long GnRH agonist protocol with rLH initiated at the beginning of the stimulation with rFSH, although the number of retrieved oocytes, and fertilization and implantation rates were increased, there was no difference in pregnancy and live birth rates

[21]. Nevertheless, systematic reviews and meta-analyses have provided evidence that the addition of LH to FSH or the use of a urinary preparation containing LH activity does not have any advantage irrespective of the use of an agonist or an antagonist in the treatment protocol [22;23]. It should be noted that there are not many studies looking at live birth rate. In the most recent meta-analysis [24], live birth rate was reported in only four studies with no significant difference between rFSH and its combination with rLH (odds ratio [OR] 1.32, 95% confidence interval [CI] 0.85–2.06), but there was a very low quality of evidence. In the same study, there was no difference between the two treatments regarding the occurrence of OHSS (6 studies) or miscarriage rate (13 studies). Studies have also been conducted to investigate whether LH activity, contained in the form of a urinary FSH preparation, might improve the clinical outcome in unselected population compared with rFSH. A comparison between rFSH and human menopausal gonadotropin (hMG) performed in the context of a meta-analysis of studies published from 2002 to 2007 has shown that with high purity (HP) hMG, the ongoing pregnancy/live birth rate was significantly higher in the hMG arm than the rFSH in IVF (OR 1.31, 95% CI 1.02–1.60) but not in intracytoplasmic sperm injection cycles [23]. A subsequent Cochrane systematic review showed no significant differences in live birth rate between rFSH and all urinary FSH preparations,

that is, hMG, P-FSH, and HP-FSH [18]. It is known that hCG has biological activity of LH. Whether supplementation with low doses of hCG during ovarian stimulation with rFSH may provide extra benefit is not known. In a well-designed but small RCT, no improvement in clinical pregnancy and live birth rates was found when daily doses of hCG from 50 to 150 IU were added to rFSH from the beginning of the ovarian stimulation [25]. In the same study, there was no difference in the total dose of FSH and in the number of oocytes retrieved. It is interesting to note that there seems to be no difference in the endocrinological and follicular profiles between rFSH and urinary preparations, as on the day of triggering with hCG similar serum estradiol concentrations and number of follicles of different diameter categories have been reported [26]. Regarding the luteal phase of superovulated cycles, endogenous LH secretion is markedly suppressed by the high levels of ovarian steroids [27]. Nevertheless, due to its short half-life, in such cases exogenous LH is not used, but either GnRH agonists to stimulate endogenous LH secretion or various commercially available progesterone preparations are preferred [28;29]. By inference, from the existing data, it becomes evident that supplementation with exogenous LH during ovarian stimulation is not justified in unselected population, although the evidence to encourage or discourage this process is of low to very low quality (Table 21.1).

Table 21.1 Main studies on LH supplementation during ovarian stimulation in unselected population

Author	Study	Results
Tarlatzis et al., 2006 [19]	Prospective RCT (rLH in late stimulation phase) – GnRH long agonist	No difference in clinical outcome
Kolibianakis et al., 2007 [22]	Systematic review and meta-analysis	No difference in live birth rate
Mochtar et al., 2007 [30]	Cochrane database systematic review	No difference in clinical and ongoing pregnancy rates
NyboeAndersen et al., 2008 [20]	Prospective RCT, multicenter (LH from midfollicular phase) – GnRH long agonist	No difference in ongoing live gestation 10–12 weeks
Franco et al., 2009 [21]	Matched case–control study (LH from the beginning of stimulation) – GnRH long agonist	No difference in clinical outcome – more oocytes and embryos and higher implantation rate
van Wely et al., 2011 [18]	Cochrane database systematic review (rFSH vs. urinary hMG, P-FSH, HP-FSH)	No difference in live birth rate or OHSS
Mochtar et al., 2017 [24]	Cochrane database systematic review	No difference in live birth rate, OHSS, and miscarriage rate

RCT = randomized controlled trial; P = purified; HP = highly purified; OHSS = ovarian hyperstimulation syndrome.

Poor Ovarian Responders

Poor ovarian responders are a difficult group of infertile women with regard to ovarian stimulation for IVF as their ovaries will eventually provide a small number of oocytes per cycle. Supplementation with exogenous LH has been attempted in an effort to increase androgen drive and enhance the number of maturing follicles. Evidence was first provided by a Cochrane systematic review that the pooled pregnancy estimates of trials including women with poor ovarian response showed a significant increase when rLH was added to FSH [30]. Subsequent RCTs have shown conflicting results. When the age was taken into account as the main denominator, it was shown that in women 35 years and above in a long GnRH agonist protocol live birth rate was marginally increased after the addition of LH [31]. This, however, was not confirmed in two subsequent RCTs using GnRH antagonists. In the first of them, which included women 36–39 years old, only the implantation rate increased significantly [32], while in the second including women 35 years and above no difference was seen between the two groups, despite that serum LH levels on the day of hCG were significantly higher in the rLH group [33]. A concurrent meta-analysis of seven RCTs demonstrated a significant increase in implantation and clinical pregnancy rates in the combination group, but live birth rate was not reported [34]. Nevertheless, a more recent meta-analysis has confirmed that the addition of rLH to rFSH increased the clinical pregnancy and ongoing pregnancy rates, but not the live birth rate [35]. The debate on supplementation with LH continued in the most recent RCT using a long GnRH agonist protocol and including the high number of 477 women in the rFSH plus rLH group and 462 women in the rFSH group [36]. That study has shown no differences in clinical and ongoing pregnancy rates or in live birth rate between the two groups, but in the combination group the total pregnancy outcome failure was significantly lower. Regarding the time of onset of supplementation with LH, it has been shown that there is no difference in ongoing/delivered pregnancies between an early start (day 1) and a late start (day 7) of the stimulation [37]. It becomes clear from the above discussion that regarding the use of rLH as a supplement to FSH for ovarian stimulation in women with poor ovarian response there are variable results. Overall, there seems to be some benefit in terms of implantation and pregnancy rates, but there is no ultimate benefit translated into live birth rate. On the other hand, during ovarian stimulation any gonadotropin, urinary or recombinant, that is, with or without LH activity, can be used from the beginning of stimulation. However, regarding supplementation of FSH with LH in poor ovarian responders further research is needed (Table 21.2).

Hypogonadotropic Hypogonadism

This condition is characterized by extremely low circulating concentrations of LH and FSH as a result of minimal or no secretion of these two gonadotropins from the pituitary. The classical way of treating these patients seeking pregnancy without any other infertility causes is ovulation induction with the use of both FSH and LH, usually in the form of an hMG preparation from the beginning of the treatment [38]. The starting dose is usually 150 IU of FSH and LH, although with the recombinant preparations 75 IU of LH is considered sufficient. The administration of hCG for triggering final follicle maturation is necessary, as the positive feedback cannot be activated in such patients due to the lack of pituitary gonadotropin reserves. It is also important to note that the luteal phase should be supported with estradiol and progesterone and possibly with small dosages of hCG [38]. In case there are also other causes of infertility, such as tubal or male factor, which indicate the need for IVF treatment, a much higher starting dose of hMG or rFSH/rLH should be given for ovarian stimulation than for ovulation induction [39;40].

LH Instead of FSH

The administration of LH is unable to initiate follicle growth in women without the co-administration of FSH. Priming of women with rLH for a whole week before starting ovarian stimulation with FSH has been attempted with the expectation to increase androgen production from the theca cells [41]. Nevertheless, this approach has provided no clinical benefit following IVF treatment. In contrast, following the selection of a single follicle under the exogenous

Table 21.2 Main studies on LH supplementation during ovarian stimulation in poor-responder women

Author	Study	Results
Mochtar et al., 2007 [30]	Cochrane database systematic review	Higher pregnancy rate
Matorras et al., 2009 [31]	Single-center, randomized, parallel group, comparative study (women 35–39 years) – LH from cycle day 6 – GnRH long agonist	Higher implantation and live birth rates (intention to treat analysis)
Bosch et al., 2011 [32]	RCT (rLH from stimulation day 1) – GnRH antagonist	Higher implantation rate in women 36–39 years
Revelli et al., 2012 [37]	Prospective RCT – GnRH long agonist (poor responders) – rLH from stimulation day 1 vs. from day 7	No difference in clinical outcome
Hill et al., 2012 [34]	Systematic review and meta-analysis (women ≥ 35 years)	Higher implantation and clinical pregnancy rates
König et al., 2013 [33]	Multicenter RCT (women ≥ 35 years) – GnRH antagonist – rLH from stimulation day 6	No difference in implantation, clinical pregnancy, and ongoing pregnancy rates
Lehert et al., 2014 [35]	Systematic review and meta-analysis (poor responders)	Higher clinical and ongoing pregnancy rates, but not live birth rate
Humaidan et al., 2017 [36]	RCT (poor responders) – GnRH long agonist	Lower rate of total pregnancy outcome failure

RCT = randomized controlled trial.

administration of FSH, follicle growth can be maintained with the administration of LH alone in a way similar to the FSH alone [42]. In clinical practice, treatment always starts with FSH with or without the administration of LH.

LH Ceiling Effect

In the normal gonadotropin profile, during the normal menstrual cycle, there is a trend for gradually increasing levels of LH from the early follicular phase until the midcycle LH surge, while FSH levels decline. It seems, however, that for optimal follicle development in the second half of the follicular phase there is a threshold level of LH, above which follicle atresia will happen. In vitro experiments have demonstrated that low doses of LH can stimulate steroidogenesis with no effect on DNA synthesis, while high doses can increase the production of progesterone, suppress aromatase activity, and inhibit cell growth [43]. It is likely that, as each follicle has a specific FSH threshold for initiation of growth during cyclic recruitment, it also has an LH threshold and if that is exceeded follicle growth ceases. Clinical studies have provided evidence for a "ceiling

effect" in humans. Especially, experiments have been performed in women having very low or normal LH and FSH levels with the exogenous administration of these two gonadotropins [44]. Compared with conventional doses of LH, higher dosages can reduce the number of dominant follicles that would become preovulatory. From a practical point of view, this might be important, as with the use of different dosages of exogenous LH, an optimal number of more synchronized follicles for IVF or monofollicular development in ovulation induction protocols can be achieved [45]. Existing evidence, however, is still preliminary and as a result there are not any specific guidelines or clinical recommendations for use.

Conclusions

It is evident that pituitary secretion of LH during ovarian stimulation for IVF can be markedly suppressed. However, apart from women with hypogonadotropic hypogonadism, it is still unclear if supplementation with exogenous LH can improve the clinical outcome following IVF treatment (Table 21.3). Further research is required particularly in women with poor ovarian response.

Table 21.3 Supplementation with exogenous LH during ovarian stimulation with FSH

Category	LH supplementation	Comments
Unselected population	Possibly not needed	Very low-quality evidence (live birth rate, ongoing pregnancy, OHSS) – based on Mochtar et al., 2017 [24]
Poor ovarian responders	Possibly needed (still debatable)	Lower total pregnancy outcome failure – based on Humaidan et al., 2017 [36]
Hypogonadotropic hypogonadism	Definitely needed	Without LH during stimulation with FSH serum estradiol levels remain very low
Experimental	Ceiling effect	May be helpful for monofollicular development in ovulation induction programs or for better synchronization of follicle maturation in controlled ovarian hyperstimulation

OHSS = ovarian hyperstimulation syndrome.

References

1. Gougeon A. Dynamics of follicular growth in the human: a model from preliminary results. *Hum Reprod* 1986;**1**:81–87.

2. Messinis IE, Messini CI, Dafopoulos K. The role of gonadotropins in the follicular phase. *Ann N Y Acad Sci* 2010;**1205**:5–11.

3. Messinis IE. Mechanisms of follicular development: the role of gonadotrophins. In: Rizk B, Garcia-Velasco J, Sallam H, Makrigiannakis A., eds. *Infertility and Assisted Reproduction.* Cambridge: Cambridge University Press; 2008:3–24.

4. van Santbrink EJ, Hop WC, van Dessel TJ, de Jong FH, Fauser BC. Decremental follicle-stimulating hormone and dominant follicle development during the normal menstrual cycle. *Fertil Steril* 1995;**64**:37–43.

5. Mihm M, Baker PJ, Ireland JL, et al. Molecular evidence that growth of dominant follicles involves a reduction in follicle-stimulating hormone dependence and an increase in luteinizing hormone dependence in cattle. *Biol Reprod* 2006;**74**:1051–1059.

6. Hillier SG. Gonadotropic control of ovarian follicular growth and development. *Mol Cell Endocrinol* 2001;**179**:39–46.

7. Garg D, Tal R. The role of AMH in the pathophysiology of polycystic ovarian syndrome. *Reprod Biomed Online* 2016;**33**:15–28.

8. Erickson GF, Shimasaki S. The role of the oocyte in folliculogenesis. *Trends Endocrinol Metab* 2000;**11**:193–198.

9. Messinis IE, Templeton AA. Pituitary response to exogenous LHRH in superovulated women. *J Reprod Fertil* 1989;**87**:633–639.

10. Messinis IE, Milingos S, Zikopoulos K, et al. Luteinizing hormone response to gonadotrophin-releasing hormone in normal women undergoing ovulation induction with urinary or recombinant follicle stimulating hormone. *Hum Reprod* 1998;**13**:2415–2420.

11. Messinis IE, Messini CI, Anifandis G, Garas A, Daponte A. Gonadotropin surge-attenuating factor: a nonsteroidal ovarian hormone controlling GnRH-induced LH secretion in the normal menstrual cycle. *Vitam Horm* 2018;**107**:263–286.

12. Cedrin-Durnerin I, Bidart JM, Robert P, et al. Consequences on gonadotrophin secretion of an early discontinuation of gonadotrophin-releasing hormone agonist administration in short-term protocol for in-vitro fertilization. *Hum Reprod* 2000;**15**:1009–1014.

13. Borm G, Mannaerts B. Treatment with the gonadotrophin-releasing hormone antagonist ganirelix in women undergoing ovarian stimulation with recombinant follicle stimulating hormone is effective, safe and convenient: results of a controlled, randomized, multicentre trial. The European Orgalutran Study Group. *Hum Reprod* 2000;**15**:1490–1498.

14. Felberbaum RE, Albano C, Ludwig M, et al. Ovarian stimulation for assisted reproduction with HMG and concomitant midcycle administration of the GnRH antagonist cetrorelix according to the multiple dose protocol: a prospective uncontrolled phase III study. *Hum Reprod* 2000;**15**:1015–1020.

15. Propst AM, Hill MJ, Bates GW, et al. Low-dose human chorionic gonadotropin may improve in vitro fertilization cycle outcomes in patients with low luteinizing hormone levels after

gonadotropin-releasing hormone antagonist administration. *Fertil Steril* 2011;**96**:898–904.

16. Fleming R, Lloyd F, Herbert M, *et al*. Effects of profound suppression of luteinizing hormone during ovarian stimulation on follicular activity, oocyte and embryo function in cycles stimulated with purified follicle stimulating hormone. *Hum Reprod* 1998;**13**:1788–1792.

17. Bosch E, Vidal C, Labarta E, *et al*. Highly purified hMG versus recombinant FSH in ovarian hyperstimulation with GnRH antagonists: a randomized study. *Hum Reprod* 2008;**23**:2346–2351.

18. van Wely M, Kwan I, Burt AL, *et al*. Recombinant versus urinary gonadotrophin for ovarian stimulation in assisted reproductive technology cycles. *Cochrane Database Syst Rev* 2011;**2**: CD005354.

19. Tarlatzis B, Tavmergen E, Szamatowicz M, *et al*. The use of recombinant human LH (lutropin alfa) in the late stimulation phase of assisted reproduction cycles: a double-blind, randomized, prospective study. *Hum Reprod* 2006;**21**:90–94.

20. NyboeAndersen A, Humaidan P, Fried G, *et al*.; Nordic LH study group. Recombinant LH supplementation to recombinant FSH during the final days of controlled ovarian stimulation for in vitro fertilization. A multicentre, prospective, randomized, controlled trial. *Hum Reprod* 2008;**23**:427–434.

21. Franco JG Jr., Baruffi RL, Oliveira JB, *et al*. Effects of recombinant LH supplementation to recombinant FSH during induced ovarian stimulation in the GnRH-agonist protocol: a matched case-control study. *Reprod Biol Endocrinol* 2009;**7**:58.

22. Kolibianakis EM, Kalogeropoulou L, Griesinger G, *et al*. Among patients treated with FSH and GnRH analogues for in vitro fertilization, is the addition of recombinant LH associated with the probability of live birth? A systematic review and meta-analysis. *Hum Reprod Update* 2007;**13**:445–452.

23. Al-Inany HG, Abou-Setta AM, Aboulghar MA, Mansour RT, Serour GI. Highly purified hMG achieves better pregnancy rates in IVF cycles but not ICSI cycles compared with recombinant FSH: a meta-analysis. *Gynecol Endocrinol* 2009;**25**:372–378.

24. Mochtar MH, Danhof NA, Ayeleke RO, Van der Veen F, van Wely M. Recombinant luteinizing hormone (rLH) and recombinant follicle stimulating hormone (rFSH) for ovarian stimulation in IVF/ICSI cycles. *Cochrane Database Syst Rev* 2017;**5**:CD005070.

25. Thuesen LL, Loft A, Egeberg AN, *et al*. A randomized controlled dose-response pilot study of addition of hCG to recombinant FSH during controlled ovarian stimulation for in vitro fertilization. *Hum Reprod* 2012;**27**:3074–3084.

26. Requena A, Cruz M, Ruiz FJ, García-Velasco JA. Endocrine profile following stimulation with recombinant follicle stimulating hormone and luteinizing hormone versus highly purified human menopausal gonadotropin. *Reprod Biol Endocrinol* 2014;**12**:10.

27. Messinis IE, Templeton AA. Disparate effects of endogenous and exogenous oestradiol on luteal phase function in women. *J Reprod Fertil* 1987;**79**:549–554.

28. Martins WP, Ferriani RA, Navarro PA, Nastri CO. GnRH agonist during luteal phase in women undergoing assisted reproductive techniques: systematic review and meta-analysis of randomized controlled trials. *Ultrasound Obstet Gynecol* 2016;**47**:144–151.

29. van der Linden M, Buckingham K, Farquhar C, Kremer JA, Metwally M. Luteal phase support for assisted reproduction cycles. *Cochrane Database Syst Rev* 2015;**7**:CD009154.

30. Mochtar MH, Van der Veen F, Ziech M, van Wely M. Recombinant luteinizing hormone (rLH) for controlled ovarian hyperstimulation in assisted reproductive cycles. *Cochrane Database Syst Rev* 2007;**2**:CD005070.

31. Matorras R, Prieto B, Exposito A, *et al*. Mid-follicular LH supplementation in women aged 35-39 years undergoing ICSI cycles: a randomized controlled study. *Reprod Biomed Online* 2009;**19**:879–887.

32. Bosch E, Labarta E, Crespo J, *et al*. Impact of luteinizing hormone administration on gonadotropin-releasing hormone antagonist cycles: an age-adjusted analysis. *Fertil Steril* 2011;**95**:1031–1036.

33. König TE, van der Houwen LE, Overbeek A, *et al*. Recombinant LH supplementation to a standard GnRH antagonist protocol in women of 35 years or older undergoing IVF/ICSI: a randomized controlled multicentre study. *Hum Reprod* 2013;**28**:2804–2812.

34. Hill MJ, Levens ED, Levy G, *et al*. The use of recombinant luteinizing hormone in patients undergoing assisted reproductive techniques with advanced reproductive age: a systematic review and meta-analysis. *Fertil Steril* 2012;**97**:1108.e1–1114.e1.

35. Lehert P, Kolibianakis EM, Venetis CA, *et al*. Recombinant human follicle-stimulating hormone (r-hFSH) plus recombinant luteinizing

hormone versus r-hFSH alone for ovarian stimulation during assisted reproductive technology: systematic review and meta-analysis. *Reprod Biol Endocrinol* 2014;**12**:17.

36. Humaidan P, Chin W, Rogoff D, *et al.*; ESPART Study Investigators. Efficacy and safety of follitropin alfa/lutropin alfa in ART: a randomized controlled trial in poor ovarian responders. *Hum Reprod* 2017;**32**:544–555.

37. Revelli A, Chiado' A, Guidetti D, *et al.* Outcome of in vitro fertilization in patients with proven poor ovarian responsiveness after early vs. mid-follicular LH exposure: a prospective, randomized, controlled study. *J Assist Reprod Genet* 2012;**29**:869–875.

38. Messinis IE, Bergh T, Wide L. The importance of human chorionic gonadotropin support of the corpus luteum during human gonadotropin therapy in women with anovulatory infertility. *Fertil Steril* 1988;**50**:31–35.

39. Lewit N, Kol S. The low responder female IVF patient with hypogonadotropic hypogonadism: do not give up! *Fertil Steril* 2000;**74**:401–402.

40. Pandurangi M, Tamizharasi M, Reddy NS. Pregnancy outcome of assisted reproductive technology cycle in patients with hypogonadotropic hypogonadism. *J Hum Reprod Sci* 2015;**8**:146–150.

41. Durnerin CI, Erb K, Fleming R, *et al.*; Luveris Pretreatment Group. Effects of recombinant LH treatment on folliculogenesis and responsiveness to FSH stimulation. *Hum Reprod* 2008;**23**:421–426.

42. Sullivan MW, Stewart-Akers A, Krasnow JS, Berga SL, Zeleznik AJ. Ovarian responses in women to recombinant follicle-stimulating hormone and luteinizing hormone (LH): a role for LH in the final stages of follicular maturation. *J Clin Endocrinol Metab* 1999;**84**:228–232.

43. Yong EL, Baird DT, Yates R, Reichert LE Jr., Hillier SG. Hormonal regulation of the growth and steroidogenic function of human granulosa cells. *J Clin Endocrinol Metab* 1992;**74**:842–849.

44. Loumaye E, Engrand P, Shoham Z, Hillier SG, Baird DT. Clinical evidence for an LH 'ceiling' effect induced by administration of recombinant human LH during the late follicular phase of stimulated cycles in World Health Organization type I and type II anovulation. *Hum Reprod* 2003;**18**:314–322.

45. Baird DT. Is there a place for different isoforms of FSH in clinical medicine? IV. The clinician's point of view. *Hum Reprod* 2001;**16**:1316–1318.

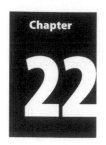

Chapter

22

Ovulation Induction for Hypogonadotropic Hypogonadism

Lina El-Taha, Botros Rizk, Chantal Farra, and Johnny Awwad

Introduction

Reproduction in humans is contingent upon the pulsatile secretion of gonadotropin-releasing hormone (GnRH) from the hypothalamus. This neuroendocrine activity results in the production and release of follicle-stimulating hormone (FSH) and luteinizing hormone (LH), and is essential therefore for proper steroidogenesis and gametogenesis within gonads.

Hypogonadotropic hypogonadism (HH) is a rare disorder of reproductive function characterized by failure of gonadal/ovarian function secondary to the absence of normal hypothalamic–pituitary synchronous activity. It represents a heterogeneous list of diseases (congenital, neoplastic, infiltrative, traumatic, or idiopathic) with the common hallmark of central gonadotropin deficiency (Table 22.1). Suboptimal FSH and LH production results in a hypoestrogenic state; arrested folliculogenesis; and consequently a symptom complex of anovulation, amenorrhea, and infertility despite preserved end-organ gonadal function and competence [1]. The origin of the disease may rest in either the pituitary gland disrupting the secretion of LH and FSH or, more commonly, in the hypothalamus interrupting the pulsatile release of GnRH critical for reproductive integrity [2]. The congenital form of HH is referred to as idiopathic, with Kallmann syndrome accounting for approximately 40–60 percent of all cases.

An interesting theory central to ovarian function is the two-cell two-gonadotropin hypothesis stressing their physiologically synergistic action in the reproductive cascade [2;3]. According to this theory, both FSH and LH are necessary for ovarian follicular maturation and the production of ovarian steroids. In addition to its role in recruiting and promoting follicular growth, FSH stimulates the granulosa cells to increase expression of the cytochrome P450 enzyme aromatase. LH increases ovarian granulosa cells' sensitivity to FSH and promotes the production of androgens from cholesterol and pregnenolone by stimulating 17-alpha hydroxylase activity in the thecal cells [4]. These androgens then diffuse to the granulosa cells, where they are converted to estrogens by the activity of the aromatase enzyme [5]. Adequate estrogen levels in the follicle are essential to facilitate FSH induction of LH receptors on the granulosa cells, allowing the follicle to respond to the ovulatory surge of LH levels. Thus, the LH surge is absolutely required for successful ovulation, oocyte maturation, fertilization, and implantation within the female reproductive tract [6;7]. Women with HH do not have the cyclic threshold level of gonadotropins (FSH and LH) necessary to accomplish optimal follicular development, and steroidogenesis necessary for a receptive endometrium. Essentially, ovulation induction is the treatment of choice to achieve fertility in these women irrespective of the etiology of the underlying hypogonadotropic hypogonadal dysfunction.

Ovulation Induction Protocols in Hypogonadotropic Hypogonadism

Background

Gonadotropin treatment for induction of ovulation in anovulatory women began in the 1960s [8] and is currently considered as one of the recommended therapies for ovulation induction in women with HH, also defined as type 1 amenorrhea according to the World Health Organization (WHO) Classification [9]. The three conditions included in WHO Group 1 anovulation include congenital hypogonadotropic hypogonadism (HH), hypothalamic amenorrhea (HA), and hypopituitarism (HP). Before treatment begins, various causes of infertility including other hormonal or structural abnormalities of the genitourinary tract of the couple should be excluded.

Table 22.1 Classification of hypogonadotropic hypogonadism caused by disorders of the hypothalamic–hypopituitary unit

Functional hypothalamic disorder

Stress (psychogenic or physical)

Nutrition-related (dieting, malnutrition)
Eating disorders (anorexia nervosa, bulimia)

Vigorous exercise

Chronic illness

Post-traumatic stress disorder
Chronic anabolic steroid use/glucocorticoid therapy

Congenital/genetic causes

Kallmann syndrome (mutation in the *KAL* [anosmin] gene), with hyposmia or anosmia or without anosmia

Leptin and leptin-receptor mutations

Congenital adrenal hypoplasia (mutation in the *DAX1* gene)

Mutations in the gene coding for the gonadotropin-releasing hormone (GnRH) receptor

Isolated luteinizing hormone (LH) deficiency

Isolated follicle-stimulating hormone (FSH) deficiency

Mutations in the *PROP*, *LHX3*, and *HESX1* genes
Prader–Willi syndrome, Laurence–Moon syndrome, Bardet–Biedl syndrome

Acquired/anatomical/vascular abnormalities

Craniopharyngioma

Germinoma, meningioma

Hypothalamic and optic glioma

Astrocytoma

Pituitary tumors

Infiltrative diseases: thesaurismosis (sarcoidosis, histiocytosis X, tuberculosis, lymphocytic hypophysitis, Gaucher disease)
Iron overload (transfusion-dependent thalassemia)

Postinfectious lesions of the CNS

Vascular abnormalities of the CNS

Radiation therapy

Endocrine disorders

Hypothyroidism, Cushing syndrome, hyperprolactinemia, polycystic ovary syndrome, congenital adrenal hyperplasia, multiple endocrine neoplasia

Miscellaneous

Idiopathic hypogonadotropic hypogonadism (IHH)

Adapted from Xekouki and Tolis [86].

A baseline transvaginal ultrasonography is prudent to exclude ovarian cysts that might be confused with new follicular growth, taking into consideration reports that some hypogonadotropic patients have an ovarian ultrasound appearance similar to that seen in patients with polycystic ovary syndrome (PCOS) [10;11]. Women with HH on hormone replacement therapy are expected to have a normal size uterus in contrast to infantile uterus with thin endometrial lining anticipated in the absence of estrogen and progesterone supplementation. Hysterosalpingography to evaluate the uterine cavity and the patency of the fallopian tubes, as well as a semen analysis to rule out an associated male factor, are also recommended to confirm the feasibility of natural conception.

The occurrence of regular sexual intercourse should be evaluated and advice on the optimal timing of sexual encounters during the process of ovulation induction provided. Timed intercourse in the course of ovulation induction remains the first line of treatment for these women in the absence of associated factors which may preclude natural conception. The ultimate goal of ovulation induction therapy in women with HH is single follicle development to avoid multiple pregnancies.

Gonadotropin Treatment Protocols for Ovulation Induction

Gonadotropin therapy has been established as a feasible and well-tolerated approach for ovulation induction in women with HH with reported good reproductive outcome. Gonadotropin products available for human use are derived from urinary extracts or recombinant technology. There is a lot of debate in the literature on whether urinary gonadotropins should be replaced by recombinant gonadotropins [12]. Based on the current literature there are no confirmed differences in safety or chemical efficacy among various available urinary or recombinant gonadotropin formulations [13–15]. Similarly, a meta-analysis of 42 trials involving 9606 women undergoing ovarian stimulation for various infertility etiologies demonstrated comparable live birth rates between different gonadotropic therapies and concluded that the choice of gonadotropin should be best guided by availability, convenience, and costs [16].

In women with hypogonadotropic amenorrhea, optimal clinical results are achieved by the combined administration of FSH and LH, which may be accomplished by administration of human menopausal gonadotropin (hMG) or a combination of recombinant FSH and LH [17]. Alternatively, low-dose human chorionic gonadotropin (hCG) may be used to supplement LH activity [17]. Earlier studies have shown that women with HH who were treated with FSH-only preparations required more menotropin ampoules while exhibiting fewer preovulatory follicles, lower estradiol (E_2) levels, decreased endometrial thickness, and reduced ovulation events [18]. Since most women with HH do not secrete sufficient endogenous LH, they require a complement of exogenous LH to stimulate local production of androgen substrates by theca cells, which facilitates the production of E_2 by the dominant follicle. Physiological E_2 levels promote optimal endometrial development and cervical mucus production needed for sperm entry and embryo implantation. LH supplementation during ovulation induction appears more significant in a subpopulation of women with profound LH deficiency [19]. An interesting observation is that women with a basal serum LH of less than 1.2 IU/L, suggestive of a more severe deficiency, would benefit most from LH supplementation [20;21].

Although various stimulation protocols have been used so far, there are no universally established gonadotropin regimens for ovulation induction in hypogonadotropic women and no large prospective randomized studies to assess treatment outcomes with various gonadotropin dosages and combinations. The European Recombinant Human LH Study Group using a dose-finding approach, determined the optimal gonadotropin daily dose for ovulation induction in women with HH to be 150 IU for rhFSH and 75 IU for rhLH.

Ovulation stimulation in women with HH may be started randomly or following hormone replacement therapy withdrawal bleeding. Anticipation of ovarian response in these women may be particularly challenging, especially with inherent interpretation limits of commonly used markers of ovarian reserve such as antral follicle count (AFC) and basal FSH/E_2 levels. Previous studies have reported conflicting results with respect to tests of ovarian reserve in women with HH. Significantly lower AFC values were found in women with isolated HH. Reduced AFC in this subpopulation of women is believed to be linked to a persistent and profound FSH deficit leading to diminished ovarian volume. Conversely, women with acquired functional HA display a more inconsistent and often conflicting spectrum of findings, ranging from an ultrasound background of polycystic to small-size ovaries. Diminished ovarian volume with a few detectable antral follicles is more commonly found in cases of severe anorexia. Although anti-Müllerian hormone (AMH) levels are preferred for predicting ovarian response in women with HH, knowledge on its clinical applicability for these patients is lacking and larger studies are needed to better define thresholds and limits [22;23]. It should be noted that even when AMH levels are in the high-normal range, women with HH require higher gonadotropin doses and longer durations of stimulation [22].

To avoid multiple follicular development during ovulation induction, the ovarian sensitivity to FSH (FSH threshold) should be identified and the lowest effective dose should be used. Treatment is individualized and monitored by serum E_2 measurements and ultrasound scans of the ovaries.

Conventional ovulation induction protocols aim at using the minimum effective gonadotropin dose while defining the threshold dose for ovarian response. Typically, an initial dose of 75–150 IU/day (higher doses may be necessary with higher body mass index values) are sufficient, and may be used with a step-up approach of increasing the dose by 33 percent every five to seven days until follicular growth is achieved [24]. When recombinant gonadotropin preparations are utilized, an FSH:LH ratio of 2:1 is preferred [24].

Optimal response to gonadotropin therapy is considered if three criteria are met during the stimulation cycle, that is, having at least one follicle with a mean diameter of 17 mm or more, a preovulatory serum E_2 level of 400 pmol/L or more, and a midluteal phase progesterone level of 25 nmol/L or more [24]. When follicular response is adequate, ovulation is triggered by a single intramuscular injection of 10 000 IU of hCG [24]. Luteal support after ovulation induction is clearly indicated and recommended in women with HH whose endogenous gonadotropin secretion may be inadequate to support normal luteal function. Therefore, supplemental exogenous progesterone during the luteal phase of these cycles is suggested by many to decrease rate of luteal phase defect and improve pregnancy outcome [24–27].

Defining the Optimum LH Dosage and Regimen

In an effort to define the optimum LH dosage, a number of studies have been performed [18–21;28;29]. The European Recombinant Human LH Study Group randomly assigned 38 hypogonadotropic women (LH ≤ 1.2 IU/L) to receive 0, 25, 75, or 225 IU rhLH once daily in addition to 150 IU rhFSH once daily for up to 20 days [7]. Patients who received 75 and 225 IU of rhLH were more sensitive to FSH than patients who received no rhLH or a lower dose of rhLH. It should be noted that, although not statistically significant, the group that received 225 IU rhLH had a lower number of growing follicles than the group who received 75 IU rhLH/day. This observation could be interpreted on the basis of a LH ceiling effect, whereby some secondary follicles may undergo atresia due to their high sensitivity to LH [7;19]. Pregnancy rates ranging from 20% per cycle with a dose of 225 IU rhLH to 29% per cycle with a dose of 75 IU rhLH were

comparable to those from previous studies where hMG was used for ovulation induction in HH women [7].

In a double-blinded randomized pilot study, Loumaye et al. tested the hypothesis that overdosing with rhLH during the late follicular phase would suppress follicular development "ceiling effect." Twenty HH women were randomized to receive either rhFSH and 225 IU/day rhLH (eight women) or rhLH alone (six women) or rhFSH alone (six women). No women exhibited follicular growth arrest in the rhFSH group versus one in the rhFSH/LH group and four in the rhLH alone group. These findings stressed that rhLH alone can trigger follicular growth arrest particularly in the late preovulatory follicular maturation, adding more evidence in favor of an "LH ceiling" [30].

In a multicenter study of 31 hypogonadotropic hypogonadal women, a fixed dose of lutropin alfa 75 IU was used in combination with an individualized dose of follitropin alfa at the recommended starting dose of 75–150 IU [28]. This dose was adjusted up to a maximum of 225 IU according to ovarian response [28]. The main advantages of this particular approach were that patients could undergo additional cycle treatment up to a total of three cycles and adjustment of follitropin dose was permitted according to individual patient response in the previous cycle. The dose-adjustment protocol was associated with an elevated patient response rate (87.1%), a low cycle cancellation rate, and a satisfactory pregnancy rate (74.1%) after three treatment cycles [28]. Despite the open-label, non-comparative nature of the study design, it provides valuable insight into the use of LH as part of a more flexible dosage regimen that could minimize the risk of cycle cancellation due to either stimulation failure or over-response.

Shoham et al., in a randomized, double-blind, placebo-controlled trial, confirmed the validity of the 1.2 IU/L cut-off and the efficacy of 75 IU as the effective dose for LH supplementation for patients with profound LH deficiency [29]. In fact, two-thirds of patients given lutropin alfa 75 IU/day achieved follicular development compared with only 20 percent of patients receiving placebo ($p = 0.023$). The improvement in follicular development was maintained even when an over-response was treated as a failed treatment response ($p = 0.034$). A 1.5-fold increase in antral follicle number and a threefold increase in serum

E_2 levels were detected in patients treated with lutropin alfa. The authors suggested that LH-related increase in E_2 levels may also facilitate endometrial support of implantation and pregnancy, particularly in older patients (over 35 years).

In a prospective controlled non-randomized pilot study, Awwad et al. investigated whether split daily doses of rhLH were more effective than a single daily dose in supporting follicular development and ovulation [31]. The rationale stemmed from the pharmacodynamics and pharmacokinetics of LH [32], accounting for its body distribution and short half-life. Twenty-seven women with primary HH received 150 IU rhFSH fixed daily subcutaneous dose, and 75 IU daily dose of rhLH given either as a single dose or as four equally divided doses. Ovulation was defined by three efficacy end points: having at least one follicle with a mean diameter of 17 mm or more, a preovulatory serum E_2 level of 400 pmol/L or more, and a midluteal phase progesterone level of 25 nmol/L or more. Despite a lack of statistical significance, a clinical improvement in ovulation rates was observed in the group receiving split-dose rhLH compared with single daily dose (72.2% vs. 55.6%). The split-dose protocol was also associated with higher serum E_2 concentrations per follicle (median 600 vs. 592), more growing follicles (median 2 vs. 1), and thicker endometrium (median 9.5 vs. 8) [31]. Despite the limited sample size and the non-randomized study design, these findings call for high-quality studies to explore the value of splitting the daily dose of LH in order to achieve a better reproductive outcome in hypogonadotropic hypogonadal women.

Using a prospective self-controlled study design, Balasch et al. evaluated the effects of rhLH pretreatment on the pattern of follicular response to FSH stimulation in women with HH [33]. The sequential approach to induce complete follicular development by using rhLH (300 units daily administered for seven days) preceding rhFSH administration resulted in a significantly lower threshold dose of FSH and also a lower, albeit not statistically different, total FSH dosage required. However, no beneficial effect of rhLH pretreatment in terms of follicular dynamics during the later FSH treatment phase was detected [33]. Of interest, five women with intact pituitary glands (i.e., idiopathic HH) manifested higher mean serum LH concentrations during the course of rhFSH ovarian stimulation in cycles pretreated with rhLH compared with mean serum levels at screening ($p < 0.05$) [33]. The increases in LH levels and biological activity were further evidenced by the rise in serum androstenedione concentrations (a direct secretory product of LH action on theca cells) observed throughout the study period in those five patients. A possible effect of LH-FSH priming on pituitary LH secretion in idiopathic HH patients was proposed, and is believed to be operational through ovarian expression and secretion of kisspeptins, potent elicitors of gonadotropin secretion [33].

Treatment Outcomes with Gonadotropin Administration in HH

The clinical reproductive outcomes of hMG or rhFSH/LH therapy for ovulation induction in women with HH have been underreported in recent years. It may be difficult to extrapolate results from earlier studies, since in many of them a proper differentiation between various etiologies of anovulation has not been properly made. Also, in addition to small sample size, these studies are mostly observational in nature further limiting the interpretability of results. A study of 77 women with HH and 20 women with HA showed a cumulative pregnancy rate of 82.1% after 12 cycles of treatment in the HH group and 95.0% in the HA group. The overall miscarriage rates were 22.9% in the HH group and 32.3% in the HA group. It should also be noted that the cumulative pregnancy rate of 89% after six ovulatory cycles has been reported following menotropin ovulation induction in two small series [34;35]. Findings from fourteen studies showed significant inconsistencies in reproductive outcomes and wide variations in conception rates ranging from 16 to 78 percent per cycle.

It is observed that ovarian stimulation of HH women undergoing assisted reproduction is associated with significantly higher gonadotropin requirements and longer stimulation period [33]. In some studies, however, these women appear to have higher fertilization (89% vs. 80%, $p = 0.03$) and implantation rates (36.5% vs. 13%, $p < 0.0001$) [36;37] after accounting for age. A small observational retrospective study suggested that the oocyte quality, embryo quality, and pregnancy outcome are not affected in HH even when the duration of ovarian stimulation duration was prolonged [38]. Similarly, a retrospective study comparing reproductive outcomes in 33 women with HH to 47 women with male factor infertility found no differences in peak E_2 levels, endometrial thickness, total number of retrieved oocytes, number of mature oocytes, and pregnancy outcomes despite significantly higher duration of stimulation in HH women [39].

Controversy exists on whether a GnRH analogue is required for pituitary suppression in women with HH undergoing assisted reproduction. In a retrospective multicenter cohort study by Mumusoglu *et al.* in 2017, women with congenital HH who underwent intracytoplasmic sperm injection (ICSI) were compared to age-matched controls with tubal factor infertility. While live birth rates per started cycle were comparable between groups, women with HH who received a GnRH antagonist or a long GnRH agonist protocol for pituitary suppression had significantly lower embryo implantation rates (21.6% vs. 52.6%, $p = 0.03$) than those receiving exogenous gonadotropin stimulation alone [40]. The investigators suggested that pituitary suppression during ovarian stimulation may be associated with a detrimental effect on implantation in women with congenital HH. This hypothesis was contested by other investigators, however. In fact, the findings of an observational retrospective cohort study by Cecchino *et al.* in 2019, in which women with HH who underwent assisted reproductive technology were compared with age-matched counterparts with tubal or male factor infertility, were found to be in sharp contrast. Fertilization rates and live birth rates per cycle were found to be similar between comparison groups irrespective of the use of a GnRH analogue for pituitary suppression [41].

Complications of Gonadotropin Treatment

Multifetal gestation resulting from a multifollicular response is the most frequent complication of ovulation induction in women with HH. To minimize the risk of multiple pregnancy and associated maternal and fetal morbidities, criteria for cycle cancellation have been established. Cycle cancellation should be seriously considered when three or more mature follicles (> 16–17 mm) or a large number of intermediate-sized follicles (10–15 mm) are observed, or

when the serum E_2 concentration exceeds 1000–1500 pg/ml [17]. Alternatively, in vitro fertilization (IVF) with the transfer of a limited number of embryos in fresh and/or vitrified-warmed cycles may be employed to prevent the risk of multiple pregnancies. In a retrospective publication, the outcome of freeze-all embryos was investigated in 135 vitrified-warmed single embryo transfers after hormone replacement therapy in 77 HH women. The clinical pregnancy rate was 34.6% in cleavage-stage embryo transfer cycles versus 65.1% in blastocyst embryo transfer. The cumulative live birth rates were 55.7% (44.6–66.2, 95% confidence interval [CI]) after the first oocyte retrieval and 83.1% (70.1–91.1%, 95% CI) after the third oocyte retrieval. Although lacking a fresh embryo transfer comparator group, these findings were very favorable in reducing the incidence of multiple conception in HH women while maintaining a good reproductive efficacy [42].

Ovarian hyperstimulation syndrome (OHSS) is the most serious iatrogenic complication associated with ovarian stimulation. The incidence of OHSS in the literature is difficult to estimate due to different classification criteria used historically, and to the varying incidence between treatments and patient groups. In a report from Finland, the rate of hospitalization for OHSS following ovulation induction was 0.04% per cycle, whereas the one following IVF was 0.9% [43]. Mild manifestations of OHSS are relatively common and include: transient lower abdominal discomfort, mild nausea, vomiting, diarrhea, and abdominal distension (observed in up to one-third of super ovulation cycles) [44]. Onset of symptoms typically occurs soon after ovulation (in super ovulation cycles) or after oocyte retrieval in assisted reproductive technology cycles, but may also be delayed [44]. Progression of illness is recognized when symptoms persist, worsen, or include ascites that may be demonstrated by increasing abdominal girth or ultrasound evaluation [45]. Serious illness exists when pain is accompanied by one or more of the following: rapid weight gain, tense ascites, hemodynamic instability (orthostatic hypotension, tachycardia), respiratory difficulty (tachypnea), progressive oliguria, or laboratory abnormalities [45]. The pathophysiology of OHSS is characterized by increased capillary permeability, leading to leakage of fluid from the vasculature, third-space fluid accumulation, and intravascular dehydration [45]. In severe cases, the process can produce multisystem dysfunction, with a tendency to thrombosis, renal and hepatic dysfunction, and pulmonary edema. Vascular endothelial growth factor (VEGF), also known as vascular permeability factor, has emerged as one of the factors most likely involved in the pathophysiology of OHSS, and VEGF levels correlate with the severity of OHSS [45]. In women undergoing ovarian stimulation with gonadotropins, hCG is the usual trigger for OHSS. Risk factors for OHSS are young age, low body weight, PCOS, high doses of exogenous gonadotropins, high absolute or rapidly rising serum E_2 levels, and previous episodes of OHSS [35]. The keys to prevention of OHSS are experience with ovulation induction therapy and recognition of risk factors for OHSS. Ovulation induction regimens should be highly individualized, carefully monitored, and use the minimum dose and duration of gonadotropin therapy necessary to achieve the therapeutic goal [44;46]. Caution is indicated when any of the following indicators are present: rapidly rising serum E_2 levels, E_2 concentration > 2500 pg/ml for IVF/ICSI cycles, or a large number of intermediate-sized follicles (10–14 mm). A lower dose of hCG (e.g., 5000 IU instead of the standard 10 000 IU dosage) may be prudent for patients at high risk for OHSS although not proven to reduce the severe manifestations of the disease [44–46].

Earlier reports that ovulation induction might be associated with an increased risk for cancer of the ovary and breast have not been confirmed by subsequent studies [17].

Ovulation Induction Using Subcutaneous Pulsatile Gonadotropin-Releasing Hormone in HH

Treatment Protocols and Mode of Administration

Pulsatile GnRH can be used to recuperate periodic gonadotropin secretion. This treatment is suitable for women with a hypothalamic etiology of HH with an intact pituitary gland, namely idiopathic or stress-induced form of the disorder [24]. Another clinical application includes women with GnRH receptor mutations [24]. Pulsatile GnRH is not suitable nonetheless for ovulation induction in women with hypopituitarism. The infusion of GnRH is performed by a computerized, automated minipump at pulse intervals of about 60 to 180 minutes, with more successful outcomes reported with pulse frequencies of 90 to 120 minutes [47;48]. Although there has been some debate in favor of the intravenous route (5–10 µg/pulse) compared with the subcutaneous route (15–20 µg/pulse) [24], no prospective randomized studies are available to offer more conclusive data on this subject. Using this approach, ovulation is expected to occur following a spontaneous endogenous LH surge in response to rising estrogen levels. Pulsatile GnRH in combination with exogenous menotropins has also been suggested for women who demonstrate prolonged follicular phases. Women with profound GnRH deficit tend to have prolonged follicular phases caused by a required initial priming phase of the pituitary gland before active production and secretion of gonadotropins.

For monitoring of treatment, serum progesterone measurements could verify normal luteal phase, while ultrasound scans of the ovaries can predict the risk of multiple pregnancy. The reported pregnancy rate per GnRH treatment cycle is 25 percent, while the number of cycles required to obtain a pregnancy is 2.8 ± 1.7 [24;49]. Following six cycles of treatment, the overall ovulatory rate was 93% and the cumulative pregnancy rate was 96% [50]. Using this approach, the reported miscarriage rate was 8.2% and the multiple pregnancy rate 8.8%, although a rate as high as 17.4% has also been described [51]. In one large series involving 292 anovulatory women and 600 treatment cycles, ovulation and pregnancy rates following pulsatile intravenous GnRH administration at a dose of 1.25–2.00 µg of GnRH every 30–120 minutes was found to be higher in all types of HH women compared with other anovulatory etiologies [52]. There is no evidence that hCG is required for ovulation induction, while lower doses of GnRH are recommended during the first treatment cycle [24].

Side Effects of Pulsatile GnRH Therapy

There are several disadvantages with the use of a GnRH pump for ovulation induction in anovulatory women, some of which may be related to inconvenience and cumbersome use. In fact, the pump must be connected to the body all day long for a considerable number of days, and must be refilled at frequent intervals. Described side effects associated with it use include site-related reactions (infections, local venous thrombosis, skin reactions ...) to administration, most of which are preventable by proper skin care including adhering to sterile procedures and by changing the needle once or twice a week [51]. The development of antibodies against synthetic GnRH seems to be a rare possibility [51]. The most serious side effect nonetheless remains the risk for overstimulation and multiple pregnancies, although the rates are much lower than with gonadotropin administration [24;50–52]. Patients, who usually present with a low-grade disturbance of hypothalamic ovarian failure carry a higher risk for overstimulation and multiple births, especially in association with the initial cycle of treatment. This phenomenon may be the result of cumulative follicle development preceding the start of GnRH pulsatile administration, and may be prevented by pretreatment ovarian suppression with oral contraceptives [51].

Additional Strategies for Ovulation Induction in Women with HH

GH/IGF-1 Administration

Women with hypopituitarism constitute a challenging and difficult-to-handle group of hypogonadotropic patients. Although the majority of women with this condition experience successful ovulation induction and conception using hMG or rhFSH/LH alone, there are a number of women who fail to respond with the use of the standard protocols previously described. Fertility outcomes in women with hypopituitarism are much lower than those reported in isolated HH [53], and growth hormone deficiency (GHD) has been considered as a contributor to poor pregnancy rate [53]. The above assumption is based on our knowledge of the role of GH and insulin-like growth factor-1 (IGF-1) in female reproduction. In the female, GH has a role not only as a modulator on gonadotropins, mediated by the property of IGF-1 to amplify the action of both LH and FSH on granulosa cells; but also, through a direct GH action, on follicular maturation [54]. In vivo and in vitro studies suggest that GH stimulates growth and prevents atresia in small follicles [54]. Furthermore, it has been shown that

GH acts in conjunction with gonadotropins to stimulate later stages of folliculogenesis and luteinization. The folliculogenic effect of GH, at least in human luteinized granulosa cells, is dependent upon FSH and independent of IGF-1 [54]. GH may also facilitate ovulation by increasing sensitivity to gonadotropins and by reducing the incidence of apoptosis in preovulatory ovarian follicles [54]. IGF-1 is involved in the regulation of follicular development and potentiates the FSH responsiveness of granulosa cells from preantral follicles [54]. The addition of IGF-1 to gonadotropins in granulosa cell cultures increases gonadotropin action on the ovary by several mechanisms, including augmentation of aromatase activity, 17-beta estradiol and progesterone production, and luteinizing hormone receptor formation [54].

The possible use of GH as an adjunct to human gonadotropin (hMG) to induce ovulation has thus been the focus of extensive research. Clinical studies have shown that GH may be therapeutically useful in some, but not all, infertile women [54–59]. In particular, GH administration as a co-treatment for ovulation induction, as 24 units on alternate days or 12 units daily, to hypogonadotropic anovulatory women has been shown to reduce significantly the dosage and duration of gonadotropin treatment required for ovulation induction [54]. Furthermore, a considerable proportion of women who respond to GH fail to respond to hMG and rhFSH/LH alone [54]. GH therapy may similarly improve the success of in vitro fertilization techniques by enhancing the hyperovulatory response to menotropins [54], and such findings led to the use of GH for the improvement of the follicular response to gonadotropins in women who responded poorly during IVF [60]. In a prospective, randomized, placebo-controlled European and Australian multicenter study, Jacobs et al. demonstrated that the addition of GH to gonadotropin treatment in HH women amplified gonadotropin's action on the ovary as shown by a net reduction in gonadotropin consumption required to achieve follicular growth compared with those receiving placebo (22.3 ± 12.0 vs. 37.2 ± 18.9 ampoules; $p < 0.05$) [61]. Although the study did not define a minimum effective dose of GH for gonadotropin-stimulated ovarian induction, it demonstrated a GH dose-related amplification of gonadotropin effect. However promising these findings may be, they

215

failed to demonstrate significant improvements in pregnancy outcomes [61].

Paradoxically, in a report of 16 women with acquired pituitary insufficiency of varying degrees and etiologies (prolactinomas, Cushing syndrome, craniopharyngiomas), pregnancies were achieved without GH administration [62]. Spontaneous pregnancies in Laron-type dwarfism, a model of low IGF-1 and normal GH values, have also been reported [63]. Natural conception and successful pregnancy outcome and delivery have also been described in two women with *Prop1* gene mutations, an ideal model for the study of familial combined GH, IGF-1, prolactin, LH, and FSH deficiencies, after gonadotropins-only stimulation [64].

Based on the previous data and since GH, directly or indirectly via IGF-1, regulates reproductive functions at all levels of the hypophyseal–pituitary–gonadal axis, it should always be tested as a possible cause of unexplained infertility. Further studies are required before GH or IGF-1 administration become a standard co-treatment in certain groups of infertile women who might benefit from such therapeutic regimens (e.g., those with multiple pituitary insufficiency or poor responders to previous gonadotropin administration).

Estrogen Pretreatment

There is sparse evidence in the literature, mainly derived from case reports and non-comparative observational studies, indicating that estrogen pretreatment with or without progesterone improves success with ovulation induction in hypogonadotropic women [55;65;66]. In one study, hypogonadotropic women who failed to achieve pregnancy after six cycles of gonadotropin therapy underwent pretreatment with cyclic estrogen and progesterone before ovulation induction with hMG. Twenty-two out of 30 patients achieved pregnancy within the next four cycles [65]. The major problem with this study is the absence of a control group. The authors suggested that in the presence of a hypoestrogenic environment, hMG alone seems less effective, and that pretreatment with an estrogen–progestogen combination results in a high estrogenic status, which might enhance ovulatory rates [65]. In a case report, successful pregnancy was achieved in a patient with HH resulting from a craniopharyngioma after the addition of conjugated estrogens to hMG treatment

[66]. The patient had undergone several cycles of hMG therapy with successful follicular development but failed to become pregnant. Co-treatment with conjugated estrogens resulted in pregnancy achievement on the seventh cycle of this protocol. Although the authors suggested that supplemental estrogen improved the uterine environment which enabled successful endometrial implantation, such conclusions may not be supported except with well-designed studies [66]. In a more recent study, successful pregnancy outcome was reported in a 31-year-old woman with panhypopituitarism [55]. The patient had previously conceived with recombinant FSH and hCG and had an uncomplicated pregnancy. In her second attempt to become pregnant and after 36 days of an unsuccessful step-up stimulation protocol with the use of rhFSH, she was given a four-month treatment with GH prior to restarting gonadotropins. Transdermal E_2 was added to the gonadotropin treatment protocol. She finally had a successful ovulation induction and pregnancy after 63 days of treatment. The authors suggested that treatment with GH and estrogen may directly or indirectly benefit poor-responder patients [55]. Nevertheless, further studies are needed to elucidate the mechanism of beneficial effect, if any, of estrogen pretreatment.

Ovulation Induction in Thalassemia Patients

Advances in the primary care (pediatric and hematological) of patients with thalassemia major, including optimal blood transfusions and chelation therapies, have contributed remarkably to an improved overall survival and quality of life. Endocrine complications due to hemosiderosis – and especially HH – are common in young adults with this blood disorder, and are thought to contribute to low fertility in this population [67]. Gonadotropin insufficiency is present in around 70–80 percent of the thalassemia patient population globally [68]. Studies have shown that this HH is the most common endocrinopathy in this group of patients and is present in 40–91 percent of transfusion-dependent beta-thalassemia cases. As a result, multiple clinical manifestations have been described, including impaired growth, sexual dysfunction, and reduced fertility; with consequent psychological trauma and decreased quality of life [69].

Case reports and small published series demonstrate that successful pregnancy is possible in women with thalassemia major, even in the absence of any hormonal assistance [70–74]. Preparations of hMG/hCG have been used in most published protocols, with an initial hMG starting dose ranging from 150 to 300 IU, adjusted subsequently according to serum E_2 levels and ultrasound ovarian findings. In a review, fertility and pregnancy were evaluated in women with thalassemia major over a period of 15 years [74]. Twenty-two women completed 29 pregnancies. Of these pregnancies 16 followed spontaneous ovulation and 12 followed induction of ovulation using gonadotropins. The authors suggested maternal conception screening for cardiac insufficiency, liver dysfunction, and risks of vertical transmission of viruses in thalassemic women. They also proposed close monitoring of pregnant women with monitoring of blood sugars, thyroid function tests, and ferritin levels. Review of potentially teratogenic medication such as hypoglycemic agents, bisphosphonates, ACE inhibitors, and deferoxamine is also suggested and these should be stopped prior to ovulation induction. This multidisciplinary team approach was encouraged after describing favorable pregnancy outcomes after assisted reproductive technology derived independently from experience in London and Italy with thalassemia major patients [75;76].

Future Advances in Ovulation Induction Therapies

Kisspeptin-GPR54 Complex

Many genes have been identified in association with HH which can offer possible future therapeutic options in its management. Insights in the signaling circuits for the regulation of GnRH secretion have been found following identification of the *Kiss-1* gene and its product kisspeptin-54 or metastin [77]. This 54-amino acid peptide, originally detected in tumor cells and with antimetastatic properties [78], has been detected in the hypothalamus and the placenta [79;80]. In 2003, it was found that GPR54, a G-protein-coupled receptor of unknown significance, expressed both in brain and pituitary, has a high affinity for kisspeptin, and that mutations in the GPR54 gene in mice and adult humans cause low plasma levels of gonadotropins and sex steroids, underdeveloped gonads,

and infertility [79]. In the following years, it was documented that central and peripheral administration of kisspeptin provoked a dose-dependent rise in LH/FSH likely via activation of GnRH neurons [81]. Evidence today suggests that kisspeptin neurons found in the forebrain act as gatekeepers to awakening reproduction at puberty and coordinating reproductive activity during adulthood [79]. As such kisspeptin has been suggested to have a key role in the onset of puberty, as a mediator of metabolic factors affecting the hypothalamus and neuromodulator controlling pulsatile GnRH release.

It has been demonstrated that exogenous kisspeptin-GPR54 stimulates the hypothalamic–pituitary–gonadal axis in healthy female subjects [82]. Kisspeptin-GPR54 (at doses between 0.2 and 6.4 nmol/kg) was initially administered to women during the follicular phase of the menstrual cycle. Following injection, kisspeptin-GPR54 led to a rise in plasma LH and FSH over the 240-minute time period of the study, with progressively greater stimulation at higher doses. However, no significant rise in free E_2 index was observed [82]. Further administration of kisspeptin in women during the preovulatory and luteal phases of the menstrual cycle showed the most pronounced rise in mean plasma LH occurring during the preovulatory phase [82]. Following these observations, kisspeptin-GPR54 might be a promising fertility treatment for ovulation induction [83]. Since kisspeptin acts through upregulation of GnRH secretion to stimulate endogenous gonadotropin release [79], its treatment might carry a lower risk of OHSS. In addition, the future development of an oral GPR54 agonist might offer a practical advantage over the currently available gonadotropin injections. More studies are needed to delineate the potential role of kisspeptin administration in ovulation induction of hypogonadotropic hypogonadal women.

Key Role of ERK1 and ERK2 Activities in Ovarian Function and Fertility

The role of many other factors has been investigated in HH. ERK1 and ERK2, two extracellular signal-regulated kinases, have been defined as master regulators of fertility by mediating the effect of LH on all components of the ovulatory response: oocyte maturation, cumulus expansion, luteinization, and follicle rupture in mice [84].

A new era in identification of cellular signaling pathways that support follicle maturation and oocyte release emerged with the published work of Fan *et al.* [85]. Signal-regulated kinases 1 and 2 (ERK1 and ERK2) were identified as a critical nexus between the surge in luteinizing hormone and ovulation in mice. Particularly, ERK1 and ERK2, in response to follicular exposure to LH, phosphorylate the gap-junction proteins in the granulosa and cumulus cells of the Graafian follicle, leading to a diminution of molecules such as cyclic AMP (cAMP) both between these cells and between the cumulus cells and the oocyte [85]. Cyclic AMP is known to repress the resumption of meiosis and thus maturation of the oocyte. Consequently, a reduction of cAMP in the oocyte results in a resumption of meiosis, oocyte maturation, and finally in ovulation. However, as shown by Fan *et al.*, if the molecular pathology is restricted to the somatic cells of the ovarian follicle, the oocyte is capable of resuming meiotic maturation if physically isolated from the ovarian follicle [85]. These findings advance our understanding and may one day contribute to new treatments for infertility. Nevertheless, it remains to be seen whether ERK1 and ERK2 genes in humans mimic their orthologous genes in mice and their inactivation (e.g., by mutation) causes infertility in humans.

Conclusions

Hypogonadotropic hypogonadism remains one of the most challenging causes of infertility to treat and manage. Individualization of treatment protocol to achieve an ideal ovarian stimulation regimen balancing the risk of no response/cycle cancellation with hyperstimulation remains highly empiric. Most available evidence on the management of fertility in hypogonadotropic hypogonadal women is derived from observational retrospective studies, case reports, and small randomized trials. Although limited by the low prevalence of the condition, large-scale randomized trials are crucial to the growing knowledge on the management of fertility in affected women.

New developments in the area of pharmacology, and with evidence pointing to kisspeptin-GPR54 signaling as the principal trigger for activation of GnRH neurons and subsequent ovulation, presage a new era in the management of infertile women for which exploration is currently underway. Additionally, the kisspeptin-GPR54 complex might be used as a more natural and potent molecule for ovulation induction in those women with intact pituitary gland, and especially for those with idiopathic HH. The findings involving ERK1 and ERK2 as a critical nexus between the surge in LH and ovulation in mice also call for studies delineating the role of these kinases in hypogonadotropic hypogonadal women subfertility.

Acknowledgment

We acknowledge the contribution of Dr. Paraskevi Xekouki and late Professor George Tolis for their significant contribution to the preparation and writing of the chapter in the previous edition of this book.

References

1. The Practice Committee of the American Society for Reproductive Medicine. Current evaluation of amenorrhea. *Fertil Steril* 2008;**90**:S219–S225.

2. Bulun SE, Adashi EY. The physiology and pathology of the female reproductive axis. In: Melmed S, Polonsky KS, Larsen PR, Kronenberg HM, eds. *Williams Textbook of Endocrinology*, 13th ed. Philadelphia: Elsevier Health Sciences; 2015:590–663.

3. Fevold HL. Synergism of follicle stimulating and luteinizing hormones in producing estrogen secretion. *Endocrinology* 1941;**28**:33–36.

4. Richards JS. Hormonal control of gene expression in the ovary. *Endocr Rev* 1994;**15**:725–751.

5. Erickson GF, Magoffin DA, Dyer CA, Hofeditz C. The ovarian androgen producing cells: a review of structure/function relationships. *Endocr Rev* 1985;**6**:371–399.

6. Angelopoulos N, Goula A, Tolis G. The role of luteinizing hormone activity in controlled ovarian stimulation. *J Endocrinol Invest* 2005;**28**:79–88.

7. European Recombinant Human LH Study Group. Recombinant human luteinizing hormone (LH) to support recombinant human follicle-stimulating hormone (FSH)-induced follicular development in LH- and FSH-deficient anovulatory women: a dose-finding study. *J Clin Endocrinol Metab* 1998;**83**:1507–1514.

8. Lunenfeld B. Historical perspectives in gonadotrophin therapy. *Hum Reprod Update* 2004;**10**:453–467.

9. Rowe PJ, Comhaire FH, Hargreave TB, *et al.* WHO *Manual for the Standardized Investigation and*

Diagnosis of the Infertile Couple. Cambridge: Cambridge University Press; 1993.

10. Shoham Z, Conway GS, Patel A, Jacobs HS. Polycystic ovaries in patients with hypogonadotropic hypogonadism: similarity of ovarian response to gonadotropin stimulation in patients with polycystic ovarian syndrome. *Fertil Steril* 1992;**58**:37–45.

11. Schachter M, Balen AH, Patel A, Jacobs HS. Hypogonadotropic patients with ultrasonographically detected polycystic ovaries: endocrine response to pulsatile gonadotropin-releasing hormone. *Gynecol Endocrinol* 1996;**10**:327–335.

12. Muasher SJ, Abdallah RT, Hubayter ZR. Optimal stimulation protocols for in vitro fertilization. *Fertil Steril* 2006;**86**:267–273.

13. The Practice Committee of the American Society for Reproductive Medicine, Birmingham, Alabama. Gonadotropin preparations: past, present and future perspectives. *Fertil Steril* 2008;**90**(5 Suppl):S13–S20.

14. Al-Inany H, Aboulghar MA, Mansour RT, Proctor M. Recombinant versus urinary gonadotrophins for triggering ovulation in assisted conception. *Hum Reprod* 2006;**21**:569–570.

15. Bordewijk EM, Mol F, van der Veen F, Van Wely M. Required amount of rFSH, HP-hMG and HP-FSH to reach a live birth: a systematic review and meta-analysis. *Hum Reprod Open* 2019;**2019** (3):hoz008.

16. van Wely M, Kwan I, Burt AL, *et al.* Recombinant versus urinary gonadotrophin for ovarian stimulation in assisted reproductive technology cycles. *Cochrane Database Syst Rev* 2011;**2**: CD005354.

17. The Practice Committee of the American Society for Reproductive Medicine. Use of exogenous gonadotropins in anovulatory women: a technical bulletin. *Fertil Steril* 2008;**90**(5 Suppl):S7–S12.

18. Filicori M, Cognigni GE, Samara A, *et al.* The use of LH activity to drive folliculogenesis: exploring uncharted territories in ovulation induction. *Hum Reprod Update* 2002;**8**:543–557.

19. Krause BT, Ohlinger R, Haase A. Lutropin alpha, recombinant human luteinizing hormone, for the stimulation of follicular development in profoundly LH-deficient hypogonadotropic hypogonadal women: a review. *Biologics* 2009;**3**:337–347.

20. Shoham Z, Balen A, Patel A, Jacobs HS. Results of ovulation induction using human menopausal gonadotropin or purified follicle-stimulating

hormone in hypogonadotropic hypogonadism patients. *Fertil Steril* 1991;**56**:1048–1053.

21. O'Dea L, the US Recombinant Human LH Study Group. Recombinant LH in support of recombinant FSH in female hypogonadotropic hypogonadism-evidence of threshold effect. *Fertil Steril* 2000;**74**(Suppl 1):S36.

22. Hagen CP, Sørensen K, Anderson RA, Juul A. Serum levels of antimüllerian hormone in early maturing girls before, during, and after suppression with GnRH agonist. *Fertil Steril* 2012;**98**(5):1326–1330.

23. Sönmezer M, Özmen B, Atabekoglu CS, *et al.* Serum anti-Mullerian hormone levels correlate with ovarian response in idiopathic hypogonadotropic hypogonadism. *J Assist Reprod Genet* 2012;**29**(7):597–602.

24. Messinis IE. Ovulation induction: a mini review. *Hum Reprod* 2005;**20**:2688–2697.

25. Messinis IE, Bergh T, Wide L. The importance of human chorionic gonadotropin support of the corpus luteum during human gonadotropin therapy in women with anovulatory infertility. *Fertil Steril* 1988;**50**(1):31–35.

26. Van der Linden M, Buckingham K, Farquhar C, Kremer JA, Metwally M. Luteal phase support in assisted reproduction cycles. *Hum Reprod Update* 2012;**18**(5):473.

27. Aboulghar M. Luteal support in reproduction: when, what and how? *Curr Opin Obstet Gynecol* 2009;**21**:279–284.

28. Kaufmann R, Dunn R, Vaughn T, *et al.* Recombinant human luteinizing hormone, lutropin alfa, for the induction of follicular development and pregnancy in profoundly gonadotrophin-deficient women. *Clin Endocrinol (Oxf)* 2007;**67**:563–569.

29. Shoham Z, Smith H, Yeko T, *et al.* Recombinant LH (lutropin alfa) for the treatment of hypogonadotrophic women with profound LH deficiency: a randomized, double-blind, placebo-controlled, proof-of-efficacy study. *Clin Endocrinol (Oxf)* 2008;**69**:471–478.

30. Loumaye E, Engrand P, Shoham Z, Hillier SG, Baird DT. Clinical evidence for an LH 'ceiling' effect induced by administration of recombinant human LH during the late follicular phase of stimulated cycles in World Health Organization type I and type II anovulation. *Hum Reprod* 2003;**18**(2):314–322.

31. Awwad JT, Farra C, Mitri F, *et al.* Split daily recombinant human LH dose in hypogonadotrophic hypogonadism: a nonrandomized controlled pilot study. *Reprod Biomed Online* 2013;**26**(1):88–92.

32. le Cotonnec JY, Loumaye E, Porchet H, Beltrami V, Munafo A. Pharmacokinetic and pharmacodynamic interactions between recombinant human luteinizing hormone and recombinant human follicle-stimulating hormone. *Fertil Steril* 1998;**69**(2):201–209.

33. Balasch J, Fábregues F, Carmona F, Casamitjana R, Tena-Sempere M. Ovarian luteinizing hormone priming preceding follicle-stimulating hormone stimulation: clinical and endocrine effects in women with long-term hypogonadotropic hypogonadism. *J Clin Endocrinol Metab* 2009;**94**:2367–2373.

34. Fluker MR, Urman B, Mackinnon M, *et al.* Exogenous gonadotropin therapy in World Health Organization groups I and II ovulatory disorders. *Obstet Gynecol* 1994;**83**:189–196.

35. Tadokoro N, Vollenhoven B, Clark S, *et al.* Cumulative pregnancy rates in couples with anovulatory infertility compared with unexplained infertility in an ovulation induction programme. *Hum Reprod* 1997;**12**:1939–1944.

36. Kumbak B, Kahraman S. Women with hypogonadotropic hypogonadism: cycle characteristics and results of assisted reproductive techniques. *Acta Obstet Gynecol Scand* 2006;**85**:1453–1457.

37. Ghaffari F, Arabipoor A, Lankarani NB, Etminan Z, Tehraninejad ES. Assisted reproductive technique outcomes in hypogonadotropic hypogonadism women. *Ann Saudi Med* 2013;**33**(3):235–240.

38. Pandurangi M, Tamizharasi M, Reddy NS. Pregnancy outcome of assisted reproductive technology cycle in patients with hypogonadotropic hypogonadism. *J Hum Reprod Sci* 2015;**8**(3):146–150.

39. Yilmaz S, Ozgu-Erdinc AS, Yumusak O, *et al.* The reproductive outcome of women with hypogonadotropic hypogonadism undergoing in vitro fertilization. *Syst Biol Reprod Med* 2015;**61**(4):228–232.

40. Mumusoglu S, Ata B, Turan V, *et al.* Does pituitary suppression affect live birth rate in women with congenital hypogonadotrophic hypogonadism undergoing intra-cytoplasmic sperm injection? A multicenter cohort study. *Gynecol Endocrinol* 2017;33(9):728–732.

41. Cecchino GN, Canillas GM, Cruz M, García-Velasco JA. Impact of hypogonadotropic hypogonadism on ovarian reserve and response. *J Assist Reprod Genet* 2019;**36**(11):2379–2384.

42. Kuroda K, Ezoe K, Kato K, *et al.* Infertility treatment strategy involving combined freeze-all embryos and single vitrified-warmed embryo transfer during hormonal replacement cycle for in vitro fertilization of women with hypogonadotropic hypogonadism. *J Obstet Gynaecol Res* 2018;**44**(5):922–928.

43. Klemetti R, Sevon T, Gissler M, Hemm E. Complications of IVF and ovulation induction. *Hum Reprod* 2005;**20**:3293–3300.

44. Aboulghar M. Symposium: Update on prediction and management of OHSS. Prevention of OHSS. *Reprod Biomed Online* 2009;**19**:33–42.

45. The Practice Committee of the American Society for Reproductive Medicine. Ovarian hyperstimulation syndrome. *Fertil Steril* 2008;**90**(5 Suppl):S188–S193.

46. Mathur R, Kailasam C, Jenkins J. Review of the evidence base of strategies to prevent ovarian hyperstimulation syndrome. *Hum Fertil* 2007;**10**:75–85.

47. Letterie GS, Coddington CC, Collins RL, Merriam GR. Ovulation induction using s.c. pulsatile gonadotrophin-releasing hormone: effectiveness of different pulse frequencies. *Hum Reprod* 1996;**11**:19–22.

48. Homburg R, Eshel A, Armar NA, *et al.* One hundred pregnancies after treatment with pulsatile luteinizing hormone releasing hormone to induce ovulation. *Br Med J* 1989;**298**:809–812.

49. Braat DD, Ayalon D, Blunt SM, *et al.* Pregnancy outcome in luteinizing hormone-releasing hormone induced cycles: a multicentre study. *Gynecol Endocrinol* 1989;**3**:35–44.

50. Martin KA, Hall JE, Adams JM, Crowley WF Jr. Comparison of exogenous gonadotropins and pulsatile gonadotropin-releasing hormone for induction of ovulation in hypogonadotropic amenorrhea. *J Clin Endocrinol Metab* 1993;**77**(1):125–129.

51. Mattle V, Leyendecker G, Wildt L. Side effects of pulsatile GnRH therapy for induction of ovulation. *Expert Rev Endocrinol Metab* 2008;3:535–538.

52. Filicori M, Flamigni C, Dellai P, *et al.* Treatment of anovulation with pulsatile gonadotropin-releasing hormone: prognostic factors and clinical results in 600 cycles. *J Clin Endocrinol Metab* 1994;**79**(4):1215–1220.

53. Hall R, Manski-Nankervis J, Goni N, Davies MC, Conway GS. Fertility outcomes in women with hypopituitarism. *Clin Endocrinol* 2006;**65**:71–74.

54. Hull KL, Harvey S. Growth hormone: roles in female reproduction. *J Endocrinol* 2001;**168**:1–23.

55. Park JK, Murphy AA, Bordeaux BL, Dominguez CE, Session DR. Ovulation induction

in a poor responder with panhypopituitarism: a case report and review of the literature. *Gynecol Endocrinol* 2007;**23**:82–86.

56. Homburg R, West C, Torresani T, Jacobs HS. Cotreatment with human growth hormone and gonadotropins for induction of ovulation: a controlled clinical trial. *Fertil Steril* 1990;**53**:254–260.

57. Giampietro A, Milardi D, Bianchi A, *et al.* The effect of treatment with growth hormone on fertility outcome in eugonadal women with growth hormone deficiency: report of four cases and review of the literature. *Fertil Steril* 2009;**91** (3):930.e7–930.e11.

58. Daniel A, Ezzat S, Greenblatt E. Adjuvant growth hormone for ovulation induction with gonadotropins in the treatment of a woman with hypopituitarism. *Case Rep Endocrinol* 2012;**20**:12.

59. Salle A, Klein M, Pascal-Vigneron V, *et al.* Successful pregnancy and birth after sequential cotreatment with growth hormone and gonadotropins in a woman with panhypopituitarism: a new treatment protocol. *Fertil Steril* 2000;**74**:1248–1250.

60. Harper K, Proctor M, Hughes E. Growth hormone for in vitro fertilization. *Cochrane Database Syst Rev* 2003;**3**:CD000099.

61. Jacobs HS, Shoham Z, Schachter M, *et al.* Cotreatment with growth-hormone and gonadotropin for ovulation induction in hypogonadotropic patients-a prospective, randomized, placebo-controlled, dose-response study. *Fertil Steril* 1995;**64**(5):917–923.

62. Curran AJ, Peacey SR, Shalet SM. Is maternal growth hormone essential for a normal pregnancy? *Eur J Endocrinol* 1998;**139**:54–58.

63. Menashe Y, Sack J, Mashiach S. Spontaneous pregnancies in two women with Laron-type dwarfism: are growth hormone and circulating insulin-like growth factor mandatory for induction of ovulation? *Hum Reprod* 1991;**6**:670–671.

64. Voutetakis A, Sertedaki A, Livadas S, *et al.* Ovulation induction and successful pregnancy outcome in two patients with Prop1 gene mutations. *Fertil Steril* 2004;**82**:454–457.

65. Yildirim M, Noyan V, Tiras MB. Estrogen-progestagen pre-treatment before HMG induction in hypogonadotropic patients. *Int J Gynaecol Obstet* 2000;**71**:249–250.

66. Hayashi M, Tomobe K, Hoshimoto K, Ohkura T. Successful pregnancy following gonadotropin therapy in a patient with hypogonadotropic hypogonadism resulting from

craniopharyngioma. *Int J Clin Pract* 2002;**56**:149–151.

67. Toumba M, Sergis A, Kanaris C, Skordis N. Endocrine complications in patients with thalassaemia major. *Pediatr Endocrinol Rev* 2007;**5**:642–648.

68. Chatterjee R, Bajoria R. Critical appraisal of growth retardation and pubertal disturbances in thalassemia. *Ann N Y Acad Sci* 2010;**1202** (1):100–114.

69. Poggi M, Sorrentino F, Pugliese P, *et al.* Longitudinal changes of endocrine and bone disease in adults with β-thalassemia major receiving different iron chelators over 5 years. *Ann Hematol* 2016;**95**(5):757–763.

70. Pafumi C, Farina M, Pernicone G, *et al.* At term pregnancies in transfusion-dependent beta-thalassemic women. *Clin Exp Obstet Gynecol* 2000;**27**:185–187.

71. Skordis N, Christou S, Koliou M, Pavlides N, Angastiniotis M. Fertility in female patients with thalassemia. *J Pediatr Endocrinol Metab* 1998;**11** (Suppl 3):935–943.

72. Karagiorga-Lagana M. Fertility in thalassemia: the Greek experience. *J Pediatr Endocrinol Metab* 1998;**11**(Suppl 3):945–951.

73. Cunningham MJ, Macklin EA, Muraca G, Neufeld EJ. Successful pregnancy in thalassemia major women in the Thalassemia Clinical Research Network. *Pediatr Res* 2004;**55**:294A.

74. Tuck SM. Fertility and pregnancy in thalassemia major. *Ann N Y Acad Sci* 2005;**1054**:300–307.

75. Bajoria R, Chatterjee R. Current perspectives of fertility and pregnancy in thalassemia. *Hemoglobin* 2009;**33**(Suppl 1):S131–S135.

76. Origa R, Piga A, Quarta G, *et al.* Pregnancy and β-thalassemia: an Italian multicenter experience. *Haematologica* 2010;**95**(3):376–381.

77. Dungan HM, Clifton DK, Steiner RA. Minireview: kisspeptin neurons as central processors in the regulation of gonadotropin-releasing hormone secretion. *Endocrinology* 2006;**147**:1154–1158.

78. Lee JH, Miele ME, Hicks DJ, *et al.* KiSS-1, a novel human malignant melanoma metastasis-suppressor gene. *J Natl Cancer Inst* 1996;**88**:1731–1737.

79. Tena-Sempere M. Kisspeptin signaling in the brain: recent developments and future challenges. *Mol Cell Endocrinol* 2010;**314**:164–169.

80. Reynolds RM, Logie JJ, Roseweir AK, McKnight AJ, Millar RP. A role for kisspeptins in pregnancy: facts and speculations. *Reproduction* 2009;**138**:1–7.

81. Thompson EL, Patterson M, Murphy KG, *et al.* Central and peripheral administration of kisspeptin-10 stimulates the hypothalamic-pituitary-gonadal axis. *J Neuroendocrinol* 2004;**16**:850–858.

82. Dhillo WS, Chaudhri OB, Thompson EL, *et al.* Kisspeptin-54 stimulates gonadotropin release most potently during the preovulatory phase of the menstrual cycle in women. *J Clin Endocrinol Metab* 2007;**92**:3958–3966.

83. Roa J, Aguilar E, Dieguez C, Pinilla L, Tena-Sempere M. New frontiers in kisspeptin/GPR54 physiology as fundamental gatekeepers of reproductive function. *Front Neuroendocrinol* 2008;**29**:48–69.

84. Dekel N. Master regulators of female infertility. *N Engl J Med* 2009;**361**:718–719.

85. Fan HY, Liu Z, Shimada M, *et al.* MAPK3/1 (ERK1/2) in ovarian granulosa cells are essential for female fertility. *Science* 2009;**324**:938–941.

86. Xekouki P, Tolis G. Ovulation induction for hypogonadotropic hypogonadism. In: Aboulghar M, Rizk B, eds. *Ovarian Stimulation.* Cambridge: Cambridge University Press; 2011:162–172.

Chapter

23

Hyperprolactinemia

Botros Rizk, Natalie L. Shammas, Shima AlBakhit, Ahmet Helvacioglu, and Shannon Gilmore

Introduction

Prolactin is a polypeptide hormone that was discovered more than 70 years ago and is also known as the lactogenic hormone, lactotropin, luteotropic hormone, or luteotropin [1]. It was initially thought that it is only produced by the anterior pituitary gland and mainly involved with lactation, but increasing evidence suggests that there are other sources of prolactin and that it is involved in diverse essential biological activities [2].

Embryology of Lactotrophs

Prolactin is mainly produced by the pituitary lactotrophs, which comprise 15–25 percent of the anterior pituitary [3]. During embryological development, the anterior pituitary (adenohypophysis) arises from Rathke's pouch (named after the German embryologist and anatomist Martin Heinrich Rathke 1793–1860). Rathke's pouch is an ectodermal outpouching of the floor of the primitive mouth that grows upwards and later fuses with the posterior pituitary (neurohypophysis) that develops as a downward extension from the neuroectoderm of the diencephalon [4;5].

Several homeodomain transcription factors are released during the development of the anterior pituitary and are important in the gene activation and cell-lineage differentiation. The most important is Pit-1, which is necessary

for the activation of prolactin (PRL), growth hormone (GH), growth hormone-releasing hormone (GHRH), and thyroid-stimulating hormone (TSH) genes. Modulation of Pit-1 via acetylation or phosphorylation can increase or decrease PRL expression on lactotrophs [6]. Congenital absence of Pit-1 gene causes a syndrome characterized by deficiency of lactotrophs, somatotrophs, and thyrotrophs [3;7;8].

Prolactin Biosynthesis

PRL is a 199-amino acid single polypeptide chain with a very similar structure to that of GH and hPL (human placental lactogen). It is encoded by a single gene located on the short arm of chromosome 6 that has an overall length of approximately 10 kb and consists of five exons separated by four introns. Recently, an additional exon 1a has been described (Figure 23.1).

PRL gene belongs to the PRL/GH/hPL group of genes that are structurally similar to each other and are known as group I helix bundle protein hormones. It is believed that all of these protein hormones evolved from a common ancestral gene by duplication [9;10]. For example, although GH and hPL share an 85% sequence homology, these two hormones only share a 21% and 22% homology with hPRL (human prolactin), respectively [11]. The low sequence homologies between

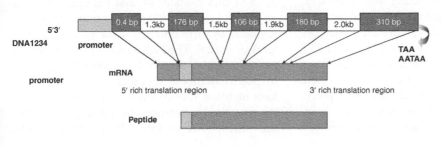

Figure 23.1 Prolactin gene transcription.

hPRL and GH or hPL yield unique chemical binding surfaces for other molecules to bind to these lactogens [11].

Recently, the PRL/GH/hPL family was also linked to another extended family of proteins known as the hematopoietic cytokines, which triggered a controversy on whether PRL should be considered as a cytokine or a hormone. This is based on the fact that the PRL structure is very similar to the hematopoietic cytokines and its receptor, as will be mentioned later, belongs to the cytokine receptor superfamily, along with the fact that there is evidence that PRL seems to have an immune modulatory effect [5;12].

The 5′ flanking region contains two independent promoter regions. The proximal 5000-bp region is known as a pituitary promoter, which directs pituitary-specific expression, while a more upstream promoter region of 3000 bp is known as the extrapituitary promoter and is responsible for extrapituitary expression [13;14]. Various hormones can bind to and consequently alter the rate of PRL gene expression such as estrogen, DA (dopamine), TRH (thyrotropin-releasing hormone), VIP (vasoactive intestinal peptide), and so on. The mature PRL mRNA is only 1 kb long, which undergoes translation to yield the final PRL molecule [15;16]. Further posttranslational modifications occur (cleavage, glycosylation, phosphorylation, and polymerization), which are usually detrimental to the PRL molecule as they lead to reduced bioavailability and accelerated proteolytic cleavage [17].

Prolactin Structure

PRL is an all-α-helix protein. The protein consists of four long helices folded into a parallel bundle with an up-up-down-down pattern [11]. As mentioned above, this type of three-dimensional structure places hPRL into a group with the long-helix-bundle cytokines, which include GH and hPL. The three-dimensional structure of hPRL was recently recognized using the homology-modeling approach, based on the crystallographic coordinates of porcine GH (Figure 23.2) [4;10;18].

There is a wide heterogeneity in the final PRL product, but it is mostly in a monomeric form (90%), less commonly diametric (8%), or seldom polymeric (2%). It appears that the most potent biological form of PRL is the 23-kD non-glycosylated form, while usually the larger polymers

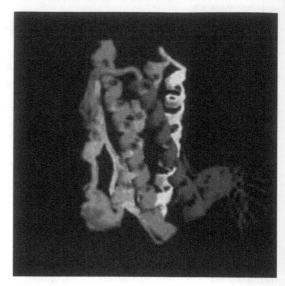

Figure 23.2 Prolactin molecule.

have reduced receptor affinity and lower bioactivity. Macroprolactinemia refers to the condition when most of the elevated prolactin is due to the presence of these large polymers also known as big PRL (50 kD) or big-big PRL (> 150 kD) [17]. The high molecular weight PRL consists of an antigen–antibody complex of monomeric PRL and IgG [19]. Even though these polymers have reduced in vivo activity, they are still detected by the conventional laboratory assays that explain the normal reproductive functions in many women with macroprolactinemia. Macroprolactinemia is a common condition reported in 10–46 percent of patients with hyperprolactinemia, which will be expanded on later in the chapter [20–22].

Prolactin Receptors

The PRL receptor is a transmembrane receptor belonging to class 1 of the cytokine receptor superfamily composed of three major domains: extracellular, transmembrane, and intracellular [11]. It is encoded by a gene on chromosome 5p13-14 that contains at least ten exons and has an overall length of 100 kb. It is transcriptionally regulated by three different tissue-specific promoter regions [20]. The PRL receptor exists in several isoforms, which are produced via RNA splicing, or posttranslational modifications. All isoforms have identical transmembrane domains, whereas the structural differences are witnessed in either the extracellular or intracellular domains [11].

Single amino acid mutations of the PRL receptor are associated with functional changes [11].

The receptor has close gross structural similarity to GH receptors and is composed of an extracellular region (that binds PRL), a single transmembrane region, and a cytoplasmatic region [21]. Numerous PRL receptor isoforms have been described in different tissues. Splicing of the intracellular domain creates the long-form activating receptor and at least eight other short variants, which usually vary in the length and composition of their cytoplasmic domain while their extracellular domain is usually identical [12,22]. These various forms of the receptor occur due to alternative splicing of pre-mRNA. In addition to the membrane-anchored PRL receptors, there is a soluble isoform (known as PRL receptor-binding protein) that is generated by proteolytic cleavage of membrane-bound PRL receptor [23;24]. Extracellular domains have been found in the blood, and are suggested to buffer fast changes in free hPRL concentration [11].

PRL receptors can also bind GH and hPL, which might explain the less severe phenotypes observed in PRL knockout mice compared to PRL receptor knockout mice [25].

PRL receptors are widely expressed by different cells including the pituitary, breast, liver, pancreas, brain, adrenal cortex, lungs, prostate, epididymis, ovary, and lymphocytes [26].

Prolactin Secretion

PRL release does not depend entirely on the nursing stimulus but is also affected by other stimuli such as light, stress, olfaction, and audition. It is released in a pulsatile pattern with pulse frequency ranging between 14 pulses per day in the late follicular phase to 9 pulses per day in the late luteal phase. Each pulse normally lasts for approximately 70 minutes, with interpulse interval of approximately 90 minutes [27].

PRL is produced in both the anterior pituitary and in numerous tissues throughout the human body. It can be generated in the endometrium, brain, breast, skin, lymphocytes, and adipocytes. Due to its widespread production throughout the body, it has been shown to function in many processes such as reproduction, metabolism, immunology, and pathologically in cancer. Hormones, cytokines, and steroids all modulate PRL expression throughout tissues in the body [6]. The PRL level in the body is a combination of positive and negative feedback systems throughout many organ systems.

There is also a diurnal variation, with the lowest levels occurring midmorning after the subject awakes and the highest levels during sleep. Levels starts to rise one hour after the onset of sleep and continue to rise until peak values are reached between 5:00 A.M. and 7:00 A.M. (Figure 23.3). Most of the rise occurs in REM sleep and then falls again prior to the next period of REM sleep. This circadian rhythm is generated by the suprachiasmatic nuclei of the hypothalamus. The pulse amplitude of PRL appears to increase from early to late follicular and luteal phases due to increased levels of estrogens, which promote the release of PRL [28].

PRL secretion could also be induced by acute stress and exercise just as adrenocorticotropic hormone and GH are. The stress-induced rise usually doubles or triples the PRL basal level for a short period of time and then drops back again

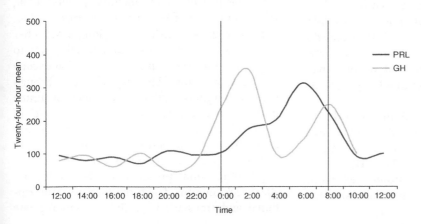

Figure 23.3 Circadian rhythm of PRL versus GH.

within 1–2 hours. On the contrary, chronic stress and high exercise level do not result in chronic elevation of the PRL basal levels [29;30].

Due to such variability of secretion along with the inherent limitations of radioimmunoassay, any elevated levels should always be rechecked and specimens should preferably be drawn mid-morning and not after stress, venipuncture, breast stimulation, or physical examination, which all increase PRL levels.

Neuroendocrine Regulation of Prolactin Secretion

PRL has unique features that separate it from other hormones released from the anterior pituitary. In contrast to other anterior pituitary hormones, which are controlled by hypothalamic releasing factors, PRL is normally under the tonic inhibitory effect of DA, which is known as the PRL inhibitory factor (PIF) [31]. PRL also targets numerous cell types, whereas most hormones have a specific neuroendocrine target.

Prolactin secretion is regulated by the tuberoinfundibular, tuberohypophyseal, and periventricular hypophyseal dopaminergic neurons in the hypothalamus. DA, otherwise known as PIF, circulates through the pituitary portal blood vessels where it eventually binds to type-2 DA receptors on lactotrophs, and inhibits PRL secretion from the anterior pituitary [32].

PRL also acts as a negative feedback on its own secretion, either directly through inhibiting the lactotrophs on dopaminergic neurons or indirectly through stimulating the neuroendocrine dopaminergic neurons. They also can stimulate gene expression and/or phosphorylation of tyrosine hydroxylase, which is the rate-limiting enzyme in DA production in dopaminergic neurons [33].

One other hormone that could have an inhibitory effect on the secretion of PRL is gonadotropin-releasing hormone (GnRH)-associated peptide (GAP), a 56-amino acid peptide chain derived from the carboxyterminal region of the GnRH precursor [34].

In addition to the tonic inhibition by PIF, PRL secretion is positively regulated by other hormones known as the PRL-releasing factors (PRFs): estrogens, TRH, GnRH, GHRH, VIP, angiotensin II, and peptide histidine methionine, which is a VIP precursor with similar structure [35–38].

Estrogens are key regulators of PRL production as they enhance the growth of PRL-producing cells and stimulate PRL production either directly through activating the PRL gene or indirectly through suppressing DA. It also seems that the stimulatory effect of GnRH on PRL is dependent on the estrogen level. It has been shown that peak PRL release from lactotrophs occurs during the periovulatory period. Analysis of PRL and luteinizing hormone (LH) secretory pulses showed a high degree of concordance, suggesting a common stimulus that is probably GnRH [39;40].

Serotonin likely mediates the nocturnal surge of PRL along with participating in the suckling-induced rise in PRL through the ascending serotonergic pathways from the dorsal raphe nucleus [37–41].

VIP has both a paracrine and an autocrine effect on PRL. VIP is synthesized in the paraventricular nucleus of the hypothalamus and is transported via the neuronal axons to the median eminence where it promotes PRL secretion (paracrine effect). The autocrine effect is achieved by VIP that is synthesized by the anterior pituitary itself [38].

Recent studies also revealed the presence of a 31-amino acid peptide, which results in PRL release and hence is called PRL-releasing peptide [28]. This peptide is released from neurons in the paraventricular and supraoptic nuclei of the hypothalamus and transported via nerve axons to the median eminence [42].

Primary Effect of Prolactin

PRL exerts many physiological functions, perhaps the most prominent of which is inducing lobuloalveolar growth of the mammary gland along with stimulation of lactogenesis or milk production after giving birth. PRL, along with other hormones such as cortisol and insulin, acts to induce the transcription of the genes that encode for milk proteins. This is achieved through increased arginase activity, stimulated ornithine decarboxylase activity, and enhanced rate of transport of polyamines into the mammary gland. All result in increased spermine and spermidine synthesis (polyamines), which are required for milk production. The polyamines stabilize membrane structures, increase transcriptional and translational activities, and regulate enzymes. PRL also elicits increased synthesis of casein, lactose, and phospholipids, which are all required for lactation [43;44].

During pregnancy, progesterone interferes with PRL's action at the receptor level. While estrogen and progesterone are required to attain full activity of the PRL receptor, progesterone antagonizes the positive action of PRL on its receptor by inhibiting upregulation of the PRL receptor, reducing estrogen binding (lactogenic activity), and competing for binding at the glucocorticoid receptors. Lactation occurs after birth due to the release of progesterone inhibition, which is more rapidly cleared from the maternal serum after delivery in contrast to PRL. It takes approximately seven days for PRL to reach nonpregnant levels, while estrogen and progesterone elevations are cleared in three to four days postpartum [45;46].

In males, PRL seems to provide the body with sexual gratification after sexual acts and is responsible for the male's refractory period. It is believed that PRL represses the effect of DA, which is normally responsible for sexual arousal. Accordingly, the amount of PRL could be used as an indicator for the amount of sexual satisfaction and relaxation [47].

PRL is also thought to have trophic effects on the male prostate gland, which includes proliferative and differentiation effects, and regulatory effects on the secretory activity of the prostate gland [48]. It is found in high concentrations in semen and is very important for spermatozoa metabolism, which includes glucose oxidation, fructose utilization, and glycolysis [49;50].

Other Sources and Functions of Prolactin

PRL is secreted by a broad range of other cells in the body, including mammary glands, immune cells, different brain cells, and the decidua of the pregnant uterus. Still, these tissues are probably modulated rather than strictly dependent on PRL.

The pituitary gland increases in size during pregnancy secondary to multiplying lactotrophs in the anterior lobe. Serum PRL levels markedly increase in the first trimester of pregnancy, up to 10 times higher than the levels when the mother is at term. It is postulated that the elevated PRL levels are due to extremely increased serum estradiol concentration [51].

The decidual cells produce large amounts of PRL during pregnancy. The PRL level in the amniotic fluid is usually 10- to 100-fold higher than the maternal serum level. The exact function of PRL during this time is not entirely clear; however, there is evidence that it may contribute to the osmoregulation of the amniotic fluid, uterine contractility, and immune modulation during pregnancy [52;53].

In addition to uptaking PRL from the blood, the mammary epithelial cells of lactating animals also synthesize PRL. Experimental studies on rats have shown that approximately 20 percent of the PRL ingested in milk passes to the neonatal circulation and that milk PRL participates in the maturation of their neuroendocrine and immune systems.

PRL acts as a cytokine and plays an important role in the immune system. It is produced by lymphocytes, which suggests that it may act as an autocrine or paracrine modulator of immune activity [54–56]. Increased stress in early pregnancy suppresses production of progesterone and PRL. This can potentially alter the protective cytokines and immune response that occurs in pregnancy [57].

Immunoreactivity studies have shown that PRL is also produced by different parts of the brain such as the hypothalamus, brain stem, cerebellum, spinal cord, caudate putamin, amygdala, hippocampus, and the choroid plexus, though its exact role is not clear yet [58].

It had long been known that PRL, GH, and hPL all have in vivo and in vitro angiogenic effects, but what is more surprising is that the proteolytic fragments of native PRL have antiangiogenic properties. This antiangiogenic activity is inherent to both the N-terminal 16-kD fragment and the 14-kD fragment. These fragments were shown to bind to certain sites on the capillary endothelium and prevent angiogenesis [59–61].

Some studies showed that the number of PRL receptors is increased in breast and prostate cancer cells. This suggests that PRL plays a role in tumor growth [62–65].

Currently, this 16-kD PRL and its protease (cathepsin) are being investigated in breast cancer research [66].

Hyperprolactinemia and Infertility

PRL excess can have a detrimental effect on the reproductive potential both in men and women through its effect on various points of the hypothalamic–pituitary–gonadal axis. In women, PRL values vary widely [67]. Increased PRL levels usually present with menstrual irregularities, galactorrhea, or simply infertility in the absence of the former two symptoms. In men, it can cause impotence, diminished libido, galactorrhea, or abnormal semen analysis (decreased count and increased abnormal morphology). Elevated levels of PRL decrease the pulsatile release of GnRH from the hypothalamic neurons by binding to PRL receptors on these neurons. Consequently, this results in reduced pulsatile LH release from the anterior pituitary. Hyperprolactinemia also decreases the numbers of GnRH receptors on the gonadotropins, and interferes with the positive estrogen feedback loop [68–70].

At the level of the gonads, the role of PRL is more obscure. Experimental studies have shown that PRL exerts a trophic effect on the corpus luteum of rats' ovaries, which does not seem to be the case in humans. Still, it is believed that normal levels of PRL are essential for estrogen and progesterone synthesis. On the contrary, PRL excess has a direct suppressive effect on estrogen synthesis through antagonizing the stimulatory effect of follicle-stimulating hormone (FSH) on aromatase activity [71–73].

PRL is also important for progesterone synthesis. Studies showed that when bromocriptine was given to euprolactinemic women, it resulted in a shorter luteal phase with a lower progesterone level than their controls. This seems to be due to the PRL stimulatory effect on progesterone synthesis through the induction of 3β-hydroxysteroid dehydrogenase, which is an essential enzyme in the progesterone synthesis pathway. However, many women with hyperprolactinemia were also found to have a short luteal phase [74;75].

Men with hyperprolactinemia show abnormal semen analysis secondary to PRL's effects on spermatogenesis. PRL receptors present on Sertoli and Leydig cells in the testes are inappropriately stimulated, producing hypogonadism and infertility [76]. The increased PRL levels can also cause abnormal histological structure of the testicles with distorted seminiferous tubules and abnormal Sertoli cells [77].

Hyperprolactinemia is also frequently reported in patients with polycystic ovarian syndrome (PCOS; 9–17%) [78]. Though the association between the two conditions is not clear, one study hypothesized that the pathogenesis of PCOS may be secondary to a central deficiency in dopaminergic activity at the level of the hypothalamus [79]. It is also believed that androgen excess in PCOS patients leads to higher free estradiol ratio due to reduced sex hormone-binding globulin (even though the total estradiol is not elevated), which in turn leads to PRL elevation. However, some studies argue against this association stating that such hyperprolactinemia is usually mild and transient and is probably coincidental rather than a pathogenically related phenomenon [79].

Causes of Hyperprolactinemia

The upper normal value for serum PRL in most laboratories is about 20 ng/ml (20 μg/L SI units). Many physiological and/or pathological changes involving lactotroph cells can result in hyperprolactinemia.

Physiological Causes

Basal serum PRL concentrations parallel the increase in serum estradiol concentrations throughout pregnancy, beginning at around seven to eight weeks of gestation and reaching a peak at delivery. The magnitude of the increase is quite variable, ranging from 35 to 600 ng/ml [80]. The mechanism for increased PRL levels in pregnancy is secondary to suppression of DA and direct stimulation of gene transcription in the pituitary by the high levels of estrogen [81;82]. Regardless of whether or not a mother breast-feeds, estradiol secretion decreases by six weeks postpartum, and the basal serum PRL concentration returns to normal. For this reason, contraception should begin as early as the third week postpartum. Nipple stimulation increases serum PRL concentrations via a neural pathway. Due to the preexisting lactotroph hyperplasia secondary to high estrogen levels during pregnancy, the serum PRL concentration increases up to a few hundred ng/ml above baseline in response to suckling in the first weeks of the postpartum phase. Several months after delivery, the lactotroph hyperplasia resolves, and the change in PRL due to suckling is less than 10 ng/ml [80]. Physical or psychological stress can also cause smaller increases in the serum PRL concentration, though values rarely exceed 40 ng/ml.

Women have greater increases than men, presumably due to the effect of their higher serum estradiol concentrations on the lactotroph cells.

Pathological Causes

Tumors of the lactotroph cell (prolactinomas), decreased dopaminergic inhibition of PRL secretion, and decreased clearance of PRL will all cause pathological hyperprolactinemia. Serum PRL concentrations in patients who have lactotroph adenomas can range from minimal elevation to 50 000 ng/ml; in hyperprolactinemia due to other causes, the concentrations rarely exceed 200 ng/ml [83].

Prolactinomas

Lactotroph adenomas otherwise known as prolactinomas are true neoplasms of the anterior pituitary. They arise from monoclonal expansion of a single cell that has undergone a somatic mutation [84;85]. The pituitary tumor-transforming gene is overexpressed in most lactotroph adenomas [86]. This gene appears to play a role in tumor invasiveness since its expression is increased in tumors that invade the sphenoid bone [86]. A truncated form of the receptor for fibroblast growth factor-4 has been identified in human pituitary adenomas. Transgenic mice that express this mutation develop lactotroph adenomas [87]. The majority of prolactinomas contain only lactotroph cells and produce excess PRL. About 10 percent of prolactinomas are made of both lactotroph and either somatotroph or somatomammotroph cells and secrete growth hormone as well [88].

Lactotroph adenomas are relatively common, accounting for approximately 30–40 percent of all clinically recognized pituitary adenomas and 10 percent of all intracranial neoplasms. The diagnosis is made more frequently in women than in men, especially in women of reproductive age [89] due to menstrual irregularities. However, adenomas that do occur in men are usually larger at the time of diagnosis, in part due to the lack of symptoms or delay in seeking medical attention for symptoms such as erectile dysfunction [90]. Most lactotroph adenomas are sporadic, but they can rarely occur as part of the multiple endocrine neoplasia type 1 syndrome [91]. There seems to be an association between female patients with prolactinomas and Hashimoto's thyroiditis [92]. A study suggested that PRL activates complement and antibody-dependent cytotoxicity, which may lead to a more rapid progression of Hashimoto's thyroiditis [92]. Almost all lactotroph tumors are benign but rarely can be malignant and metastasize [93]. PRL secretion by lactotroph adenomas varies with the adenoma size. Adenomas less than 1 cm in diameter are typically associated with serum PRL values below 200 ng/ml; 1.0–2.0 cm in diameter with values between 200 and 1000 ng/ml; and those greater than 2.0 cm in diameter with values above 1000 ng/ml. In less well-differentiated and largely cystic lactotroph adenomas, the size of the adenoma may not correlate well with the level of PRL. Due to an artifact in the immunoradiometric assay for PRL, the reported serum PRL concentration may be disproportionately low to the large size of the adenoma. This artifact, called the "hook effect," can be obviated by dilution of the sera, which will allow a true assessment of the PRL concentration [94–96].

CNS Causes

As pointed out earlier, PIF is normally released from the hypothalamic nuclei and inhibits PRL secretion. Any disease in or near the hypothalamus or pituitary that interferes with the secretion of DA or its delivery to the pituitary gland can cause hyperprolactinemia [83]. These include tumors of the hypothalamus, both benign (e.g., craniopharyngiomas) and malignant (e.g., metastatic breast carcinoma), infiltrative diseases of the hypothalamus (e.g., sarcoidosis), section of the hypothalamic–pituitary stalk (e.g., due to head trauma or surgery), and adenomas of the pituitary other than lactotroph adenomas.

Medications

A number of drugs cause hyperprolactinemia (Table 23.1). Many of these drugs raise serum PRL levels by functioning as DA D_2 receptor antagonists. These include antipsychotic drugs such as risperidone, phenothiazines, haloperidol [97], butyrophenones [98], metoclopramide [99], sulpiride [100], and domperidone [101]. Serum PRL concentrations increase within hours after acute administration of these drugs and return to normal within two to four days after cessation of chronic therapy [99]. The magnitude of the elevation varies according to the administered drug, that is, 17 ng/ml with the use of haloperidol compared to 80 ng/ml with risperidone [97].

Table 23.1 Pharmacological agents causing hyperprolactinemia

Typical antipsychotics	Gastrointestinal drugs
Phenothiazines	Metoclopramide
Thioridazine	Cimetidine
Clomipramine	
Fluphenazine	
Pimozide	
Prochlorperazine	
Atypical antipsychotics	**Antihypertensive agents**
Risperidone	Methyldopa
Olanzapine	Verapamil
Molindone	Reserpine
Antidepressant agents	**Opiates**
Clomipramine	Codeine
Desipramine	Morphine
Amitriptyline	
	Monoamine oxidase inhibitors
	Pargyline
	Clorgyline

Antihypertensive drugs such as methyldopa and reserpine increase PRL secretion by a similar mechanism. Methyldopa inhibits DA synthesis [102], while reserpine depletes DA stores [103]. Verapamil may raise serum PRL concentrations [104], but other calcium channel blockers do not [105]. The mechanism of this verapamil-induced increase is not known. The elevated serum PRL concentration returns to normal in all patients after the drug is stopped.

Selective serotonin reuptake inhibitors cause little if any increase in the serum PRL concentration. In one study [106], 20 mg of paroxetine a day did not increase the serum PRL concentration after one week but did cause a slight increase – only to high normal – after three weeks. In another study, patients who received fluoxetine chronically had a mean basal serum PRL concentration that was no different from that of untreated patients with similar diseases [107]. These drugs, in short, do not appear to cause clinically significant hyperprolactinemia.

Other Causes

TRH is a potent stimulant of PRL and could be labeled as PRF. Hypothyroidism predisposes to hyperprolactinemia due to elevated levels of TRH. However, basal serum PRL concentrations are normal in most hypothyroid patients [108], and only the serum PRL response to stimuli, such as TRH, is increased [109]. In the few hypothyroid patients who have elevated basal serum PRL concentrations, the values return to normal when the hypothyroidism is corrected [110;111]. It is important to recognize hypothyroidism as a potential cause of an enlarged pituitary gland (due to thyrotroph hyperplasia, lactotroph hyperplasia, or both) and hyperprolactinemia and not to confuse this entity with a lactotroph adenoma.

Chest wall injuries, such as severe burns, increase PRL secretion, presumably due to a neural mechanism similar to that of suckling [112]. The serum PRL concentration is high in patients who have chronic renal failure and returns to normal after renal transplantation [113]. The major mechanism is a threefold increase in PRL secretion, and a one-third decrease in metabolic clearance rate [114].

Occasionally, serum PRL concentration in some patients would range between 20 and 100 ng/ml, with no identifiable cause. Some studies showed that these patients may have microadenomas not visible on imaging studies and that in most of them the serum PRL concentrations change little during follow-up for several years [115–117] or even spontaneously decline during follow-up (in about 20 percent) [117].

Approximately 10 percent of elevated PRL levels are caused by macroprolactinemia due to decreased clearance of PRL. The elevated serum PRL concentration in these patients can be distinguished from hyperprolactinemia of other causes by gel filtration or polyethylene glycol precipitation [118–120].

Macroprolactinemia rarely has any effect on the reproductive potential of the patient. A study examined 1163 women that attended an infertility clinic during a period of one year. Symptoms related to elevated PRL levels were seen in 40–50 percent of women with macroprolactinomas, and up to 80–90 percent of patients with monomeric hyperprolactinemia [19]. Although patients with true hyperprolactinemia are more likely to present with oligomenorrhea, macroprolactinemic patients could not be differentiated from true hyperprolactinemic patients in this study [19]. It has been postulated that because of its larger size and decreased biological activity, a macroprolactinoma is less likely to cross the vascular endothelium and cause symptoms [19]. Thus, macroprolactinemia appears to be a benign clinical condition, and the only clinical significance of macroprolactinemia is when it is misdiagnosed and treated as ordinary hyperprolactinemia [121]. This can be avoided by asking the laboratory to pretreat the serum with polyethylene glycol to precipitate the macroprolactin before the immunoassay for PRL.

One study suggests that macroprolactin causes hyperprolactinemia secondary to its slow clearance rate rather than increased PRL production [19].

Clinical Manifestations and Diagnosis of Hyperprolactinemia

Infertility, oligomenorrhea, amenorrhea, galactorrhea, hot flashes, vaginal dryness, headaches, and visual changes are the clinical manifestations of hyperprolactinemia in premenopausal women. Hyperprolactinemia accounts for approximately 10–20 percent of cases of amenorrhea in nonpregnant women [122;123].

Hypogonadism

The release of GnRH is inhibited in hyperprolactinemia, causing decreased LH and FSH secretion, resulting in low serum gonadotropin concentrations and secondary hypogonadism.

The symptoms of hypogonadism due to hyperprolactinemia in premenopausal women directly correlate with the level of PRL. A serum PRL level above 15–20 ng/ml in most laboratories is considered high in women of reproductive age.

Levels above 100 ng/ml are typically associated with overt hypogonadism, causing amenorrhea, hot flashes, and vaginal dryness. Serum PRL levels of 50–100 ng/ml cause either amenorrhea or oligomenorrhea. Serum PRL levels of 20–50 ng/ml may cause only insufficient progesterone secretion, and, therefore, a short luteal phase of the menstrual cycle [124;125]. About 20 percent of those evaluated for infertility have luteal phase defect caused by subtle elevations of PRL, causing infertility even when there is no abnormality of the menstrual cycle.

Long-term negative health effects of hyperprolactinemia in women with amenorrhea include osteopenia and osteoporosis [126;127]. Decreased bone mass should be promptly diagnosed and managed, especially in adolescents with prolactinomas. Improvement in bone density after DA agonist therapy may not be enough alone to improve osteopenia [128]. Patients need close monitoring of bone density with appropriate supplementation of calcium, vitamin D, and rarely bisphosphonates.

Galactorrhea

Hyperprolactinemia in premenopausal women can cause galactorrhea, but most premenopausal women who have hyperprolactinemia do not have galactorrhea. In contrast, many women who have galactorrhea have normal serum PRL concentrations [94].

Elevated PRL levels are relatively difficult to diagnose in men and in postmenopausal women due to lack of clear and specific symptoms associated with hyperprolactinemia. Headaches or impaired vision due to the large size of lactotroph adenoma usually leads to the diagnosis of hyperprolactinemia in postmenopausal women. Because these women are markedly hypoestrogenemic, galactorrhea is rare.

Hyperprolactinemia in Men

Decreased libido, impotence, infertility, gynecomastia, and rarely galactorrhea [129;130] are the signs and symptoms of hyperprolactinemia in men caused by hypogonadotropic hypogonadism. As in women, there is a rough correlation between the presence of any of these symptoms and the degree of hyperprolactinemia. Hyperprolactinemia causes decreased testosterone secretion and low serum testosterone concentrations that are not associated with an increase in LH secretion [129]. As in women, the effect of prolactin is on the hypothalamic–pituitary centers. The consequences of the hypogonadism include, in the short term, decreased energy and libido, and in the long term, decreased muscle mass, body hair, and osteoporosis [131].

Hyperprolactinemia also causes erectile dysfunction in some men by a mechanism unrelated to hypogonadism because correcting the hyperprolactinemia with a DA agonist drug corrects the impotence, while correcting the hypogonadism by the administration of testosterone does not [131]. Hyperprolactinemia can infrequently cause infertility in men by decreasing LH and FSH secretions [130]. Men with hyperprolactinemia may develop galactorrhea although less often than in women. This is because the glandular breast tissue in men has not been made sensitive to PRL by precedent stimulation of estrogen and progesterone.

Evaluation

Oligomenorrhea, amenorrhea, infertility, or galactorrhea in women and hypogonadism, impotence, or infertility in men call for serum PRL determination. The evaluation is aimed at exclusion of pharmacological or extrapituitary causes of hyperprolactinemia and neuroradiological evaluation of the hypothalamic–pituitary region [132]. The usual normal range for serum PRL is 5–20 ng/ml (5–20 µg/L). The measurement can be performed at any time, but it is preferred to be done early in the morning since PRL concentrations may increase slightly during sleep, strenuous exercise, and occasionally as a result of emotional or physical stress, intense breast stimulation, and high-protein meals. A slightly high value (21–40 ng/ml) should be confirmed before the patient is considered to have hyperprolactinemia. A persistently elevated serum PRL value of any magnitude needs proper evaluation for etiology.

Serum PRL values between 20 and 200 ng/ml can be found in patients with any cause of hyperprolactinemia. Serum PRL values above 200 ng/ml usually indicate the presence of a lactotroph adenoma.

When there is a macroadenoma and the reported PRL levels are between 20 and 200 ng/ml, the assay should be repeated using a 1:100 dilution of serum. This is due to the fact that very high serum levels of PRL, for example, 5000 ng/ml produced by a large tumor, saturates both the capture and signal antibodies used in immunoradiometric and chemiluminescent assays, preventing the binding of the two in a "sandwich." The result is artifactually low values of PRL concentration due to this "hook effect" [94–96].

History

Pregnancy (physiological hyperprolactinemia), medications that can cause hyperprolactinemia (such as estrogen, neuroleptic drugs, metoclopramide, antidepressant drugs, cimetidine, methyldopa, reserpine, verapamil, and risperidone), headache, visual symptoms, symptoms of hypothyroidism, and a history of renal disease should be included in the history.

Physical Examination

Visual field examination to test for a chiasmal syndrome (e.g., bitemporal field loss), chest wall injury, and signs of hypothyroidism or hypogonadism should be evaluated.

Laboratory/Imaging Tests

TSH, BUN (blood urea nitrogen), creatinine, and creatinine clearance should be checked to test for hypothyroidism and renal insufficiency. Magnetic resonance imaging (MRI) of the head should be performed in patients with significant hyperprolactinemia to diagnose pituitary adenomas, except if the patient is taking a medication known to cause hyperprolactinemia, such as an antipsychotic drug, which typically causes the magnitude of the PRL elevation. There are no stimulatory or suppressive endocrine tests that distinguish among the causes of hyperprolactinemia.

If a mass lesion is found in the region of the sella turcica, secretion of other pituitary hormones should also be evaluated. Only a pituitary adenoma can cause hypersecretion of other pituitary hormones, but any mass lesion in the area of the sella can cause hyposecretion of one or more pituitary hormones.

If the MRI shows normal hypothalamic–pituitary anatomy and there is no other identifiable secondary cause of hyperprolactinemia, the diagnosis of idiopathic hyperprolactinemia is made. This syndrome may, in some patients, be due to microadenomas, which are too small to be seen on imaging.

Galactorrhea without Hyperprolactinemia

In almost half of the women who present with galactorrhea, the serum PRL concentration is going to be normal [83]. These women will have regular menses. Galactorrhea in the absence of hyperprolactinemia is not the result of any ongoing disease. Often it represents persistent milk secretion following correction of elevated PRL, most commonly after nursing or drug-induced hyperprolactinemia.

The first step in diagnosis is to be sure the breast secretion is clear or milky. If so, the next step is to measure the serum PRL concentration. If the PRL is elevated, the cause should be sought. If the PRL is not elevated, and there is no ongoing disease, then no further tests are needed. Green or black or bloody fluid is a reason for referral for evaluation of a breast tumor.

Galactorrhea in the absence of hyperprolactinemia does not need treatment. If galactorrhea occurs spontaneously and to a degree that causes staining of the clothes, treatment with a low dose of DA agonist, such as 0.25 mg of cabergoline twice a week, will reduce the PRL concentration to below normal and reduce or eliminate the galactorrhea.

Treatment of Hyperprolactinemia

DA agonists usually decrease both the secretion and size of lactotroph adenomas and, therefore, are the treatment of choice to achieve fertility, to relieve breast discomfort, reduce galactorrhea, and to restore ovarian function [115]. Surgery is recommended when a tumor continues to grow and cause visual impairment, despite treatment with DA agonists.

Lactotroph adenoma is called a microadenoma when it is less than 1 cm in diameter. Treatment of asymptomatic microadenomas is not necessary. Microadenomas rarely grow during pregnancy, very rarely progress to macroadenoma, recur significantly if operated upon, and maintain a natural course even if treated [115;133]. Unsuspected adenomas are found in almost 30 percent of pituitary glands in autopsy specimens [134–136]. If microadenoma size remains unchanged at one, two, and five years upon MRI assessments, no further studies are necessary but approximately 5 percent do enlarge during follow-up and these patients should be treated.

A lactotroph adenoma greater than 1 cm is called a macroadenoma. Once macroadenoma is diagnosed, a follow-up MRI should be ordered at six months, one, two, and five years. When the adenoma extends outside of the sella and compresses the optic chiasm or invades the cavernous or sphenoid sinuses or the clivus, treatment is needed. These patients will have neurological symptoms, such as visual impairment or headache. Lesions of this size are likely to continue to grow and eventually cause neurological symptoms.

Treatment of hyperprolactinemia is also indicated when it causes hypogonadism.

Medical Treatment

A DA agonist drug is first-line treatment for patients with hyperprolactinemia secondary to any cause, including lactotroph adenomas of all sizes [137]. The purpose of medical treatment is to normalize PRL levels, decrease the tumor mass, and reinstate eugonadism in the patient [138]. The DA agonists are generally split into two categories: ergot derivatives such as bromocriptine and cabergoline, and non-ergot derivatives such as quinagolide [138]. Following are the available DA agonists to treat hyperprolactinemia.

Bromocriptine

Bromocriptine mesylate is marketed under the trade name Parlodel, which comes in 5 mg capsule and 2.5 mg tablet forms. Therapeutic dosing varies between 2.5 and 15 mg/day [138]. However, most patients require 7.5 mg or less per day to attain a therapeutic response [138]. It has a shorter half-life than cabergoline, so it may need to be dosed multiple times per day, depending on the dose required.

Bromocriptine belongs to the class of antiparkinsonian and DA agonist drugs, and has been used for approximately two decades for treatment of hyperprolactinemia. Bromocriptine mesylate is a DA D_2 receptor agonist that activates the postsynaptic DA receptors to inhibit PRL secretions. It also stimulates DA receptors in the corpus striatum to improve motor functions. However, it also contains D_1 receptor antagonist features [138]. It is 90–96 percent protein bound and is completely metabolized. It is excreted 84.6 percent in the feces and 2.5–5.5 percent in urine.

Side effects of bromocriptine include headache, nausea, vomiting, and postural hypotension [138]. The starting dose is usually one-fourth of the maintenance dose to decrease the incidence of adverse effects. Once the patient becomes accustomed to the drug, the dose can be slowly titrated upward. Patients taking bromocriptine should be monitored for blood pressure and renal, liver, and hematopoietic functions. In peptic ulcer patients, signs and symptoms for gastrointestinal bleeding must be watched [137]. Bromocriptine is listed as category B during pregnancy and is excreted in small amounts in milk. The drug is contraindicated in postpartum women with coronary artery disease or other severe cardiovascular conditions and in patients with uncontrollable hypertension.

Cabergoline

Cabergoline is marketed under the trade name Dostinex and comes in 0.5 mg oral tablets. It is a long-acting selective DA receptor agonist, and unlike bromocriptine, which exhibits antagonistic properties to the D_1 receptor, cabergoline is a selective D_2 receptors agonist. It has low affinity for D_1, α_1 and α_2 adrenergic, and serotonin receptors. It inhibits the synthesis and release of PRL from the anterior pituitary by directly stimulating the D_2 receptors of the pituitary lactotrophs in a dose-related fashion.

The elimination half-life is between 63 and 69 hours, so it is generally dosed two times per week. The liver mainly metabolizes cabergoline. Sixty percent of the drug is excreted in the feces, 22 percent in the urine, and 4 percent is unchanged. The drug is considered as a category B during pregnancy and is secreted in milk in small amounts. Cabergoline is contraindicated in patients with uncontrolled hypertension. Patients need to be monitored with serial serum PRL measurements, blood pressure checks, and periodic liver function tests. Dose adjustment is needed in liver failure. It is administered once or twice a week and has much less tendency to cause nausea than bromocriptine and pergolide [139]. It may be effective in patients resistant to bromocriptine [140]. For patients with macroprolactinomas, treatment with cabergoline should be started at very low doses, 0.25 mg/week, to avoid rapid tumor shrinking and tumor hemorrhage [138].

Recently, researchers used cabergoline for prevention of ovarian hyperstimulation syndrome (OHSS). This condition can occur during ovulation induction therapy. A certain degree of ovarian hyperstimulation is required during induction therapy; however, excess ovarian stimulation leads to increased vascular permeability of the ovary and significant third spacing of fluid leading to pleural effusions, ascites, oliguria, and hypovolemia [136]. Cabergoline has been shown to prevent OHSS by inhibiting vascular endothelial growth factor receptor 2 phosphorylation, and vascular permeability (see Chapter 15 for the details of clinical trials) [141]. A prospective, randomized trial found that oocyte donors at high risk of developing moderate to severe OHSS were significantly less likely to develop OHSS when they received 0.5 mg cabergoline daily compared with placebo [142]. This study showed that patients who received cabergoline therapy showed significantly less ascites formation at different time points with a similar ovarian response compared with patients receiving the placebo [142].

Furthermore, a meta-analysis of eight randomized controlled trials demonstrated that cabergoline reduces the risk of OHSS, and does not negatively impact the number of retrieved oocytes [143]. It seems that the use of a DA receptor agonist provides a simple, safe, and effective alternative to mediate the risk of OHSS development during ovulation induction therapy.

Pergolide

Pergolide mesylate is marketed under the trade name Permax and comes as 0.05 mg, 0.25 mg, and 1 mg oral tablets. The FDA approved pergolide for the treatment of Parkinson's disease, but not for hyperprolactinemia [144]. It belongs to the antiparkinsonian and DA agonist class of drugs. Pergolide mesylate is an ergot derivative and a D_1 and D_2 receptor agonist, exerting direct stimulation on the postsynaptic DA receptors in the nigrostriatal system in patients with Parkinson's disease. It inhibits PRL secretion and causes a transient elevation in GH concentration and a reduced LH concentration. It is 90 percent protein bound and excreted 55 percent by the kidneys. The usual dosing for treatment of hyperprolactinemia is 0.025–0.6 mg PO once daily. Unlike bromocriptine, it can be taken once a day. It also costs about one-sixth as much as cabergoline. For example, a one-month starting-dose supply of pergolide costs $35 versus $235 for cabergoline, and $85 for bromocriptine.

Recently, the use of the DA agonists including pergolide and cabergoline was associated with an increased risk of newly diagnosed cardiac-valve regurgitation. The frequency of valve regurgitation was significantly higher in patients taking pergolide or cabergoline when compared with control subjects [145;146]. Such increased risk was not reported in patients taking non-ergot-derived DA agonists [147]. It is believed that because of the high affinity for the 5-HT (2B) serotonin receptors, which are expressed in heart valves, ergot-derived DA agonists can mediate mitogenesis leading to proliferation of fibroblasts. This ultimately causes fibrotic changes, thickening, retraction, and stiffening of valves, which result in incomplete leaflet coaptation and clinically significant regurgitation [148]. Further studies are needed to reveal whether these changes are reversible and whether they are dose or duration dependent. Due to these side effects on cardiac valves, pergolide was taken off the market in 2007 [138].

Quinagolide

Quinagolide is marketed under the trade name Norprolac and comes as 0.025 mg, 0.05 mg, 0.075 mg, and 1.5 mg oral tablets. It is a non-ergot DA agonist with selective affinity for the D_2 receptor [138]. It is given once daily, and is considered as effective as bromocriptine therapy [138]. A Cochrane review found that quinagolide is as effective as cabergoline as well [149]. This review also found that there is no association between the non-ergot derivatives, such as quinagolide, and cardiac-valve destruction [149]. These non-ergot derivatives may be useful alternatives in this regard. Quinagolide is approved for treatment of prolactinomas in Canada and some European countries. However, it is not available in the United States for this purpose.

Common Side Effects

Other side effects common to all DA agonist drugs include nausea, postural hypotension, mental fogginess, nasal congestion, depression, Raynaud phenomenon, alcohol intolerance, and constipation. Side effects are more likely to occur once treatment is initiated or when the dose is increased. They can be avoided in most patients by starting with a small dose such as 1.25 mg bromocriptine daily or 0.25 mg cabergoline twice a week and then gradually increasing the dose from there. Some patients experience side effects even at the lowest doses. Other formulations of bromocriptine were created in the hope of decreasing adverse effects. These included intramuscular injections, intranasal sprays, and vaginal creams [138]. Some studies suggest that nausea can be avoided by intravaginal administration [150;151]. Unfortunately, none of these bromocriptine formulas are currently available.

However, nausea is less frequently encountered with cabergoline compared with bromocriptine. Rare side effects include cerebrospinal fluid rhinorrhea during DA agonist treatment [149]. This typically only occurs for large lactotroph adenomas that extend inferiorly and invade the floor of the sella [152].

Therapeutic Efficacy

DA agonists decrease PRL secretion (Figure 23.4) and reduce the size of the lactotroph adenoma in more than 90 percent of patients. Both effects are mediated by binding of the drug to cell surface DA receptors, leading to reductions in the synthesis and secretion of PRL and in adenoma cell size. Cabergoline is better than bromocriptine in decreasing the serum PRL concentration [139;140;153]. If bromocriptine fails to normalize PRL levels, then the medication should be switched to cabergoline. Cabergoline treatment of individuals who have already been treated with bromocriptine or quinagolide has been shown to cause more shrinkage of a prolactinoma [138]. This was also seen in patients who were deemed resistant to DA agonists [138]. For example, at a median dose of 1 mg cabergoline weekly, 70 percent of the patients with visual field abnormalities returned to normal, and pituitary tumor size decreased in 67 percent of the 190 patients who had macroadenomas or microadenomas before treatment. The dose was later reduced to 0.5 mg weekly in 25 percent of patients with no increase in serum PRL concentrations. Cabergoline has also been shown to improve the fertility of male patients. It normalizes the sperm quality and improves sexual function in men [138]. Quinagolide appears to have equivalent therapeutic effects in reducing serum PRL and

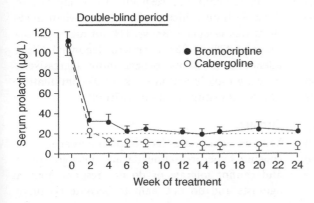

Figure 23.4 The effect of DA agonist drugs on serum prolactin concentration.

adenoma size [154;155]. The effect on adenoma size is most apparent in patients with lactotroph macroadenomas. The fall in serum PRL occurs within the first two to three weeks of therapy with a DA agonist [139]. The decrease in adenoma size, however, may take six weeks to six months [156]. Overall, the greater the decrease in serum PRL concentration, the greater the decrease in adenoma size, although there is considerable variation from patient to patient. Vision usually begins to improve within days after the initiation of treatment [156;157]. Women recover menses and fertility, and men regain testosterone secretion, sperm count, and erectile function [137;139;158–160]. Hypothyroid and/or hypoadrenal with macroadenomas may also recover these functions [161]. The therapeutic efficacy of DA agonists may be blunted by the concurrent use of drugs known to raise serum PRL concentrations, including neuroleptic drugs, metoclopramide, sulpiride, domperidone, methyldopa, reserpine, verapamil, and cimetidine.

Cabergoline is useful because it is most likely to be effective and least likely to cause side effects. The initial dose is 0.25 mg twice a week (the FDA-approved dose) or 0.5 mg once a week (a dose also reported to be effective). Although bromocriptine has classically been used for the treatment of infertility [162], data to date suggests that cabergoline is also safe in early pregnancy [163;164].

If the serum PRL concentration fails to return to normal and the patient has not experienced side effects, the DA agonist dose is gradually increased to 1.5 mg of cabergoline two or three times per week or 5 mg of bromocriptine twice a day. If the patient cannot tolerate the first DA agonist administered, another can be tried. If none of these approaches is effective, transsphenoidal surgery or ovulation induction with clomiphene (clomifene) citrate or gonadotropins can be considered. If fertility is not desired, estrogen and progesterone replacement can be considered.

Duration of Treatment

In cases of microadenoma, if the patient tolerates the DA agonist and the serum PRL eventually returns to normal, the drug should be continued until the patient becomes pregnant. After approximately one year, the dose can often be decreased. If the PRL has been normal for two or more years and no adenoma is seen on MRI, discontinuation of the drug can be considered and PRL monitored.

After menopause, the drug can be discontinued. Imaging should be performed if the value rises above 200 ng/ml to determine if the adenoma has enlarged. If so, drug therapy should be resumed.

In macroadenomas, visual field exam should be reassessed within one month of onset of therapy if vision was abnormal. Improvement may occur within a few days. An MRI should be repeated in 6–12 months to determine if the size of the adenoma has decreased. If the serum PRL concentration has been normal for at least one year and the adenoma has decreased markedly in size, the dose of the DA agonist can be decreased gradually, as long as the serum PRL remains normal [165]. Patients with an initial size of macroadenomas less than 1.5 cm, whose serum PRL concentrations have been normal for more than two years, and whose adenomas can no longer be visualized by MRI, may stop treatment. In contrast, discontinuation should not be considered if the adenoma was initially greater than 2 cm, if it is still visualized by MRI during treatment, or if the PRL level has normalized during treatment. The DA agonist should not be discontinued entirely, even after menopause, because hyperprolactinemia will probably recur and the adenoma may increase in size [166;167].

Withdrawal of Therapy

The risk of recurrent hyperprolactinemia or adenoma regrowth following discontinuation of the drug is low during two to five years of observation [166–168]. After two to five years of observation, hyperprolactinemia recurred in 24, 31, and 36 percent of patients with idiopathic hyperprolactinemia, microadenomas, and macroadenomas, respectively. In patients with adenomas, hyperprolactinemia was more likely to recur if an adenoma remnant was seen on MRI compared to those with no evidence of remnance when treatment was stopped (78% vs. 33% for macroadenomas and 42% vs. 26% for microadenomas). Giant adenomas (> 3 cm) behave more aggressively, growing rapidly within weeks of discontinuation of DA agonist medication [167;168].

Estrogen

Women who have lactotroph microadenomas causing hyperprolactinemia and hypogonadism and cannot tolerate or do not respond to DA agonists and do not want to become pregnant can be treated with estrogen and progestin. In reproductive age women, oral contraceptive pills, contraceptive patches, or contraceptive rings are possible options. In postreproductive age women, either hormone replacement therapy or non-hormonal bone-building medications should be considered. Estrogen is also a reasonable option for women with hyperprolactinemia and amenorrhea due to antipsychotic agents. Since estrogen treatment might pose a slight risk of increasing the size of the adenoma, the serum PRL concentration should be measured periodically in these patients. Estrogen should not be used as the sole treatment for lactotroph macroadenomas.

Surgical Treatment

Transsphenoidal surgery is indicated if the patient cannot tolerate medical treatment, or when DA agonists fail to lower serum PRL concentration or reduce the size of the adenoma. When a woman with a giant lactotroph adenoma (> 3 cm) wishes to become pregnant, even if the adenoma responds to a DA agonist, surgery should be considered to prevent aggressive growth of the adenoma during pregnancy.

Surgery is usually successful in substantially reducing serum PRL concentrations in patients with prolactinomas [169–171]. Cure rates with surgery can reach 80 to 90 percent for microadenomas, but are less than 50 percent for larger macroadenomas [171]. The lower cure rate for macroadenomas suggests an incomplete excision of the adenoma tissue [171]. Cure rates and safety outcomes are highly dependent on a surgeon's skill and experience [171]. When performed by experienced neurosurgeons, associated mortality is low at 0.2 percent, and complications such as, cerebrospinal fluid leak is also low at 1.4 percent [172]. Recurrence of the adenoma (50 percent at four years) and hyperprolactinemia (39 percent at five years) seems to be a shortcoming of surgical therapy [171;172]. A serum PRL concentration at or below 5 ng/ml on the first postoperative day suggests that the patient will be cured from the prolactinoma.

Radiation Therapy

Supervoltage radiation decreases the size and secretion of lactotroph adenomas, but normalization of PRL levels may take many years after treatment [173]. Radiation treatment is primarily used to prevent regrowth of a residual tumor in a patient with a very large macroadenoma after transsphenoidal debulking. Complications of radiation therapy include transient nausea, lassitude, loss of taste and smell, loss of scalp hair, possible damage to the optic nerve, and neurological dysfunction [173]. There is also a 50 percent chance of loss of anterior pituitary hormone secretion during the subsequent 10 years [173]. The risk of hypopituitarism is increased if the patient is treated with radiation therapy while also on medical therapy as well. It is advised that patients discontinue all medical treatment for prolactinomas one month prior to beginning radiation therapy [173].

Treatment of Hyperprolactinemia due to Other Causes

Treatment of hyperprolactinemia due to an abnormality other than a lactotroph adenoma varies depending on the cause. If hyperprolactinemia is the result of hypothyroidism, treatment of hypothyroidism will correct the problem. If hyperprolactinemia is a result of drug use, and the drug cannot be discontinued because it is essential and no substitute can be found, the resulting hypogonadism can be treated with the appropriate sex steroid. In women where antipsychotic medication use is the cause of hypogonadism, one should use a DA agonist cautiously because it might counteract the DA antagonist property of the antipsychotic drug. Another potential solution is to discuss with the treating psychiatrist the use of an antipsychotic drug that does not raise PRL, such as quetiapine (Seroquel).

References

1. Davis JR. Prolactin and reproductive medicine. *Curr Opin Obstet Gynecol* 2004;4:331–337.

2. Treier M, Gleiberman AS, O'Connell SM, *et al.* Multistep signaling requirements for pituitary organogenesis in vivo. *Genes Dev* 1998;**12** (11):1691–1704. http://www.genesdev.org/cgi/doi/10.1101/gad.12.11.1691.

3. Sharp ZD. Rat Pit-1 stimulates transcription in vitro by influencing pre-initiation complex assembly. *Biochem Biophys Res Commun* 1995;**206**(1):40–45.

4. Goffin V, Shiverick KT, Kelly PA, Martial JA. Sequence-function relationships within the expanding family of prolactin, growth hormone, placental lactogen and related proteins in mammals. *Endocr Rev* 1996;**17**(4):385–410.

5. Horseman ND, Yu-Lee LY. Transcriptional regulation by the helix bundle peptide hormones: growth hormone, prolactin, and hematopoietic cytokines. *Endocr Rev* 1994;**15**(5):627–649.

6. Featherstone K, White MR, Davis RJ. The prolactin gene: a paradigm of tissue-specific gene regulation with complex temporal transcription dynamics. *J Neuroendocrinol* 2012;**24**:977–990.

7. Cohen LE, Wondisford FE, Radovick S. Role of Pit-1 in the gene expression of growth hormone, prolactin, and thyrotropin. *Endocrinol Metab Clin North Am* 1996;**25**(3):523–540. https://linkinghub.elsevier.com/retrieve/pii/S088985290570339X.

8. González-Parra S, Chowen JA, Segura LMG, Argente J. Ontogeny of pituitary transcription factor-1 (Pit-1), growth hormone (GH) and prolactin (PRL) mRNA levels in male and female rats and the differential expression of Pit-1 in lactotrophs and somatotrophs. *J Neuroendocrinol* 1996;**8**(3):211–225. https://onlinelibrary.wiley.com/doi/abs/10.1046/j.1365-2826.1996.04526.x.

9. Nicoll CS, Mayer GL, Russell SM. Structural features of prolactins and growth hormones that can be related to their biological properties. *Endocr Rev* 1986;**7**(2):169–203. https://academic.oup.com/edrv/article-lookup/doi/10.1210/edrv-7-2-169.

10. Teilum K, Hoch JC, Goffin V, *et al.* Solution structure of human prolactin. *J Mol Biol* 2005;**351**(4):810–823.

11. Brooks CL. Molecular mechanisms of prolactin and its receptor. *Endocr Rev* 2012;**33**(4):504–525. https://academic.oup.com/edrv/article-lookup/doi/10.1210/er.2011-1040.

12. Bazan JF. Structural design and molecular evolution of a cytokine receptor superfamily. *Proc Natl Acad Sci U S A* 1990;**87**(18):6934–6938.

13. Berwaer M, Monget P, Peers B, *et al.* Multihormonal regulation of the human prolactin gene expression from 5000 bp of its upstream sequence. *Mol Cell Endocrinol* 1991;**80**(1–3):53–64.

14. Berwaer M, Martial JA, Davis JR. Characterization of an up-stream promoter directing extrapituitary expression of the human prolactin gene. *Mol Endocrinol* 1994;**8**(5):635–642.

15. Peers B, Voz ML, Monget P, *et al.* Regulatory elements controlling pituitary-specific expression of the human prolactin gene. *Mol Cell Biol* 1990;**10**(9):4690–4700.

16. Truong AT, Duez C, Belayew A, *et al.* Isolation and characterization of the human prolactin gene. *EMBO J* 1984;**3**(2):429–437. http://doi.wiley.com/10.1002/j.1460-2075.1984.tb01824.x.

17. Sinha YN. Structural variants of prolactin: occurrence and physiological significance. *Endocr Rev* 1995;**16**(3):354–369.

18. Keeler C, Dannies PS, Hodsdon ME. The tertiary structure and backbone dynamics of human prolactin. *J Mol Biol* 2003;**328**(5):1105–1121.

19. Thirunavakkarasu K, Dutta P, Sridhar S, *et al.* Macroprolactinemia in hyperprolactinemic infertile women. *Endocrine* 2013;**44**(3):750–755.

20. Bazan JF. Haemopoietic receptors and helical cytokines. *Immunol Today* 1990;**11**(11):350–354. https://linkinghub.elsevier.com/retrieve/pii/016756999090139Z.

21. Rizk B. Genetics of ovarian hyperstimulation syndrome. In: Rizk B, ed. *Ovarian Hyperstimulation Syndrome.* Cambridge: Cambridge University Press; 2006:79–91.

22. Schuler LA, Nagel RM, Gao J, Horseman ND, Kessler MA. Prolactin receptor heterogeneity in bovine fetal and maternal tissues. *Endocrinology* 1997;**138**(8):3187–3194.

23. Kline JB, Roehrs H, Clevenger CV. Functional characterization of the intermediate isoform of the human prolactin receptor. *J Biol Chem* 1999;**274**(50):35461–35468.

24. Trott J, Hovey R, Koduri S, Vonderhaar B. Alternative splicing to exon 11 of human prolactin receptor gene results in multiple isoforms including a secreted prolactin-binding protein. *J Mol Endocrinol* 2003;**30**:31–47. https://jme.bioscientifica.com/view/journals/jme/30/1/31.xml.

25. Herman A, Bignon C, Daniel N, Grosclaude J, Gertler A. Functional heterodimerization of prolactin and growth hormone receptors by ovine placental lactogen. *J Biol Chem* 2000;**275**:6295–301.

26. Bole-Feysot C, Goffin V, Edery M, Binart N, Kelly PA. Prolactin (PRL) and its receptor: actions, signal transduction pathways and phenotypes observed in PRL receptor knockout mice. *Endocr Rev* 1998;**19**(3):225–268. https://academic.oup.com/edrv/article-lookup/doi/10.1210/edrv.19.3.0334.

27. Veldhuis JD, Johnson ML. Operating characteristics of the hypothalamo-pituitary-gonadal axis in men: circadian, ultradian, and pulsatile release of prolactin and its temporal coupling with luteinizing hormone. *J Clin Endocrinol Metab* 1988;**67**(1):116–123.

28. Veldhuis JD, Evans WS, Stumpf PG. Mechanisms that subserve estradiol's induction of increased prolactin concentrations: evidence of amplitude modulation of spontaneous prolactin secretory

bursts. *Am J Obstet Gynecol* 1989;**161** (5):1149–1158.

29. Freeman ME, Kanyicska B, Lerant A, Nagy G. Prolactin: structure, function, and regulation of secretion. *Physiol Rev* 2000;**80**(4):1523–1631.

30. Van den Berghe G, de Zegher F, Veldhuis JD, *et al.* Thyrotrophin and prolactin release in prolonged critical illness: dynamics of spontaneous secretion and effects of growth hormone-secretagogues. *Clin Endocrinol (Oxf)* 1997;**47**(5):599–612.

31. Ben-Jonathan N. Dopamine: a prolactin-inhibiting hormone. *Endocr Rev* 1985;6 (4):564–589. https://academic.oup.com/edrv/ article-lookup/doi/10.1210/edrv-6-4-564.

32. Grattan DR, Kokay IC. Prolactin: a pleiotropic neuroendocrine hormone. *J Neuroendocrinol* 2008;**20**(6):752–763.

33. Grattan DR. The actions of prolactin in the brain during pregnancy and lactation. In: *Progress in Brain Research*, Vol. 133. Amsterdam: Elsevier; 2001:153–171.

34. Vacher P, Mariot P, Dufy-Barbe L, *et al.* The gonadotropin-releasing hormone associated peptide reduces calcium entry in prolactin-secreting cells. *Endocrinology* 1991;128 (1):285–294.

35. Steele MK. The role of brain angiotensin II in the regulation of luteinizing hormone and prolactin secretion. *Trends Endocrinol Metab* 1992;3 (8):295–301.

36. Steele MK, McCann SM, Negro-Vilar A. Modulation by dopamine and estradiol of the central effects of angiotensin II on anterior pituitary hormone release. *Endocrinology* 1982;111 (3):722–729. https://academic.oup.com/endo/ article-lookup/doi/10.1210/endo-111-3-722.

37. Ayala ME, Velázquez DE, Mendoza JL, *et al.* Dorsal and medial raphe nuclei participate differentially in reproductive functions of the male rat. *Reprod Biol Endocrinol* 2015;**13**(1):132. http:// www.rbej.com/content/13/1/132.

38. Dalcik H, Phelps CJ. Median eminence-afferent vasoactive intestinal peptide (VIP) neurons in the hypothalamus: localization by simultaneous tract tracing and immunocytochemistry. *Peptides* 1993;**14**(5):1059–1066.

39. Braund W, Roeger DC, Judd SJ. Synchronous secretion of luteinizing hormone and prolactin in the human luteal phase: neuroendocrine mechanisms. *J Clin Endocrinol Metab* 1984;**58** (2):293–297.

40. Christiansen E, Veldhuis JD, Rogol AD, Stumpf P. Evans WS. Modulating actions of estradiol on gonadotropin-releasing hormone-stimulated prolactin secretion in postmenopausal individuals. *Am J Obstet Gynecol* 1987;**157**(2):320–325.

41. De V, Kar LD, Bethea CL. Pharmacological evidence that serotonergic stimulation of prolactin secretion is mediated via the dorsal raphe nucleus. *Neuroendocrinology* 1982;**35**(4):225–230.

42. Takahashi K, Yoshinoya A, Arihara Z, *et al.* Regional distribution of immunoreactive prolactin-releasing peptide in the human brain. *Peptides* 2000;**21**(10):1551–1555.

43. Barber MC, Clegg RA, Finley E, Vernon RG, Flint DJ. The role of growth hormone, prolactin and insulin-like growth factors in the regulation of rat mammary gland and adipose tissue metabolism during lactation. *J Endocrinol* 1992;**135**(2):195–202.

44. Tucker HA. Hormones, mammary growth, and lactation: a 41-year perspective. *J Dairy Sci* 2000;**83** (4):874–884. https://www.researchgate.net/ publication/246637154_Lactation_and_its_ Hormonal_Control.

45. Whitworth N. Lactation in humans. *Psychoneuroendocrinology* 1988;13(1–2):171–188. https://linkinghub.elsevier.com/retrieve/pii/ 0306453088900133.

46. Speroff L, Glass RH, Kase NG. *Clinical Gynecologic Endocrinology and Infertility*, 6th ed. Baltimore, MD: Lippincott Williams & Wilkins; 1999.

47. Kruger TH, Haake P, Haverkamp J, *et al.* Effects of acute prolactin manipulation on sexual drive and function in males. *J Endocrinol* 2003;**179** (3):357–365.

48. Costello LC, Franklin RB. Effect of prolactin on the prostate. *Prostate* 1994;**24**(3):162–166.

49. Sheth AR, Mugatwala PP, Shah GV. Occurrence of prolactin in human semen. *Fertil Steril* 1975;26 (9):905–907.

50. Shah GV, Desai RB, Sheth AR. Effect of prolactin on metabolism of human spermatozoa. *Fertil Steril* 1976;**27**(11):1292–1294.

51. Soma-Pillay P, Nelson-Piercy C, Tolppanen H, *et al.* Physiological changes in pregnancy. *Cardiovasc J Afr* 2016;27(2):89–94.

52. Hernandez-Andrade E, Villanueva-Diaz C, Ahued-Ahued JR. Growth hormone and prolactin in maternal plasma and amniotic fluid during normal gestation. *Rev Invest Clin* 2005;**57** (5):671–675.

53. Shennan DB. Regulation of water and solute transport across mammalian plasma cell membranes by prolactin. *J Dairy Res* 1994;**61** (1):155–166.

54. Prolactin autoantibodies. In: *Autoantibodies*. E-book. Elsevier; 1996:400–402. https://linkin

ghub.elsevier.com/retrieve/pii/
B9780444823830500613.

55. Neidhart M. Prolactin in autoimmune diseases. *Exp Biol Med* 1998;**217**(4):408–419. http://ebm.sagepub.com/lookup/doi/10.3181/00379727-217-44251.

56. Walker SE, Allen SH, McMurray RW. Prolactin and autoimmune disease. *Trends Endocrinol Metab* 1993;**4**(5):147–151.

57. Egli M, Leeners B, Kruger TH. Prolactin secretion patterns: basic mechanisms and clinical implications for reproduction. *Reproduction* 2010;**140**(5):643–654.

58. Roky R, Paut-Pagano L, Goffin V, *et al.* Distribution of prolactin receptors in the rat forebrain. Immunohistochemical study. *Neuroendocrinology* 1996;**63**(5):422–429.

59. Clapp C, Martial JA, Guzman RC, Rentier-Delrue F, Weiner RI. The 16-kilodalton N-terminal fragment of human prolactin is a potent inhibitor of angiogenesis. *Endocrinology* 1993;**133** (3):1292–1299.

60. Clapp C, Torner L, Gutiérrez-Ospina G, *et al.* The prolactin gene is expressed in the hypothalamic-neurohypophyseal system and the protein is processed into a 14-kDa fragment with activity like 16-kDa prolactin. *Proc Natl Acad Sci U S A* 1994;**91**(22):10384–10388.

61. Clapp C, Weiner RI. A specific, high affinity, saturable binding site for the 16-kilodalton fragment of prolactin on capillary endothelial cells. *Endocrinology* 1992;**130**(3):1380–1386.

62. Lissoni P, Mandala M, Rovelli F, *et al.* Paradoxical stimulation of prolactin secretion by L-dopa in metastatic prostate cancer and its possible role in prostate-cancer-related hyperprolactinemia. *Eur Urol* 2000;**37**:569–572.

63. Leav I, Merk FB, Lee KF, *et al.* Prolactin receptor expression in the developing human prostate and in hyperplastic, dysplastic, and neoplastic lesions. *Am J Pathol* 1999;**154**(3):863–870. https://linkin ghub.elsevier.com/retrieve/pii/S0002944010653333.

64. Touraine P, Martini J-F, Zafrani B, *et al.* Increased expression of prolactin receptor gene assessed by quantitative polymerase chain reaction in human breast tumors versus normal breast tissues. *J Clin Endocrinol Metab* 1998;**83** (2):667–674. https://academic.oup.com/jcem/article/83/2/667/2865659.

65. Wennbo H, Gebre-Medhin M, Gritli-Linde A, *et al.* Activation of the prolactin receptor but not the growth hormone receptor is important for induction of mammary tumors in transgenic mice. *J Clin Invest* 1997;**100**(11):2744–2751.

66. Goffin V, Touraine P, Pichard C, Bernichtein S KP. Should prolactin be reconsidered as a therapeutic target in human breast cancer? *Mol Cell Endocrinol* 1999;**151**(1–2):79–87.

67. Eniola OW, Adetola AA, Abayomi BT. A review of female infertility; important etiological factors and management. *J Microbiol Biotechnol Res* 2017;**2** (3):379–385.

68. Cheung CY. Prolactin suppresses luteinizing hormone secretion and pituitary responsiveness to luteinizing hormone-releasing hormone by a direct action at the anterior pituitary. *Endocrinology* 1983;**113**(2):632–638.

69. Milenkovic L, D'Angelo G, Kelly PA, Weiner RI. Inhibition of gonadotropin hormone-releasing hormone release by prolactin from GIT neuronal cell lines through prolactin receptors. *Proc Natl Acad Sci U S A* 1994;**91**(4):1244–1247.

70. Glass MR, Shaw RW, Butt WR, Edwards RL, London DR. An abnormality of oestrogen feedback in amenorrhoea-galactorrhoea. *BMJ* 1975;**3**(5978):274–275. http://www.bmj.com/cgi/doi/10.1136/bmj.3.5978.274.

71. McNeilly KP, Glasier A, Jonassen J. Evidence for direct inhibition of ovarian function by prolactin. *J Reprod Fert* 1982;**65**:559–569.

72. Dorrington JH, Gore-Langton RE. Antigonadal action of prolactin: further studies on the mechanism of inhibition of follicle stimulating hormone-induced aromatase activity in rat granulosa cell cultures. *Endocrinology* 1982;**110** (5):1701–1707.

73. McNatty KP, Sawers RS, McNeilly AS. A possible role for prolactin in control of steroid secretion by human graffian follicle. *Nature* 1974;**250** (5468):653–655.

74. Del Pozo E, Wyss H, Tolis G, *et al.* Prolactin and deficient luteal function. *Obstet Gynecol* 1979;**53** (3):282–286.

75. Feltus FA, Groner B, Melner MH. Stat5-mediated regulation of the human type II 3a hydroxysteroid dehydrogenase isomerase gene activation by prolactin. *Mol Endocrinol* 1999;**13**(7):1084–1093.

76. Singh P, Singh M, Cugati G, Singh A. Hyperprolactinemia: an often missed cause of male infertility. *J Hum Reprod Sci* 2011;**4** (2):102–103.

77. Cameron DF, Murray FT, Drylie DD. Ultrastructural lesions in testes from hyperprolactinemic men. *J Androl* 1984;**5**(4):283–293.

78. Lee DY, Oh YK, Yoon BK, Choi D. Prevalence of hyperprolactinemia in adolescents and young women with menstruation-related problems. *Am J Obstet Gynecol* 2012;**206**(3):213.e1–213.e5.

79. Minakami H, Abe N, Oka N, *et al.* Prolactin release in polycystic ovarian syndrome. *Endocrinol Jpn* 1988;**35**(2):303–310.

80. Tyson JB, Ito P, Guyda H. Studies of prolactin in human pregnancy. *Am J Obstet Gynecol* 1972;**113**:14–20.

81. Tyson JE, Friesen HG. Factors influencing the secretion of human prolactin and growth hormone in menstrual and gestational women. *Am J Obstet Gynecol* 1973;**116**:377–387.

82. Barberia JM, Abu-Fadil S, Kletzky OA, Nakamura RM, Mishell DR Jr. Serum prolactin patterns in early human gestation. *Am J Obstet Gynecol* 1975;**121**:1107–1110.

83. Kleinberg DL, Noel GL, Frantz AG. Galactorrhea: a study of 235 cases, including 48 with pituitary tumors. *N Engl J Med* 1977;**296**(11):589–600. http://www.nejm.org/doi/abs/10.1056/NEJM197703172961103.

84. Alexander JM, Biller BMK, Bikkal H. Clinically nonfunctioning pituitary tumors are monoclonal in origin. *J Clin Invest* 1990;**86**(1):336–340.

85. Herman V, Fagin J, Gonsky R. Clonal origin of pituitary adenomas. *J Clin Endocrinol Metab* 1990;**71**(6):1427–1433.

86. Zhang X, Horwitz GA, Heaney AP. Pituitary tumor transforming gene (PTTG) expression in pituitary adenomas. *J Clin Endocrinol Metab* 1999;**84**(2):761–767.

87. Ezzat S, Zheng L, Zhu XF. Targeted expression of a human pituitary tumor-derived isoform of FGF receptor-4 recapitulates pituitary tumorigenesis. *J Clin Invest* 2002;**109**(1):69–78.

88. Corenblum B, Sirek AMT, Horvath E. Human mixed somatotrophic and lactotrophic pituitary adenomas. *J Clin Endocrinol Metab* 1976;**42**(5):857–863.

89. Mindermann T, Wilson CB. Age-related and gender-related occurrence of pituitary adenomas. *Clin Endocrinol (Oxf)* 1994;**41**(3):359–364. http://doi.wiley.com/10.1111/j.1365-2265.1994.tb02557.x.

90. Delgrange E, Trouillas J, Maiter D. Sex-related difference in the growth of prolactinomas: a clinical and proliferation marker study. *J Clin Endocrinol Metab* 1997;**82**(7):2102–2107.

91. Prosser PR, Karam JH, Townsend JJ, Forsham PH. Prolactin-secreting pituitary adenomas in multiple endocrine adenomatosis, type 1. *Ann Intern Med* 1979;**91**(1):41–44.

92. Elenkova A, Atanasova I, Kirilov G, *et al.* Autoimmune hypothyroidism is three times more frequent in female prolactinoma patients compared to healthy women: data from a cross-sectional case-control study. *Endocrine* 2017;**57**:486–493.

93. Walker JD, Grossman A, Anderson JV. Malignant prolactinoma with extracranial metastases: a report of three cases. *Clin Endocrinol (Oxf)* 1993;**38**(4):411–419.

94. Petakov MS, Damjanović SS, Nikolić-Durović MM, *et al.* Pituitary adenomas secreting large amounts of prolactin may give false low values in immunoradiometric assays. The hook effect. *J Endocrinol Invest* 1998;**21**(3):184–188. http://link.springer.com/10.1007/BF03347299.

95. St-Jean E, Blain F, Comtois R. High prolactin levels may be missed by immunoradiometric assay in patients with macroprolactinomas. *Clin Endocrinol (Oxf)* 1996;**44**(3):305–309.

96. Barkan AL, Chandler WF. Giant pituitary prolactinoma with falsely low serum prolactin: the pitfall of the "high-dose hook effect." *Neurosurgery* 1998;**42**(4):913–915.

97. David SR, Taylor CC, Kinon BJ, Breier A. The effects of olanzapine, risperidone, and haloperidol on plasma prolactin levels in patients with schizophrenia. *Clin Ther* 2000;**22**(9):1085–1096.

98. Rivera JL, Lal S, Ettigi P, *et al.* Effect of acute and chronic neuroleptic therapy on serum prolactin levels in men and women of different age groups. *Clin Endocrinol (Oxf)* 1976;**5**(3):273–282.

99. McCallum RW, Sowers JR, Hershman JM, Sturdevant RA. Metoclopramide stimulates prolactin secretion in man. *J Clin Endocrinol Metab* 1976;**42**(6):1148–1152.

100. Mancini AM, Guitelman A, Vargas CA, Debeljuk L, Aparicio NJ. Effect of sulpiride on serum prolactin levels in humans. *J Clin Endocrinol Metab* 1976;**42**(1):181–184. https://academic.oup.com/jcem/article-lookup/doi/10.1210/jcem-42-1-181.

101. Sowers JR, Sharp B, McCallum RW. Effect of domperidone, an extracerebral inhibitor of dopamine receptors, on thyrotropin, prolactin, renin, aldosterone, and 18-hydroxycorticosterone secretion in man. *J Clin Endocrinol Metab* 1982;**54**(4):869–871.

102. Steiner J, Cassar J, Mashiter K, *et al.* Effects of methyldopa on prolactin and growth hormone. *BMJ* 1976;**1**(6019):1186–1188. http://www.bmj.com/cgi/doi/10.1136/bmj.1.6019.1186.

103. Lee PA, Kelly MR, Wallin JD. Increased prolactin levels during reserpine treatment of hypertensive patients. *JAMA* 1976;**235**(21):2316–2317.

104. Fearrington EL, Rand CH, Rose JD. Hyperprolactinemia-galactorrhea induced by verapamil. *Am J Cardiol* 1983;**51**(8):1466–7. https://linkinghub.elsevier.com/retrieve/pii/0002914983903363.

105. Veldhuis JD, Borges JLC, Drake CR, *et al.* Divergent influences of the structurally dissimilar calcium entry blockers, diltiazem and verapamil, on the thyrotropin-and gonadotropin-releasing hormone-stimulated anterior pituitary hormone secretion in man. *J Clin Endocrinol Metab* 1985;**60**(1):144–149.

106. Cowen PJ, Sargent PA. Changes in plasma prolactin during SSRI treatment: evidence for a delayed increase in 5-HT neurotransmission. *J Psychopharmacol* 1997;**11**(4):345–348. http://journals.sagepub.com/doi/10.1177/026988119701100410.

107. Meltzer H, Bastani B, Jayathilake K, Maes M. Fluoxetine, but not tricyclic antidepressants, potentiates the 5-hydroxytryptophan-mediated increase in plasma cortisol and prolactin secretion in subjects with major depression or with obsessive compulsive disorder. *Neuropsychopharmacology* 1997;**17**(1):1–11.

108. Honbo KS, van Herle AJ, Kellett KA. Serum prolactin levels in untreated primary hypothyroidism. *Am J Med* 1978;**64**(5):782–787.

109. Snyder PJ, Jacobs LS, Utiger RD, Daughaday WH. Thyroid hormone inhibition of the prolactin response to thyrotropin-releasing hormone. *J Clin Invest.* 1973;**52**(9):2324–2329.

110. Groff TR, Shulkin BL, Utiger RD, Talbert LM. Amenorrhea-galactorrhea, hyperprolactinemia, and suprasellar pituitary enlargement as presenting features of primary hypothyroidism. *Obstet Gynecol* 1984;**63**(3 Suppl):86S–89S.

111. Grubb MR, Chakeres D, Malarkey WB. Patients with primary hypothyroidism presenting as prolactinomas. *Am J Med* 1987;**83**(4):765–769.

112. Morley JE, Hodgkinson DH, Kalk WJ. Galactorrhea and hyperprolactinemia associated with chest wall injury. *J Clin Endocrinol Metab* 1977;**45**(5):931–935.

113. Lim VS, Kathpalia SC, Frohman LA. Hyperprolactinemia and impaired pituitary response to suppression and stimulation in chronic renal failure: reversal after transplantation. *J Clin Endocrinol Metab* 1979;**48**(1):101–107.

114. Sievertsen GD, Lim VS, Nakawatase C, Frohman LA. Metabolic clearance and secretion rates of human prolactin in normal subjects and patients with chronic renal failure. *J Clin Endocrinol Metab* 1980;**50**(5):846–852.

115. Schlechte J, Dolan K, Sherman B, Chapler F, Luciano A. The natural history of untreated hyperprolactinemia: a prospective analysis. *J Clin Endocrinol Metab* 1989;**68**(2):412–418. https://academic.oup.com/jcem/article-lookup/doi/10.1210/jcem-68-2-412.

116. Martin TL, Kim M, Malarkey WB. The natural history of idiopathic hyperprolactinemia. *J Clin Endocrinol Metab* 1985;**60**:855–888.

117. Sluijmer AV, Lappöhn LR. Clinical history and outcome of 59 patients with idiopathic hyperprolactinemia. *Fertil Steril* 1992;**58**(1):72–77.

118. Carlson HE, Markoff E, Lee DW. On the nature of serum prolactin in two patients with macroprolactinemia. *Fertil Steril* 1992;**58**:78–87.

119. Vallette-Kasic S, Morange-Ramos I, Selim A, *et al.* Macroprolactinemia revisited: a study on 106 patients. *J Clin Endocrinol Metab* 2002;**87**(2):581–588. https://academic.oup.com/jcem/article-lookup/doi/10.1210/jcem.87.2.8272.

120. Olukoga AO, Kane JW. Macroprolactinaemia: validation and application of the polyethylene glycol precipitation test and clinical characterization of the condition. *Clin Endocrinol (Oxf)* 1999;**51**(1):119–126.

121. Gibney J, Smith TP, McKenna TJ. Clinical relevance of macroprolactin. *Clin Endocrinol (Oxf)* 2005;**62**(6):633–643. http://doi.wiley.com/10.1111/j.1365-2265.2005.02243.x.

122. Gomez F, Reyes FI, Faiman C. Nonpuerperal galactorrhea and hyperprolactinemia. Clinical findings, endocrine features and therapeutic responses in 56 cases. *Am J Med* 1977;**62**(5):648–660.

123. Schlechte J, Sherman B, Halmi N, *et al.* Prolactin-secreting pituitary tumors in amenorrheic women: a comprehensive study. *Endocr Rev* 1980;**1**(3):295–308. https://academic.oup.com/edrv/article-lookup/doi/10.1210/edrv-1-3-295.

124. Seppälä M, Ranta T, Hirvonen E. Hyperprolactinæmia and luteal insufficiency. *Lancet* 1976;**307**(7953):229–230. https://linkinghub.elsevier.com/retrieve/pii/S014067367691343X.

125. Corenblum B, Pairaudeau N, Shewchuk AB. Prolactin hypersecretion and short luteal phase defects. *Obstet Gynecol* 1976;**47**(4):486–488.

126. Biller BM, Baum HB, Rosenthal DI, *et al.* Progressive trabecular osteopenia in women with hyperprolactinemic amenorrhea. *J Clin Endocrinol Metab* 1992;**75**(3):692–697. https://academic.oup.com/jcem/article-lookup/doi/10.1210/jcem.75.3.1517356.

127. Schlechte J. A longitudinal analysis of premenopausal bone loss in healthy women and women with hyperprolactinemia. *J Clin Endocrinol Metab* 1992;**75**(3):698–703. http://press.endocrine.org/doi/10.1210/jcem.75.3.1517357.

128. Colao A, Di Somma C, Loche S, Di Sarno, *et al.* Prolactinomas in adolescents: persistent bone

loss after 2 years of prolactin normalization. *Clin Endocrinol (Oxf)* 2000;**52**(3):319–327. http://doi.wiley.com/10.1046/j.1365-2265.2000.00902.x.

129. Carter JN, Tyson JE, Tolis G. Prolactin-secreting tumors and hypogonadism in 22 men. *N Engl J Med* 1978;**299**(16):847–852.

130. Segal S, Yaffe H, Laufer N, Ben-David M. Male hyperprolactinemia: effects on fertility. *Fertil Steril* 1979;**32**(5):556–561.

131. Somma C, Colao A, Di Sarno A. Marker and bone density responses to dopamine agonist therapy in hyperprolactinemic males. *J Clin Endocrinol Metab* 1998;**83**(3):807–813.

132. Casanueva FF, Molitch ME, Schlechte JA, et al. Guidelines of the Pituitary Society for the diagnosis and management of prolactinomas. *Clin Endocrinol (Oxf)* 2006;**65**(2):265–273.

133. Sisam DA, Sheehan JP, Sheeler LR. The natural history of untreated microprolactinomas. *Fertil Steril* 1987;**48**(1):67–71. https://linkinghub.elsevier.com/retrieve/pii/S0015028216592929.

134. Costello RT. Subclinical adenoma of the pituitary gland. *Am J Pathol* 1936;**12**(2):205–216.1.

135. Kraus HE. Neoplastic diseases of the human hypophysis. *Arch Pathol* 1945;**39**:343–349.

136. Burrow GN, Wortzman G, Rewcastle NB, Holgate RC, Kovacs K. Microadenomas of the pituitary and abnormal sellar tomograms in an unselected autopsy series. *N Engl J Med* 1981;**304**(3):156–158. http://www.nejm.org/doi/abs/10.1056/NEJM198101153040306.

137. Vance ML. Drugs five years later. Bromocriptine. *Ann Intern Med* 1984;**100**(1):78–91. http://annals.org/article.aspx?doi=10.7326/0003-4819-100-1-78.

138. Colao A, Savastano S. Medical treatment of prolactinomas. *Nat Rev Endocrinol* 2011;**7**(5):267–278.

139. Webster J, Piscitelli G, Polli A, et al. A comparison of cabergoline and bromocriptine in the treatment of hyperprolactinemic amenorrhea. *N Engl J Med* 1994;**331**(14):904–909. http://www.nejm.org/doi/abs/10.1056/NEJM199410063311403.

140. Verhelst J, Abs R, Maiter D, et al. Cabergoline in the treatment of hyperprolactinemia: a study in 455 patients. *J Clin Endocrinol Metab* 1999;**84**(7):2518–2522. https://academic.oup.com/jcem/article-lookup/doi/10.1210/jcem.84.7.5810.

141. Rizk B. Treatment of ovarian hyperstimulation syndrome. In: Rizk B, ed. *Ovarian Hyperstimulation Syndrome*. Cambridge: Cambridge University Press; 2006:200–226.

142. Garcia-Velasco JA. How to avoid ovarian hyperstimulation syndrome: a new indication for dopamine agonists. *Reprod Biomed Online* 2009;**18**:S71–S75. https://linkinghub.elsevier.com/retrieve/pii/S147264831060452X.

143. Leitao VMS, Moroni RM, Seko LMD, Nastri CO, Martins WP. Cabergoline for the prevention of ovarian hyperstimulation syndrome: systematic review and meta-analysis of randomized controlled trials. *Fertil Steril* 2014;**101**(3):664.e7–675.e7. https://linkinghub.elsevier.com/retrieve/pii/S0015028213032585.

144. Kleinberg DL, Boyd AE, Wardlaw S, et al. Pergolide for the treatment of pituitary tumors secreting prolactin or growth hormone. *N Engl J Med* 1983;**309**(12):704–709. http://www.nejm.org/doi/abs/10.1056/NEJM198309223091205.

145. Schade R, Andersohn F, Suissa S, Haverkamp W, Garbe E. Dopamine agonists and the risk of cardiac-valve regurgitation. *N Engl J Med* 2007;**356**(1):29–38.

146. Zanettini R, Antonini A, Gatto G, et al. Valvular heart disease and the use of dopamine agonists for Parkinson's disease. *N Engl J Med* 2007;**356**(1):39–46. http://www.nejm.org/doi/abs/10.1056/NEJMoa054830.

147. Simonis G, Fuhrmann JT. Strasser RH. Meta-analysis of heart valve abnormalities in Parkinson's disease patients treated with dopamine agonists. *Mov Disord* 2007;**22**(13):1936–1942.

148. Antonini A, Poewe W. Fibrotic heart-valve reactions to dopamine-agonist treatment in Parkinson's disease. *Lancet Neurol* 2007;**6**(9):826–829. https://linkinghub.elsevier.com/retrieve/pii/S1474442207702181.

149. Mann WA. Treatment for prolactinomas and hyperprolactinaemia: a lifetime approach. *Eur J Clin Invest* 2011;**41**(3):334–342. http://doi.wiley.com/10.1111/j.1365-2362.2010.02399.x.

150. Kletzky OA, Vermesh M. Effectiveness of vaginal bromocriptine in treating women with hyperprolactinemia. *Fertil Steril* 1989;**51**(2):269–272.

151. Motta T, de Vincentiis S, Marchini M, Colombo N, D'Alberton A. Vaginal cabergoline in the treatment of hyperprolactinemic patients intolerant to oral dopaminergics. *Fertil Steril* 1996;**65**(2):440–442. https://linkinghub.elsevier.com/retrieve/pii/S0015028216581138.

152. Leong KS, Foy PM, Swift AC, et al. CSF rhinorrhoea following treatment with dopamine agonists for massive invasive prolactinomas. *Clin Endocrinol (Oxf)* 2000;**52**(1):43–49. http://doi.wiley.com/10.1046/j.1365-2265.2000.00901.x.

153. Biller BM, Molitch ME, Vance ML, et al. Treatment of prolactin-secreting macroadenomas with the once-weekly dopamine agonist cabergoline. *J Clin Endocrinol Metab* 1996;**81**(6):2338–2343. https://academic.oup.com/jcem/article-lookup/doi/10.1210/jcem.81.6.8964874.

154. Van der Lely AJ, Brownell J, Lamberts SW. The efficacy and tolerability of CV 205-502 (a nonergot dopaminergic drug) in macroprolactinoma patients and in prolactinoma patients intolerant to bromocriptine. *J Clin Endocrinol Metab* 1991;**72**(5):1136–1141.

155. Molitch ME. Macroprolactinoma size reduction with dopamine agonists. *Endocrinologist* 1997;**7**(5):390–398.

156. Molitch ME, Elton RL, Blackwell RE, et al. Bromocriptine as primary therapy for prolactin secreting macroadenomas: results of a prospective multicenter study. *J Clin Endocrinol Metab* 1985;**60**(4):698–705.

157. Moster ML, Savino PJ, Schatz NJ, et al. Visual function in prolactinoma patients treated with bromocriptine. *Ophthalmology* 1985;**92**(10):1332–1341.

158. De Rosa M, Colao A, Di Sarno A, et al. Cabergoline treatment rapidly improves gonadal function in hyperprolactinemic males: a comparison with bromocriptine. *Eur J Endocrinol* 1998;**138**(3):286–293. https://eje.bioscientifica.com/view/journals/eje/138/3/286.xml.

159. De Rosa M, Zarrilli S, Vitale G, et al. Six months of treatment with cabergoline restores sexual potency in hyperprolactinemic males: an open longitudinal study monitoring nocturnal penile tumescence. *J Clin Endocrinol Metab* 2004;**89**(2):621–625. https://academic.oup.com/jcem/article-lookup/doi/10.1210/jc.2003-030852.

160. Colao A, Vitale G, Cappabianca P, et al. Outcome of cabergoline treatment in men with prolactinoma: effects of a 24-month treatment on prolactin levels, tumor mass, recovery of pituitary function, and semen analysis. *J Clin Endocrinol Metab* 2004;**89**(4):1704–1711.

161. Warfield A. Bromocriptine treatment of prolactin-secreting pituitary adenomas may restore pituitary function. *Ann Intern Med* 1984;**101**(6):783–785. http://annals.org/article.aspx?doi=10.7326/0003-4819-101-6-783.

162. Turkalj I, Braun P, Krupp P. Surveillance of bromocriptine in pregnancy. *JAMA* 1982;**247**(11):1589–1591. http://jama.jamanetwork.com/article.aspx?doi=10.1001/jama.1982.03320360039028.

163. Robert E, Musatti L, Piscitelli G, Ferrari CI. Pregnancy outcome after treatment with the ergot derivative, cabergoline. *Reprod Toxicol* 1996;**10**(4):333–337. https://linkinghub.elsevier.com/retrieve/pii/0890623896000639.

164. Bajwa S, Mohan P, Bajwa SS, Singh A. Management of prolactinoma with cabergoline treatment in a pregnant woman during her entire pregnancy. *Indian J Endocrinol Metab* 2011;**15**(Suppl 3):S267–S270. http://www.ijem.in/text.asp?2011/15/7/267/84883.

165. Liuzzi A, Dallabonzana D, Oppizzi G, et al. Low doses of dopamine agonists in the long-term treatment of macroprolactinomas. *N Engl J Med* 1985;**313**(11):656–659. http://www.nejm.org/doi/abs/10.1056/NEJM198509123131103.

166. Colao A, Di Sarno A, Cappabianca P, et al. Withdrawal of long-term cabergoline therapy for tumoral and nontumoral hyperprolactinemia. *N Engl J Med* 2003;**349**(21):2023–2033. http://www.nejm.org/doi/abs/10.1056/NEJMoa022657.

167. Thorner MO, Perryman RL, Rogol AD, et al. Rapid changes of prolactinoma volume after withdrawal and reinstitution of bromocriptine. *J Clin Endocrinol Metab* 1981;**53**(3):480–483.

168. Van't Verlaat JW, Croughs RJM. Withdrawal of bromocriptine after long-term therapy for macroprolactinomas; effect on plasma prolactin and tumour size. *Clin Endocrinol (Oxf)* 1991;**34**(3):175–178. http://doi.wiley.com/10.1111/j.1365-2265.1991.tb00289.x.

169. Passos VQ, Souza JJ, Musolino NR, Bronstein MD. Long-term follow-up of prolactinomas: normoprolactinemia after bromocriptine withdrawal. *J Clin Endocrinol Metab* 2002;**87**(8):3578–3582.

170. Feigenbaum SL, Downey DE, Wilson CB, Jaffe RB. Transsphenoidal pituitary resection for preoperative diagnosis of prolactin-secreting pituitary adenoma in women: long term follow-up. *J Clin Endocrinol Metab* 1996;**81**(5):1711–1719. https://academic.oup.com/jcem/article-lookup/doi/10.1210/jcem.81.5.8626821.

171. Randall RV, Laws JE, Abboud CF, et al. Transsphenoidal microsurgical treatment of prolactin-producing pituitary adenomas. Results in 100 patients. *Mayo Clin Proc* 1983;**58**(2):108–121. https://www.ncbi.nlm.nih.gov/pubmed/6681646.

172. Klibanski A. Prolactinomas. *N Engl J Med* 2010;**362**(13):1219–1226. http://www.nejm.org/doi/abs/10.1056/NEJMcp0912025.

173. Loeffler JS, Shih HA. Radiation therapy in the management of pituitary adenomas. *J Clin Endocrinol Metab* 2011;**96**(7):1992–2003.

Chapter 24

Ovarian Cautery for Polycystic Ovary Syndrome

Gabor T. Kovacs

History

The term "polycystic ovary syndrome" (PCOS) has replaced the term Stein–Leventhal syndrome. Stein and Leventhal not only were the first to describe the condition but also developed and reported on a treatment, reporting on a successful series of 108 women treated by "wedge resection" [1]. In fact until the availability of clomiphene (clomifene) citrate (CC) in 1961 [2], this was the only option available to treat the infertility of women with this condition; characterized by obesity, oligomenorrhea, and anovulation. However, as treatment required laparotomy, and often resulted in periovarian adhesion formation, once medical treatment was available, initially CC, then human pituitary gonadotropins (hPG) [3], then urinary human menopausal gonadotropin (hMG) [4], wedge resection lost popularity, unless it was performed in conjunction with another surgical procedure that already required laparotomy.

With the development of laparoscopy, a window of opportunity arose using minimally invasive surgery to undertake a surgical approach to the ovary as an option to treat anovulation in PCOS. With the development of Palmer forceps, ovarian grasping and burning became possible using laparoscopic access. Palmer and Cohen described the first pregnancies after ovarian biopsy and electrocautery back in 1972 [5]. A very detailed early history of laparoscopic ovarian surgery (LOS) was recorded by the late Jean Cohen in 2007 [6]. While the reader is directed to Jean Cohen's landmark chapter, I will summarize the early reports reviewed by him.

By 1972, Cohen and colleagues had reported 41 pregnancies obtained after 51 successive ovarian biopsies and electrocautery [5]. They concluded that ovarian biopsy had a therapeutic effect on some ovarian infertility, confirmed by several French workers [6]. However, there was little interest in this form of therapy until the

report of Gjönnaess [7], who was responsible for a renewed interest in surgical treatment of anovulation in women with polycystic ovaries. Gjönnaess described a series of 62 women who were treated by laparoscopic ovarian unipolar diathermy, with an ovulation rate of 92 percent. Published reports over the next decade were summarized by Cohen (Table 24.1) [6].

Methods of Drilling

The original French reports described purely biopsying the ovary to induce ovulation. Gjönnaess described unipolar ovarian cautery, and this has been the most commonly used method, as it is readily available and can be performed by any laparoscopically trained operating gynecologist. Initially Semm forceps were used. This was not ideal as it was difficult to grasp the enlarged ovary with forceps with a narrow jaw opening, something that could be compared to trying to grasp a football with ice-tongs. Consequently an insulated needle (Corson needle) that could easily pierce the ovarian capsule and burn the cortex has been developed. Also atraumatic forceps have been designed to grasp the ovarian pedicle, to decrease the risk of hemorrhage, as the conventional forceps can easily damage the fragile veins in the ovarian pedicle. While bipolar diathermy is safer as the current only passes between the two jaws of the forceps, it is difficult to use for ovarian cautery, because again the opening and separation of the two jaws is limited.

Laser

With the application of laser technology to laparoscopic surgery, some workers reported on the effect of laser ovarian drilling. The use of a carbon dioxide (CO_2) laser in PCOS was first described by

Table 24.1 Laparoscopic ovarian biopsy and drilling: initial reports

Author	Year	Technique	Number of women	Spontaneous ovulation (%)	Pregnancies (%)
Cohen et al. [5]	1972	Biopsy	51		41
Gjönnaess [7]	1984	Cautery	62	92	84
Greenblatt and Casper	1987	Cautery	6	71	56
Huber et al.	1988	Laser	8	42	
Cohen [6]	1989	Cautery	778		32
Daniell and Miller [8]	1989	Laser	85	84	67
Gadir et al.	1990	Cautery	29	26	44
Tasaka et al.	1990	Cautery	11	91	36
Utsonomiya et al.	1990	Biopsy	16	94	50
Gurgan et al.	1991	Cautery	40	71	57
Kovacs et al.	1991	Cautery	10	70	20
Gurgan et al.	1992	Laser	40	70	50
Ostrzenski	1992	Laser	12	92	92
Pellicer and Remohi	1992	Cautery	131	67	53
Armar and Lachelin	1993	Cautery	50	86	66
Campo et al.	1993	Resection	23	56	56
Gjönnaess	1994	Cautery	252	92	84

Modified from Cohen [6].

Daniell and Miller [8]. They used a 25 W continuous-mode laser to destroy some of the subcapsular cysts, recommending 25 to 40 vaporization sites in each ovary. They postulated that laser vaporization would cause fewer adhesions. Experimental support for this suggestion came from a study on sheep by Petrucco [9]. In contrast, Keckstein reported that three of seven women treated by CO_2 laser ovarian drilling did develop adhesions [10], so it was no perfect approach.

The use of the holmium:YAG (Ho:YAG) laser was reported by Asada and colleagues [11]. The Ho:YAG laser has a wavelength of 2.14 μm and is approximately 100 times more highly absorbed in water than the Nd:YAG laser. Ho:YAG laser energy is transmitted by a standard quartz fiberoptic light guide, and achieves a controlled penetration depth in tissue of around 0.5 mm. Ho:YAG energy produces a consistent zone of thermal necrosis of less than 1.0 mm, and the thermal damage is independent of pigmentation.

These authors reported on eight women with CC-resistant PCOS-related anovulation who were treated with laparoscopic ovarian drilling (LOD) using the Ho:YAG laser at the

Saiseikai Kanagawaken Hospital, Yokohama. Postoperatively, ovulation occurred spontaneously in all the patients. The cumulative probability of conception at 6, 12, and 13 months after surgery was 37.5%, 75%, and 87.5%, respectively. The authors concluded that LOD using the Ho:YAG laser may be an effective treatment in CC-resistant anovulatory women with PCOS.

Various laser types (KTP, Nd:YAG [12], and argon [13]) have all been used. The initial Cochrane review [14] concluded that "None of the studied modalities of drilling technique had any obvious advantages." There has not been any new evidence to define the superiority of any method. Using laser of course is far more expensive, can be performed by fewer clinicians, and is possibly more dangerous.

Unilateral or Bilateral

Balen and Jacobs [15] reported a novel modification of the technique where they compared the cautery of one ovary at only four sites with the more radical method of multiple cautery to both ovaries. Surprisingly, they showed no difference in efficacy. Supportive evidence for such a conservative unilateral approach comes from the work of Roy and colleagues [16], who reported a prospective, randomized study of 44 patients, half of whom underwent bilateral ovarian drilling, and the other half unilateral. The number of drilling sites in each ovary was limited to five. Outcomes during a follow-up period of one year were compared. The clinical and biochemical response, ovulation, and pregnancy rates were similar in both groups. No adhesions were found in a single case in either group following assessment of 16 (36.3%) of the patients. Supportive evidence that unilateral ovarian drilling by electrocautery is equally effective comes from a study from Youssef and Atallah [17]. They compared unilateral and bilateral ovarian drilling in 87 PCOS women in a prospective randomized clinical study. Ovulation, pregnancy, and miscarriage rates were similar in both groups.

Transvaginal Hydrolaparoscopy

A relatively recent modification to ovarian cautery is the transvaginal approach using hydrolaparoscopy (THL). Hydrolaparoscopy was first described by Gordts et al. in 1998 to explore the pelvic cavity by a transvaginal approach using a saline solution medium [18]. Since then several reviews have validated the concept of THL and compared it to laparoscopy, the "gold standard." The failure rate to obtain satisfactory views was similar to conventional laparoscopy, and complications of bowel perforation were well below one percent [19].

Subsequently, THL has been used for ovarian drilling in polycystic ovary syndrome, and Gordts and colleagues reported on 39 PCOS patients with previously failed ovulation induction who underwent drilling of the ovarian capsule using THL, using a 5-Fr bipolar needle (Karl Storz, Tüttlingen, Germany), creating 10–15 holes to a depth of 1–2 mm ± 0.20 mm in each ovary [20]. In total, 25 out of 33 patients (76%) – six lost to follow-up – became pregnant, with a mean duration between procedure and onset of pregnancy of 7.2 months (SD ±5.4). They concluded that the transvaginal approach for ovarian capsule drilling offers a valuable alternative to the standard laparoscopic procedure.

Ultrasound-Guided Transvaginal Ovarian Needle Drilling

Badawy and colleagues reported the outcome of ovarian needle drilling using transvaginal ultrasound guidance as an alternative to the tradiional laparoscopic electrosurgical drilling for patients with PCOS in a randomized, controlled, prospective trial [21]. The study comprised 163 patients with CC-resistant PCOS randomly allocated to either treatment with ultrasound-guided transvaginal needle ovarian drilling (UTND; $n = 82$) or laparoscopic electrosurgery ovarian drilling ($n = 81$). There were no significant differences between the two groups with regard to resumption of normal menstruation, hirsutism, acne, ovulation, and pregnancy. UTND resulted in significant improvement in ovulation, pregnancy, hirsutism, and acne. UTND has the advantage that it can be adopted as an outpatient office procedure with ease of scheduling, reduced costs, and rapid recovery.

Zhu and colleagues modified UTND by applying laser energy. Since 2006 they published three reports of treatment of anovulatory women with CC-resistant PCOS [22–24]. The authors suggested that intraovarian coagulation be created at a spot 10 mm in diameter away from the ovarian surface; the coagulation was kept to at least 5 mm from the surface so that there was minimal damage to the ovarian surface.

Api had a number of reservations about this technique [25]. He agreed that transvaginal, ultrasound-guided ovarian interstitial laser treatment seems to prevent ovarian surface damage, and that it might have a theoretical advantage of preventing postoperative adhesion formation over laparoscopic ovarian drilling. However, he was concerned that as the intraovarian vessels and main blood supply enter the ovary from the hilum, there was a potential risk of damaging the cortical blood supply by intraovarian coagulation. He was also concerned about the risk of unrecognized inadvertent hemorrhage from the ovary, and adjacent pelvic organ damage, because the technique is not under direct visualization.

Additionally, he pointed out that as the fiberoptic cable is 400 μm in diameter and is not easily visualized using ultrasound, there is the risk of unrecognized ovarian surface perforation if the cable is inserted more than the intended distance. Because the procedure is performed without general anesthesia, any unintentional movement of the patient during the procedure may potentially cause inadvertent needle movements inside the ovary, with catastrophic consequences if the fiberoptic cable tip reaches beyond the ovarian surface when the laser energy is activated.

Furthermore, transvaginal, ultrasound-guided ovarian interstitial laser treatment does not allow direct visualization of pelvic organs to assess the tuboovarian relationship, tubal patency, adhesions, and endometriosis. He concluded that this novel treatment method has not yet been investigated thoroughly, and that further studies for its efficacy and safety should be undertaken.

Laparoscopic Ovarian Multi-needle Intervention

A new, specially designed laparoscopic device and technique was described by Kaya and colleagues [26]. Thirty-five infertile CC-resistant women with PCOS were studied. Seventeen women underwent laparoscopic ovarian multi-needle intervention (LOMNI), and 18 women received ovulation induction treatment. There was no significant difference in outcomes, but the cost of LOMNI was significantly ($p < 0.001$) lower than the ovulation induction treatment. They concluded that LOMNI may be a safe, inexpensive, and effective procedure for the treatment of CC-resistant infertility in patients with PCOS. It seems to preserve the beneficial effects yet probably omits the unwanted effects (such as adhesion formation) of LOD.

Possible Complications of Ovarian Cautery/Drilling

Intraoperative and early postoperative complications for ovarian drilling with electrocautery or laser are similar to those experienced after operative laparoscopy, and are shown in Table 24.2.

Postoperative – Delayed

The complications specific to ovarian drilling with possible effects on future fertility include the risk of ovarian adhesions and possible reduction of ovarian reserve.

Pelvic/Ovarian Adhesions

Varying incidence of postoperative ovarian adhesions between 0 and 100 percent have been

Table 24.2 Complications of surgical laparoscopy/ovarian drilling

- Anesthetic complications
- Laparoscopic injury at insertion
- Gas complication – CO_2 embolism
- Mis-insufflation into tissues
- Trauma to viscus or vessel
- Heat damage at time of drilling
- Bowel, bladder, or vessel damage

reported [6]. In a published study, Mercorio and colleagues reported on 96 women who were randomized into two study groups of 48 women each, one group treated with 6 punctures on the left ovary and 12 on the right, and the other treated with 6 punctures on the right ovary and 12 on the left [27]. A short-term, second-look minilaparoscopy was performed to evaluate postsurgical adhesion formation. They detected adhesion formation in 54 of the 90 women (60%) and in 83 of the 180 ovaries treated (46%). Dense adhesions were more likely to develop on the left ovary to a statistically significant extent, and independently of the number of ovarian punctures performed. Logistic regression analysis showed that the incidence of ovarian adhesions was independent of both number of punctures and side. They concluded that the incidence of ovarian adhesion formation after LOD was high, and that their extent and severity was not influenced by the number of ovarian punctures; however, the left ovary appeared more prone to develop severe adhesions than the right one.

Premature Ovarian Failure

Api reviewed the available literature on whether LOD is harmful on the ovarian reserve markers [28]. He found four articles that specifically reported on the ovarian reserve tests. Among these, three compared before and after drilling values, and one of them compared ovarian reserve markers among different groups of subjects: those with LOD, those with PCOS without LOD, and normal ovulatory controls. He found that there were statistically significant differences between day-3 follicle-stimulating hormone (FSH), inhibin B levels, ovarian volume, and antral follicle count (AFC) before and after LOD in some of the reports. Although the post-LOD values were found to be lower than the pre-LOD values by means of ovarian reserve markers, the post-LOD values stayed higher than normal when compared with normal women without PCOS. He concluded that there was no concrete evidence of a decreased ovarian reserve nor premature ovarian failure associated with LOD in women with PCOS. Most of the changes in the ovarian reserve markers observed after LOD could be interpreted as normalization of ovarian function rather than as a reduction of ovarian reserve.

Weerakiet and colleagues evaluated ovarian reserve assessed by hormones and sonography in 21 women with PCOS undergoing LOD, and compared these with those of PCOS women who did not undergo LOD (the PCOS group) and those of normal ovulatory women (the control group) [29]. In this study of ovarian reserve assessed by anti-Müllerian hormone levels, day-3 FSH, and AFC, inhibin B levels seemed to be lower in the LOD than in the PCOS group. The PCOS women both with and without LOD had significantly greater ovarian reserve than the age-matched controls having normal ovulatory menstruation.

Hendriks and colleagues carried out experimental comparisons of damage from CO_2 laser, monopolar electrocoagulation, and bipolar electrocoagulation on bovine ovaries [30]. They found that bipolar electrocoagulation resulted in significantly more destruction per burn than the CO_2 laser and monopolar electrocoagulation (287.6 vs. 24.0 and 70.0 mm^3, respectively). They concluded that ovarian drilling, especially bipolar electrocoagulation, causes extensive destruction of the ovary. Given the same clinical effectiveness of the various procedures, they recommended that the least destructive method should be used and that the first choice should be CO_2 laser or monopolar electrocoagulation

As a possible mechanism of ovarian damage is through impairment of blood supply, the study by Vizer and colleagues, using three-dimensional color power angiography (CPA) to evaluate and quantify intraovarian blood flow before and after LOD and comparing this with hormonal changes, is of interest [31]. They found that ovarian volume decreased, and three-dimensional CPA showed increased intraovarian flow intensity after laparoscopic electrocautery. Serum luteinizing hormone (LH) and testosterone levels, and ratios of urinary steroids after laparoscopic ovarian electrocautery, in 10 women with polycystic ovary reflecting 5-alpha-reductase enzyme activity, and androgen to cortisol metabolites decreased; serum FSH

levels increased one week after laparoscopy and correlated well with changes in three-dimensional sonographic features. Seven patients ovulated regularly after surgery, and five pregnancies were conceived within one year. They concluded that three-dimensional ultrasonography may be a useful adjunct and non-invasive method for correlating clinical parameters with the blood flow alterations in PCOS patients.

Reassurance comes from a 15- to 25-year follow-up of nearly 150 women after ovarian wedge resection which shows that regular menstrual patterns lasting up to 25 years after surgery were restored in 88 percent of patients with a cumulative pregnancy/live birth rate of 78 percent [32].

Cost Analysis

We compared the cost of LOD using electrocautery with the cost of ovulation induction using injectable FSH in the Australian private health system [33]. The cost of LOD using unipolar diathermy was 84 percent of the cost of one cycle of ovulation induction using FSH, including the cost of hormones, biochemistry, medical costs, and ultrasound.

Mechanism of Action

How wedge resection of the ovaries, as described by Stein and Leventhal [1], worked was never understood, although they postulated a decrease in crowding of the cortex, thus enabling the growth of normal follicles to the surface. Gjönnaess postulated that the benefit of drilling was either non-specific stromal destruction or the discharge of the contents of subcapsular cysts [7], while Daniell and Miller hypothesized that by opening the follicular capsules by laser energy, follicular fluid containing androgens was released, thus removing the block to ovulation [8]. While the mechanism of action is still not understood, various hormones have been measured before and after ovarian surgery. Campo reviewed data regarding 1803 anovulatory PCOS patients, 679 of them treated by classical ovarian resection after laparotomy, 720 by laparoscopic electrocauterization, 322 by laparoscopic laser vaporization, and 82 by laparoscopic multiple biopsies [34]. He found that hormone variations after surgery consisted of a remarkable fall in serum androgen levels (androstenedione and testosterone), an FSH increase, reduced biological activity, and reduced amplitude of LH pulses, and an LH/FSH ratio trending toward normal levels. We reported that there was a significant and persistent fall in serum testosterone levels, and a transient fall with subsequent rise in inhibin [35]. However, a study by Amer and colleagues of 50 anovulatory women with PCOS who underwent LOD found no statistically significant change in inhibin B after LOD in the overall group of women with PCOS or in the subgroup of non-obese PCOS women with higher preoperative inhibin B [36]. They concluded that it was unlikely that inhibin had any role to play in the mechanism of action of LOD.

Seow and colleagues confirmed that the reduction of serum androgen level is the possible mechanism of LOD to improve spontaneous ovulation and promote fertility in women with PCOS [37]. In addition, LOD may cause a significant reduction in serum LH and insulin levels.

Vizer and colleagues, in addition to their study of intraovarian blood flow with three-dimensional CPA histogram analysis before and after laparoscopic ovarian electrocautery, also compared the hormonal effects of surgery with three-dimensional sonographic findings [31]. They also found that serum LH and testosterone levels, ratios of urinary steroids reflecting 5-alpha-reductase enzyme activity, and androgen to cortisol metabolites decreased; serum FSH levels increased one week after laparoscopy and correlated well with changes in three-dimensional sonographic features.

Efficacy Compared with FSH Ovulation Induction

Individual Expert Opinion

In a recent review looking at strategies to induce ovulation in PCOS, Palomba and colleagues concluded that in CC-resistant PCOS patients, a CC and metformin combination, and LOD, in selected cases, should be considered before gonadotropin administration [38].

Consensus Expert Opinion

A group of international experts gathered in Thessaloniki in Greece in 2007 to draft some consensus statements on various aspects of the management of PCOS [39]. With respect to the site of LOS they concluded that:

- LOS can achieve unifollicular ovulation with no risk of ovarian hyperstimulation syndrome or high-order multiples
- Intensive monitoring of follicular development is not required after LOS
- LOS is an alternative to gonadotropin therapy for CC-resistant anovulatory PCOS
- The treatment is best suited to those for whom frequent ultrasound monitoring is impractical
- LOS is a single treatment using existing equipment
- The risks of surgery are minimal and include the risk of laparoscopy, adhesion formation, and destruction of normal ovarian tissue. Minimal damage should be caused to the ovaries. Irrigation with an adhesion barrier may be useful, but there is no evidence of efficacy from prospective studies. Surgery should be performed by appropriately trained personnel
- LOS should not be offered for non-fertility indications

Evidence-Based "Meta-analyses"

Five Cochrane reviews on the role of ovarian drilling have been published, the latest in 2012 [14;40–43].

Although in their first review Farquhar and colleagues stated that "the value of laparoscopic ovarian drilling as a primary treatment for subfertile patients with anovulation (failure to ovulate) and polycystic ovarian syndrome (PCOS) is undetermined" [14], by the time of their 2005 review they changed the conclusion to "there was no evidence of a difference in the live birth rate and miscarriage rate in women with clomiphene resistant PCOS undergoing LOD compared to gonadotropin treatment" [41]. In all the reviews they highlighted the benefit of lack of multiple pregnancies with ovarian drilling. In 2000 they stated that none of the studied modalities of drilling technique had any obvious advantages [14]. Their conclusions after the 2012 review were similar [43]: "There was no evidence of a significant difference in rates of clinical pregnancy, live birth or miscarriage in women with clomiphene-resistant PCOS undergoing LOD compared to other medical treatments. The reduction in multiple pregnancy rates in women undergoing LOD makes this option attractive. However, there are ongoing concerns about the long-term effects of LOD on ovarian function."

More recently, the International evidence-based guideline for the assessment and management of polycystic ovary syndrome was produced in 2018. This guideline was authored by Helena Teede, Marie Misso, Michael Costello, Anuja Dokras, Joop Laven, Lisa Moran, Terhi Piltonen, and Robert Norman on behalf of the International PCOS Network in collaboration with funding, partner, and collaborating organizations [44].

These guidelines produced a detailed review of the literature and analyzed in detail the comparisons between surgical treatment of PCO-related anovulation and the use of metformin, CC without and with metformin, and against aromatase inhibitors. Their evidence for comparison of LOD against FSH ovulation induction was the Cochrane review of 2012 [43].

Laparoscopic Ovarian Surgery versus Metformin

Two medium-quality randomized controlled trials (RCTs) (level II) (published across three papers) compared LOS to metformin and found that there was insufficient evidence to make a recommendation about LOS compared to metformin for live birth rate per patient, ovulation rate per cycle, pregnancy rate per cycle, pregnancy rate per patient, multiple pregnancies, miscarriage rate per pregnancy, adverse effects, and quality of life [45;46]. The two studies showed conflicting results. Both were medium-quality single-center studies, with a small sample size and moderate risk of bias.

Laparoscopic Ovarian Surgery versus Clomiphene Citrate

Two high-quality RCTs (level II) with a low risk of bias compared LOS with CC [47;48] and found that there was no difference between LOS and CC for live birth rate per patient and pregnancy rate per patient, ovulation rate per patient, and miscarriage rate per pregnancy.

This comparison is rather irrelevant, as it is agreed by most that LOS is not a first-line treatment

but should be considered for women who fail to ovulate with CC.

Laparoscopic Ovarian Surgery Versus Clomiphene Citrate plus Metformin

The guidelines referred to three studies included in the 2012 Cochrane review [43]. The conclusion was that there was insufficient evidence to support or refute the use of LOS over CC plus metformin for ovulation rate per patient [43].

Laparoscopic Ovarian Surgery versus Aromatase Inhibitors

In the guideline review, three RCTs compared letrozole with LOS and found that there was insufficient evidence of a difference. The Cochrane review of 2012 combined these studies in meta-analysis for pregnancy rate per patient, multiple pregnancy rate per pregnancy, and miscarriage rate per pregnancy and there was no statistical difference between the two interventions [43].

Laparoscopic Ovarian Surgery versus Gonadotropins

Again, referenced from the 2012 Cochrane review [43], the guidelines quoted one high-quality systematic review of RCTs comparing LOS with FSH and found that there was no difference between the interventions for live birth rate per patient and pregnancy rate per patient, ovulation rate per patient, and miscarriage rate per pregnancy, but LOS was better than FSH for avoiding multiple pregnancy rate [43].

I will conclude this chapter with the four recommendations from the guidelines with respect to the role of laparoscopic ovarian surgery in women with clomiphene-resistant anovulation due to PCO [44]:

1. Laparoscopic ovarian surgery could be second line therapy for women with PCOS, who are clomiphene citrate resistant, with anovulatory infertility and no other infertility factors.
2. Laparoscopic ovarian surgery could potentially be offered as first line treatment if laparoscopy is indicated for another reason in women with PCOS with anovulatory infertility and no other infertility factors.
3. Risks need to be explained to all women with PCOS considering laparoscopic ovarian surgery.

4. Where laparoscopic ovarian surgery is to be recommended, the following need to be considered:

   - comparative cost
   - expertise required for use in ovulation induction
   - intra-operative and post-operative risks are higher in women who are overweight and obese
   - there may be a small associated risk of lower ovarian reserve or loss of ovarian function
   - periadnexal adhesion formation may be an associated risk.

References

1. Stein FI, Leventhal ML. Amenorrhoea associated with bilateral polycystic ovaries. *Am J Obstet Gynecol* 1935;**29**:181–191.

2. Greenblatt RB. Chemical induction of ovulation. *Fertil Steril* 1961;**60**:766–769.

3. Kovacs GT, Pepperell RJ, Evans JH. Induction of ovulation with human pituitary gonadotrophin (HPG): the Australian experience. *Aust N Z J Obstet Gynaecol* 1989;**29**:315–318.

4. Lunenfeld B, Sulimovici S, Rabau E. L'Induction de l'ovulation les amenorhees hypophysaires par un trait-mentcombine de gonadotrophines urinaeres menopausiques et de gonadotrophines chorioniques. *Compt Rendus Soc Fr Gynecol* 1962;**5**:287.

5. Cohen J, Audebert A, De Brux J, Giorgi H. Les stérilités poar dysovulation: rôle pronotisque et thérapeutique de la biopsie ovairenne percoelioscopique. *J Gynécol Obstet Biol Reprod (Paris)* 1972;**1**:657–671.

6. Cohen J. Laparoscopic surgical treatment of infertility related to PCOS revisited. In: Kovacs GT, Norman R, eds. *Polycystic Ovary Syndrome*. Cambridge: Cambridge University Press; 2007:159–176.

7. Gjönnaess H. Polycystic ovarian syndrome treated by ovarian electrocautery through the laparoscope. *Fertil Steril* 1984;**41**:20–25.

8. Daniell JF, Miller W. Polycystic ovaries treated by laparoscopic laser vaporization. *Fertil Steril* 1989;**51**:232–236.

9. Petrucco OM. Laparoscopic CO_2 laser drilling of sheep ovaries-interval assessment of histological changes and adhesion formation. *Abstracts of the Seventh Annual Scientific Meeting of The Fertility Society of Australia*, Newcastle;1988:21.

10. Keckstein J. Laparoscopic treatment of polycystic ovarian syndrome. In: Sutton CJG, ed. *Bailliere's Clinical Obstetrics and Gynaecology. Laparoscopic Surgery* Vol. 3 Iss. 3; 1989:563–581.

11. Asada H, Kishi I, Kaseda S, *et al.* Laparoscopic treatment of polycystic ovaries with the holmium: YAG laser. *Fertil Steril* 2002;**77**:852–853.

12. Gürgan T, Yarali H, Urman B. Laparoscopic treatment of polycystic ovarian disease. *Hum Reprod* 1994;**9**:573–577.

13. Heylen SM, Puttemans PJ, Brosens IA. Polycystic ovarian disease treated by laparoscopic argon laser capsule drilling: comparison of vaporization versus perforation technique. *Hum Reprod* 1994;**9**:1038–1042.

14. Farquhar C, Vandekerckhove P, Arnot M, Lilford R. Laparoscopic "drilling" by diathermy or laser for ovulation induction in anovulatory polycystic ovary syndrome. *Cochrane Database Syst Rev* 2000;**2**:CD001122.

15. Balen AH, Jacobs HS. A prospective study comparing unilateral and bilateral laparoscopic ovarian diathermy in women with the polycystic ovary syndrome. *Fertil Steril* 1994;**62**:921–925.

16. Roy KK, Baruah J, Moda N, Kumar S. Evaluation of unilateral versus bilateral ovarian drilling in clomiphene citrate resistant cases of polycystic ovarian syndrome. *Arch Gynecol Obstet* 2009;**280**:573–578.

17. Youssef H, Atallah MM. Unilateral ovarian drilling in polycystic ovarian syndrome: a prospective randomized study. *Reprod Biomed Online* 2007;**15**:457–462.

18. Gordts S, Campo R, Rombauts L, Brosens I. Transvaginal hydrolaparoscopy as an outpatient procedure for infertility investigation. *Hum Reprod* 1998;**13**:99–103.

19. Daraï E, Coutant C, Dessolle L, Ballester M. Transvaginal hydrolaparoscopy. *Minerva Chir* 2009;**64**:365–372.

20. Gordts S, Gordts S, Puttemans P, *et al.* Transvaginal hydrolaparoscopy in the treatment of polycystic ovary syndrome. *Fertil Steril* 2009;**91**:2520–2526.

21. Badawy A, Khiary M, Ragab A, Hassan M, Sherief L. Ultrasound-guided transvaginal ovarian needle drilling (UTND) for treatment of polycystic ovary syndrome: a randomized controlled trial. *Fertil Steril* 2009;**91**:1164–1167.

22. Zhu W, Li X, Chen X, Lin Z, Zhang L. Ovarian interstitial YAG-laser: an effective new method to manage anovulation in women with polycystic ovary syndrome. *Am J Obstet Gynecol* 2006;**195**:458–463.

23. Zhu WJ, Li XM, Chen XM, Lin Z, Zhang L. Transvaginal, ultrasound-guided, ovarian, interstitial laser treatment in anovulatory women with clomifene-citrate-resistant polycystic ovary syndrome. *BJOG* 2006;**113**:810–816.

24. Zhu W, Fu Z, Chen X, *et al.* Transvaginal ultrasound-guided ovarian interstitial laser treatment in anovulatory women with polycystic ovary syndrome: a randomized clinical trial on the effect of laser dose used on the outcome. *Fertil Steril* 2010;**94**:268–275.

25. Api M. Could transvaginal, ultrasound-guided ovarian interstitial laser treatment replace laparoscopic ovarian drilling in women with polycystic ovary syndrome resistant to clomiphene citrate? *Fertil Steril* 2009;**92**:2039–2040.

26. Kaya H, Sezik M, Ozkaya O. Evaluation of a new surgical approach for the treatment of clomiphene citrate-resistant infertility in polycystic ovary syndrome: laparoscopic ovarian multi-needle intervention. *J Minim Invasive Gynecol* 2005;**12**:355–358.

27. Mercorio F, Mercorio A, Di Spiezio Sardo A, *et al.* Evaluation of ovarian adhesion formation after laparoscopic ovarian drilling by second-look minilaparoscopy. *Fertil Steril* 2007;**88**:894–899.

28. Api M. Is ovarian reserve diminished after laparoscopic ovarian drilling? *Gynecol Endocrinol* 2009;**25**:159–165.

29. Weerakiet S, Lertvikool S, Tingthanatikul Y, *et al.* Ovarian reserve in women with polycystic ovary syndrome who underwent laparoscopic ovarian drilling. *Gynecol Endocrinol* 2007;**2**:1–6.

30. Hendriks M-L, van der Valk P, Lambalk CB, *et al.* Extensive tissue damage of bovine ovaries after bipolar ovarian drilling compared to monopolar electrocoagulation or carbon dioxide laser. *Fertil Steril* 2010;**93**:969–975.

31. Vizer M, Kiesel L, Szabó I, *et al.* Assessment of three-dimensional sonographic features of polycystic ovaries after laparoscopic ovarian electrocautery. *Fertil Steril* 2007;**88**:894–899.

32. Lunde O, Djoseland O, Grottum P. Polycystic ovarian syndrome: a follow-up study on fertility and menstrual pattern in 149 patients 15-25 years after ovarian wedge resection. *Hum Reprod* 2001;**16**:1479–1485.

33. Kovacs GT, Clarke S, Burger HG, Healy DL, Vollenhoven B. Surgical or medical treatment of polycystic ovary syndrome: a cost-benefit analysis. *Gynecol Endocrinol* 2002;**16**:53–55.

34. Campo S. Ovulatory cycles, pregnancy outcome and complications after surgical treatment of polycystic ovary syndrome. *Obstet Gynecol Surv* 1998;**53**:297–308.

35. Kovacs G, Buckler H, Bangah M, *et al.* Treatment of anovulation due to polycystic ovarian syndrome by laparoscopic ovarian electrocautery. *Br J Obstet Gynaecol* 1991;**98**:30–35.

36. Amer SA, Laird S, Ledger WL, Li TC. Effect of laparoscopic ovarian diathermy on circulating inhibin B in women with anovulatory polycystic ovary syndrome. *Hum Reprod* 2007;**22**:389–394.

37. Seow KM, Juan CC, Hwang JL, Ho LT. Laparoscopic surgery in polycystic ovary syndrome: reproductive and metabolic effects. *Semin Reprod Med* 2008;**26**:101–110.

38. Palomba S, Falbo A, Zullo F. Management strategies for ovulation induction in women with polycystic ovary syndrome and known clomifene citrate resistance. *Curr Opin Obstet Gynecol* 2009;**21**:465–473.

39. Thessaloniki ESHRE/ASRM-sponsored PCOS Consensus Workshop Group. Consensus on infertility treatment related to polycystic ovary syndrome. *Hum Reprod* 2008;**23**:462–477.

40. Farquhar C, Vandekerckhove P, Lilford R. Laparoscopic "drilling" by diathermy or laser for ovulation induction in anovulatory polycystic ovary syndrome. *Cochrane Database Syst Rev* 2001;**4**:CD001122.

41. Farquhar C, Lilford RJ, Marjoribanks J, Vandekerckhove P. Laparoscopic "drilling" by diathermy or laser for ovulation induction in anovulatory polycystic ovary syndrome. *Cochrane Database Syst Rev* 2005;**3**:CD001122.

42. Farquhar C, Lilford RJ, Marjoribanks J, Vandekerckhove P. Laparoscopic 'drilling' by diathermy or laser for ovulation induction in anovulatory polycystic ovary syndrome. *Cochrane Database Syst Rev* 2007;**3**:CD001122.

43. Farquhar C, Brown J, Marjoribanks J. Laparoscopic drilling by diathermy or laser for ovulation induction in anovulatory polycystic ovary syndrome. *Cochrane Database Syst Rev* 2012;**6**:CD001122.

44. International evidence-based guideline for the assessment and management of polycystic ovary syndrome. Copyright Monash University, Melbourne Australia 2018.

45. Hamed H, Hasan AF, Ahmed OG, Ahmed MA. Metformin versus laparoscopic ovarian drilling in clomiphene- and insulin-resistant women with polycystic ovary syndrome. *Int J Gynecol Obstet* 2010;**108**:143–141.

46. Palomba S, Orio F Jr., Nardo LG, *et al.* Metformin administration versus laparoscopic ovarian diathermy in clomiphene citrate-resistant women with polycystic ovary syndrome: a prospective parallel randomized double-blind

placebo-controlled trial. *J Clin Endocrinol Metab* 2004;**89**:4801–4809.

47. Abu Hashim H, Foda O, Ghayaty E, Elawa A. Laparoscopic ovarian diathermy after clomiphene failure in polycystic ovary syndrome: is it worthwhile? A randomized controlled trial. *Arch Gynecol Obstet* 2011;**284**:1303–1309.

48. Amer S, Li TC, Metwally M, Emarh M, Ledger WL. Randomized controlled trial comparing laparoscopic ovarian diathermy with clomiphene citrate as a first-line method of ovulation induction in women with polycystic ovary syndrome. *Hum Reprod* 2009;**24**:219–225.

Chapter 25

Elective Freeze-All Embryos Policy

Mehmet Cihat Unlu and Ahmet Yigit Cakiroglu

Introduction

Allowing infertile couples to fulfill their longings of having children, assisted reproductive techniques (ART) have progressed rapidly day by day since 1978, the time when they were first introduced. Advances and improvements in the existing techniques and interventions in medicine (ovulation induction, embryo culture techniques and the selection criteria, culture media, and advanced techniques for embryo manipulation) lead the achievements in this area to progress further every day.

The medication protocols administered during controlled ovarian stimulation (COS) have long been discussed in regards to their long-term effects on the endometrium and ovaries. In addition, the introduction of gonadotropin-releasing hormone (GnRH) antagonist protocols to the daily clinical practice created further discussion on the use of GnRH agonist triggering interventions for ovarian hyperstimulation syndrome (OHSS) prevention [1]. At this stage, embryo transfer policies may provide benefits after cycle segmentation and cryopreservation of all embryos. Furthermore, there are several concerns about the potentially unfavorable effects of the triggering day elevated progesterone levels on pregnancy outcomes. Again, cryopreservation of all embryos and their transfer in the following cycle has been described as a treatment strategy to be employed against these concerns [2]. Depending on the indication, genetic screening of embryos and the transfer of the genetically healthy embryos are also included in the clinical practice [3]. As obtaining the genetic test results will take longer, the transfer of embryos in the same cycle will not be possible. Therefore, the transfer will be scheduled to be performed in the following months after freezing all embryos, from which biopsy samples were collected. Indeed, all these interventions have been made possible owing to the advances and improvements in laboratory facilities. Especially, the introduction of the vitrification technique to the routine clinical practice at the freezing step provided a more positive view toward the freeze-all policy [4]. One of the points in introducing this technique is that it does not lead to increased risks as it is devoid of significantly negative effects on the pregnancy outcomes in the prenatal period.

Not performing the embryo transfer in the same cycle of stimulation and deferring it to the proceeding months reflects the underlying point of view that the transfer will be made to an endometrium free of the negative effects arising due to the COS. All hypotheses here suggest that the applied stimulation will not impinge negative effects on the embryo. Therefore, in regards to the future of this policy, it is critical to find out which patient groups will benefit from this process and when the benefits will occur.

Elective Freeze-All Policy: Why?

Effect of COS on Endometrial Receptivity and Gene Expression

During COS cycles, higher amounts of exogenous gonadotropins are used to increase the number of collected oocytes. This leads to the development of a higher number of follicles, synthesizing estrogen and progesterone reaching supraphysiological levels. Both animal and human research have suggested that the "receptive window" is affected in the process of embryo implantation [5]. The histological modifications in the endometrium lead to alterations in the expression of several mediators of implantation [6]. It has been demonstrated that the expression of the specific integrins involved in the implantation window was altered following hyperstimulation [7]. This process may disrupt embryo–endometrial synchrony, resulting in changes at the receptor level. If this process takes longer than three days, it may lead to implantation failure [8]. Even if implantation occurs, it will not mean that the entire process has been completed and healthy as placental anomalies or fetal developmental abnormalities potentially may occur during the pregnancy [9].

It may be suggested that the changes in endometrial genes in COS may affect the implantation process. Horcajadas *et al.* evaluated the human chorionic gonadotropin (hCG)+7 and luteinizing hormone (LH)+7 gene expression profile in COS using microarray analysis [10]. They demonstrated that a two-day delay in activation repression occurred in a total of 218 and 133 genes on days hCG+7 and LH+7, respectively, both of which are associated with the receptive processes in the implantation window. Liu *et al.* evaluated gene expression profiles in natural versus artificial cycles (moderate and excessive) with microarray analysis and quantitative polymerase chain reaction [11]. After comparing the stimulated cycles according to the estradiol levels, they determined twofold higher changes in a total of 411 genes expressed, which might affect endometrial receptivity in the three study groups. The same authors have also investigated the gene expression of Wnt-signaling molecules and have stated that high serum estrogen/progesterone levels may result in subendometrial development and impaired implantation [12].

Effect of COS on the Embryo

It has recently been suggested that several epigenetic mechanisms are also involved, in addition to the effects of superovulation, on embryo implantation. In mouse models, de Waal *et al.* demonstrated that these effects via the oocyte and the preimplantation embryo were associated with the impaired differentiation of the trophoblast and disordered placental development [13]. A comparison of the superovulation group with the control group revealed differences in the labyrinth zone of the mouse placenta, involved in the transfer of food. Furthermore, in the superovulation group, the study demonstrated a higher rate of Grb10, involved in fetal development.

Several epigenetic effects in the environment may cause alterations in the embryo during implantation. The methylation process starts during the development of the gamete, dependent on gender determination involving the oocyte and the sperm. Methylation occurs at different time points during sperm and oocyte development essentially [14]. Genome-wide methylation occurs in the embryo after fertilization. Mouse models have shown that superovulation causes methylation loss in imprinted genes during methylation processes both in the developing oocyte and in the developing embryo [15]. This way, ovarian stimulation affects the embryo during post-fertilization. Methylation loss leads to the occurrence of a non-physiological uterine micro window, affecting the fetal development. Therefore, the environment may induce epigenetic changes during the peri-implantation period, affecting fetal development and long-term fetal survival.

Vitrification

Embryo freezing was introduced along with the principle of storing the remaining embryos after the transfer of the selected ones obtained by COS. For this purpose, laboratory research started in 1972 with freezing mouse embryos at -196°C. Accomplishments in embryo freezing allowed the process to be applied commonly after the first human pregnancy following cryopreservation [16]. Cryopreservation, long been named as slow-freezing, became the technique used in this process; however, data showed that both the survival and fertilization rates were lower with this method [17]. The process of vitrification is based on the principle of freezing the embryos rapidly by exposing them to high concentrations of cryoprotectants followed by an ultra-rapid cooling. This method minimizes the risk of crystal formation inside the cells, which is the superiority of vitrification over slow freezing showing results with a survival rate greater than 95 percent [18].

The frequencies of live births have improved along with the introduction of safer cryopreservation methods like the vitrification process, resulting in the transfer of a reduced number of embryos and a reduced frequency of high-order multiple pregnancies [19].

Elective Freeze-All Policy: to Whom?

Agonist Trigger and Elective Freeze-All Policy

Ovarian hyperstimulation syndrome is one of the major complications that might occur due to the stimulation of ovaries during ART. In order to prevent this highly critical complication, agonist triggering was introduced first, to be followed by standard treatment to support the luteal phase. This way, it was aimed to prevent an early occurrence of OHSS, which may occur due to the effects of hCG. However, several endocrinological studies conducted at that time resulted in low pregnancy rates suggesting those patients might have needed a different strategy to support the luteal phase. However, an accomplished pregnancy, after a cycle combined with intensive luteal support, will not prevent a late OHSS. For this reason, segmentation of the cycle may appear an appropriate strategy [20]. Agonist triggering after COS and embryo freezing so it can be transferred in the following cycle may be employed as an approach, which will also eliminate the need for luteal support.

Antagonist Protocol

Agonist triggering was first introduced in 1991 by Itskovitz *et al.* in order to prevent OHSS; however, it was not employed commonly because of the available agonist protocols [21]. Antagonist protocols started to be used commonly in clinical practice at the beginning of the 2000s [22]. At this stage, agonist triggering was reintroduced due to the short half-life of antagonists and their ability to rapidly dissociate from the receptors as specified in the agonist protocol. Hence, agonist triggering results in a lower frequency of OHSS, instead of triggering with hCG, which has a longer half-life [23]. The meta-analysis conducted by Al-Inany *et al.* compared the agonist- and hCG-triggered cycles in respect to the rates of live births, and no statistically significant differences were observed [24]. When these two groups were compared with respect to the occurrence of OHSS, the OHSS rates were found to be approximately 50 percent lower, favoring the antagonist group.

Agonist Trigger

Human chorionic gonadotropin has long been administered to achieve the LH effect in order to accomplish final oocyte maturation. While its long half-life is useful in providing luteal support by means of its beneficial effects on the hormonal levels at the luteal phase during implantation, it increases the risk of OHSS, which is especially increased in the high-risk

patients. The European Society of Human Reproduction and Embryology (ESHRE) reports the incidence of OHSS to be 0.18–1.40 percent in the couples receiving treatment for infertility in general [25]. Although the concept of total freezing following hCG triggering reduces the risk of late OHSS significantly, the risk of early OHSS remains. GnRH agonist triggering, which has been used more commonly in recent years, may be an effective strategy at this point acting via a different pathophysiological process. Agonist triggering requires the accomplishment of an antagonist cycle primarily. A GnRH agonist is found to be 2–50 times more effective than endogenous GnRH on the basis of its effects at the level of GnRH receptors. Moreover, the shorter half-life will allow for a shorter luteotropic effect on the corpus luteum, especially in comparison to the administration of hCG (6–10 days vs. 33 hours, respectively) [26]. The association of the higher level of hCG with the higher number of follicles, oocytes, and corpus luteum observed in OHSS processes may lead to the secretion of vascular endothelial growth factor for a longer duration. The agonist's short half-life allows for the oocyte maturation to be completed following the secretion of LH and follicle-stimulating hormone (FSH) shortly after the agonist administration. Then, its effect is terminated. While this short-term effect requires intense luteal phase support in fresh embryo transfers following agonist triggering, this requirement is eliminated in cycles with total freezing following agonist triggering. Despite the remarkable likelihood of reduced incidences of OHSS after GnRH agonist triggering, there are some case reports available in the literature [27;28]. In these cases, mutations might be involved in association with the development of OHSS, or GnRH, FSH, or LH receptor polymorphisms might be present.

Premature Progesterone Elevation and Elective Freeze-All Policy

Although its mechanism of action has not been clarified yet, the elevated levels of serum progesterone in the follicular phase have long been a significant subject of debate. Despite the absence of a consensus on a defined cut-off point, serum progesterone levels > 1.5 ng/ml on the day of hCG trigger have been shown to be associated with statistically significant lower rates of ongoing pregnancies [29].

The strategies to be employed in the presence of high progesterone levels include corticosteroid administration, giving tapered doses of gonadotropins by the end of the stimulation process or transferring blastocysts; however, no strategies have been established yet. Freeze-all and cycle segmentation strategies at this stage may increase the chance of eliminating the endometrial changes at the receptive level [30]. One of the major issues to be considered in these circumstances is that a variety of outcomes may occur in the presence of various particularities associated with different medical centers, including the conditions of embryo cryopreservation, laboratory standards, and the techniques used in preparing the embryo.

Preimplantation Genetic Screening and Elective Freeze-All Policy

Preimplantation genetic screening is a strategy based on the higher likelihood of achieving implantation with a chromosomally normal embryo. It is a screening program, recommended for a number of indications including advanced age, recurrent implantation failure, and recurrent pregnancy loss. Fluorescence in situ hybridization method was the first technique used for this purpose. Later, other methods were introduced to the clinical practice, including polymerase chain reaction, single-nucleotide polymorphism, comparative genomic hybridization techniques, and next-generation sequencing technologies [31].

Biopsy samples are collected from the embryos after sperm have fertilized the oocytes obtained after COS. Two different strategies may be applied after collecting the biopsy samples from the embryos on the fifth day. The first strategy is to freeze all embryos after the biopsy process and to schedule a frozen-thawed transfer in the proceeding cycle. In the second strategy, biopsies are performed on the fifth-day embryo early in the morning and the transfer is performed on the sixth day in the afternoon depending on the test results [32]. This may enable inclusion of all blastocysts in the embryo biopsy process and inclusion of more patients to the embryo transfer.

Elective Freeze-All Policy: How?

Endometrial Preparation

With the advances in technology in frozen-thawed embryo transfer (FET) cycles, the strategy of freezing a number of embryos to be transferred in the proceeding cycles is employed more frequently. Probably the most important feature of this process is the ability to make the embryo transfer at an appropriate time when the endometrial environment is ready.

In general, three principles are involved in the endometrial preparation [33]: The first is the principle of ovulation induction in an anovulating patient or ovulation induction during the natural cycle in an ovulating patient. The second principle includes the preparation of the endometrium with exogenous estrogen and progesterone in the presence or absence of suppression with the GnRH in the previous cycle. The third principle includes ovulation induction with oral medications or gonadotropins, followed by hCG administration. The latter principle is almost never applied today.

Embryo Transfer in a Natural (Spontaneous) Cycle

Natural cycle FET is achieved owing to the synthesis of endogenous steroids from the follicles during the cycle of endometrial preparation. Embryo transfer can be performed with a spontaneous LH surge or with the administration of hCG to enable luteinization. Determining the ovulation time and estimating the endometrial receptivity precisely are critical predictors of thawing and transfer.

Monitoring of ovulation can be accomplished by following up the levels of LH in the urine or in the blood during a natural cycle FET. The LH surge in the urine occurs 21 hours after the LH surge in the blood and ovulation occurs 36–40 hours after the LH surge. The measurements should be made every day or twice a day primarily with the purpose of determining the urinary LH levels accurately. Furthermore, false negativity is an issue as the threshold levels of urinary LH show variations depending on the types of kits used in the tests [34]. Under these circumstances, interpretation of patient results and scheduling an ideal date of transfer may be difficult. In order to overcome these disadvantages in LH quantification, it has been suggested that hCG is used in ovulation induction. This process is called a "modified natural cycle" and does not require LH to be monitored; however, it requires monitoring of the development of the dominant follicle with ultrasound. The general criterion is to administer hCG when the follicle reaches a size of 18–20 mm so that ovulation and oocyte maturation are induced [35]. It is estimated that ovulation occurs in the 34th to 36th hour after the injection. Ovulation may occur earlier than expected in some of the cycles, in which transfer cannot be made [36]. Transfer can be scheduled depending on the time of the freezing of the embryos after hCG administration. However, hCG administration for ovulation induction, even during the natural cycles, may affect the ongoing pregnancy rates negatively [37].

In natural cycle FETs a combination of diagnostic methods can be used including ultrasound examinations and the quantification of LH, estradiol, and progesterone levels. A comparison of natural cycles with modified cycles revealed no differences in the rates of clinical pregnancies and live births [38]. Saito *et al.* compared pregnancy outcomes between natural ovulatory cycle (NC)-FET ($n = 29\ 760$) and hormone replacement cycle (HRC)-FET ($n = 75\ 474$) cycles. The pregnancy rate (32.1% vs. 36.1%) and the live birth rate among pregnancies (67.1% vs. 71.9%) in HRC-FET cycles were significantly lower than those in NC-FET cycles. A multiple logistic regression analysis showed that pregnancies after HRC-FET had increased odds of hypertensive disease of pregnancy (adjusted odds ratio [aOR] 1.43, 95% confidence interval [CI] 1.14–1.80) and placenta accreta (aOR 6.91, 95% CI 2.87–16.66) and decreased odds for gestational diabetes mellitus (aOR 0.52, 95% CI 0.40–0.68) in comparison to pregnancies after NC-FET [39].

Artificial Endometrium Preparation by the Exogenous Administration of Estrogen-Progesterone

Similar to the pattern observed in a normal menstrual cycle, estrogen and progesterone are administered consecutively in the artificial cycle FET. Estrogen administration in the first phase of the cycle provides a similar effect to that of the endogenous estrogen, which is synthesized from the granulosa cells in the growing follicle in the follicular phase, inducing endometrial proliferation. Estrogen can be given orally or in the form of transdermal bands or transvaginal rings. The most commonly used form is either the oral or the transdermal mode of administration. Estrogen induces endometrial proliferation on the one hand and inhibits the development of the growing dominant follicle on the other. Progesterone is included in the treatment to induce secretory changes usually when the endometrial thickness reaches 7–9 mm in the ultrasound examination [40]. This way, the transition from estrogen to progesterone is simulated as it occurs in the midcycle after ovulation. Then, the duration of progesterone support and the time of transfer are scheduled depending on the time of embryo freezing.

Although estrogen administration usually inhibits follicular growth, spontaneous luteinization occurs in the follicle under some circumstances, leading to an early exposure of the endometrium to progesterone. This changes the implantation window and the duration of receptivity. GnRH agonists have been introduced at this stage to induce pituitary downregulation. When pituitary suppression is induced at the end of the preceding cycle, the development of the follicle will be inhibited too. But this intervention can be accepted as a physiological treatment only at a lesser degree as it requires the administration of both hormone replacing medications and agonists. The ability to schedule the embryo transfer time at this stage accurately can be accepted as an advantage of this method owing to the longer hormone replacement treatment.

It has been demonstrated that there are no differences in the rates of clinical pregnancy and live births in artificial cycles when the GnRH agonist-triggered cycles are compared with the cycles without GnRH administration. A meta-analysis revealed similar results with no differences upon the comparison of natural cycles with artificial endometrial preparation cycles.

Pregnancy Rates

Pregnancy outcomes have been evaluated separately by a randomized controlled study on ovulating women and in women with polycystic ovary syndrome (PCOS) [41]. In PCOS, higher rates of pregnancy were achieved with FET cycles at the cleavage phase compared with fresh embryo transfer cycles (49.3% vs. 42.0%; ratio 1.17, 95% CI 1.05–1.31; $p = 0.004$), accompanied with a lower risk of OHSS (1.3% vs. 7.1%; ratio 0.19, 95% CI 0.10–0.37; $p < 0.001$). Furthermore, the percentage of pregnancy losses was found to be lower in FET cycles (22.0% vs. 32.7%, ratio 0.67, 95% CI 0.54–0.83; $p < 0.001$). Another randomized controlled study compared FET cycles with fresh embryo transfer cycles [42]. The two groups were compared with each other in terms of implantation, clinical pregnancy rates, pregnancy losses, rates of ongoing pregnancies, and live births; however, no differences were observed. Similar to the findings of the previous study, OHSS risk was found to be significantly lower in the FET cycles (0.6% vs. 2.0%; relative risk [RR] 0.32, 95% CI 0.14–0.74; $p = 0.005$). The most recent randomized controlled study comparing the pregnancy rates reported that frozen-thawed transfer cycles provided no superiorities in terms of ongoing pregnancy or live birth rates in couples without a diagnosis of PCOS [43].

The comparison of frozen-thawed transfer cycles with fresh embryo transfer cycles revealed lower rates of ectopic pregnancies per clinical pregnancy (odds ratio [OR] 0.31, 95% CI 0.24–0.39) [44]. When FETs are compared on the basis of whether the transferred embryo was in the cleavage or blastocyst phase, it was found that the incidence of ectopic pregnancies was statistically significantly lower in blastocyst transfers (0.8% vs. 1.8%; $p = 0.002$). When the incidence of heterotopic pregnancies was compared between FET cycles and fresh embryo transfer cycles in a large cohort of patients, no differences were observed [45].

Perinatal Outcomes

The rates of clinical pregnancies, as well as the process of pregnancy, the rate of live births, and the long-term effects, have recently received gradually increasing attention in the interpretation of the data associated with ART. Perinatal and obstetric outcomes of pregnancies achieved by ART have recently raised several concerns in recent years. Different studies have reported a higher likelihood of negative outcomes with ART, including especially preterm delivery (PTB), gestational age (small for gestational age [SGA]), low birth weight (LBW), and perinatal mortality, compared with natural pregnancies [46]. In addition, the common use of freezing-thawing cycles allowed for a comparison of the perinatal outcomes of ART. A meta-analysis included a total of 26 studies to compare the perinatal outcomes and found that singleton pregnancies achieved after FET cycles were associated with a lower relative risk of PTB (RR 0.90, 95% CI 0.84–0.97), LBW (RR 0.72, 95% CI 0.67–0.77), and being SGA (RR 0.61, 95% CI 0.56–0.67) [47]. Furthermore, the same meta-analysis determined that FET cycles were associated with a higher relative risk of hypertensive diseases of pregnancy (HDP) (RR 1.29, 95% CI 1.07–1.56), being large for gestational age (LGA) (RR 1.54, 95% CI 1.48–1.61), and high birth weight (RR 1.85, 95% CI 1.46–2.33). FET cycles were associated with a relative risk of 3.16 for placenta accrete; however, no significantly increased risks of congenital anomalies were identified compared with fresh transfers [48;49].

Gu *et al.* compared perinatal outcomes of vitrified embryo transfer with slow-FET in singletons; vitrification was non-inferior ($p > 0.05$) to the slow-freezing method in terms of the occurrence of preterm birth (OR 0.68, 95% CI 0.35–1.31), LBW (OR 1.19, 95% CI 0.61–2.32), macrosomia (OR 0.94, 95% CI 0.48–1.86), SGA (OR 1.55, 95% CI 0.91–2.64), and LGA (OR 0.78, 95% CI 0.42–1.45) [50].

A Nordic study included 3650 children born after transfer of vitrified blastocysts, 8123 children born after transfer of slow-frozen cleavage stage embryos, and 4469 children born after transfer of fresh blastocysts during 2002–2015. A higher risk of PTB was noted in the vitrified blastocyst group compared with the slow-frozen cleavage stage group (aOR 1.33, 95% CI 1.09–1.62). No significant differences were observed for LBW, SGA, macrosomia, and LGA when comparing the vitrified blastocyst with the slow-frozen cleavage stage group. For maternal outcomes, no significant difference was seen in the risk of HDP, placenta previa, placental abruption and postpartum hemorrhage (PPH) in the vitrified blastocyst versus the slow-frozen cleavage stage group. Furthermore, comparing vitrified and fresh blastocysts, there were higher risks of macrosomia (aOR 1.77, 95% CI 1.35–2.31) and LGA (aOR 1.48, 95% CI 1.18–1.84). Further, the risks of HDP (aOR 1.47, 95% CI 1.19–1.81) and PPH (aOR 1.68, 95% CI 1.39–2.03) were higher in singletons born after vitrified compared with fresh blastocyst transfer while the risks of SGA (aOR 0.58, 95% CI 0.44–0.78) and placenta previa (aOR 0.35, 95% CI 0.25–0.48) were lower [51].

Conclusion

In conclusion, pregnancy rates are reported to be increasing day by day along with the growing body of experience and advancing technologies in the freezing-thawing cycles. Especially the elective freeze-all policy plays a remarkably significant role in preventing OHSS, which is the most concerning issue in ART. Establishing proper laboratory conditions and performing an optimal cryopreservation program are critical at this stage, especially accompanied with the cycle segmentation strategy.

References

1. Fatemi HM, Garcia-Velasco J. Avoiding ovarian hyperstimulation syndrome with the use of gonadotropin-releasing hormone agonist trigger. *Fertil Steril* 2015;**103**:870–873.

2. Basile N, Garcia-Velasco JA. The state of "freeze-for-all" in human ARTs. *J Assist Reprod Genet* 2016;**33**:1543–1550.

3. Coates A, Kung A, Mounts E, *et al.* Optimal euploid embryo transfer strategy, fresh versus frozen, after preimplantation genetic screening with next generation sequencing: a randomized controlled trial. *Fertil Steril* 2017;**107**:723–730.

4. Sparks AE. Human embryo cryopreservation-methods, timing, and other considerations for optimizing an embryo cryopreservation program. *Semin Reprod Med* 2015;**33**:128–144.

5. Weinerman R, Mainigi M. Why we should transfer frozen instead of fresh embryos: the translational rationale. *Fertil Steril* 2014;**102**:10–18.

6. Shapiro BS, Daneshmand ST, Garner FC, *et al.* Evidence of impaired endometrial receptivity after ovarian stimulation for in vitro fertilization: a prospective randomized trial comparing fresh and frozen-thawed embryo transfer in normal responders. *Fertil Steril* 2011;**96**:344–348.

7. Meyer WR, Novotny DB, Fritz MA, *et al.* Effect of exogenous gonadotropins on endometrial maturation in oocyte donors. *Fertil Steril* 1999;**71**:109–114.

8. Ubaldi F, Bourgain C, Tournaye H, *et al.* Endometrial evaluation by aspiration biopsy on the day of oocyte retrieval in the embryo transfer cycles in patients with serum progesterone rise during the follicular phase. *Fertil Steril* 1997;**67**:521–526.

9. Cha J, Sun X, Dey SK. Mechanisms of implantation: strategies for successful pregnancy. *Nat Med* 2012;**18**:1754–1767.

10. Horcajadas JA, Mínguez P, Dopazo J, *et al.* Controlled ovarian stimulation induces a functional genomic delay of the endometrium with potential clinical implications. *J Clin Endocrinol Metab* 2008;**93**:4500–4510.

11. Liu Y, Lee KF, Ng EH, Yeung WS, Ho PC. Gene expression profiling of human peri-implantation endometria between natural and stimulated cycles. *Fertil Steril* 2008;**90**:2152–2164.

12. Liu Y, Kodithuwakku SP, Ng PY, *et al.* Excessive ovarian stimulation up-regulates the Wnt-signaling molecule DKK1 in human endometrium and may affect implantation: an in vitro co-culture study. *Hum Reprod* 2010;**25**:479–490.

13. de Waal E, Vrooman LA, Fischer E, *et al.* The cumulative effect of assisted reproduction procedures on placental development and epigenetic perturbations in a mouse model. *Hum Mol Genet* 2015;**24**:6975–6985.

14. Denomme MM, Mann MR. Genomic imprints as a model for the analysis of epigenetic stability during assisted reproductive technologies. *Reproduction* 2012;**144**:393–409.

15. Market-Velker BA, Zhang L, Magri LS, Bonvissuto AC, Mann MR. Dual effects of superovulation: loss of maternal and paternal imprinted methylation in a dose-dependent manner. *Hum Mol Genet* 2010;**19**:36–51.

16. Trounson A, Mohr L. Human pregnancy following cryopreservation, thawing and transfer of an eight-cell embryo. *Nature* 1983;**305**:707–709.

17. Yu L, Jia C, Lan Y, *et al.* Analysis of embryo intactness and developmental potential following slow freezing and vitrification. *Syst Biol Reprod Med* 2017;**63**:285–293.

18. Cobo A, de los Santos MJ, Castelló D, *et al.* Outcomes of vitrified early cleavage-stage and blastocyst-stage embryos in a cryopreservation program: evaluation of 3,150 warming cycles. *Fertil Steril* 2012;**98**:1138–1146.

19. Devine K, Connell MT, Richter KS, *et al.* Single vitrified blastocyst transfer maximizes liveborn children per embryo while minimizing preterm birth. *Fertil Steril* 2015;**103**:1454–1460.

20. Zech J, Brandao A, Zech M, *et al.* Elective frozen-thawed embryo transfer (FET) in women at risk for ovarian hyperstimulation syndrome. *Reprod Biol* 2018;**18**:46–52.

21. Itskovitz J, Boldes R, Levron J, et al. Induction of preovulatory luteinizing hormone surge and prevention of ovarian hyperstimulation syndrome by gonadotropin-releasing hormone agonist. *Fertil Steril* 1991;**56**:213–220.

22. Albano C, Smitz J, Camus M, et al. Comparison of different doses of gonadotropin-releasing hormone antagonist cetrorelix during controlled ovarian hyperstimulation. *Fertil Steril* 1997;**67**:917–922.

23. Engmann L, Benadiva C, Humaidan P. GnRH agonist trigger for the induction of oocyte maturation in GnRH antagonist IVF cycles: a SWOT analysis. *Reprod Biomed Online* 2016;**32**:274–285.

24. Al-Inany HG, Youssef MA, Ayeleke RO, et al. Gonadotrophin-releasing hormone antagonists for assisted reproductive technology. *Cochrane Database Syst Rev* 2016;**4**:CD001750.

25. European IVF-Monitoring Consortium (EIM); European Society of Human Reproduction and Embryology (ESHRE); Kupka MS, D'Hooghe T, Ferraretti AP, et al. Assisted reproductive technology in Europe, 2011: results generated from European registers by ESHRE. *Hum Reprod* 2016;**31**:233–248.

26. Yen SS, Llerena O, Little B, Pearson OH. Disappearance rates of endogenous luteinizing hormone and chorionic gonadotropin in man. *J Clin Endocrinol Metab* 1968;**28**:1763–1767.

27. Fatemi HM, Popovic-Todorovic B, Humaidan P, et al. Severe ovarian hyperstimulation syndrome after gonadotropin-releasing hormone (GnRH) agonist trigger and "freeze-all" approach in GnRH antagonist protocol. *Fertil Steril* 2014;**101**:1008-1011.

28. Ling LP, Phoon JW, Lau MS, et al. GnRH agonist trigger and ovarian hyperstimulation syndrome: relook at 'freeze-all strategy'. *Reprod Biomed Online* 2014;**29**:392–394.

29. Venetis CA, Kolibianakis EM, Papanikolaou E, et al. Is progesterone elevation on the day of human chorionic gonadotrophin administration associated with the probability of pregnancy in in vitro fertilization? A systematic review and meta-analysis. *Hum Reprod Update* 2007;**13**:343–355.

30. Fatemi HM, Van Vaerenbergh I. Significance of premature progesterone rise in IVF. *Curr Opin Obstet Gynecol* 2015;**27**:242–248.

31. Handyside AH. 24-chromosome copy number analysis: a comparison of available technologies. *Fertil Steril* 2013;**100**:595–602.

32. Sermon K, Capalbo A, Cohen J, et al. The why, the how and the when of PGS 2.0: current practices and expert opinions of fertility specialists, molecular biologists, and embryologists. *Mol Hum Reprod* 2016;**22**:845–857.

33. Kalem Z, Kalem MN, Gürgan T. Methods for endometrial preparation in frozen-thawed embryo transfer cycles. *J Turk Ger Gynecol Assoc* 2016;**17**:168–172.

34. O'Connor KA, Brindle E, Miller RC, et al. Ovulation detection methods for urinary hormones: precision, daily and intermittent sampling and a combined hierarchical method. *Hum Reprod* 2006;**21**:1442–1452.

35. Andersen AG, Als-Nielsen B, Hornnes PJ, Franch Andersen L. Time interval from human chorionic gonadotrophin (HCG) injection to follicular rupture. *Hum Reprod* 1995;**10**:3202–3205.

36. Al-Azemi M, Kyrou D, Kolibianakis EM, et al. Elevated progesterone during ovarian stimulation for IVF. *Reprod Biomed Online* 2012;**24**:381–388.

37. Fatemi HM, Kyrou D, Bourgain C, et al. Cryopreserved-thawed human embryo transfer: spontaneous natural cycle is superior to human chorionic gonadotropin-induced natural cycle. *Fertil Steril* 2010;**94**:2054–2058.

38. Weissman A, Horowitz E, Ravhon A, et al. Spontaneous ovulation versus HCG triggering for timing natural-cycle frozen–thawed embryo transfer: a randomized study. *Reprod Biomed Online* 2011;**23**:484–489.

39. Saito K, Kuwahara A, Ishikawa T, et al. Endometrial preparation methods for frozen-thawed embryo transfer are associated with altered risks of hypertensive disorders of pregnancy, placenta accreta, and gestational diabetes mellitus. *Hum Reprod* 2019;**34** (8):1567–1575.

40. El-Toukhy T, Coomarasamy A, Khairy M, et al. The relationship between endometrial thickness and outcome of medicated frozen embryo replacement cycles. *Fertil Steril* 2008;**89**:832–839.

41. Chen ZJ, Shi Y, Sun Y, et al. Fresh versus frozen embryos for infertility in the polycystic ovary syndrome. *N Engl J Med* 2016;**375**:523–533.

42. Shi Y, Sun Y, Hao C, et al. Transfer of fresh versus frozen embryos in ovulatory women. *N Engl J Med* 2018;**378**:126–136.

43. Vuong LN, Dang VQ, Ho TM, et al. IVF transfer of fresh or frozen embryos in women without polycystic ovaries. *N Engl J Med* 2018;**378**:137–147.

44. Zhang X, Ma C, Wu Z, et al. Frozen-thawed embryo transfer cycles have a lower incidence of ectopic pregnancy compared with fresh embryo transfer cycles. *Reprod Sci* 2018;**25**:1431–1435.

45. Xiao S, Mo M, Hu X, *et al.* Study on the incidence and influences on heterotopic pregnancy from embryo transfer of fresh cycles and frozen-thawed cycles. *J Assist Reprod Genet* 2018;**35**:677–681.

46. Spijkers S, Lens JW, Schats R, Lambalk CB. Fresh and frozen-thawed embryo transfer compared to natural conception: differences in perinatal outcome. *Gynecol Obstet Invest* 2017;**82**:538–546.

47. Maheshwari A, Pandey S, Amalraj Raja E, *et al.* Is frozen embryo transfer better for mothers and babies? Can cumulative meta-analysis provide a definitive answer? *Hum Reprod Update* 2018;**24**:35–58.

48. Maheshwari A, Raja EA, Bhattacharya S. Obstetric and perinatal outcomes after either fresh or thawed frozen embryo transfer: an analysis of 112,432 singleton pregnancies recorded in the Human Fertilisation and Embryology Authority anonymized dataset. *Fertil Steril* 2016;**106**:1703–1708.

49. Ishihara O, Araki R, Kuwahara A, *et al.* Impact of frozen-thawed single-blastocyst transfer on maternal and neonatal outcome: an analysis of 277,042 single-embryo transfer cycles from 2008 to 2010 in Japan. *Fertil Steril* 2014;**101**:128–133.

50. Gu F, Li S, Zheng L, *et al.* Perinatal outcomes of singletons following vitrification versus slow-freezing of embryos: a multicenter cohort study using propensity score analysis. *Hum Reprod* 2019;**34**(9):1788–1798.

51. Ginström Ernstad E, Spangmose AL, Opdahl S, *et al.* Perinatal and maternal outcome after vitrification of blastocysts: a Nordic study in singletons from the CoNARTaS group. *Hum Reprod* 2019;**34**(11):2282–2289.

Chapter

26

Ultrasound Monitoring for Ovulation Induction: Pitfalls and Problems

Mona M. Aboulghar and Yomna Islam

Ovulation induction using stimulation drugs has now been in practice for over 40 years. Until the introduction of ultrasound, monitoring of follicular growth was a difficult task. Transvaginal ultrasound is now the routine for ovulation induction monitoring. Transvaginal probes have a much higher frequency reaching 4–9 MHz, and have wider angles up to 180° and depths that could reach 16 cm, facilitating the procedure of monitoring.

Pretreatment Evaluation

All infertile patients, especially those scheduled for in vitro fertilization (IVF), should have a basic infertility scan, which ideally is best done in the early follicular phase and should be performed using transvaginal ultrasound. It should include:

- *Assessment of the uterus* – site, size, mobility, texture of myometrium, uniformity of the endometrium, assessment of the cervix, and cervical canal
- *Assessment of the ovaries* – confirm the presence of the ovaries, measure volume, texture including antral follicle count (AFC), and detection of abnormalities
- *Assessment of pelvic peritoneum and tubes* – detection of hydrosalpinges and peritoneal cysts

The Uterus

A retroverted flexed uterus which is fixed and shows no mobility on pressure by vaginal probe suggests pelvic adhesions, especially common in endometriosis. Abnormalities of the uterus, causing increase in size and change in texture, include the following.

Fibroids

The incidence has been reported to vary greatly, occurring in 5.4–77 percent of women of

reproductive age [1]; however, it is known to increase in the late reproductive period and that is why it is common in infertile patients. Ultrasound detection of myoma has a high sensitivity of 99 percent and specificity of 86 percent [2], which increases even more if sonohysterography is added to the examination [3].

Fibroids appear as hypoechoic areas arising from within the myometrium causing attenuation of the ultrasound beam and distal shadowing. They usually have a well-defined outline formed by the capsule. The size and number of the fibroids should be recorded. The site is of special importance in IVF patients. **According to the FIGO (2018) abnormal uterine bleeding classification system, uterine fibroids are subclassified into Submucous and Others [4].**

Submucous includes

Type 0: Intracavitary lesions attached to the endometrium by a narrow stalk

Types 1 and 2: A portion of the lesion is intramural – with Type 1 having less than 50% involvement and Type 2 at least 50%

Others include

Type 3: Lesions are totally intramural, contacting endometrium

Type 4: Lesions are intramural that are entirely within the myometrium, with no extension to the endometrial surface or to the serosa

Subserosal (*Types 5–7*) represent the mirror image of the submucosal fibroids

Type 5: Being at least 50% intramural

Type 6: Less than 50% intramural

Type 7: Attached to the serosa by a stalk

An additional category, *Type 8*: Fibroids that do not relate to the myometrium at all, and would include cervical lesions, those that exist in the

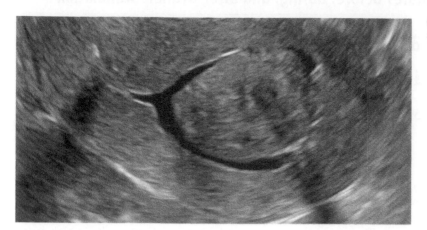

Figure 26.1 Submucous fibroid seen with sonohysterography.

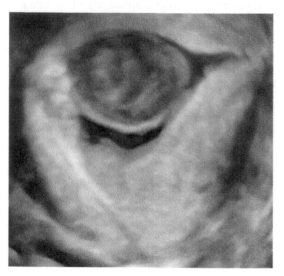

Figure 26.2 Three-dimensional sonohysterography of submucous fibroid.

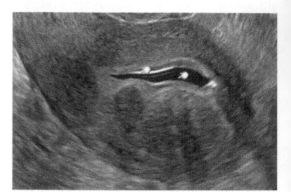

Figure 26.3 Sonohysterography showing posterior intramural fibroids.

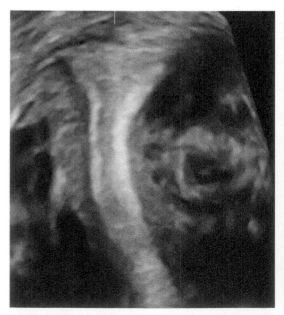

Figure 26.4 Three-dimensional intramural fibroid with normal cavity.

round or broad ligaments without direct attachment to the uterus, and other so-called "parasitic" lesions

Ultrasound criteria of submucous fibroids include central position and distortion of the endometrial–myometrial interface. Confirmation of the submucous variant is essentially performed by adding sonohysterography to the examination (Figure 26.1) or three-dimensional ultrasound (Figure 26.2), which adds to the accuracy of diagnosis [5]. Also, normal intact cavity is confirmed by sonohysterography (Figure 26.3) or three-dimensional ultrasound (Figure 26.4).

Effect of Fibroids on IVF Programs

The presence of non-cavity-distorting fibroids appears to negatively affect clinical pregnancy and live birth rates. The deleterious effect of fibroids on live birth rates was significant in women with two or more fibroids and in women with fibroids of ≥ 30 mm in diameter. Conversely, in women with single fibroids of < 30 mm in diameter, no difference in pregnancy outcomes was identified [6]. In a study assessing the effect of uterine leiomyomas on the endometrium using molecular markers of endometrial receptivity, a decrease in HOX gene expression throughout the endometrium and not simply over a submucosal myoma was found. This observation implies that impairment of fertility may be attributed to a global effect and not simply a focal change of the endometrium overlying the myoma [7]. A meta-analysis was performed that explored the impact of non-cavity-distorting intramural fibroids on the efficacy of IVF-embryo transfer (IVF-ET) treatment, and suggests that non-cavity-distorting intramural fibroids would significantly reduce the implantation rate, clinical pregnancy rate, and live birth rate and significantly increase miscarriage after IVF treatment, but it would not significantly increase the ectopic pregnancy rate [8].

Submuous fibroids should be removed hysteroscopically, while subserous fibroid removal is not recommended. There is fair evidence to recommend against myomectomy in women with intramural fibroids (hysteroscopically confirmed intact endometrium) and otherwise unexplained infertility, regardless of their size. If the patient has no other options, the benefits of myomectomy should be weighed against the risks, and management of intramural fibroids should be individualized [9]. In our practice, prior to IVF we usually advise removal of intramural fibroids that are not distorting the cavity if > 4 cm.

The size of the fibroids could make monitoring of ovulation and examination of the ovaries difficult as they obscure the ovaries by posterior acoustic shadowing.

Adenomyosis

A report on ultrasound diagnosis of adenomyosis gave sensitivity, specificity, positive predictive value (PPV), and negative predictive value (NPV) of 76.4%, 92.8%, 73.8%, and 88.8%, respectively, which was not different from MRI [10]. Most recent ultrasound descriptors for adenomyosis follow the Morphological Uterus Sonographic Assessment (MUSA) descriptors which have been published in the MUSA consensus statement [11]. The MUSA features typical of a uterus with adenomyosis include an enlarged globular uterus, asymmetrical thickening of the myometrium (Figure 26.5), myometrial cysts, echogenic subendometrial lines and buds, hyperechogenic islands, fan-shaped shadowing, an irregular or interrupted junctional zone (Figure 26.6), and translesional vascularity on color Doppler ultrasound examination. When adenomyosis is found, the location, the number, and the site have to be described. Focal from global adenomyosis has to be differentiated.

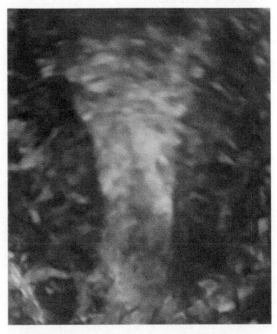

Figure 26.6 Interrupted junctional zone in adenomyosis.

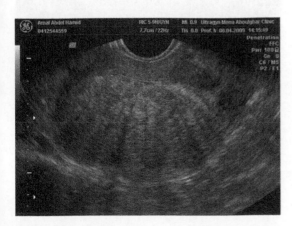

Figure 26.5 Adenomyosis.

Differentiation from fibroids is mainly by the absence of lesion margin and the presence of hypoechoic lacunae.

A meta-analysis in 2014 studying the effect of adenomyosis on IVF/intracytoplasmic sperm injection (ICSI) outcome included nine studies in a pooled analysis and all the presented studies in IVF/ICSI women. Based on a total of 1865 women, 306 of whom were diagnosed with adenomyosis, it was concluded that adenomyosis adversely affects the probability of clinical pregnancy and increases the risk of early pregnancy loss [12]. Women with adenomyosis had a lower clinical pregnancy rate after IVF-ET [13]. Adenomyosis has a detrimental effect on IVF clinical outcomes. Pretreatment with the use of long-term gonadotropin-releasing hormone (GnRH) agonist or long protocol could be beneficial [14]. In women with diminished ovarian reserve, immediate IVF or ICSI with long protocol or oocyte retrieval can be followed by frozen embryo transfer after GnRH agonist treatment is performed. There is limited evidence for an improved outcome after surgery, and surgery should only be an option for symptomatic women with repeated IVF/ICSI failure in validated studies [15].

Similar to large fibroids, adenomyosis poses difficulties during monitoring of ovulation due to acoustic shadowing.

Müllerian Anomalies

The incidence of Müllerian anomalies in infertile patients is higher than the general population; in a recent report it reached 8 percent [16] and canalization defect is the most common uterine anomaly in women with infertility (3 percent).

Therefore, Müllerian anomalies could have an impact on infertility and its treatment. Ultrasound was recommended as the first diagnostic tool to be used owing to its high PPV (96.3%) and NPV (100%). The recommendation of the most recent ESHRE/ESGE Thessaloniki Consensus (2013) on the diagnosis of female genital anomalies is that three-dimensional ultrasound is the diagnostic tool of choice owing to its high sensitivity (98.3%), specificity (99.4%), PPV (99.2%), NPV (93.9%), and accuracy (97.6%). The three-dimensional image gives the coronal view of the uterus, which allows a simultaneous view of the uterine cavity and the fundal myometrium and consequently will allow accurate diagnosis of the type of Müllerian anomaly (Figures 26.7, 26.8, and 26.9 show Müllerian anomalies).

The recent ESHRE classification [17] shown in Figures 26.10 and 26.11 is mainly based on the measurement of the uterine muscle distortion rather than the examination of the uterine cavity itself and cervical and vaginal anomalies are classified in independent supplementary subclasses.

Precycle diagnosis of the type of Müllerian anomaly is essential for counseling and assessing the effect on cycle success. No consensus exists on removal of septae versus leaving them prior to an IVF cycle. However, a review of literature on all the available international guidelines in order to propose a management strategy for infertile patients with a uterine septum concluded that hysteroscopic septum incision seems to improve natural conception rates in the year following surgery. Moreover, it improves IVF outcomes when performed before the embryo transfer, by improving embryo implantation rates. In cases of recurrent implantation failure or recurrent pregnancy loss following IVF, hysteroscopic resection

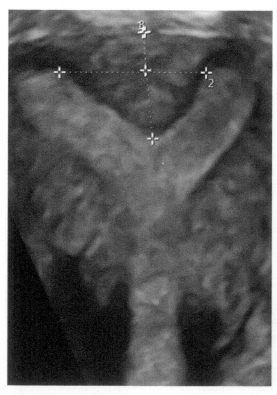

Figure 26.7 Subseptate uterus.

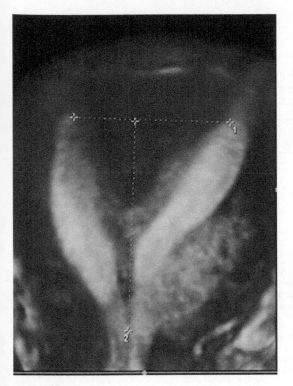

Figure 26.8 Septate uterus.

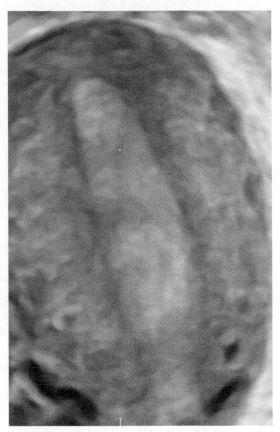

Figure 26.9 Unicornuate uterus.

could be proposed [18]. There is an ongoing multicenter randomized controlled trial (TRUST) aiming to assess whether hysteroscopic septum resection improves reproductive outcome in women with a septate uterus. The live birth rates will be compared, but results have not been published yet [19].

Endometrium

Ultrasound examination of the endometrium is essential to confirm uniformity of the uterine cavity. In the early follicular phase, it is thin, ranging in thickness from 4 to 8 mm, increasing in thickness as the cycle advances into the secretory phase measuring 8 to 14 mm, changing into the typical triple line (echogenic) appearance.

Measurement is done at the maximal thickness of the echogenic endometrial–myometrial interphase in the sagittal plane of the uterus (Figure 26.12).

B-mode examination gives a good image; however, three-dimensional imaging provides the coronal view of the endometrial cavity, with the site of tubal insertion and fundal myometrium in the same view (Figure 26.13).

Abnormalities detected during examination of the endometrium that should be excluded and managed before embryo transfer include polyps, submucous fibroids, and intrauterine synechiae.

Polyps

Polyps appear as persistent hyperechogenic areas, and can be mistaken for the normal thickness of the endometrium, especially if the scan is done in the luteal phase. It is therefore advisable to repeat examination in the early follicular phase, or perform sonohysterography (Figure 26.14) and, if available, perform three-dimensional examination (Figure 26.15). A helpful tool for confirming polyps with B-mode ultrasound is using color Doppler to detect the feeding vessel (Figure 26.16), which was found to have a high PPV for intracavitary pathology [20].

Intrauterine Synechiae

Ultrasound criteria for diagnosis of intrauterine synechiae include failure to visualize a uniform

ESHRE/ESGE classification
Female genital tract anomalies

	Uterine anomaly		Cervical / Vaginal anomaly	
Main class		Sub-class	Co-existent class	
U0	Normal uterus		C0	Normal cervix
U1	Dysmorphic uterus	a. T-shaped	C1	Septate cervix
		b. Infantilis		
		c. Others	C2	Double "normal" cervix
U2	Septate uterus	a. Partial	C3	Unilateral cervical aplasia
		b. Complete		
			C4	Cervical Aplasia
U3	Bicorporeal uterus	a. Partial		
		b. Complete		
		c. Bicorporeal septate	V0	Normal Vagina
U4	Hemi-uterus	a. With rudimentary cavity (communicating or not horn)	V1	Longitudinal non-obstructing vaginal septum
		b. Without rudimentary cavity (horn without cavity / no horn)	V2	Longitudinal obstructing vaginal septum
U5	Aplastic	a. With rudimentary cavity (bi- or unilateral horn)	V3	Transverse vaginal septum and/or imperforate hymen
		b. Without rudimentary cavity (bi- or unilateral uterine remnants/Aplasia)	V4	Vaginal aplasia
U6	Unclassified Malformations			
U			C	V

Figure 26.10 Scheme for the classification of female genital tract anomalies according to the new ESHRE/ESGE classification system.

endometrial lining, and a thin and echogenic endometrium with interruption of the lining (Figure 26.17).

Using sonohysterography will show failure of distension of the cavity with saline. Three-dimensional imaging is highly suggestive when an irregular cavity is seen (Figure 26.18).

Sonohysterography

Sonohysterography is a technique which entails saline injection into the uterine cavity under ultrasound guidance. It is an easy and cheap technique performed in the clinic and does not need concomitant antibiotic or analgesic therapy. It aids in confirmation of doubtful findings during B-mode examination. It is our routine to perform sonohysterography on all our patients with suspected lesions using B-mode ultrasound. An embryo transfer catheter is used for injection, a tenaculum is rarely needed, and only a small amount of saline is injected, not exceeding 10 ml. The most common

lesions detected by adding sonohysterography to the ultrasound examination include polyps, submucous myomas, and intramural myomas with intracavitary extension. In a study comparing transvaginal ultrasound and sonohysterography, sonohysterography demonstrated high specificity (92.8%) in the detection of uterine polyps, and high sensitivity (92.9%) and specificity (96.8%) in the diagnosis of endometrial hyperplasia. In addition it shows high sensitivity (90%), specificity (99%), PPV (92.2%), and NPV (99%) for detection of submucous myomas. Finally, sonohysterography shows high PPV (100%) and NPV (100%) for synechiae assessment [21].

A three-dimensional volume added to sonohysterography will minimize time of examination, therefore reducing pain perceived by the patient and the volume stored can be studied later with no need for the presence of the patient. Comparing three-dimensional sonohysterography and hysteroscopy, specificity and sensitivity for three-dimensional sonohysterography were 67% and 100%, respectively, and for hysteroscopy 67% and

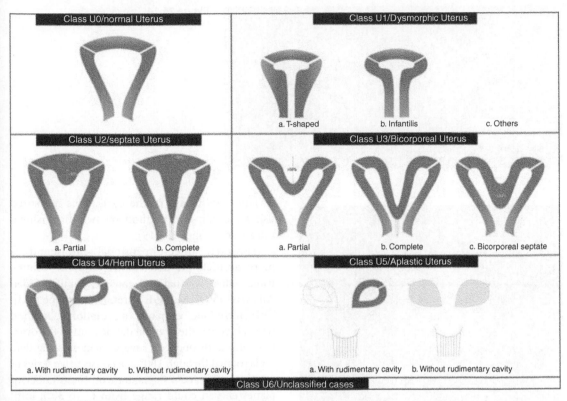

Figure 26.11 ESHRE/ESGE classification of uterine anomalies.

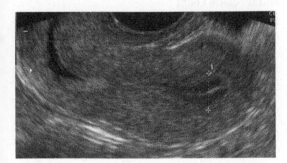

Figure 26.12 Measurement of midcyclic endometrium.

98%, respectively. In addition, the PPV and NPV were 98% and 100%, respectively, for three-dimensional sonohysterography, while for diagnostic hysteroscopy they were 98% and 67%, respectively [22].

Assessment of the Ovaries

Assessment of the ovaries is an essential part of this basic scan, in an attempt to predict the response of the patient to ovulation induction. It is essential to confirm the presence of the ovaries.

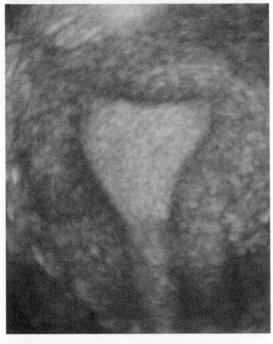

Figure 26.13 Normal three-dimensional image of endometrial cavity.

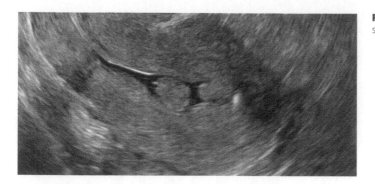

Figure 26.14 Two-dimensional sonohysterography image of a polyp.

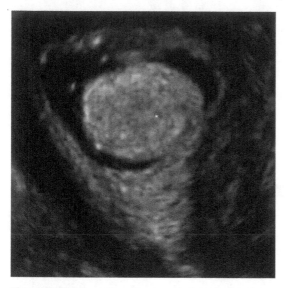

Figure 26.15 Three dimensional sonohysterography of endometrial polyp.

Some ovaries are laterally or upwardly displaced due to pelvic adhesions. This requires marked angulation of the probe and abdominal pressure for proper visualization. Ovaries are easier to visualize when stimulated; however, it is much better to be prepared and note the site of the ovaries prior to the start of cycle treatment. Mobility of the ovaries is tested by gentle pressure using the vaginal probe, which will show sliding of the ovaries against the surface of the uterus.

Evaluation of Normal Ovaries

Evaluation should be performed in the early follicular phase.

Ovarian Volume

Normal mean volume of a premenopausal unstimulated ovary is 5.4 cm^3 (4–7 cm^3). This shows variation with days of the cycle. It is measured using the ellipsoid method by two-dimensional ultrasound (Figure 26.19).

However, three-dimensional ultrasound is more accurate in determining ovarian volume using the Virtual Organ Computer-Aided Analysis (VOCAL, GE Kretz) technique [23]. This technique employs a rotational method which involves the manual delineation of the ovarian volume throughout several planes as the data set is rotated through 180° in a consecutive series of rotations (the angle dependent on the number of planes chosen could range from 6° to 30°), until a calculated volume is generated (Figure 26.20).

Antral Follicle Count

Basal AFC shows 5–11 small follicles < 10 mm in diameter. The number of follicles in the early follicular phase has been reported to be a good test for prediction of ovarian response [20;21].

Technique of AFC Measurement

All follicles 2–10 mm are measured using two-dimensional transvaginal ultrasound with a minimum of 7 MHz probe. The number of follicles in two planes, longitudinal and transverse, should be determined and the average diameter calculated. If the follicle is rounded one measurement is sufficient; if it is oval the mean should be determined by two perpendicular diameters [24].

Two-dimensional cine loops could help as well in calculating accurately the AFC.

In the three-dimensional manual mode the volume of the entire ovary is acquired, then using the multiplanar view, AFC counting can be performed while visualizing three perpendicular planes simultaneously (Figure 26.21).

Three-dimensional techniques are more accurate, reproducible, and less time-consuming.

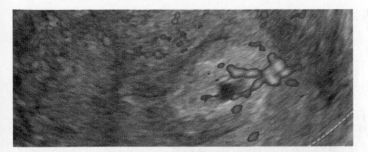

Figure 26.16 Feeding vessel of endometrial polyp.

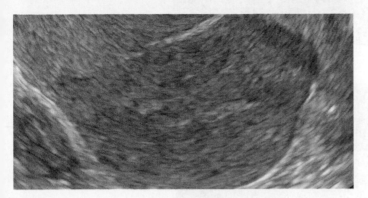

Figure 26.17 Two-dimensional image interrupted endometrium, intrauterine synechiae.

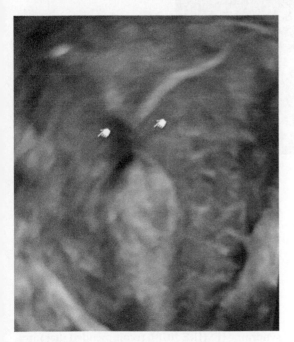

Figure 26.18 Three-dimensional image of midcavity intrauterine synechiae.

Automated follicle count [25;26] can be done. Using the software (SonoAVC; GE), the volume of each follicle can be automatically calculated based on the anechoic intrafollicular areas in the scanner. The software gives a mean diameter and volume of the

hypoechoic areas within the ovary representing the follicles, it will then color-code each follicle differently allowing study of each one separately. Three-dimensional technology can measure more follicles than two-dimensional, this is particularly important and relevant in ovaries with more than 20 follicles. The better estimation of AFCs by three-dimensional ultrasound was also detected regarding a different group of patients such as obese polycystic ovary syndrome (PCOS) patients. The predictive value of AFC and anti-Müllerian hormone (AMH) were similar for both clinical pregnancy and live birth. To predict the live birth, age ≤ 41, AFC > 3 and total retrieved oocytes > 6 appeared to be meaningful [27]. Poor response was defined as cycles that were canceled due to inadequate ovarian response or the number of retrieved oocytes being less than four [28]. Both AMH and AFC were good predictors of ovarian response, even though it seems that AFC was a better predictor. Both had poor predictive ability for clinical pregnancy and live birth rates [29].

Abnormalities of the Ovaries

Polycystic Ovaries

According to a consensus meeting of Amsterdam in 2012, three of the Rotterdam criteria should be included for the diagnosis of PCOS, which are

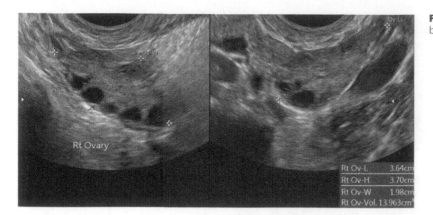

Figure 26.19 Ovarian volume by two-dimensional ultrasound.

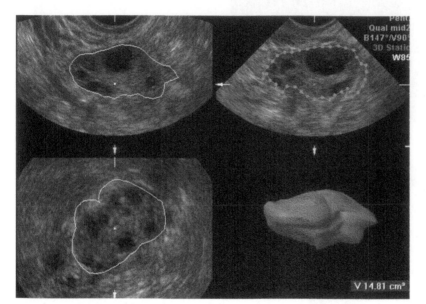

Figure 26.20 Ovarian volume by three-dimensional VOCAL.

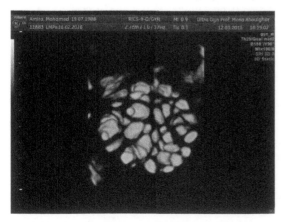

Figure 26.21 Three-dimensional counting of AFC.

chronic anovulation, clinical or biochemical hyperandrogenism, and polycystic ovary appearance. Polycystic morphology is defined as > 12 follicles with diameter of 2–9 mm in ovaries or ovarian volume of > 10 ml on pelvic ultrasonography (Figure 26.22). However, the more recent International evidence-based guideline for the assessment and management of polycystic ovary syndrome (ESHRE 2018), recommended that ultrasound should not be used in diagnosing PCOS within eight years of menarche, due to the high incidence of multifollicular ovaries in this life stage [30]. After that it is recommended to use endovaginal ultrasound transducers with a frequency bandwidth that includes 8 MHz, the threshold for

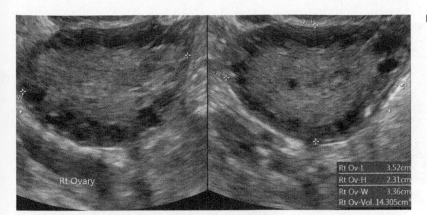

Figure 26.22 Polycystic ovaries.

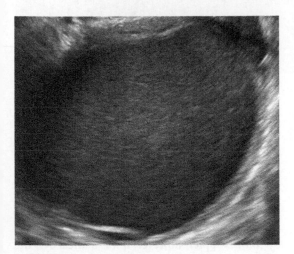

Figure 26.23 Endometrioma.

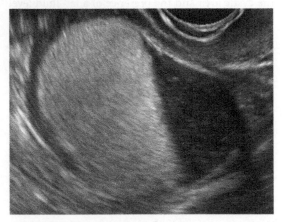

Figure 26.24 Dermoid cyst.

PCOS should be on either ovary, a follicle number per ovary of > 20 and/or an ovarian volume ≥ 10 ml, ensuring no corpora lutea, cysts, or dominant follicles are present. If abdominal ultrasound is to be used relying on ovarian volume of > 10 ml is better due to difficulty in assessing AFC abdominally.

Endometriomas

Endometriomas appear as unilocular cysts with low echogenic content (ground glass appearance). They can reach large sizes and cause limited ovarian mobility, especially if associated with pelvic adhesions. Kissing ovaries are described when both are situated in the Douglas pouch posterior to the uterus. Endometriomas show minimal vascularity by color Doppler (Figure 26.23) [31]. Ultrasound evaluation using gray-scale and Doppler with standardized examination and standardized definitions (described as pattern recognition) by an experienced ultrasonographer for diagnosis of endometriomas gave a sensitivity of 77% and specificity ranges from 94% to 100% [32]. Ultrasound prediction of associated pelvic adhesions (fixation of ovary to the uterus) had a good sensitivity and specificity of 89% and 90%, respectively [33]. In addition, ultrasound diagnosis of endometriomas has been shown to be reproducible and has good agreement between sonographers [33].

Dermoid Cysts

Dermoid cysts are very common, making up about 20 percent of ovarian tumors; the ultrasound characteristics of dermoid cysts are highly variable, ranging from predominantly cystic to uniformly dense. The most distinctive feature is the presence of a discrete highly echogenic focus, with posterior shadowing (Rokitansky protuberance). Other characteristics considered pathognomonic are fine, echogenic bands (representing hair) within

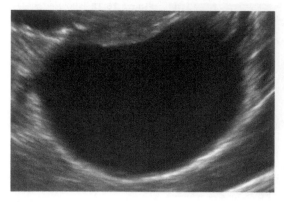

Figure 26.25 Functional clear cyst.

the cystic area and the presence of a fat–fluid level (Figure 26.24) and no evidence of vascularity by color Doppler [31]. Other reported ultrasound features for dermoid cysts include multiple floating balls in a cyst [34]. Similar to previously described ultrasound examination of endometrioma, pattern recognition gave an even higher sensitivity of 86% and specificity ranging from 94% to 100% [32]. Inter- and intraobserver agreement between sonographers for diagnosis of dermoid cysts was found to be less than that for endometriomas and serous cysts [33].

Functional Cysts

With ultrasound these appear as unilocular cysts with a uniform non-vascular wall, hypoechoic clear content and are small in size (< 5 cm) (Figure 26.25). The reported specificity using pattern recognition [32] is high (94–100%), albeit with a low sensitivity of 14%. Small functional cysts are commonly seen in patients in the luteal phase at the start of GnRH agonist treatment. It is our general practice to leave small cysts, as the majority disappears under the effect of the GnRH analogue, while larger cysts are better postponed till they resolve either spontaneously or with hormonal treatment. Some cysts appear after intake of GnRH analogues. Due to the flare effect, this may result in delay of downregulation and failure of the estradiol level to drop. In these cases prolongation of GnRH analogue treatment or transvaginal cyst aspiration is our usual practice. An ovarian cyst formation during the GnRH agonist suppression period negatively affects oocyte quality, fertilization rate, and high-quality embryos. Cyst aspiration before gonadotropin stimulation does not improve the IVF outcome. No statistically significant differences in implantation and clinical

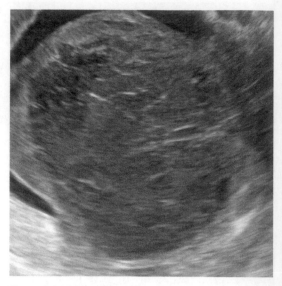

Figure 26.26 Hemorrhagic cyst.

pregnancy rates were determined between those who had aspiration and those who did not [35].

Hemorrhagic Cysts

Hemorrhagic cysts are unilocular, basically clear, but contain echogenic thread-like strands representing fibrin strands (clotted blood) and could give a star-shaped or cobweb-like appearance (Figure 26.26) [36]. Usually they appear avascular by color Doppler; however, if it is a luteal cyst the typical circular vascularity using color Doppler will appear all around the cyst.

The use of three-dimensional ultrasound adds to the correct diagnosis of all previous benign lesions, especially in confirming the benign nature of the lesion [37]; however, two- and three-dimensional power Doppler do not seem to add much to gray-scale imaging [38].

Similarly to clear cysts, they are commonly seen at the luteal phase with the start of GnRH agonist treatment and do not necessitate postponement of the treatment as they usually disappear spontaneously.

Para-ovarian Cysts

Para-ovarian cysts are clear cysts seen outside and separate from the normal ovarian tissue. They appear as clear hypoechoic cysts, usually small in size, and are avascular by color Doppler. They have no effect on the process of induction of ovulation and ovarian response.

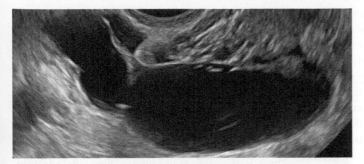

Figure 26.27 Hydrosalpinx with incomplete septations.

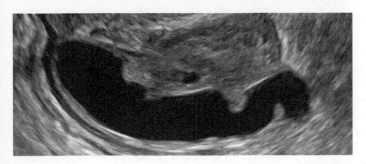

Figure 26.28 Hydrosalpinx with "cogwheel" appearance.

Hydrosalpinges

In patients with severe pelvic adhesions, history of surgeries, or complaining of continuous vaginal discharge denoting a communicating hydrosalpinx, proper ultrasound assessment is mandatory to look for visible hydrosalpinges that take different appearances by ultrasound.

It could appear as a tubular cystic structure separate from the ovary, with incomplete septations, or contains internal projections giving a cogwheel or beads-on-a-string appearance (Figures 26.27 and 26.28) [31]. The reported sensitivity and specificity using pattern recognition [32] is high, at 86% and 94–100%, respectively.

Visible hydrosalpinges by ultrasound should be removed by laparoscopic salpingectomy [39] or disconnection of the tubes. Management of hydrosalpinx by laparoscopic salpingectomy and laparoscopic proximal tubal occlusion or disconnection yielded the same effect on the improvement of the pregnancy outcome after IVF. The hysteroscopic placement of Essure devices to treat hydrosalpinx before IVF produces inferior pregnancy outcomes compared with those following the laparoscopic approach but sometimes it is the only method that can be done in cases with extensive pelvic adhesions. Laparoscopic disconnection or hysteroscopic occlusion is our usual practice in such cases [40].

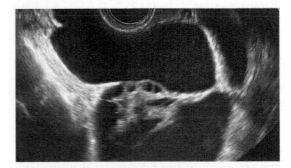

Figure 26.29 Peritoneal cyst.

Peritoneal or Pseudoperitoneal Cysts

These appear as irregular cysts with internal mobile septae which might contain the ovary centrally; there is no evident vascularity by color Doppler.

These cysts are very common in patients with previous pelvic surgeries and pelvic adhesions. They should be differentiated from ovarian cysts or multiple follicles (Figure 26.29).

Ultrasound Methods of Monitoring Ovulation

Transvaginal two-dimensional ultrasound is the routine used for monitoring ovulation. This is done by manual counting of the follicles and measurement of two to three diameters of each follicle, taking the average of measured diameters to give final follicle measurement. Measurement of follicles is more difficult during stimulation as they attain an ellipsoid shape. Despite good correlation between volume obtained from the mean diameter of the follicles, it is less accurate [41] than three-dimensional volume calculation, but that takes a much longer time to acquire.

The SonoAVC software is available on certain three-dimensional machines, it relies on volume calculation using three-dimensional VOCAL techniques and on color-coding each follicle (SonoAVC, GE) [25]. A three-dimensional volume is obtained from the stimulated ovary, and the software will give mean diameter and volume of the hypoechoic areas within the ovary representing the follicles. It will then color-code each follicle allowing them to be separately studied. It was found that the number of retrieved oocytes, number and rate of mature oocytes, fertilization rate, and clinical pregnancy rate were similar for two-dimensional sonography and three-dimensional SonoAVC. Follicle tracking with three-dimensional sonographic follicular volume measurements does not achieve better fertility outcomes than standard two-dimensional sonography. Mature oocytes were retrieved if the follicular volume was found to be over 0.6 ml on the day of human chorionic gonadotropin (hCG) injection [42]. It is still important to note that it needs the availability of three-dimensional ultrasound machines in the IVF unit, expertise in three-dimensional ultrasound, and manipulation of volumes.

Timing of Monitoring

First, ultrasound monitoring is performed one week after the start of human menopausal gonadotropin (hMG) injections, usually at day 8. Follow-up is determined by size of the follicles and serum estradiol levels, based on the fact that the follicle grows by 2–3 mm daily.

Earlier monitoring on day 5 or 6 of hMG injections is advised in patients with anticipated hyper-response or if using the antagonist protocol to start the antagonist injections when the leading follicle is 14 mm.

The mean diameter of the growing follicles is recorded in a special chart including all patient data.

Use of Doppler in Ovulation Induction Monitoring

Perifollicular Blood Flow (PFBF)

There is some evidence that well-vascularized follicles yielded high percentages of good-quality embryos, a well-vascularized endometrium, high follicular fluid EG-VEGF (endocrine gland-derived vascular endothelial growth factor) levels, and high clinical pregnancy rates. In addition, pregnant women had an increased percentage of well-vascularized follicles, a well-vascularized endometrium, and elevated follicular fluid insulin-like growth factor-1 and serum EG-VEGF levels [43]. A systemic review demonstrated an important prognostic value of perifollicular Doppler analysis on the pregnancy rate after IVF. PFBF also showed a positive correlation with embryo quality. An indirect influence of PFBF on the pregnancy rate is assumed through formation of a more mature follicle, a more resistant oocyte, and a better embryo cleavage potential. However, there is a need to investigate the role for PFBF assessment by Power Doppler in ART in randomized controlled trials [44].

The Role of Three-Dimensional Power Doppler Ultrasound Parameters on Endometrial Receptivity

Controversial data exist on the use of three-dimensional power Doppler ultrasound for assessing endometrial blood flow in IVF cycles. Some published data show that good endometrial blood flow on the day of embryo transfer might be associated with high pregnancy success with a GnRH long protocol, because this is indicative of endometrial receptivity in fresh IVF cycles. The pregnant group had higher endometrial vascularization index (VI), flow index (FI), and vascularization flow index (VFI) scores than the non-pregnant group. By contrast, neither subendometrial region VI, FI, and VFI scores, nor uterine artery pulsatility index (PI), resistance index (RI), or systolic/diastolic ratio (S/D) scores differed between groups [45]. However, these findings are inconsistent with a more recent study including 435 patients in their first IVF cycle, following a standard long GnRH agonist long ovarian stimulation regimen, and who had two highest scoring embryos transferred on day 3. Patients in both the pregnant group and non-pregnant group, and miscarriage and ongoing pregnant group did not show a significant difference in endometrial thickness, endometrial volume, endometrial pattern, uterine PI, RI, and S/D, endometrial and subendometrial VI, FI, and VFI. In the relative thin endometrium group, pregnant patients had similar endometrial thickness, endometrial volume, endometrial pattern, uterine PI, RI, and S/D, endometrial and subendometrial VI, FI, and VFI to non-pregnant patients. So, it was concluded that three-dimensional power Doppler ultrasound parameters of endometrium measured on the hCG day were not good predictors of pregnancy in IVF treatment, neither good predictors of ongoing pregnancy [46].

Problems Encountered during Monitoring of Ovulation

Failure to Visualize the Ovaries

This is the most difficult situation during ovulation monitoring; it occurs when there is abnormal position of the ovaries or in non-stimulated ovaries. The first is very common in patients with a history of pelvic surgeries or adhesions from endometriosis where the normal anatomy becomes distorted, ovaries are more laterally situated, or need abdominal pressure to be guided into view. In very rare situations the ovaries are not seen except by abdominal ultrasound; proper measurement of follicular diameter and determination of the count becomes a difficult task in that situation.

In the case of unstimulated ovaries, the ovaries are seen to contain small follicles; this could be anticipated in patients with poor ovarian reserve as assessed prior to the cycle by low AMH and low AFC and those with previous poor ovarian response.

Maternal habitus and high body mass index pose difficulties during examination, in spite of performing the examination transvaginally, due to manipulation of the probe and need for abdominal pressure.

Retroverted flexed uteri and uterine abnormalities such as large fibroids and adenomyosis pose additional difficulties as they cause posterior acoustic shadowing that distorts the view of the ovaries. Also endometriomas and other types of cysts sometimes mask surrounding follicles due to shadowing or may be mistaken as follicles.

Conclusion

It is without doubt that IVF programs and ovulation induction cannot be performed without the use of transvaginal ultrasound for monitoring of follicular growth and endometrium. Its application in these two fields is essential and has many uses and advantages before cycle start and during monitoring.

References

1. Stewart EA, Cookson CL, Gandolfo RA, *et al.* Epidemiology of uterine fibroids: a systematic review. *BJOG* 2017;**124**(10):1501–1512.
2. Dueholm M, Lundorf E, Hansen ES, *et al.* Accuracy of magnetic resonance imaging and transvaginal ultrasonography in the diagnosis, mapping, and measurement of uterine myomas. *Am J Obstet Gynecol* 2002;**186**(3):409–415.
3. Becker E Jr., Lev-Toaff AS, Kaufman EP, *et al.* The added value of transvaginal sonohysterography over transvaginal sonography alone in women with known or suspected leiomyoma. *J Ultrasound Med* 2002;**21**:237–247.
4. Munro MG, Critchley HOD, Fraser IS; FIGO Menstrual Disorders Committee. The two FIGO systems for normal and abnormal uterine bleeding symptoms and classification of causes of abnormal uterine bleeding in reproductive years: 2018 revisions. *Int J Gynaecol Obstet* 2018;**143**(3):393–408.
5. Sylvestre C. A prospective study to evaluate the efficacy of two- and three-dimensional sonohysterography in women with intrauterine lesions. *Fertil Steril* 2003;**79**:1222–1225.
6. Van der Veen F. Fibroids and IVF: retrospective studies or randomised clinical trials? *BJOG* 2017;**124**(4):622.
7. Rackow BW, Taylor HS. Submucosal uterine leiomyomas have a global effect on molecular determinants of endometrial receptivity. *Fertil Steril* 2010;**93**(6):2027–2034.
8. Wang X, Chen L, Wang H, *et al.* The impact of noncavity-distorting intramural fibroids on the efficacy of in vitro fertilization-embryo transfer: an updated meta-analysis. *Biomed Res Int* 2018;**2018**:8924703.
9. Carranza-Mamane B, Havelock J, Hemmings R. The management of uterine fibroids in women with otherwise unexplained infertility. *J Obstet Gynaecol Can* 2015;**37**(3):277–285.
10. Bazot M, Cortez A, Darai E, *et al.* Ultrasonography compared with magnetic resonance imaging for the diagnosis of

adenomyosis: correlation with histopathology. *Hum Reprod* 2001;**16**:2427–2433.

11. Van den Bosch T, Dueholm M, Leone FPG, *et al.* Terms, definitions and measurements to describe sonographic features of myometrium and uterine masses: a consensus opinion from the Morphological Uterus Sonographic Assessment (MUSA) group. *Ultrasound Obstet Gynecol* 2015;**46**:284–298.

12. Vercellini P, Consonni D, Dridi D, *et al.* Uterine adenomyosis and in vitro fertilization outcome: a systematic review and meta-analysis. *Hum Reprod* 2014;**29**:964–77.

13. Mavrelos D, Holland TK, Khalaf Y, *et al.* The impact of adenomyosis on the outcome of IVF-embryo transfer. *Reprod Biomed Online* 2017;**35**(5):549–554.

14. Younes G, Tulandi T. Effects of adenomyosis on in vitro fertilization treatment outcomes: a meta-analysis. *Fertil Steril* 2017;**108**(3):483.e3–490.e3.

15. Tsui KH, Lee FK, Seow KM, *et al.* Conservative surgical treatment of adenomyosis to improve fertility: controversial values, indications, complications, and pregnancy outcomes. *Taiwan J Obstet Gynecol* 2015;**54**:635–640.

16. Chan YY, Jayaprakasan K, Zamora J, *et al.* The prevalence of congenital uterine anomalies in unselected and high-risk populations: a systemic review. *Hum Reprod Update* 2011;**17**(6):761–771.

17. Grimbizis GF, Gordts S, Di Spiezio Sardo A, *et al.* The ESHRE/ESGE consensus on the classification of female genital tract congenital anomalies. *Hum Reprod* 2013;**28**(8):2032–2044.

18. Corroenne R, Legendre G, May-Panloup P, *et al.* Surgical treatment of septate uterus in cases of primary infertility and before assisted reproductive technologies. *J Gynecol Obstet Hum Reprod* 2018;**47**(9):413–418.

19. Rikken JFW, Kowalik CR, Emanuel MH, *et al.* The randomised uterine septum transection trial (TRUST): design and protocol. *BMC Womens Health* 2018;**18**(1):163.

20. Timmerman D, Verguts J, Konstantinovic ML, *et al.* The pedicle artery sign based on sonography with color Doppler imaging can replace second-stage tests in women with abnormal vaginal bleeding. *Ultrasound Obstet Gynecol* 2003;**22**:166–171.

21. La Sala GB, Blasi I, Gallinelli A, *et al.* Diagnostic accuracy of sonohysterography and transvaginal sonography as compared with hysteroscopy and endometrial biopsy: a prospective study. *Minerva Ginecol* 2011;**63**(5):421–427.

22. Nieuwenhuis LL, Hermans FJ, Bij de Vaate AJM, *et al.* Three-dimensional saline infusion sonography compared to two-dimensional saline infusion sonography for the diagnosis of focal intracavitary lesions. *Cochrane Database Syst Rev* 2017;**5**:CD011126.

23. Raine-Fenning NJ. The interobserver reliability of ovarian volume measurement is improved with three dimensional ultrasound, but dependent upon technique. *Ultrasound Med Biol* 2003;**29**:1685–1690.

24. Coelho Neto MA, Ludwin A, Borrell A, *et al.* Counting ovarian antral follicles by ultrasound: a practical guide. *Ultrasound Obstet Gynecol* 2018;**51**(1):10–20.

25. Raine-Fenning N, Jayaprakasan K, Clewes J, *et al.* SonoAVC: a novel method of automatic volume calculation. *Ultrasound Obstet Gynecol* 2008;**31**:691–696.

26. Peres Fagundes PA, Chapon R, Olsen PR, *et al.* Evaluation of three-dimensional SonoAVC ultrasound for antral follicle count in infertile women: its agreement with conventional two-dimensional ultrasound and serum levels of anti-Müllerian hormone. *Reprod Biol Endocrinol* 2017;**15**(1):96.

27. Lee Y, Kim TH, Park JK, *et al.* Predictive value of antral follicle count and serum anti-Müllerian hormone: which is better for live birth prediction in patients aged over 40 with their first IVF treatment? *Eur J Obstet Gynecol Reprod Biol* 2018;**221**:151–155.

28. Mutlu MF, Erdem M, Erdem A, *et al.* Antral follicle count determines poor ovarian response better than anti-Müllerian hormone but age is the only predictor for live birth in in vitro fertilization cycles. *J Assist Reprod Genet* 2013;**30**(5):657–665.

29. Ashrafi M, Hemat M, Arabipoor A, *et al.* Predictive values of anti-müllerian hormone, antral follicle count and ovarian response prediction index (ORPI) for assisted reproductive technology outcomes. *J Obstet Gynaecol* 2017;**37**(1):82–88.

30. International evidence-based guideline for the assessment and management of polycystic ovary syndrome 2018. ESHRE guidelines.

31. Timmerman D, Valentin L, Bourne TH, *et al.*, International Ovarian Tumor Analysis (IOTA) Group. Terms, definitions and measurements to describe the sonographic features of adnexal tumors: a consensus opinion from the International Ovarian Tumor Analysis (IOTA) Group. *Ultrasound Obstet Gynecol* 2000;**16**:500–505.

32. Sokalska A, Timmerman D, Testa AC, *et al.* Diagnostic accuracy of transvaginal ultrasound examination for assigning a specific diagnosis to adnexal masses. *Ultrasound Obstet Gynecol* 2009;**34**:462–470.

33. Guerriero S, Ajossa S, Garau N, *et al.* Diagnosis of pelvic adhesions in patients with endometrioma: the role of transvaginal ultrasonography. *Fertil Steril* 2009;**94**:742–746.

34. Gürel H, Gürel SA. Ovarian cystic teratoma with a pathognomonic appearance of multiple floating balls: a case report and investigation of common characteristics of the cases in the literature. *Fertil Steril* 2008;**90**:2008.e17–2008.e19.

35. Eryılmaz OG, Sarıkaya E, Aksakal FN, *et al.* Ovarian cyst formation following gonadotropin-releasing hormone-agonist administration decreases the oocyte quality in IVF cycles. *Balkan Med J* 2012;**29** (2):197–200.

36. Jain KA. Sonographic spectrum of hemorrhagic ovarian cysts. *J Ultrasound Med* 2002;**21**:879–886.

37. Geomini PM, Coppus SF, Kluivers KB, *et al.* Is three-dimensional ultrasonography of additional value in the assessment of adnexal masses? *Gynecol Oncol* 2007;**106**:153–159.

38. Jokubkiene L, Sladkevicius P, Valentin L. Does three-dimensional power Doppler ultrasound help in discrimination between benign and malignant ovarian masses? *Ultrasound Obstet Gynecol* 2007;**29**:215–225.

39. Strandell A, Lindhard A, Waldenström U, Thorburn J. Hydrosalpinx and IVF outcome: cumulative results after salpingectomy in a randomized controlled trial. *Hum Reprod* 2001;**16**:2403–2410.

40. Xu B, Zhang Q, Zhao J, *et al.* Pregnancy outcome of in vitro fertilization after Essure and laparoscopic management of hydrosalpinx: a systematic review and meta-analysis. *Fertil Steril* 2017;**108**(1):84.e5–95.e5.

41. Amer A. Three-dimensional versus two-dimensional ultrasound measurement of follicular volume: are they comparable? *Arch Gynecol Obstet* 2003;**268**:155–157.

42. Wertheimer A, Nagar R, Oron G, *et al.* Fertility treatment outcomes after follicle tracking with standard 2-dimensional sonography versus 3-dimensional sonography-based automated volume count: prospective study. *J Ultrasound Med* 2018;**37**(4):859–866.

43. Vural F, Vural B, Doğer E, *et al.* Perifollicular blood flow and its relationship with endometrial vascularity, follicular fluid EG-VEGF, IGF-1, and inhibin-a levels and IVF outcomes. *J Assist Reprod Genet* 2016; **33**(10):1355–1362.

44. Huyghe S, Verest A, Thijssen A, *et al.* The prognostic value of perifollicular blood flow in the outcome after assisted reproduction: a systematic review. *Facts Views Vis Obgyn* 2017;**9**(3):153–156.

45. Kim A, Jung H, Choi WJ, *et al.* Detection of endometrial and subendometrial vasculature on the day of embryo transfer and prediction of pregnancy during fresh in vitro fertilization cycles. *Taiwan J Obstet Gynecol* 2014;**53** (3):360–365.

46. Zhang T, He Y, Wang Y, *et al.* The role of three-dimensional power Doppler ultrasound parameters measured on hCG day in the prediction of pregnancy during in vitro fertilization treatment. *Eur J Obstet Gynecol Reprod Biol* 2016;**203**:66–71.

27

The Use of GnRH Agonists to Trigger Final Oocyte Maturation during Controlled Ovarian Stimulation

Anastasia Salameh, Sara Faour, and Johnny Awwad

Introduction

Gonadotropin-releasing hormone (GnRH) is secreted from the medial basal hypothalamus and controls pituitary function via the hypothalamic tuberoinfundibular system [1]. Follicle-stimulating hormone (FSH) and luteinizing hormone (LH) are synthesized and secreted by the anterior pituitary gland in response to GnRH pulse activity. Physiological modulation of GnRH pulse amplitude and frequency determines the fine interplay between various gonadotropin players during the menstrual cycle [2;3]. The midcycle LH surge represents the temporal landmark that defines key follicular events, namely the resumption of meiosis in arrested oocytes and the luteinization of granulosa/theca cells [4]. LH therefore plays a key role in preserving corpus luteum activity for the next 12 to 14 days that follow ovulation. This gland produces 25 to 50 mg of progesterone daily during the first 10 weeks of pregnancy until the placenta assumes its full endocrine functions [5]. Destruction of the corpus luteum prior to seven weeks of pregnancy is likely to result in the interruption of gestation.

GnRH agonists are the product of single amino acid substitutions in the native decapeptide yielding molecules with higher potency and longer half-life. The administration of GnRH agonists is associated with an initial flare characterized by an increase in gonadotropin synthesis and secretion for the next five to seven days. Prolonged administration, however, is associated with receptor downregulation and paradoxical pituitary gonadotropin suppression. This dual property has been used in practice during ovarian stimulation in assisted reproductive technology (ART) cycles in order to downregulate the pituitary and prevent an early LH surge. Alternatively, a GnRH agonist may also be utilized to induce an endogenous LH surge. The implementation of GnRH agonists as ovulation triggering agents

became possible following the introduction of GnRH antagonists for pituitary suppression in controlled ovarian stimulation cycles [6;7].

Ovarian hyperstimulation syndrome (OHSS) is probably the most feared medical complication of controlled ovarian stimulation. It is iatrogenic and may be associated with life-threatening events. It is characterized by a protein-rich fluid shift from the intravascular space into third spaces resulting in hemoconcentration, hypercoagulability, and end-organ failure in its severe form [8]. Known risk factors include the use of a GnRH agonist for pituitary suppression and human chorionic gonadotropin (hCG) for ovulation triggering, in addition to polycystic ovary syndrome (PCOS), young age and low body mass index. The overall incidence of OHSS is about 30 percent with the severe form estimated to occur in 2 percent of cases [9;10]. Multiple strategies have been proposed to reduce the risk of OHSS, of which the use of a GnRH agonist for ovulation triggering instead of hCG in GnRH antagonist cycles has gained much attention over the past several years.

The Physiology of the GnRH Agonist-Induced Gonadotropin Surge

While the duration of the physiological LH surge in a natural cycle has been estimated at 48–50 hours, its lifespan is short-lived following GnRH agonist trigger and ranges from 24 to 36 hours [6;11]. The direct result of this suboptimal gonadotropin surge is a significant reduction in follicle LH exposure which does not seem to impede the process of oocyte maturation, but rather appears to yield a defective corpus luteum [12]. This gonadotropin surge is also characterized by the release of endogenous FSH mimicking midcycle events occurring during the natural cycle [13]. Midcycle

FSH is believed to promote the formation of LH receptors on luteinizing granulosa cells, the resumption of meiosis, and the expansion of the cumulus oophorous [14;15].

The short-lived LH activity associated with the GnRH agonist trigger affects negatively corpus luteum support resulting in its early demise [11]. As a consequence, vasoactive peptides such as vascular endothelial growth factor, soluble vascular endothelial cadherin, and angiopoietin 1 and 2 are markedly decreased [16;17], which significantly reduces the risk of OHSS [18–20]. A case–control study conducted on women with a previous history of severe OHSS showed that the use of GnRH agonist to trigger final oocyte maturation prevented the development of OHSS in the next cycle [21]. The protective effect of the GnRH agonist trigger against OHSS was also confirmed by a meta-analysis [22;23]. Although isolated cases of OHSS have been sporadically reported after this method of ovulation triggering in GnRH antagonist downregulated cycles, the overall risk remains very low compared with conventional hCG [24].

Formulations and Methods of GnRH Agonist Triggering of Final Oocyte Maturation

Various types of GnRH agonists have been utilized with great success to trigger ovulation during ART cycles. When various protocols of GnRH agonists were compared with hCG for their reproductive efficiency, the choice of the agonist (triptorelin vs. leuprolide vs. buserelin vs. nafarelin), the mode of administration (intranasal vs. subcutaneously), and the frequency of intake (once vs. twice vs. thrice) did not affect final outcome [25]. Using two different doses of leuprolide acetate, Pabuccu et al. found comparable mature oocyte yields (13.5 [3.0–40.0] vs. 12.0 [5.0–20.0]) and clinical pregnancy rates (CPRs) (42.1% [27.9–57.8] vs. 38.5% [24.9–54.1]) irrespective of whether 1 or 2 mg boluses were administered [26]. In a randomized controlled study, Vuong et al. also evaluated various subcutaneous triptorelin boluses in oocyte donors, namely 0.4 mg, 0.3 mg, and 0.2 mg. The three groups had similar numbers of metaphase II (MII) oocytes retrieved (16.0 ± 8.5, 15.9 ± 7.8, and 14.7 ± 8.4, respectively), and equivalent numbers of good-quality embryos obtained (3.8 ± 0.9, 3.6 ± 3.0, and 4.1 ± 3.0, respectively) [27].

On the other hand, the use of multiple GnRH agonist boluses for triggering of final oocyte maturation was reported by Lanzone et al. who gave three doses of buserelin 12 hours apart to induce ovulation [28]. All patients had ovulation documented by sonographic findings and serum progesterone rise. There was no reporting of pregnancy outcome, however [28]. This same approach was tested in high-risk women undergoing gonadotropin ovulation induction for intrauterine insemination [29]. Three repeated doses of triptorelin subcutaneously at 12-hour intervals resulted in a 30.3% take-home pregnancy rate and a 20% miscarriage rate. An elevated multiple pregnancy rate of 26.7% was the main limitation of the suggested protocol [29].

Oocyte Efficiency Parameters in GnRH Agonist-Triggered Cycles

Several studies reported an overall improvement in oocyte efficiency parameters when a GnRH agonist was used instead of hCG to trigger final oocyte maturation. After GnRH agonist trigger, enhanced oocyte maturation has been shown to be associated with FSH rise and increased follicular epidermal growth factor-like peptide levels in women [30]. In a randomized controlled study, Humaidan et al. demonstrated a higher MII oocyte yield in the GnRH agonist trigger group compared with the hCG group [31]. Similarly, more oocytes were collected in oocyte donors [32] and better-quality embryos obtained [33] when triggering of ovulation was achieved using a GnRH agonist. Krishna et al. also confirmed higher oocyte yield, improved fertilization rates, and enhanced embryo quality after the same triggering approach [34].

It should be noted nonetheless that incidents of partial or complete failure of oocyte collection have been reported after GnRH agonist triggering of ovulation. Empty follicle syndrome (EFS) has been described in clinical situations known to be associated with profound downregulation of the hypothalamic axis [35]. In a retrospective study, Kummer et al. demonstrated a positive correlation between the number of oocytes collected and peak estradiol levels as well as post-trigger LH and progesterone levels. EFS was more likely to occur when post-trigger LH levels were less than 15 IU/L and progesterone levels less than 3.5 ng/ml [36]. These findings were further confirmed in a prospective study design [37].

A retrospective evaluation of risk factors associated with suboptimal follicle response to a GnRH agonist trigger shed the light on women with suppressed FSH and LH levels on the second day of the cycle and decreased LH levels on the day of the trigger as possible candidates [38]. These women were more likely to require a more prolonged duration of ovarian stimulation and an increased dose of gonadotropins. In addition, women maintained on long-term oral contraception appear to represent a particularly vulnerable group for suboptimal LH response [38]. In the event of EFS resulting from failed LH surge following GnRH agonist trigger, hCG administration and deferred oocyte collection were shown to yield successful results [35;36].

The Physiology of the Luteal Phase in GnRH Agonist-Triggered Cycles

It is now established that the use of a GnRH agonist to trigger final oocyte maturation is associated with profound dysfunction of the luteal phase, namely defective steroid production and shorter cycle duration. Earlier studies demonstrated that the corpus luteum of primates does not achieve its full developmental potential when the duration of the LH surge fails to attain 48 hours [11]. In humans, this has been confirmed as well by decreased progesterone, inhibin A, and pro-alpha C serum levels during the luteal phase of women in whom a GnRH agonist was used to trigger ovulation [39]. It is therefore believed that this type of trigger is associated with demise of the corpus luteum resulting in a profoundly defective luteal phase. Comparing leuprolide (500 µg) to hCG (5000 IU) for ovulation triggering, Segal and Casper also demonstrated significantly lower estradiol and progesterone levels in the luteal phase of the GnRH agonist group. Moreover, 8 percent of women in the same group had a clinically short luteal phase despite the use of vaginal progesterone for luteal phase support (LPS) [7]. These findings emphasize the inadequacy of standard LPS in managing the dysfunction of the corpus luteum in these cycles.

Tesarik et al. have previously shown that hCG administration in women with low LH serum levels enhanced endometrial growth, increased endometrial thickness, and improved implantation rates in embryo transfer cycles [40]. This observation is in line with data supporting a positive role of LH in enhancing endometrial receptivity. Given that the LH surge after GnRH agonist triggering is short lived, a deleterious effect on the endometrium may then be expected despite standard luteal supplementation [41]. The genes activated during the window of implantation in natural and stimulated cycles have been investigated using molecular array studies. Simon et al. for instance showed differences in endometrial gene expression in relation to the type of trigger. When LH/hCG was added to the luteal phase of GnRH agonist trigger cycles, endometrial expression patterns resembled very closely hCG-triggered cycles [42]. This study highlighted the fact that standard luteal support approaches alone may not be sufficient to overcome luteal deficiency in GnRH agonist-triggered cycles.

Conventional Luteal Phase Support

Using a prospective randomized design, Humaidan et al. compared the use of buserelin (0.5 mg) with hCG (10 000 IU) for final oocyte maturation in normogonadotropic women undergoing in vitro fertilization (IVF) treatment cycles [31]. The study was prematurely discontinued due to a very high rate of early pregnancy loss (EPL) in the GnRH agonist trigger group. It should be noted that all patients received micronized progesterone 90 mg vaginally and estradiol 4 mg orally on a daily basis for luteal support. LPS was discontinued in all cases on the day of the pregnancy test. In a similar study, Kolibianakis et al. compared the use of triptorelin (0.2 mg) with hCG (10 000 IU) for ovulation triggering in normo-responding women. The ongoing pregnancy rate (OPR) was 2.9 percent and EPL 83.3 percent in the GnRH agonist arm [41]. Luteal support consisted of daily vaginal progesterone 600 mg and oral estradiol 4 mg, which was discontinued at seven weeks of pregnancy. It soon became apparent that conventional LPS used for hCG-triggered IVF/ICSI cycles is not suitable for cycles in which a GnRH agonist is used for triggering of ovulation.

A systematic review also confirmed lower CPR (odds ratio [OR] 0.22, 95% confidence interval [CI] 0.05–0.85) and higher EPL (OR 11.5, 95%

CI 0.95–138.98) in association with the use of conventional LPS in GnRH agonist-triggered cycles compared with hCG [33]. These findings strongly suggest an urgent need for a paradigm shift in the management of the luteal phase in women receiving a GnRH agonist for ovulation triggering. Different strategies have been published for this purpose, including the use of intensive LPS [20;43–45] and the use of low-dose hCG rescue to salvage the corpus luteum [36;45–49].

Luteal phase insufficiency with elevated rates of EPL was found to be the principal barrier to the widespread use of GnRH agonists as triggers of final oocyte maturation. Two strategies were proposed to overcome this shortcoming: (i) intensive LPS consisting of high exogenous progesterone and estrogen supplementation until 10–12 weeks of pregnancy; and (ii) corpus luteum rescue using a low-dose hCG bolus to supplement standard LPS.

Intensive Luteal Phase Support

The use of intensive estrogen and progesterone supplementation to overcome a profoundly deficient luteal phase has been the subject of much debate in GnRH agonist-triggered cycles.

Engmann et al. conducted a prospective randomized controlled trial (RCT) on high-responder women with PCOS who received either a GnRH agonist or hCG to trigger final oocyte maturation [20]. The GnRH agonist group received for LPS a daily dose of 50 mg of progesterone intramuscularly in combination with 0.3 mg of transdermal estrogen patches every other day until 10 weeks of gestation. LPS was dose adjusted in order to maintain serum progesterone levels above 20 ng/ml and estradiol levels above 200 pg/ml. There were no significant differences in implantation (36.0% vs. 31.0%; $p < 0.05$) and OPRs (53.3% vs. 48.3%; $p < 0.05$) between the GnRH agonist and hCG groups, respectively [20]. While no cases of OHSS were observed in the GnRH agonist group, 31 percent of women in the hCG group developed manifestations of the clinical syndrome.

Iliodromiti et al., in a retrospective review of women at risk of OHSS, reported comparable live birth rates when GnRH agonist versus hCG were used for ovulation triggering (29.8% vs. 29.2%; $p = 0.69$). Intensive LPS comprised 50 mg IM progesterone given daily, and twice daily administration

of 90 mg vaginal progesterone and 6 mg of oral estradiol valerate were used until seven weeks of gestation [45]. Compared with a 7 percent incidence of OHSS in the hCG group, only one case of late-onset OHSS was documented in the GnRH agonist group. Similar findings were reported by another retrospective study on high responders as well [50].

Low-Dose hCG Luteal Rescue

Another proposed strategy to improve the reproductive success of cycles following a GnRH agonist trigger consists of salvaging the corpus luteum by administering a low hCG dose concurrently at the time of the ovulation trigger or at oocyte collection. The purpose of the luteal hCG rescue is to circumvent the demise of the corpus luteum for the purpose of maintaining endogenous hormone production.

Low-dose hCG rescue administered at the time of oocyte retrieval. The administration of a single bolus of hCG (1500 IU) at the time of oocyte retrieval in GnRH agonist trigger cycles has been suggested in order to maintain corpus luteum function and enhance implantation.

In a randomized controlled design, Humaidan et al. evaluated a GnRH agonist trigger protocol with modified hCG luteal support (1500 IU at oocyte retrieval) in normogonadotropic women. Progesterone and estradiol were supplemented until the date of the pregnancy test. No significant differences were observed in OPR and EPL when compared with the hCG trigger group [47]. This strategy was found to be associated with a low overall incidence of OHSS, with cases described mostly in women with a high number of developing follicles (≥ 25 follicles) [45;51]. The safety of this protocol in high responders however has yet to be established. In a retrospective cohort study, Seyhan et al. showed that high responders have a 26.1 percent risk of developing severe OHSS when a GnRH agonist trigger was administered followed by a bolus of hCG 35 hours later [52]. In 2014, a Cochrane review concluded that women receiving a GnRH agonist for oocyte maturation had a similar reproductive outcome compared with those triggered with hCG only when LH stimulation was used to support the luteal phase [53]. In 2016, the same group released a letter in which they showed that even cycles having modified LPS with LH had fewer take-home-baby rates

(OR 0.63, 95% CI 0.40–0.98) compared with hCG cycles [54].

Low-dose hCG administered at the time of the GnRH agonist trigger. In a proof-of-concept study, dual triggering of final oocyte maturation using 1000 to 2500 IU of hCG at the time of the GnRH agonist trigger has been shown to be effective in achieving an encouraging OPR of 53.3% and EPL of 17.2% [32].

In order to evaluate the reproductive performance of the GnRH agonist/hCG dual trigger, Kummer *et al.* conducted a retrospective study in high responders, revealing significantly higher LBR (52.9% vs. 30.9%) in the dual trigger compared with the GnRH agonist alone group. Both groups received intensive LPS consisting of 50 mg IM progesterone daily and 0.3 mg transdermal estradiol patches every other day [36]. The concept of dual trigger (GnRH agonist + 6500 IU hCG) was also successfully evaluated retrospectively in normal responders receiving daily progesterone (50 mg IM and 300 mg vaginally) for luteal support [55].

It should be noted nonetheless that one retrospective study demonstrated a higher incidence of early OHSS in association with the use of the dual trigger compared with GnRH agonist alone (8.6% vs. 0%) [56].

Progesterone-Free Luteal Support

Luteal support using repeated daily doses of 100 µg of nasal buserelin three times per day was evaluated in a randomized prospective study in GnRH agonist-triggered cycles by Pirard *et al.*, in which luteal progesterone levels were found to be comparable to cycles receiving hCG triggering with standard LPS [57]. Bar-Hava *et al.* also studied the use of daily intranasal nafarelin for LPS started on the evening after ovum pickup in high responders in the absence of progesterone supplementation. The OPR was 52.1 percent with no cases of OHSS reported [58]. Well-designed randomized studies are nonetheless needed to confirm these findings.

In a proof-of-concept study, Kol *et al.* evaluated the concept of "luteal costing" in a case series [59]. Following GnRH agonist trigger and ovum pickup, patients received hCG boluses (1500 IU) in an adjusted manner in line with daily measurements of luteal progesterone and estradiol serum levels. The new strategy was associated with a pregnancy

rate of 43% and a relatively high miscarriage rate of 33%, mostly in the form of chemical losses. This latter finding was explained in relation to the late timing of hCG administration after ovum pickup. Vanetik *et al.*, in a retrospective study, evaluated the reproductive efficiency of GnRH agonist-triggered cycles supplemented with 1500 IU hCG two days after ovum pickup compared with the conventional hCG trigger. While live birth rates were comparable between groups, both luteal estradiol and progesterone serum levels were significantly higher in the GnRH agonist group, a finding explained by a robust luteal phase response to luteal hCG rescue [60]. Despite very promising prospects, luteal costing still needs to be explored via well-designed RCTs, namely that current studies suffer from small sample sizes, retrospective design, and lack of randomization.

Segmentation of IVF Cycles and Freeze-All Policy

In view of controversies surrounding the reproductive efficiency of intensive luteal support and the safety of hCG luteal rescue in GnRH agonist-triggered cycles, several investigators favored a complete dissociation between follicular and endometrial events [61]. The proposed strategy, designated as cycle segmentation, consists of cryopreservation of all embryos with the aim of replacing them in a subsequent cryo-warmed embryo transfer cycle. In addition to circumventing the risk of late-onset OHSS, the process of transferring embryos in a subsequent cycle seems to be associated with a reproductive advantage by circumventing the detrimental effects of GnRH agonist triggering and high steroid levels on endometrial receptivity [61–63]. Unfortunately, no well-designed randomized studies are available to confirm the benefit of this approach compared with strategies involving fresh embryo transfer.

Conclusion

There is growing interest in the use of GnRH agonists for the triggering of final oocyte maturation in women undergoing ovarian stimulation with the ultimate goal of achieving an OHSS-free IVF clinic. Despite a high safety record, the occurrence of severe cases of OHSS in high-risk women after GnRH agonist trigger has been reported, namely when hCG luteal rescue protocols have been utilized. Lower live births and higher EPL have been consistently reported in GnRH agonist-triggered cycles following fresh embryo transfers, irrespective of the luteal phase management protocol utilized. Cycle segmentation with replacement of cryo-warmed embryos in subsequent cycles remains a very attractive strategy for IVF centers with very successful cryopreservation programs.

References

1. Balasubramanian R, Dwyer A, Seminara SB, et al. Human GnRH deficiency: a unique disease model to unravel the ontogeny of GnRH neurons. *Neuroendocrinology* 2010;**92**:81–99.

2. Belchetz PE, Plant TM, Nakai Y, et al. Hypophysial responses to continuous and intermittent delivery of hypothalamic gonadotropin-releasing hormone. *Science* 1978;**202**:631–633.

3. Wetsel WC, Valenca MM, Merchenthaler I, et al. Intrinsic pulsatile secretory activity of immortalized luteinizing hormone-releasing hormone-secreting neurons. *Proc Natl Acad Sci U S A* 1992;**89**:4149–4153.

4. Richards JS. Genetics of ovulation. *Semin Reprod Med* 2007;**25**(4):235–242.

5. Duncan WC. The human corpus luteum: remodeling during luteolysis and maternal recognition of pregnancy. *Rev Reprod* 2000;**5**:12–17.

6. Itskovitz J, Boldes R, Levron J, et al. Induction of preovulatory luteinizing hormone surge and prevention of ovarian hyperstimulation syndrome by gonadotropin-releasing hormone agonist. *Fertil Steril* 1991;**56**:213–220.

7. Segal S, Casper RF. Gonadotropin-releasing hormone agonist versus human chorionic gonadotropin for triggering follicular maturation in in vitro fertilization. *Fertil Steril* 1992;**57**(6):1254–1258.

8. Aboulghar MA, Mansour RT. Ovarian hyperstimulation syndrome: classifications and critical analysis of preventive measures. *Hum Reprod Update* 2003;**9**(3):275–289.

9. Macklon NS, Stouffer RL, Giudice LC, et al. The science behind 25 years of ovarian stimulation for in vitro fertilization. *Endocr Rev* 2006;**27**(2):170–207.

10. Engmann L, Claudio B, Humaidan P. GnRH agonist trigger for the induction of oocyte maturation in GnRH antagonist IVF cycles: a SWOT analysis. *Reprod Biomed Online* 2016;**32**(3):274–285.

11. Chandrasekher YA, Hutchison JS, Zelinski-Wooten MB, et al. Initiation of periovulatory events in primate follicles using recombinant and native human luteinizing hormone to mimic the midcycle gonadotropin surge. *J Clin Endocrinol Metab* 1994;**79**(1):298–306.

12. Chandrasekher YA, Brenner RM, Molskness TA, et al. Titrating luteinizing hormone surge requirements for ovulatory changes in primate follicles. II. Progesterone receptor expression in luteinizing granulosa cells. *J Clin Endocrinol Metab* 1991;**73**(3):584–589.

13. Gonen Y, Balakier H, Powell W, et al. Use of gonadotropin-releasing hormone agonist to trigger follicular maturation for in vitro fertilization. *J Clin Endocrinol Metab* 1990;**71**(4):918–922.

14. Oktay K, Türkçüoğlu I, Rodriguez-Wallberg KA. GnRH agonist trigger for women with breast cancer undergoing fertility preservation by aromatase inhibitor/FSH stimulation. *Reprod Biomed Online* 2010;**20**(6):783–788.

15. Andersen CY, Leonardsen L, Ulloa-Aguirre A, et al. FSH-induced resumption of meiosis in mouse oocytes: effect of different isoforms. *Mol Hum Reprod* 1999;**5**(8):726–731.

16. Fraser HM. Regulation of the ovarian follicular vasculature. *Reprod Biol Endocrinol* 2006;**4**:18

17. Molskness TA, Stouffer RL, Burry KA, et al. Circulating levels of total angiopoietin-2 and the soluble Tie-2 receptor in women during ovarian stimulation and early gestation. *Fertil Steril* 2006;**86**:1531–1533.

18. Cerrillo M, Rodriguez S, Mayoral M, et al. Differential regulation of VEGF after final oocyte maturation with GnRH agonist versus hCG: a rationale for OHSS reduction. *Fertil Steril* 2009;**91**:1526–1528.

19. Bodri D, Sunkara SK, Coomarasamy A. Gonadotropin releasing hormone agonists versus antagonists for controlled ovarian hyperstimulation in oocyte donors: a systematic review and meta-analysis. *Fertil Steril* 2011;**95**:164–169.

20. Engmann L, DiLuigi A, Schmidt D, et al. The use of gonadotropin-releasing hormone (GnRH) agonist to induce oocyte maturation after cotreatment with GnRH antagonist in high-risk patients undergoing in vitro fertilization prevents the risk of ovarian hyperstimulation syndrome: a prospective randomized controlled study. *Fertil Steril* 2008;**89**:84–91.

21. Lewit N, Kol S, Manor D, et al. Comparison of gonadotrophin-releasing hormone analogues and human chorionic gonadotrophin for the induction

of ovulation and prevention of ovarian hyperstimulation syndrome: a case-control study. *Hum Reprod* 1996;**11**(7):1399–1402.

22. Fatemi HM, Garcia-Velasco J. Avoiding ovarian hyperstimulation syndrome with the use of gonadotropin-releasing hormone agonist trigger. *Fertil Steril* 2015;**103**(4):870–873.

23. Mourad S, Brown J, Farquhar C. Interventions for the prevention of OHSS in ART cycles: an overview of Cochrane reviews. *Cochrane Database Syst Rev* 2017;**1**:CD012103.

24. Gurbuz AS, Gode F, Ozcimen N, *et al.* Gonadotrophin-releasing hormone agonist trigger and freeze-all strategy does not prevent severe ovarian hyperstimulation syndrome: a report of three cases. *Reprod Biomed Online* 2014;**29**(5):541–544.

25. Parneix I, Emperaire JC, Ruffie A, *et al.* Comparison of different protocols of ovulation induction, by GnRH agonists and chorionic gonadotropin. *Gynecol Obstet Fertil* 2001;**29**(2):100–105.

26. Pabuccu EG, Pabuccu R, Caglar GS, *et al.* Different gonadotropin releasing hormone agonist doses for the final oocyte maturation in high-responder patients undergoing in vitro fertilization/intra-cytoplasmic sperm injection. *J Hum Reprod Sci* 2015;**8**(1):25–29.

27. Vuong TN, Ho MT, Ha TD, *et al.* Gonadotropin-releasing hormone agonist trigger in oocyte donors co-treated with a gonadotropin-releasing hormone antagonist: a dose-finding study. *Fertil Steril* 2016;**105**(2):356–363.

28. Lanzone A, Fulghesu AM, Apa R, *et al.* LH surge induction by GnRH agonist at the time of ovulation. *Gynecol Endocrinol* 1989;**3**(3):213–220.

29. Awwad JT, Hannoun AB, Khalil A, *et al.* Induction of final follicle maturation with a gonadotropin-releasing hormone agonist in women at risk of ovarian hyperstimulation syndrome undergoing gonadotropin stimulation and intrauterine insemination: proof-of-concept study. *Clin Exp Obstet Gynecol* 2012;**39**(4):436–439.

30. Humaidan P, Westergaard LG, Mikkelsen AL, *et al.* Levels of the epidermal growth factor-like peptide amphiregulin in follicular fluid reflect the mode of triggering ovulation: a comparison between gonadotrophin-releasing hormone agonist and urinary human chorionic gonadotrophin. *Fertil Steril* 2011;**95**(6):2034–2038.

31. Humaidan P, Ejdrup Bredkjaer H, Bungum L, *et al.* GnRH agonist (buserelin) or hCG for ovulation induction in GnRH antagonist IVF/ICSI cycles: a prospective randomized study. *Hum Reprod* 2005;**20**(5):1213–1220.

32. Shapiro BS, Daneshmand ST, Garner FC, *et al.* Gonadotropin-releasing hormone agonist

combined with a reduced dose of human chorionic gonadotropin for final oocyte maturation in fresh autologous cycles of in vitro fertilization. *Fertil Steril* 2008;**90**(1):231–233.

33. Griesinger G, Diedrich K, Devroey P, *et al.* GnRH agonist for triggering final oocyte maturation in the GnRH antagonist ovarian hyperstimulation protocol: a systematic review and meta-analysis. *Hum Reprod Update* 2005;**12**(2):159–168.

34. Krishna D, Dhoble S, Praneesh G, *et al.* Gonadotropin-releasing hormone agonist trigger is a better alternative than human chorionic gonadotropin in PCOS undergoing IVF cycles for an OHSS Free Clinic: a randomized control trial. *J Hum Reprod Sci* 2016;**9**(3):164–172.

35. Asada Y, Itoi F, Honnma H, *et al.* Failure of GnRH agonist-triggered oocyte maturation: its cause and management. *J Assist Reprod Genet* 2013;**30**(4):581–585.

36. Kummer NE, Feinn RS, Griffin DW, *et al.* Predicting successful induction of oocyte maturation after gonadotropin-releasing hormone agonist (GnRHa) trigger. *Hum Reprod* 2012;**28**(1):152–159.

37. Chen SL, Ye DS, Chen X, *et al.* Circulating luteinizing hormone level after triggering oocyte maturation with GnRH agonist may predict oocyte yield in flexible GnRH antagonist protocol. *Hum Reprod* 2012;**27**(5):1351–1356.

38. Meyer L, Murphy LA, Gumer A, *et al.* Risk factors for a suboptimal response to gonadotropin-releasing hormone agonist trigger during in vitro fertilization cycles. *Fertil Steril* 2015;**104**(3):637–642.

39. Nevo O, Eldar-Geva T, Kol S, *et al.* Lower levels of inhibin A and pro-alpha C during the luteal phase after triggering oocyte maturation with a gonadotropin-releasing hormone agonist versus human chorionic gonadotropin. *Fertil Steril* 2003;**79**(5):1123–1128.

40. Tesarik J, Hazout A, Mendoza C. Luteinizing hormone affects uterine receptivity independently of ovarian function. *Reprod Biomed Online* 2003;**7**(1):59–64.

41. Kolibianakis EM, Schultze-Mosgau A, Schroer A, *et al.* A lower ongoing pregnancy rate can be expected when GnRH agonist is used for triggering final oocyte maturation instead of HCG in patients undergoing IVF with GnRH antagonists. *Hum Reprod* 2005;**20**(10):2887–2892.

42. Bermejo A, Cerrillo M, Ruiz-Alonso M, *et al.* Impact of final oocyte maturation using gonadotropin-releasing hormone agonist triggering and different luteal support protocols on endometrial gene expression. *Fertil Steril* 2014;**101**(1):138.e3–146.e3.

43. Engmann L, Siano L, Schmidt D, *et al.* GnRH agonist to induce oocyte maturation during IVF in patients at high risk of OHSS. *Reprod Biomed Online* 2006;**13**(5):639–644.

44. Imbar T, Kol S, Lossos F, *et al.* Reproductive outcome of fresh or frozen–thawed embryo transfer is similar in high-risk patients for ovarian hyperstimulation syndrome using GnRH agonist for final oocyte maturation and intensive luteal support. *Hum Reprod* 2012;**27**(3):753–759.

45. Iliodromiti S, Blockeel C, Tremellen KP, *et al.* Consistent high clinical pregnancy rates and low ovarian hyperstimulation syndrome rates in high-risk patients after GnRH agonist triggering and modified luteal support: a retrospective multicentre study. *Hum Reprod* 2013;**28**(9):2529–2536.

46. Humaidan P. Luteal phase rescue in high-risk OHSS patients by GnRHa triggering in combination with low-dose HCG: a pilot study. *Reprod Biomed Online* 2009;**18**(5):630–634.

47. Humaidan P, Bredkjær HE, Westergaard LG, *et al.* 1,500 IU human chorionic gonadotropin administered at oocyte retrieval rescues the luteal phase when gonadotropin-releasing hormone agonist is used for ovulation induction: a prospective, randomized, controlled study. *Fertil Steril* 2010;**93**(3):847–854.

48. Humaidan P, Polyzos NP, Alsbjerg B, *et al.* GnRHa trigger and individualized luteal phase hCG support according to ovarian response to stimulation: two prospective randomized controlled multi-centre studies in IVF patients. *Hum Reprod* 2013;**28**(9):2511–2521.

49. Shapiro BS, Daneshmand ST, Garner FC, *et al.* Comparison of "triggers" using leuprolide acetate alone or in combination with low-dose human chorionic gonadotropin. *Fertil Steril* 2011;**95**(8):2715–2717.

50. Christopoulos G, Vlismas A, Carby A, *et al.* GnRH agonist trigger with intensive luteal phase support vs. human chorionic gonadotropin trigger in high responders: an observational study reporting pregnancy outcomes and incidence of ovarian hyperstimulation syndrome. *Hum Fertil* 2016;**19**(3):199–206.

51. Radesic B, Tremellen K. Oocyte maturation employing a GnRH agonist in combination with low-dose hCG luteal rescue minimizes the severity of ovarian hyperstimulation syndrome while maintaining excellent pregnancy rates. *Hum Reprod* 2011;**26**(12):3437–3442.

52. Seyhan A, Ata B, Polat M, *et al.* Severe early ovarian hyperstimulation syndrome following GnRH agonist trigger with the addition of 1500 IU hCG. *Hum Reprod* 2013;**28**(9):2522–2528.

53. Youssef MA, Van der Veen F, Al-Inany HG, *et al.* Gonadotropin-releasing hormone agonist versus HCG for oocyte triggering in antagonist assisted reproductive technology cycles. *Cochrane Database of Syst. Rev* 2011;**1**:CD008046.

54. Youssef MA, Van der Veen F, Al-Inany HG, *et al.* The updated Cochrane review 2014 on GnRH agonist trigger: an indispensable piece of information for the clinician. *Reprod Biomed Online* 2016;**32**(2):259–260.

55. Lin MH, Wu FS, Lee RK, *et al.* Dual trigger with combination of gonadotropin-releasing hormone agonist and human chorionic gonadotropin significantly improves the live-birth rate for normal responders in GnRH-antagonist cycles. *Fertil Steril* 2013;**100**(5):1296–1302

56. O'Neill KE, Senapati S, Maina I, *et al.* GnRH agonist with low-dose hCG (dual trigger) is associated with higher risk of severe ovarian hyperstimulation syndrome compared to GnRH agonist alone. *J Assist Reprod Genet* 2016;**33**(9):1175–1184.

57. Pirard C, Loumaye E, Laurent P, *et al.* Contribution to more patient-friendly ART treatment: efficacy of continuous low-dose GnRH agonist as the only luteal support – results of a prospective, randomized, comparative study. *Int J Endocrinol* 2015;**2015**:727569.

58. Bar-Hava I, Mizrachi Y, Karfunkel-Doron D, *et al.* Intranasal gonadotropin-releasing hormone agonist (GnRHa) for luteal-phase support following GnRHa triggering, a novel approach to avoid ovarian hyperstimulation syndrome in high responders. *Fertil Steril* 2016;**106**(2):330–333.

59. Kol S, Breyzman T, Segal L, Humaidan P. 'Luteal coasting' after GnRH agonist trigger–individualized, HCG-based, progesterone-free luteal support in 'high responders': a case series. *Reprod Biomed Online* 2015;**31**(6):747–751.

60. Vanetik S, Segal L, Breizman T, *et al.* Day two post retrieval 1500 IUI hCG bolus, progesterone-free luteal support post GnRH agonist trigger–a proof of concept study. *Gynecol Endocrinol* 2018;**34**(2):132–135.

61. Fatemi HM, Popovic-Todorovic B. Implantation in assisted reproduction: a look at endometrial receptivity. *Reprod Biomed Online* 2013;**27**(5):530–538.

62. Devroey P, Polyzos NP, Blockeel C. An OHSS-Free Clinic by segmentation of IVF treatment. *Hum Reprod* 2011;**26**(10):2593–2597.

63. Garcia-Velasco JA. Agonist trigger: what is the best approach? Agonist trigger with vitrification of oocytes or embryos. *Fertil Steril* 2012;**97**(3):527–528.

The Luteal Phase Support in In Vitro Fertilization

Biljana Popovic-Todorovic and Human Mousavi Fatemi

Introduction

The luteal phase is defined as the period between ovulation and either the establishment of a pregnancy or the onset of menses two weeks later [1]. Following ovulation, the luteal phase of a natural cycle is characterized by the formation of a corpus luteum, which secretes steroid hormones, including progesterone and estradiol (E_2). If conception and implantation occur, the developing blastocyst secretes human chorionic gonadotropin (hCG). The role of hCG produced by the embryo is to maintain the corpus luteum and its secretions [2].

The estimated onset of placental steroidogenesis (the luteoplacental shift) occurs during the fifth gestational week, as calculated by the patients' last menses [3]. Stimulated in vitro fertilization (IVF) cycles are associated with a defective luteal phase in almost all patients [4–6].

In the context of assisted reproduction techniques, luteal phase support (LPS) is the term used to describe the administration of medication aimed at supporting the implantation process. In an attempt to enhance the probability of pregnancy, different doses, durations, and types of treatments for LPS have been evaluated. There is, however, no agreement regarding the optimal supplementation scheme [1;7].

Luteal phase insufficiency is usually due to inadequate postovulatory progesterone production. The prevalence of a luteal phase defect in natural cycles in normo-ovulatory patients with primary or secondary infertility was demonstrated to be about 8.1 percent [8].

With the advent of IVF, it has been established that the luteal phase of all stimulated IVF cycles is abnormal [9]. The use of agonistic or antagonistic gonadotropin-releasing hormone (GnRH) protocols in stimulated IVF/intracytoplasmic sperm injection (ICSI) cycles causes disruptions to the luteal phase, leading to inadequate development of the endometrium and asynchrony between endometrial receptiveness and embryo transfer. The etiology of luteal phase defect in stimulated IVF cycles has been debated for a number of decades.

Initially it was thought that prolonged pituitary recovery that followed the GnRH agonist co-treatment designed to prevent spontaneous luteinizing hormone (LH) rise in stimulated cycles, resulting in lack of support of the corpus luteum, would cause a luteal phase defect [10;11].

The hypothesis that the removal of large quantities of granulosa cells during the oocyte retrieval could diminish the most important source of progesterone synthesis by the corpora lutea, leading to a defect of the luteal phase, has been disproved. Aspiration of a preovulatory oocyte in a natural cycle had no effect on the luteal phase [12].

It has also been suggested that the hCG administered for the final oocyte maturation in stimulated IVF cycles could potentially cause a luteal phase defect by suppressing the LH production via a short-loop feedback mechanism [13]. However, the administration of hCG did not downregulate the LH secretion in the luteal phase of normal, unstimulated cycles in normo-ovulatory women [14].

The introduction of GnRH antagonists in IVF raised speculation that a rapid recovery of the pituitary function would obviate the need for luteal phase supplementation [15;16]. However, studies have confirmed that luteolysis is also initiated prematurely in antagonist co-treated IVF cycles [17], resulting in a significant reduction in the luteal phase length and compromising the chances for pregnancy. Thus, luteal phase supplementation remains mandatory [18].

Today, it is clear that the main cause of the luteal phase defect in stimulated assisted reproductive technology (ART) cycles is related to the supraphysiological levels of steroids secreted by a high number of corpora lutea during the early luteal phase, which directly inhibits LH release via a negative feedback action at the hypothalamic–pituitary axis [19]. Studies in human and primates have demonstrated that the corpus luteum requires a consistent LH stimulus in order to perform its physiological function [20]. LH support during the luteal phase is entirely responsible for the maintenance and the normal steroidogenic activity of the corpus luteum [21]. Lack of LH support of the corpus luteum shortens the luteal phase due to premature luteolysis [22].

Progesterone has been recommended as a LPS when GnRH analogues are used during IVF-ART [23]. These recommendations are supported by recent systematic review, which demonstrated that LPS with progesterone is associated with higher live birth and pregnancy rates compared with placebo or no treatment [7].

The Role of Progesterone in Luteal Phase

Csapo *et al.* demonstrated the importance of progesterone during the first weeks of a pregnancy [24;25]. In their initial study, the removal of the corpus luteum prior to seven weeks of gestation led to pregnancy loss [24]. However, they found that pregnancy could be maintained even after removal of the corpus luteum by external administration of progesterone [25].

Progesterone induces a secretory transformation of the endometrium in the luteal phase [26]. By inducing this change after adequate estrogen priming, progesterone improves endometrial receptivity [6]. Endometrial receptivity is a self-limited period in which the endometrial epithelium acquires a functional and transient ovarian steroid-dependent status that allows blastocyst adhesion [27]. Decreased endometrial receptivity is considered largely responsible for the low implantation rates in IVF [28].

Progesterone also promotes local vasodilatation and uterine musculature quiescence by inducing nitric oxide synthesis in the decidua [29]. Inadequate uterine contractility may lead to ectopic pregnancies, miscarriages, retrograde bleeding with dysmenorrhea, and endometriosis [29].

The uterine-relaxing properties of progesterone were supported by a study of IVF embryo transfer outcomes by Fanchin *et al.* which indicated that a high frequency of uterine contractions

on the day of embryo transfer hindered transfer outcome, possibly by expelling embryos out of the uterine cavity [30]. A negative correlation between uterine contraction frequency and progesterone concentrations was detected underlining the benefits of progesterone in IVF [30].

Luteal Phase Support

Progesterone

Currently various routes of progesterone administration for LPS are being used with no single formulation or regimen identified as superior regarding efficacy [7;23].

Available formulations of progesterone include oral, vaginal, rectal, intramuscular (IM), and subcutaneous (SC) [7] with each route having different bioavailability and tolerability profiles [31–33].

Oral Progesterone

Oral micronized progesterone has low bioavailability due to first-pass prehepatic and hepatic metabolism [2]. This metabolic activity results in progesterone degradation to its 5- and 5β-reduced metabolites [2]. The use of oral micronized progesterone is associated with systemic adverse events such as drowsiness, dizziness, and headaches [32].

The micronized progesterone formulations which were initially manufactured for oral use, due to low bioavailability of only 10 percent, have been more commonly administered vaginally [34].

Parenteral administration (vaginal, rectal, and IM) of progesterone overcomes the metabolic consequences of orally administered progesterone [35].

Dydrogesterone, a retroprogesterone with good oral bioavailability, is a biologically active metabolite of progesterone and has an antiestrogenic effect on the endometrium, achieving the desired secretory transformation [36;37]. Hence, oral retroprogesterone has been approved for the treatment of threatened and recurrent miscarriage, if associated with proven progesterone deficiency, and infertility due to luteal phase insufficiency [38]. Recently, a phase III randomized controlled trial comparing the efficacy, safety, and tolerability of oral dydrogesterone with those of micronized vaginal progesterone for luteal support in in vitro fertilization was published reporting comparable ongoing pregnancy rates [38].

Vaginal Progesterone

The intravaginal route of progesterone supplementation in IVF has gained wide application as a first choice luteal support regimen, mainly due to patient comfort and effectiveness [39]. Following vaginal application, serum progesterone concentrations reach maximal levels after approximately 3 to 8 hours and then fall continuously over the next 8 hours. In the majority of cases, 300–600 mg of vaginal progesterone are administered daily, divided into two or three doses [32]. High uterine progesterone concentrations with low peripheral serum values are observed, due to countercurrent exchange in progesterone transport between anatomically close blood vessels [40]. Vaginally administered progesterone exerts a direct local effect on the endometrium and myometrium prior to entering the systemic circulation: the so-called first uterine pass effect whereby liver metabolization is absent [35]. Until now, the mechanism of the first uterine pass effect is not fully understood and different modes of action are discussed: absorption of progesterone into the rich venous or lymphatic vaginal system and/or possibly direct drug diffusion through the tissues or even intraluminal transfer from the uterus to the vagina, similar to sperm transport.

Vaginally administered progesterone is cleared from the circulation faster than IM progesterone and serum progesterone levels are higher after IM administration compared with vaginal gel administration [2]. Independent from the measured serum progesterone levels, adequate secretory endometrial transformation is achieved following vaginal progesterone use. In addition, endometrial progesterone levels are higher after vaginal progesterone administration compared with IM injection [1].

Micronized vaginal progesterone is usually administered as a gel or as capsules [41], with both formulations having similar efficacy for LPS [42].

The vaginal route is effective in providing sufficient LPS and has minimal side effects [41], and as such is the preferred route of progesterone administration.

IM Progesterone

Supplementation with IM progesterone is given as an injection of natural progesterone in oil [43]. The doses of IM progesterone used for LPS vary between 25 and 100 mg/day without any significant difference concerning the outcome [44].

Progesterone is rapidly absorbed after IM injection, with peak concentrations being achieved after approximately 8 hours. However, the IM application of progesterone may be painful [45], and daily injections are required to sustain sufficient progesterone concentrations. Swelling, redness, and even sterile abscess formation [46] may also be experienced at the injection site. In addition, several case reports have been published in which patients receiving IM progesterone for luteal supplementation have developed acute eosinophilic pneumonia [47;48]. This drug-induced disease shows that the use of IM progesterone can also be associated with a severe morbidity in otherwise healthy young patients [47].

Although serum progesterone levels following IM dosing are typically supraphysiological and easily maintained, serum levels do not predict subsequent progesterone levels in endometrial tissue, as vaginal dosing provides significantly higher levels in the endometrium than the IM dosing, affording lower plasma concentrations [40].

Since the administration of vaginal progesterone is comparable to administration of IM progesterone for LPS in assisted reproductive treatment, IM progesterone is not recommended as a first choice for LPS. Vaginal route of progesterone administration is preferred over IM route as an easier, less painful, less time-consuming route and is associated with less discomfort.

SC Progesterone

The recent market introduction of SC progesterone for LPS in IVF broadens the spectrum of treatment options for women undergoing IVF treatment, especially for those women who do not tolerate or who dislike vaginal formulations. Baker *et al.* compared the administration of SC progesterone with vaginally administered progesterone for LPS of IVF and reported that the SC route of administration was well-tolerated and comparable in efficacy to a vaginal insert [49]. However, the conclusions of the study are limited to the progesterone dosing regimen studied and the duration of treatment for the patient population studied [49]. Although an individual patient data meta-analysis of the phase III trials showed that SC progesterone is effective and safe for LPS in IVF [50], further studies are required prior to the implementation of the SC route of administration into routine clinical practice.

Progesterone with Estradiol

Quality of the endometrium, upon which implantation depends, is affected by both progesterone and estradiol (E_2) produced by the corpus luteum [51]. The role of progesterone as luteal support in stimulated cycles is well established [52] while the role of E_2 in the luteal phase has been debated for a number of years.

It has been shown that a proportion of patients exhibit a midluteal E_2 level decrease and that this might be associated with a concomitant decrease in pregnancy rates [53]. Not unexpectedly, research for optimizing LPS has been directed toward the addition of E_2 to progesterone supplementation [54]. Many studies have been performed so far to evaluate the concept of E_2 addition during the luteal phase showing no benefit of E_2 supplementation in LPS [55–57].

Kolibianakis *et al.* speculated that there could be a subpopulation of patients who could benefit from E_2 supplementation [57]. The assumption for estrogen supplementation is that a serum E_2 drop occurs in some patients and it is perhaps these patients who must be targeted in future trials. It might be worth establishing a cut-off E_2 level in progesterone-only supported IVF cycles, on a certain day during the luteal phase, probably around day 8, when hCG is about to disappear from circulation [57]. Patients with subnormal midluteal E_2 concentrations could potentially benefit from estrogen supplementation. However, this has not been shown to date [7].

The most recent Cochrane review found no conclusive evidence of differences between groups for any outcome of progesterone with E_2 supplementation for LPS [7]. Supplementation of progesterone with oral estrogen did not appear to influence live birth and ongoing pregnancy rates, but benefit from transdermal or oral + transdermal estrogen supplementation is suggested. Findings for supplementation of progesterone with vaginal estrogen were inconsistent. Currently, routine use of E_2 in LPS in stimulated cycles can not be recommended [7].

LPS after GnRH Agonist Triggering for Final Oocyte Maturation in GnRH Antagonist Downregulated Cycles

Ovarian stimulation in a GnRH antagonist protocol with the use of GnRH agonist for final oocyte maturation is the state-of-the-art treatment in patients with an expected or known high response to avoid or to at least reduce significantly the risk for development of ovarian hyperstimulation syndrome (OHSS) [58]. It has, however, been shown that administration of GnRH agonist to induce oocyte maturation results in a defective corpus luteum formation, early demise of the corpus luteum, or both. This is because the administration of GnRH agonist induces a rise of LH lasting only 24–36 hours [59], with subsequent pituitary desensitization and withdrawal of LH support for the development and function of the corpora lutea. Although an LH surge of around 18–24 hours duration will be adequate for oocyte maturation, it will not be of sufficient duration to induce adequate corpora lutea formation [60;61].

The intensive LPS used after GnRH agonist trigger is based on the premise that the corpus luteum is dysfunctional. Therefore, the design of the luteal phase protocol was initially derived from protocols used for oocyte recipient cycles where there are no functional corpora lutea, and which have always included both E_2 and progesterone supplementation [61]. The optimal approach to the luteal phase after GnRH agonist trigger is still under debate [61].

One option is high-dose steroid replacement using E_2 and IM progesterone (the "American" approach), another option includes variable regimens of repetitive injection of small doses of hCG in conjunction with steroid replacement (the "European" approach) [61]. Administration of hCG within 72 hours rescues the corpora lutea function; however, the so far often used 1500 IU still bear the risk for development of OHSS [62].

One could argue that GnRH agonist trigger followed by a "freeze-all" approach (cycle segmentation) would result in the "OHSS-free clinic"; however, even with this approach, OHSS cannot be completely avoided [63]. Additionally although the "freeze-all" and "cycle segmentation" policy approach is gaining momentum especially in the high-risk OHSS patient population, it may not be applicable for all patients due to legal, ethical, or economic reasons. The new concept of luteal coasting and individualization of the hCG dose could provide a solution for this OHSS high-risk population [62].

Luteal Coasting and Individualization of Human Chorionic Gonadotropin Dose

Luteolysis after GnRH agonist trigger is not always complete and may vary, indicating individual differences among patients [64]. Luteolysis will be induced if LH support is withdrawn from the corpus luteum for three days or more, hence corpus luteum function can be rescued if LH activity is reinitiated within approximately 72 hours [65] and in the appropriate dosage (hCG ≥ 1500 IU) [66].

Luteal coasting seems to reduce the risk of OHSS development in high-responder patients undergoing fresh embryo transfer, without negatively impacting the reproductive outcome. The key to this approach is daily monitoring of the progesterone level and, depending on the patient's individual degree of luteolysis, the application of a rescue hCG bolus [64]. In order to fine-tune this concept, future studies should investigate its efficacy, the predictive parameters of luteolysis, the lowest progesterone level consistent with ongoing pregnancy, and the minimum amount of hCG needed to rescue the luteal phase.

A relatively new concept is so-called "luteal coasting." To avoid premature hCG application with the risk of OHSS development, Kol et al. introduced the principle of luteal coasting into the LPS after final oocyte maturation using GnRH agonist, by transferring the experience from follicular phase coasting for OHSS prevention to the early luteal phase [67]. This approach requires daily monitoring of serum progesterone concentrations and the administration of a rescue bolus of hCG once progesterone concentrations drop below 30 nmol/L [67]. As was recently shown, the range of progesterone concentrations 48 hours after GnRH agonist trigger differs widely between patients [64]; thus, this approach requires individualization of LPS according to the patient-specific luteolysis. A proof-of-concept study by Lawrenz et al. [64] demonstrated that the hCG dosage can be individualized on the basis of progesterone levels, and, therefore, it seems that OHSS after GnRH agonist administration for final oocyte maturation can be avoided by dosage reduction of the hCG rescue bolus without impacting the chance of achieving and/or maintaining a pregnancy [62].

LPS Based on Repeated GnRH Agonist Dosing

Repeated GnRH agonist dosing may prevent luteolysis after GnRH agonist trigger as shown by Pirard et al. [68] and Bar-Hava et al. [69]. This is not a currently generally adopted approach.

Co-treatment Schemes Using Additional Agents with Progesterone for LPS

Progesterone with Ascorbic Acid

Ascorbic acid is a preeminent water-soluble antioxidant [70] that has long been associated with fertility [71]. Luteal regression is associated with ascorbate depletion and the generation of reactive oxygen species, which inhibit the action of LH and block steroidogenesis [72]. Women with unexplained infertility have a lower total antioxidant status in their peritoneal fluid [73]. Griesinger et al. conducted a prospective, randomized, placebo-controlled study to evaluate the impact of ascorbic acid of different doses (1, 5, or 10 g/day) as additional support during the luteal phase. There was no clinical evidence of any beneficial effect of ascorbic acid, defined by ongoing pregnancy rate, in stimulated IVF cycles, regardless of the dose used [74].

Progesterone with Prednisolone

One line of research has investigated whether or not immunosuppression by exogenous corticosteroids as a co-treatment for LPS can be used to improve the rates of embryo implantation and pregnancy in IVF patients [75]. The rationale underlying this approach has been that embryos might be exposed to bacteria or leukocyte infiltration if the protective coating of the zona pellucida is breached. Immunosuppression caused by glucocorticoid administration would decrease the presence of uterine lymphocytes and of peripheral immune cells, particularly of segmented neutrophils, which might invade and destroy the zona-dissected embryos. According to this line of reasoning, glucocorticoids used in conjunction with zona dissection would improve pregnancy and implantation rates in IVF patients [76].

In a prospective randomized study involving routine ICSI patients, however, Ubaldi *et al.* did not find any beneficial effect of adding low-dose prednisolone to progesterone during the luteal phase [76]. In this group of patients, pregnancy and implantation rates were unaffected by prednisolone administration [76]. This is in accordance with earlier research [77].

The most recent meta analysis on the subject confirmed no significant effect of prednisolone as routine LPS [78].

Progesterone with Aspirin

Vane *et al.* described the mechanism of action of aspirin, showing that it inhibits the enzyme cyclooxygenase, thus preventing prostaglandin synthesis [79]. Luteal regression is caused by a pulsatile release of prostaglandins from the uterus in the late luteal phase [80]. Because aspirin has also been shown to increase uterine blood flow [81], clinicians have postulated that aspirin could improve the receptiveness of the endometrium, thereby increasing implantation and birth rates.

Early studies suggested that low-dose aspirin (100 mg) could increase the implantation and pregnancy rates in women undergoing IVF [82;83]. However, recent studies have been unable to confirm any improvement in IVF outcomes of patients treated with low-dose aspirin in the luteal phase [84;85]. It seems that there is no apparent benefit in the routine use of aspirin during IVF cycles, and this practice should be abandoned.

It should be mentioned that a certain subpopulation of patients may benefit from aspirin and prednisone treatment. Combined treatment of prednisone for immunosuppression and aspirin as an antithrombotic agent, administered before ovulation induction, may improve pregnancy rate in autoantibody sero-positive patients (those with anticardiolipin antibodies, antinuclear antibodies, anti-double-stranded DNA, rheumatoid factor, and/or lupus anticoagulant) who have had repeated IVF embryo transfer failures [86].

Human Chorionic Gonadotropin

Since it was found that the corpus luteum can be rescued by the administration of hCG, this treatment has become the standard care for luteal support since the late 1980s [87]. hCG is an indirect form of luteal support by stimulating the corpora lutea. It raises E_2 and progesterone concentrations,

thus rescuing the failing corpora lutea in stimulated IVF cycles [88].

Moreover, hCG administration increases concentrations of placental protein 14 [89], integrin [90], and relaxin (luteal peptide hormone), which have been shown to increase at the time of implantation [91].

A recent Cochrane review demonstrated that hCG given during the luteal phase may be associated with higher rates of live birth or ongoing pregnancy than placebo or no treatment, but the evidence is not conclusive. hCG increased the risk of OHSS [7].

Significant increases in OHSS rates have been confirmed in several earlier studies [92;93]. Therefore, hCG should not be the first choice of LPS in stimulated ART cycles.

GnRH Agonist as Adjuvant LPS

Relatively recently GnRH agonists were introduced as a new means of providing LPS that may act upon pituitary gonadotrophs, the endometrium [94], and the embryo itself [95]. GnRH blocks the LH surge, and it was assumed that GnRH agonists might maintain their stimulatory effect throughout the luteal phase and restore LH levels – a process that would support the luteal phase [96]. It has been hypothesized that a GnRH agonist may support the corpus luteum by stimulating the secretion of LH by pituitary gonadotroph cells or by acting directly on the endometrium through the locally expressed GnRH receptors [96]. Tesarik *et al.* postulated a direct effect of GnRH agonist on the embryo, evidenced by increased β-hCG secretion [97].

Currently, available data suggest that inadvertent administration of a GnRH agonist during a conception cycle is not accompanied by an increased risk of birth defects although more data focusing particularly on the safety of the method for the children born are necessary [98;99].

A recent Cochrane review reported that the use of a GnRH agonist as an additional LPS appears to increase live birth, ongoing pregnancy, and clinical pregnancy compared with progesterone alone [7]. There was no evidence of a difference between the groups for other outcomes, though OHSS was reported in only one study [7].

The Onset of LPS

Current clinical practice involves beginning LPS on different days. Arbitrarily most centers start with the luteal supplementation on the day of oocyte retrieval.

LPS has to be initiated before the endogenous progesterone levels are decreasing or low but preovulatory exposure of the endometrium to progesterone may also have a negative impact on endometrial receptivity. Therefore, the timing of LPS is critical to treatment success. A recent systematic review suggests that there appears to be a window for progesterone start time between the evening of the oocyte retrieval and up to day 3 following oocyte retrieval in hCG-triggered cycles [100]. Interestingly five randomized controlled trials were included in this review but meta-analysis could not be performed due to a high degree of clinical heterogeneity with regard to the timing, dose, and route of progesterone [100].

The Duration of LPS

The increase in endogenous hCG level during early pregnancy makes up for any possible lack of endogenous LH that has been caused by stimulated IVF cycles. First-trimester progesterone supplementation in IVF may support early pregnancy through seven weeks by delaying a miscarriage but it does not improve live birth rates [101].

The use of progesterone supplementation after oocyte retrieval is practically universal but the optimal duration of progesterone administration remains controversial.

A meta-analysis evaluated the optimal duration of progesterone supplementation in pregnant women after IVF/ICSI. Currently available evidence suggests that progesterone supplementation beyond the first positive hCG test after IVF/ICSI might generally be unnecessary, although large-scale randomized controlled trials are needed to strengthen this conclusion [102]. A recent study confirmed this recommendation [103].

Conclusions

The cause of luteal phase defect in stimulated IVF cycles seems to be related to the supraphysiological levels of steroids. LPS with hCG or progesterone after assisted reproduction results in increased pregnancy rates. However, hCG is associated with a greater risk of OHSS. Vaginal, SC, and IM progesterone seem to have comparable outcomes. However, IM progesterone should not be the first choice due to possible side effects.

Natural micronized progesterone is not effective, if taken orally.

Further studies need to evaluate the use of oral dydrogesterone for LPS.

Ascorbic acid, aspirin, naloxone, and prednisolone, all of which have been suggested at some point to be beneficial in IVF cycles, have not been proven useful as co-treatment of luteal phase supplementation. There is no evidence to justify routine use of E_2 in LPS.

There appears to be a window for progesterone start time between the evening of oocyte retrieval and up to day 3 following oocyte retrieval in hCG-triggered cycles.

The duration of LPS in stimulated IVF cycles does not appear to be mandatory beyond the day of a positive hCG test.

The new concept of personalized LPS focuses on the luteal phase after final oocyte maturation with GnRH agonist triggering in a GnRH antagonist protocol. Personalized LPS demonstrates that the hCG dose and timing can be individualized based on an individual luteolysis pattern. It appears that OHSS after GnRH agonist administration for final oocyte maturation can be avoided by individualization of LPS and adopting the novel approach of luteal coasting in high-responder patients planning fresh embryo transfer without adversely affecting their chance of achieving pregnancy.

References

1. Fatemi HM, Popovic-Todorovic B, Papanikolaou E, Donoso P, Devroey P. An update of luteal phase support in stimulated IVF cycles *Hum Reprod Update* 2007;**13**(6):581–590.

2. Penzias AS. Luteal phase support. *Fertil Steril* 2002;**77**:318–323.

3. Scott R, Navot D, Liu HC, *et al.* A human in vivo model for the luteoplacental shift. *Fertil Steril* 1991;**56**:481–484.

4. Ubaldi F, Bourgain C, Tournaye H, *et al.* Endometrial evaluation by aspiration biopsy on the day of oocyte retrieval in the embryo transfer cycles in patients with serum progesterone rise during the follicular phase. *Fertil Steril* 1997;**67**:521–526.

5. Macklon NS, Fauser BC. Impact of ovarian hyperstimulation on the luteal phase. *J Reprod Fertil* 2000;**55**(Suppl):101–108.

6. Kolibianakis EM, Devroey P. The luteal phase after ovarian stimulation. *Reprod Biomed Online* 2002;5 (Suppl 1):26–35.

7. van der Linden M, Buckingham K, Farquhar C, Kremer JA, Metwally M. Luteal phase support for assisted reproduction cycles. *Cochrane Database Syst Rev* 2015;7:CD009154.

8. Rosenberg SM, Luciano AA, Riddick DH. The luteal phase defect: the relative frequency of, and encouraging response to, treatment with vaginal progesterone. *Fertil Steril* 1980;34:17–20.

9. Edwards RG, Steptoe PC, Purdy JM. Establishing full-term human pregnancies using cleaving embryos grown in vitro. *Br J Obstet Gynaecol* 1980;87:737–756.

10. Smitz J, Devroey P, Faguer B, *et al.* A randomized prospective study comparing supplementation of the luteal phase and early pregnancy by natural progesterone administered by intramuscular or vaginal route. *Rev Fr Gynecol Obstet* 1992;87:507–516.

11. Smitz J, Erard P, Camus M, *et al.* Pituitary gonadotrophin secretory capacity during the luteal phase in superovulation using GnRH-agonists and HMG in a desensitization or flare-up protocol. *Hum Reprod* 1992;7: 1225–1229.

12. Kerin JF, Broom TJ, Ralph MM, *et al.* Human luteal phase function following oocyte aspiration from the immediately preovular graafian follicle of spontaneous ovular cycles. *Br J Obstet Gynaecol* 1981;88:1021–1028.

13. Miyake A, Aono T, Kinugasa T, Tanizawa O, Kurachi K. Suppression of serum levels of luteinizing hormone by short- and long-loop negative feedback in ovariectomized women. *J Endocrinol* 1979;80:353–356.

14. Tavaniotou A, Devroey P. Effect of human chorionic gonadotropin on luteal luteinizing hormone concentrations in natural cycles. *Fertil Steril* 2003; 80:654–655.

15. Albano C, Smitz J, Camus M, *et al.* Hormonal profile during the follicular phase in cycles stimulated with a combination of human menopausal gonadotrophin and gonadotrophin-releasing hormone antagonist (cetrorelix). *Hum Reprod* 1996;11:2114–2118.

16. Albano C, Grimbizis G, Smitz J, *et al.* The luteal phase of nonsupplemented cycles after ovarian superovulation with human menopausal gonadotropin and the gonadotropin-releasing hormone antagonist cetrorelix. *Fertil Steril* 1998;70:357–359.

17. Beckers NG, Macklon NS, Eijkemans MJ, *et al.* Nonsupplemented luteal phase characteristics after the administration of recombinant human chorionic gonadotropin, recombinant luteinizing hormone, or gonadotropin-releasing hormone (GnRH) agonist to induce final oocyte maturation in in vitro fertilization patients after ovarian stimulation with recombinant follicle-stimulating hormone and GnRH antagonist cotreatment. *J Clin Endocrinol Metab* 2003;88:4186–4192.

18. Tarlatzis BC, Fauser BC, Kolibianakis EM, *et al.* GnRH antagonists in ovarian stimulation for IVF. *Hum Reprod Update* 2006;12:333–340.

19. Fauser BC, Devroey P. Reproductive biology and IVF: ovarian stimulation and luteal phase consequences. *Trends Endocrinol Metab* 2003;14 (5):236–242.

20. Jones GS. Luteal phase defect: a review of pathophysiology. *Curr Opin Obstet Gynecol* 1991;3:641–648.

21. Casper RF, Yen SS. Induction of luteolysis in the human with a long-acting analog of luteinizing hormone-releasing factor. *Science* 1979;205:408–410.

22. Duffy DM, Stewart DR, Stouffer RL. Titrating luteinizing hormone replacement to sustain the structure and function of the corpus luteum after gonadotropin-releasing hormone antagonist treatment in rhesus monkeys. *J Clin Endocrinol Metab* 1999;84:342–349.

23. Practice Committee of the American Society for Reproductive Medicine. Progesterone supplementation during the luteal phase and in early pregnancy in the treatment of infertility: an educational bulletin. *Fertil Steril* 2008;89:789–792.

24. Csapo AI, Pulkkinen MO, Ruttner B, Sauvage JP, Wiest WG. The significance of the human corpus luteum in pregnancy maintenance. I. Preliminary studies. *Am J Obstet Gynecol* 1972;112:1061–1067.

25. Csapo AI, Pulkkinen MO, Wiest WG. Effects of lutectomy and progesterone replacement therapy in early pregnant patients. *Am J Obstet Gynecol* 1973;115:759–765.

26. Bourgain C, Devroey P, Van Waesberghe L, Smitz J, Van Steirteghem AC. Effects of natural progesterone on the morphology of the endometrium in patients with primary ovarian failure. *Hum Reprod* 1990;5:537–543.

27. Martin J, Dominguez F, Avila S, *et al.* Human endometrial receptivity: gene regulation. *J Reprod Immunol* 2002;55:131–139.

28. Paulson RJ, Sauer MV, Lobo RA. Embryo implantation after human in vitro fertilization: importance of endometrial receptivity. *Fertil Steril* 1990;53:870–874.

29. Bulletti C, de Ziegler D. Uterine contractility and embryo implantation. *Curr Opin Obstet Gynecol* 2005;**17**:265–276.

30. Fanchin R, Righini C, Olivennes F, *et al.* Uterine contractions at the time of embryo transfer alter pregnancy rates after in-vitro fertilization. *Hum Reprod* 1998;**13**:1968–1974.

31. Simon JA, Robinson DE, Andrews MC, *et al.* The absorption of oral micronized progesterone: the effect of food, dose proportionality, and comparison with intramuscular progesterone. *Fertil Steril* 1993;**60**:26–33.

32. Tavaniotou A, Smitz J, Bourgain C, Devroey P. Comparison between different routes of progesterone administration as luteal phase support in infertility treatments. *Hum Reprod Update* 2000;**6**:139–148.

33. Sator M, Radicioni M, Cometti B, *et al.* Pharmacokinetics and safety profile of a novel progesterone aqueous formulation administered by the s.c. route. *Gynecol Endocrinol* 2013;**29**:205–208.

34. Hubayter Z, Muasher S. Luteal supplementation in in vitro fertilization: more questions than answers. *Fertil Steril* 2008;**89**(4):749–758.

35. de Ziegler D, Seidler L, Scharer E, Bouchard P. Non-oral administration of progesterone: experiences and possibilities of the transvaginal route. *Schweiz Rundsch Med Prax* 1995;**84**:127–133.

36. Whitehead MI, Townsend PT, Gill DK, Collins WP, Campbell S. Absorption and metabolism of oral progesterone. *Br Med J* 1980;**280**:825–827.

37. Chakravarty BN, Shirazee HH, Dam P, *et al.* Oral dydrogesterone versus intravaginal micronised progesterone as luteal phase support in assisted reproductive technology (ART) cycles: results of a randomised study. *J Steroid Biochem Mol Biol* 2005;**97**:416–420.

38. Tournaye H, Sukhikh G, Kuhler E, Griesinger G. A phase III randomized controlled trial comparing the efficacy, safety and tolerability of oral dydrogesterone versus micronized vaginal progesterone for luteal support in in vitro fertilization. *Hum Reprod* 2017;**32**(5):1019–1027.

39. Levine H. Luteal support in IVF using the novel vaginal progesterone gel Crinone 8%: results of an open-label trial in 1184 women from 16 US centers. *Fertil Steril* 2000;**74**:836–837.

40. Cicinelli E, Schonauer LM, Galantino P, *et al.* Mechanisms of uterine specificity of vaginal progesterone. *Hum Reprod* 2000;**15** (Suppl 1):159–165.

41. Vaisbuch E, Leong M, Shoham Z. Progesterone support in IVF: is evidence-based medicine translated to clinical practice? A worldwide web-based survey. *Reprod Biomed Online* 2012;**25**:139–145.

42. Simunic V, Tomic V, Tomic J, Nizic D. Comparative study of the efficacy and tolerability of two vaginal progesterone formulations, Crinone 8% gel and Utrogestan capsules, used for luteal phase support. *Fertil Steril* 2007;**87**:83–87.

43. Costabile L, Gerli S, Manna C, *et al.* A prospective randomized study comparing intramuscular progesterone and 17alpha-hydroxyprogesterone caproate in patients undergoing in vitro fertilization-embryo transfer cycles. *Fertil Steril* 2001;**76**:394–396.

44. Pritts EA, Atwood AK. Luteal phase support in infertility treatment: a meta-analysis of the randomized trials. *Hum Reprod* 2002;**17**:2287–2299.

45. Lightman A, Kol S, Itskovitz-Eldor J. A prospective randomized study comparing intramuscular with intravaginal natural progesterone in programmed thaw cycles. *Hum Reprod* 1999;**14**:2596–2599.

46. Propst AM, Hill JA, Ginsburg ES, *et al.* A randomized study comparing Crinone 8% and intramuscular progesterone supplementation in in vitro fertilization-embryo transfer cycles. *Fertil Steril* 2001;**76**:1144–1149.

47. Bouckaert Y, Robert F, Englert Y, *et al.* Acute eosinophilic pneumonia associated with intramuscular administration of progesterone as luteal phase support after IVF: case report. *Hum Reprod* 2004;**19**:1806–1810.

48. Veysman B, Vlahos I, Oshva L. Pneumonitis and eosinophilia after in vitro fertilization treatment. *Ann Emerg Med* 2006;**47**:472–475.

49. Baker V, Jones C, Doody K, *et al.* A randomized controlled trial comparing the efficacy and safety of aqueous subcutaneous progesterone with vaginal progesterone for luteal phase support of in vitro fertilization. *Hum Reprod* 2014;**29** (10):2210–2220.

50. Doblinger J, Cometti B, Trevisan S, Griesinger G. Subcutaneous progesterone is effective and safe for luteal phase support in IVF: an individual patient data meta-analysis of the phase III trials. *PLoS One* 2016;**11**(3):e0151388.

51. Johnson MR, Abbas AA, Irvine R, *et al.* Regulation of corpus luteum function. *Hum Reprod* 1994;**9**:41–48.

52. Maslar IA, Ansbacher R. Effect of short-duration progesterone treatment on decidual prolactin

production by cultures of proliferative human endometrium. *Fertil Steril* 1988;**50**:250–254.

53. Sharara FI, McClamrock HD. Ratio of oestradiol concentration on the day of human chorionic gonadotrophin administration to mid-luteal oestradiol concentration is predictive of in-vitro fertilization outcome. *Hum Reprod* 1999;**14**(11):2777–2782.

54. Ludwig M, Diedrich K. Evaluation of an optimal luteal phase support protocol in IVF. *Acta Obstet Gynecol Scand* 2001;**80**:452–466.

55. Fatemi HM, Camus M, Kolibianakis EM, *et al.* The luteal phase of recombinant follicle-stimulating hormone/gonadotropin-releasing hormone antagonist in vitro fertilization cycles during supplementation with progesterone or progesterone and estradiol. *Fertil Steril* 2006;**87**:504–508.

56. Fatemi HM, Kolibianakis EM, Camus M, *et al.* Addition of estradiol to progesterone for luteal supplementation in patients stimulated with GnRH antagonist/rFSH for IVF: a randomized controlled trial. *Hum Reprod* 2006;**21**:2628–2632.

57. Kolibianakis EM, Venetis CA, Papanikolaou EG, *et al.* Estrogen addition to progesterone for luteal phase support in cycles stimulated with GnRH analogues and gonadotrophins for IVF: a systematic review and meta-analysis. *Hum Reprod* 2008;**23**(6):1346–1354.

58. Lawrenz B, Samir S, Garrido N, *et al.* Luteal coasting and individualization of human chorionic gonadotropin dose after gonadotropin-releasing hormone agonist triggering for final oocyte maturation: a retrospective proof-of-concept study. *Front Endocrinol (Lausanne)* 2018;**9**:33.

59. Itskovitz J, Boldes R, Levron J, *et al.* Induction of preovulatory luteinizing hormone surge and prevention of ovarian hyperstimulation syndrome by gonadotropin-releasing hormone agonist. *Fertil Steril* 1991;**56**(2):213–220.

60. Zelinski-Wooten MB, Lanzendorf SE, Wolf DP, Chandrasekher YA, Stouffer RL. Titrating luteinizing hormone surge requirements for ovulatory changes in primate follicles. I. Oocyte maturation and corpus luteum function. *J Clin Endocrinol Metab* 1991;**73**(3):577–583.

61. Engmann L, Benadiva C, Humaidan P. GnRH agonist trigger for the induction of oocyte maturation in GnRH antagonist IVF cycles: a SWOT analysis. *Reprod Biomed Online* 2016;**32**(3):274–285.

62. Lawrenz B, Humaidan P, Kol S, Fatemi HM. GnRHa trigger and luteal coasting: a new approach for the ovarian hyperstimulation

syndrome high-risk patient? *Reprod Biomed Online* 2018;**36**(1):75–77.

63. Fatemi HM, Popovic-Todorovic B, Humaidan P, *et al.* Severe ovarian hyperstimulation syndrome after gonadotrophin-releasing hormone (GnRH) agonist trigger and 'freeze-all' approach in GnRH antagonist protocol. *Fertil Steril* 2014;**101**:1008–1011.

64. Lawrenz B, Garrido N, Samir S, *et al.* Individual luteolysis pattern after GnRH-agonist trigger for final oocyte maturation. *PLoS One* 2017;**12**: e0176600.

65. Hutchison JS, Zeleznik AJ. The corpus luteum of the primate menstrual cycle is capable of recovering from a transient withdrawal of pituitary gonadotrophin support. *Endocrinology* 1985;**117**:1043–1049.

66. Dubourdieu S, Charbonnel B, Massai MR, *et al.* Suppression of corpus luteum function by the gonadotrophin-releasing hormone antagonist Nal-Glu: effect of the dose and timing of human chorionic gonadotrophin administration. *Fertil Steril* 1991;**56**:440–512.

67. Kol S, Breyzman T, Segal L, Humaidan P. 'Luteal coasting' after GnRH agonist trigger– individualized, HCG-based, progesterone-free luteal support in 'high responders': a case series. *Reprod Biomed Online* 2015;**31**:747–751.

68. Pirard C, Donnez J, Loumaye E. GnRH agonist as novel luteal support: results of a randomized, parallel group, feasibility study using intranasal administration of buserelin. *Hum Reprod* 2005;**20**:1798–1804.

69. Bar-Hava I, Mizrachi Y, Karfunkel-Doron D, *et al.* Intranasal gonadotropin-releasing hormone agonist (GnRHa) for luteal-phase support following GnRHa triggering, a novel approach to avoid ovarian hyperstimulation syndrome in high responders. *Fertil Steril* 2016;**106**:330–333.

70. Buettner GR. The pecking order of free radicals and antioxidants: lipid peroxidation, alpha-tocopherol, and ascorbate. *Arch Biochem Biophys* 1993;**300**:535–543.

71. Millar J. Vitamin C–the primate fertility factor? *Med Hypotheses* 1992;**38**:292–295.

72. Margolin Y, Aten RF, Behrman HR. Antigonadotropic and antisteroidogenic actions of peroxide in rat granulosa cells. *Endocrinology* 1990;**127**:245–250.

73. Polak G, Koziol-Montewka M, Gogacz M, Kotarski J. Total antioxidant status of peritoneal fluid in infertile women. *Eur J Obstet Gynecol Reprod Biol* 2001;**94**:261–263.

74. Griesinger G, Franke K, Kinast C, *et al.* Ascorbic acid supplement during luteal phase in IVF. *J Assist Reprod Genet* 2002;**19**:164–168.

75. Lee KA, Koo JJ, Yoon TK, *et al.* Immunosuppression by corticosteroid has no effect on the pregnancy rate in routine in-vitro fertilization/embryo transfer patients. *Hum Reprod* 1994;**9**:1832–1835.

76. Ubaldi F, Rienzi L, Ferrero S, *et al.* Low dose prednisolone administration in routine ICSI patients does not improve pregnancy and implantation rates. *Hum Reprod* 2002;**17**:1544–1547.

77. Moffitt D, Queenan JT Jr., Veeck LL, *et al.* Low-dose glucocorticoids after in vitro fertilization and embryo transfer have no significant effect on pregnancy rate. *Fertil Steril* 1995;**63**:571–577.

78. Dan S, Wei W, Yichao S, *et al.* Effect of prednisolone administration on patients with unexplained recurrent miscarriage and in routine intracytoplasmic sperm injection: a meta-analysis. *Am J Reprod Immunol* 2015;**74**(1):89–97.

79. Vane JR, Flower RJ, Botting RM. History of aspirin and its mechanism of action. *Stroke* 1990;**21**:IV12–IV23.

80. Okuda K, Miyamoto Y, Skarzynski DJ. Regulation of endometrial prostaglandin F(2alpha) synthesis during luteolysis and early pregnancy in cattle. *Domest Anim Endocrinol* 2002;**23**:255–264.

81. Wada I, Hsu CC, Williams G, Macnamee MC, Brinsden PR. The benefits of low-dose aspirin therapy in women with impaired uterine perfusion during assisted conception. *Hum Reprod* 1994;**9**:1954–1957.

82. Weckstein LN, Jacobson A, Galen D, Hampton K, Hammel J. Low-dose aspirin for oocyte donation recipients with a thin endometrium: prospective, randomized study. *Fertil Steril* 1997;**68**:927–930.

83. Rubinstein M, Marazzi A, Polak DF. Low-dose aspirin treatment improves ovarian responsiveness, uterine and ovarian blood flow velocity, implantation, and pregnancy rates in patients undergoing in vitro fertilization: a prospective, randomized, double-blind placebo-controlled assay. *Fertil Steril* 1999;**71**:825–829.

84. Urman B, Mercan R, Alatas C, *et al.* Low-dose aspirin does not increase implantation rates in patients undergoing intracytoplasmic sperm injection: a prospective randomized study. *J Assist Reprod Genet* 2000;**17**:586–590.

85. Hurst BS, Bhojwani JT, Marshburn PB, *et al.* Low-dose aspirin does not improve ovarian stimulation, endometrial response, or pregnancy rates for in vitro fertilization. *J Exp Clin Assist Reprod* 2005;**2**:8.

86. Geva E, Amit A, Lerner-Geva L, *et al.* Prednisone and aspirin improve pregnancy rate in patients with reproductive failure and autoimmune antibodies: a prospective study. *Am J Reprod Immunol* 2000;**43**:36–40.

87. Whelan JG III, Vlahos NF. The ovarian hyperstimulation syndrome. *Fertil Steril* 2000;**73**:883–896.

88. Hutchinson-Williams KA, DeCherney AH, Lavy G, *et al.* Luteal rescue in in vitro fertilization-embryo transfer. *Fertil Steril* 1990;**53**:495–501.

89. Anthony FW, Smith EM, Gadd SC, *et al.* Placental protein 14 secretion during in vitro fertilization cycles with and without human chorionic gonadotropin for luteal support. *Fertil Steril* 1993;**59**:187–191.

90. Honda T, Fujiwara H, Yamada S, *et al.* Integrin alpha5 is expressed on human luteinizing granulosa cells during corpus luteum formation, and its expression is enhanced by human chorionic gonadotrophin in vitro. *Mol Hum Reprod* 1997;**3**:979–984.

91. Ghosh D, Stewart DR, Nayak NR, *et al.* Serum concentrations of oestradiol-17beta, progesterone, relaxin and chorionic gonadotrophin during blastocyst implantation in natural pregnancy cycle and in embryo transfer cycle in the rhesus monkey. *Hum Reprod* 1997;**12**:914–920.

92. Herman A, Ron-El R, Golan A, *et al.* Pregnancy rate and ovarian hyperstimulation after luteal human chorionic gonadotropin in in vitro fertilization stimulated with gonadotropin-releasing hormone analog and menotropins. *Fertil Steril* 1990;**53**:92–96.

93. Mochtar MH, Hogerzeil HV, Mol BW. Progesterone alone versus progesterone combined with HCG as luteal support in GnRHa/HMG induced IVF cycles: a randomized clinical trial. *Hum Reprod* 1996;**11**:1602–1605.

94. Pirard C, Donnez J, Loumaye E. GnRH agonist as novel luteal support: results of a randomized, parallel group, feasibility study using intranasal administration of buserelin. *Hum Reprod* (2005) **20**:1798–1804

95. Tesarik J, Hazout A, Mendoza-Tesarik R, Mendoza N, Mendoza C. Beneficial effect of luteal-phase GnRH agonist administration on embryo implantation after ICSI in both GnRH agonist- and antagonist-treated ovarian stimulation cycles. *Hum Reprod* 2006;**21**:2572–2579.

96. Pirard C, Donnez J, Loumaye E. GnRH agonist as luteal phase support in assisted reproduction technique cycles: results of a pilot study. *Hum Reprod* 2006;**21**(7):1894–1900.

97. Tesarik J, Hazout A, Mendoza C. Enhancement of embryo developmental potential by a single administration of GnRH agonist at the time of implantation. *Hum Reprod* 2004;**19**:1176–1180.

98. Kyrou D, Kolibianakis EM, Fatemi HM, *et al.* Increased live birth rates with GnRH agonist addition for luteal support in ICSI/IVF cycles: a systematic review and meta-analysis. *Hum Reprod Update* 2011;**17**:734–740.

99. Martins WP, Ferriani RA, Navarro PA, Nastri CO. GnRH agonist during luteal phase in women undergoing assisted reproductive techniques: systematic review and meta-analysis of randomized controlled trials. *Ultrasound Obstet Gynecol* 2016;**47**(2):144–151.

100. Connell MT, Szatkowski JM, Terry N, *et al.* Timing luteal support in assisted reproductive technology: a systematic review. *Fertil Steril* 2015;**103**:939–946.

101. Proctor A, Hurst BS, Marshburn PB, Matthews ML. Effect of progesterone supplementation in early pregnancy on the pregnancy outcome after in vitro fertilization. *Fertil Steril* 2006;**85**:1550–1552.

102. Liu XR, Mu HQ, Shi Q, Xiao XQ, Qi HB. The optimal duration of progesterone supplementation in pregnant women after IVF/ICSI: a meta-analysis. *Reprod Biol Endocrinol* 2012;**10**:107.

103. Pan SP, Chao KH, Huang CC, *et al.* Early stop of progesterone supplementation after confirmation of pregnancy in IVF/ICSI fresh embryo transfer cycles of poor responders does not affect pregnancy outcome. *PLoS One* 2018;**13**(8):e0201824.

Chapter 29

Luteal Phase Support Other than Progesterone

Dalia Khalife, Nour Assaf, and Johnny Awwad

Etiology of Luteal Phase Defect during Controlled Ovarian Stimulation

Deficiencies in luteal hormonal dynamics have been clearly documented during controlled ovarian stimulation [1]. Disruptions to the physiological secretion of luteinizing hormone (LH) by the anterior pituitary affect optimal corpus luteum (CL) function warranting some form of luteal phase support (LPS) in order to maintain optimal endometrial receptivity in stimulated cycles.

Supraphysiological serum levels of estradiol (E_2) resulting from the induction of multifollicular development inhibit LH release via a negative feedback effect on the hypothalamic–pituitary axis [2]. Pituitary suppression following gonadotropin-releasing hormone agonist (GnRHa) administration for the purpose of preventing a follicular premature LH surge [3;4] extends way into the luteal phase, interfering with CL function [5–7]. Since the normal function of the CL requires a steady LH stimulus to achieve peak physiological steroidogenic activity [8], diminished LH pulse amplitude invariably leads to a deficient luteal phase. In addition, it has been suggested that the mechanical process of follicle aspiration is associated with significant disruption to the granulosa cell population further compromising progesterone production [9].

It should also be noted that the trigger for final follicular maturation plays a major role in CL function. The conventional use of a large bolus of human chorionic gonadotropin (hCG) for the induction of the ovulatory processes directly stimulates the corpora lutea to produce progesterone. The hCG-mediated luteotropic effect however occurs during the early luteal phase and appears to be out of phase with critical midluteal implantation events [10]. This effect is followed by considerable LH suppression via both steroid and hCG-mediated negative feedback pathways [10] altering CL function in the midluteal phase.

Recently, the use of hCG to trigger final follicular maturation has been challenged by the use of a GnRHa in women co-treated with a GnRH antagonist. Although the GnRHa-induced LH surge is sufficient to induce final maturation of oocytes, it has failed to provide sufficient luteotropic stimulus to maintain normal CL function. As a result, the luteal phase of GnRHa-triggered cycles has been profoundly deficient requiring more intensive forms of luteal support.

It is now agreed that LPS is an essential component of controlled ovarian stimulation cycles for achieving better implantation and pregnancy rates. The primary choice for endometrial support has traditionally been exogenous progesterone supplementation in various forms, doses, and routes. It should be noted that research has also explored additional options to optimize the luteal phase during controlled ovarian stimulation, namely alternative agents such as hCG, GnRHa, and estrogen (E_2) which will be discussed in this chapter.

The Use of Human Chorionic Gonadotropins for Luteal Phase Supplementation

Pharmacokinetic and pharmacodynamic studies show that hCG serum levels rise above 100–150 IU/L during the first two days following the hCG trigger and decline gradually during the following five days. This peak is associated with an early luteal progesterone rise followed by considerable LH suppression and subsequently a progesterone decline at the critical time of embryo implantation. The importance of hCG use for LPS was initially acknowledged in women diagnosed with WHO anovulation group I [11] and was widely used initially to support the luteal phase during stimulated cycles. The prolonged half-life of the molecule and the strong luteotropic signal it generates have been associated nonetheless with a significant rise in the risk of ovarian hyperstimulation syndrome (OHSS). The current use of hCG for LPS is therefore a risk/benefit trade-off between the optimization of midluteal endocrine events and treatment-related health hazards.

Three randomized controlled trials (RCTs) evaluated the use of hCG alone for LPS compared with placebo or no treatment in women undergoing COH for in vitro fertilization/intracytoplasmic sperm injection (IVF/ICSI) [12–14]. When the data from all three trials encompassing 527 women were pooled together into a meta-analysis [15], a three-dose hCG protocol (1500 to 2500 IU) administered during the luteal phase significantly improved live birth rate (LBR) and ongoing pregnancy rate (OPR) compared with placebo or no treatment (odds ratio [OR] 1.76, 95% confidence interval [CI] 1.08–2.86). The hCG LPS protocol however was found to be associated with a significant increase in the risk of OHSS (OR 4.28, 95% CI 1.91–9.60) [12].

The pooled data from five other RCTs (833 women) comparing hCG alone with progesterone supplementation suggested no differences between groups in LBR and OPR (OR 0.95, 95% CI 0.65–1.38) [15]. Progesterone treatment nonetheless manifested a better safety profile and was associated with significantly lower chance of OHSS compared with hCG (OR 0.46, 95% CI 0.30–0.71). Furthermore, the addition of hCG to traditional progesterone supplementation with the aim of improving overall cycle outcome did not significantly improve OPR and LBR (OR 0.95, 95% CI 0.65–1.38), but increased OHSS risk [15].

Recently, the use of hCG for LPS has received wider interest in the context of GnRHa-triggered IVF/ICSI cycles. The use of the GnRHa to trigger final oocyte maturation in women at risk for OHSS has resulted in profound deficiency of the luteal phase as a result of premature demise of the CL. Lower pregnancies and higher pregnancy losses have been reported by earlier studies [16]. To improve the reproductive efficiency of GnRH-triggered cycles, a hCG luteal rescue dose was proposed at the time of the trigger or immediately following egg collection [17;18].

In a retrospective study of 45 patients, the administration of hCG rescue at the time of

agonist trigger was shown to be effective in maintaining OPR (53.3%) without increasing OHSS risk [19]. Similar findings were reported by other investigators [17].

On the other hand, a single hCG bolus (1500 IU) at the time of ovum pickup has also been evaluated in GnRHa-triggered cycles with the aim of maintaining adequate luteal support following embryo transfer. This strategy was portrayed in different studies by Humaidan and colleagues who demonstrated similar pregnancy outcomes between the GnRHa trigger with rescue hCG and the hCG trigger [20–22]. A randomized controlled study of 302 normogonadotropic women did not find any differences in LBR between both study groups (24% vs. 31% respectively) [20]. The safety of the hCG rescue however remains far from being established, namely that early cases of severe OHSS have been reported [23].

More recently, a growing interest in hCG for LPS in controlled ovarian stimulation cycles has re-emerged with the introduction of microdoses of hCG administration to support the CL when a GnRHa trigger is used for final oocyte maturation [20;24;25]. While previously suggested boluses of 1500 to 2500 IU were associated with serum levels exceeding 50–100 IU/L and a significant rise in OHSS risk, a shift to a smaller dose is believed to serve the main goal of adjusting LH activity to physiological range without additional health hazards [24;26;27]. A 100 IU bolus was demonstrated to achieve a serum steady state of 6–7 IU/L which is deemed sufficient to stimulate the CL and lead to optimal progesterone production [27]. It should be noted that progesterone levels of 25–35 nmol/L during natural cycles can be achieved with LH serum levels of 5–10 IU/L [28]. In clinical studies, daily microdoses of hCG have been reported to improve the clinical pregnancy outcome while reducing miscarriages and lowering the incidence of OHSS [24]. Despite these promising observations, further randomized studies are needed to confirm the virtues of the daily hCG microdose approach for LPS before it finds its way into our treatment armamentarium.

For the sake of completion, it should be noted that recombinant LH may represent an alternative option for LPS in GnRHa-triggered cycles. Papanikolaou et al. evaluated the effects of 300 IU recombinant LH administered every other day during the luteal phase on reproductive outcome [29]. Pregnancy rate did not differ when compared with that of the conventional hCG trigger group. Although a safer alternative to hCG, recombinant LH therapy is associated with elevated financial costs making this option less attractive compared to others.

The Use of Gonadotropin-Releasing Hormone Agonists for Luteal Phase Supplementation

The exact role of GnRHa in the luteal phase remains poorly comprehended. In primates, the use of GnRHa during pregnancy was associated with a luteolytic effect with disruption to embryo implantation [30]. These observations were not replicated in humans and such use failed to adversely affect pregnancy outcome or induce early abortion [31]. These findings led the way to exploring the use of GnRHa for luteal support by several investigators who have reported on its effectiveness with variable outcomes [32–34].

In 2005, Pirard et al. conducted a proof-of-concept feasibility study on 24 women undergoing intrauterine insemination who received 100 mg of GnRHa daily for luteal support. The luteal phase extended beyond 14 days, progesterone serum levels were persistently elevated, and clinical pregnancy rate (CPR) was satisfactory (28%) [35]. A number of studies also revealed that the addition of a GnRHa for luteal support in addition to conventional vaginal progesterone resulted in significant improvement in implantation rates, pregnancy rates, and LBRs [33;36]. These findings were not universally confirmed by other investigators however [37;38].

In an oocyte donation program, Tesarik et al. demonstrated significant improvement in implantation, live birth and twin delivery rates in recipients following a single injection of GnRHa six days after egg retrieval [33]. The investigators demonstrated that improved outcome after luteal GnRHa supplementation was associated with midluteal increase in serum E_2 and progesterone, as well as increase in hCG levels two weeks after egg collection [36]. The improvement in reproductive outcome observed in recipients of donor oocytes in the absence of a functional CL is intriguing and could indicate a direct effect of the GnRHa on the embryo

[33;39]. Animal studies showed the presence of GnRH receptors in the inner cell mass of mice blastocysts suggesting a role for GnRHa in the control of hCG secretion in the early stages of implantation [40]. Alternatively, it is possible that GnRHa may also act via a direct effect on the expression of GnRH receptors in the endometrium, promoting the secretion of cytokines and angiogenic factors involved in the adhesion of the embryo with a decrease in the natural killer cytotoxicity [34;41]. It should be noted that GnRH receptor expression has been shown to be highly accentuated during the luteal phase in stromal and epithelial endometrial tissues.

In a meta-analysis of 2012 patients, Kyrou et al. found a significantly higher LBR in women who received a GnRHa in addition to conventional progesterone luteal supplementation following GnRH agonist and antagonist pituitary suppression [42]. The Cochrane analysis by van der Linden also confirmed an improvement in LBR, CPR, and OPR after GnRHa luteal supplementation [15]. More recently, a third meta-analysis further revealed a significant improvement in the likelihood of OPR in association with luteal GnRHa administration with no effect on the miscarriage rate [43]. The quality of the evidence in all three meta-analyses nonetheless was deemed low.

Other investigators reported on the efficacy of using a GnRHa for LPS alone in the absence of progesterone supplementation [32;34]. A RCT by Pirard et al. compared the efficacy of intranasal buserelin for LPS to traditional progesterone supplementation in antagonist cycles. The GnRHa group had higher pregnancy rates (31.4% vs. 22.2%), implantation rates (22% vs. 15.4%), and CPR (25.7% vs. 16.7%) without nonetheless achieving statistical significance [34]. Bar Hava et al. also demonstrated a significantly higher LBR with the use of daily intranasal GnRHa as the sole preparation for luteal support in comparison with conventional vaginal progesterone [32]. It should be noted that higher endogenous serum levels of progesterone and E_2 have been detected during the midluteal phase following GnRHa administration [44].

Only few studies have reported on the use of GnRHa for luteal support in cryo-warmed cycles. The outcomes of six such studies (1137 women) were pooled into a meta-analysis, revealing higher implantation rates (OR 1.6, 95% CI 1.22–2.09), CPR (OR 1.87, 95% CI 1.41–2.48), and OPR (OR

1.55, 95% CI 1.15–2.09) in women receiving the GnRHa. A conclusive statement cannot be made nonetheless with respect to the reproductive benefit of GnRHa luteal supplementation in cryo-warmed cycles given the limited number of high-quality studies available in the medical literature. Also, study heterogeneity is another limiting factor to proper data interpretation and is the result of using different GnRHa luteal phase protocols and variable progesterone formulations and dosages. Consequently, the evidence of this meta-analyses is estimated to be low and additional research is required to confirm these findings [45].

The safety of GnRHa exposure on early embryo development has not been well established. On the one hand, animal studies did not demonstrate any teratogenic effects [46]. Also, the incidence of congenital abnormalities and birth defects in humans following inadvertent GnRHa administration in early pregnancy (2.5%) was reported to be identical to the risk identified in the general population [42;47–50]. The rate of pregnancy loss (15%) was equally comparable. It should also be noted that GnRHa depots formulations are in use as essential components of long suppression protocols in many centers around the world. The elimination half-life of these products extends beyond six weeks from administration and into early pregnancy with no relevant adverse events reported [51].

The use of GnRHa as the sole luteal support was also investigated in GnRH agonist-triggered cycles with the aim of maintaining adequate embryo implantation during fresh transfers without increasing the risk of OHSS. In 2006, Pirard *et al.* performed a pilot study on 30 women undergoing IVF/ICSI treatment who received daily GnRHa for luteal support following agonist triggering. Pregnancy outcome was found to be comparable to women who received progesterone supplementation following hCG triggering [39]. In a prospective clinical trial including 40 normal responders, the same investigators reported comparable CPRs between the group receiving intranasal GnRHa for ovulation trigger and luteal support and the group receiving hCG trigger and conventional vaginal progesterone [34]. In a retrospective cohort study, Bar-Hava *et al.* evaluated the use of daily intranasal GnRHa (nafarelin) for LPS in 46 high-responder women in the absence of any additional progesterone supplementation [52]. They could demonstrate a rise in serum progesterone levels in the midluteal phase and on the day of pregnancy test. The OPR was very promising (52.1%) with no cases of OHSS reported. Taken together, these findings suggest that GnRHa administration during the luteal phase maintains LH secretion and overcomes the GnRHa trigger-induced luteolytic process. Randomized controlled studies however are needed to confirm these findings before recommending this approach in clinical practice.

On the basis of available evidence, GnRHa addition to conventional progesterone support in the luteal phase is likely to be beneficial to OPR and LBR in both fresh and frozen cycles; yet, further prospective randomized studies are needed to assess the effect of GnRHa alone as LPS on endometrial receptivity and CL function.

The Use of Estradiol for Luteal Phase Supplementation

Over the past years, much attention has focused on E_2 luteal supplementation in IVF/ICSI treated women. This interest arises from clinical observations showing that a rise in serum E_2 in the mid to late luteal phase in fertile women may be correlated with pregnancy occurrence [53;54]. On the other hand, low midluteal E_2 levels have also been associated with endometrial delay and reduced endometrial receptivity [55]. Because of persistent pituitary suppression in controlled ovarian stimulation cycles, luteal function becomes severely compromised resulting in a sharp decline in E_2 and progesterone levels with a detrimental effect on pregnancy [56]. While E_2 priming of the endometrium in cryo-warmed embryo transfers is standard practice [57], the addition of E_2 to conventional progesterone LPS in IVF/ICSI cycles has not been well established.

Basic research has shown that E_2 promotes the expression of progesterone receptors on endometrial cells [58]. Estradiol also increases the endometrial L-selectin ligand in the luminal epithelium, a marker of endometrial receptivity [59]. Animal studies on ovariectomized rhesus monkeys however have failed to show any benefits of luteal E_2 supplementation on embryo implantation rates [60].

Several studies evaluated the possible clinical value of E_2 addition to standard progesterone supplementation in IVF/ICSI cycles with contradictory results reported [15;61–69]. In an initial meta-analysis, Pritts and Atwood evaluated the addition of oral E_2 (2 to 6 mg daily) to progesterone in three RCTs using a long GnRH agonist suppression protocol. They reported a significantly higher implantation rate in association with E_2 supplementation (relative risk [RR] 1.49, 95% CI 1.02–2.19) [70]. In a dose-finding trial, Lukaszuk et al. demonstrated an improved pregnancy outcome with 6 mg daily E_2 supplementation compared with lower doses [62].

In a prospective RCT of 200 women undergoing IVF/ICSI treatment, Fatemi et al. failed to demonstrate any significant reproductive benefits of supplementing the luteal phase of GnRH antagonist co-treated cycles with oral E_2 (4 mg/day) [66]. Likewise, Ceyhan et al. in another prospective randomized study of 60 women did not observe any beneficial effect of transdermal estrogen supplementation [67]. The meta-analysis of Kolibianakis et al., which included four RCTs, suggested that adding E_2 to progesterone for LPS does not increase the total pregnancy rate (RR 1.02, 95% CI 0.87–1.19), CPR (RR 0.94, 95% CI 0.78–1.13), and LBR (RR 0.96, 95% CI 0.77–1.21) [68]. Two additional meta-analyses confirmed these findings [71;72]. The latest meta-analysis by Huang et al., which included 15 RCTs and a total of 2406 patients, also failed to demonstrate any improvement in reproductive outcomes with the addition of E_2 for LPS in GnRH agonist or antagonist cycles [69]. The different routes (oral, vaginal, and transdermal) and doses (2, 4, and 6 mg) of E_2 administration of LPS did not influence outcome.

While numerous RCTs do not support the addition of E_2 to progesterone during the luteal phase in stimulated cycles, fewer clinical studies have demonstrated a favorable effect of E_2 luteal supplementation on reproductive outcome [61–65]. In a prospective open-labeled RCT evaluating the benefits of oral and vaginal E_2 luteal supplementation, Elgindy et al. showed that vaginal administration of 6 mg E_2 valerate for luteal support together with progesterone significantly improved pregnancy rates compared with conventional progesterone supplementation in ICSI cycles using the long agonist protocol [64]. Although the maximum E_2 levels on the day of hCG did not differ between groups, conventional progesterone-only luteal supplementation was associated with significantly lower E_2 levels on luteal days 7 and 10, and a higher magnitude of

E_2 decline in comparison with the E_2 supplementation groups. While both the oral and vaginal routes enhanced serum E_2 levels in the midluteal phase, only vaginal E_2 was associated with a favorable effect on reproductive parameters. Differences between the oral and vaginal routes may be traced to the first liver pass effect. While oral E_2 intake may be associated with rapid hepatic inactivation to estrone and other inactive metabolites, the vaginal route is associated with a more consistent effect on the endometrium as a result of the direct vaginal uterine transport. This mechanism has also been elucidated in frozen-thawed cycles, whereby Wright et al. reported improved pregnancy rate in women receiving vaginal E_2 compared with oral E_2 [73].

It should be noted that concerns have also been raised with respect to the most appropriate dose of E_2 supplementation. It is suggested that high circulating E_2 levels might suppress serum LH levels in the luteal phase leading to decreased progesterone production by the CL [74]. Also, based on uterine contractility data, high E_2 may induce some resistance to uterine quiescence at the time of implantation mediated by progesterone effect, potentially affecting outcome [75].

While a clear benefit has not been established for E_2 supplementation in the luteal phase of hCG-triggered cycles, the addition of estrogen to progesterone is essential for endometrial receptivity and embryo implantation in cycles in which a GnRHa has been used to trigger final follicle maturation. Estradiol transdermal patches in combination with progesterone intramuscular injections have been proposed to support the luteal phase of GnRHa-triggered cycles while closely monitoring serum estrogen and progesterone levels [76]. Intensive luteal support enhanced pregnancy rate in the GnRHa trigger group in comparison with the hCG group. In a cohort study of 70 women undergoing IVF/ICSI treatment, the use of a combination of 50 mg of intramuscular progesterone and 6 mg of E_2 per day was also associated with satisfactory LBRs [77].

In summary, the best available evidence suggests that adding E_2 to progesterone for LPS in hCG-triggered cycles does not improve reproductive outcome. Estradiol supplementation is a key element of LPS in GnRHa-triggered cycles and should be continued until after a positive pregnancy test.

Conclusion

The need for LPS has been thoroughly acknowledged to confer benefit to women undergoing IVF cycles. Exogenous progesterone has been the conventional option and the drug of choice to supplement the luteal phase; other options nonetheless exist, such as the addition of hCG, GnRHa, and E_2, which in specific clinical situations lend better support to embryo implantation. The addition of hCG was shown to confer a reproductive advantage mainly in GnRHa-triggered cycles, albeit with some risk of OHSS. The addition of E_2 equally is associated with improved outcome in cycles in which a GnRHa is used to trigger final oocyte maturation. The use of GnRHa during the luteal phase has shown promising results although more well-designed studies are needed to improve the quality of the evidence.

References

1. Edwards RG, Steptoe PC, Purdy JM. Establishing full-term human pregnancies using cleaving embryos grown in vitro. *BJOG* 1980;**87**(9):737–756.

2. Gardner DK, Weissman A, Howles CM, Shoham Z (eds.). *Textbook of Assisted Reproductive Techniques: Laboratory and Clinical Perspectives.* Boca Raton: CRC Press; 2016.

3. Messinis IE, Messini CI, Dafopoulos K. Luteal-phase endocrinology. *Reprod Biomed Online* 2009;**19**:15–29.

4. Pabuccu R, Akar ME. Luteal phase support in assisted reproductive technology. *Curr Opin Obstet Gynecol* 2005;**17**(3):277–281.

5. De Ziegler D, Cedars MI, Randle D, *et al.* Suppression of the ovary using a gonadotropin releasing-hormone agonist prior to stimulation for oocyte retrieval. *Fertil Steril* 1987;**48**(5):807–810.

6. Neveu S, Hedon B, Bringer J, *et al.* Ovarian stimulation by a combination of a gonadotropin-releasing hormone agonist and gonadotropins for in vitro fertilization. *Fertil Steril* 1987;**47**(4):639–643.

7. Fraser HM. Effect of oestrogen on gonadotrophin release in stumptailed monkeys (*Macaca arctoides*) treated chronically with an agonist analogue of luteinizing hormone releasing hormone. *J Endocrinol* 1981;**91**(3):525–530.

8. Fauser BC, Devroey P. Reproductive biology and IVF: ovarian stimulation and luteal phase consequences. *Trends Endocrinol Metab* 2003;**14**(5):236–242.

9. Miyake A, Aono T, Kinugasa T, Tanizawa O, Kurachi K. Suppression of serum levels of luteinizing hormone by short- and long-loop negative feedback in ovariectomized women. *J Endocrinol* 1979;**80**(3):353–356.

10. Smitz J, Devroey P, Van Steirteghem AC. Endocrinology in luteal phase and implantation. *Br Med Bull* 1990;**46**(3):709–719.

11. Messinis IE, Bergh T, Wide L. The importance of human chorionic gonadotropin support of the corpus luteum during human gonadotropin therapy in women with anovulatory infertility. *Fertil Steril* 1988;**50**(1):31–35.

12. Belaisch-Allart J, De Mouzon J, Lapousterle C, Mayer M. The effect of HCG supplementation after combined GnRH agonist/HMG treatment in an IVF programme. *Hum Reprod* 1990;**5**(2):163–166.

13. Kuperminc MJ, Lessing JB, Amit A, *et al.* A prospective randomized trial of human chorionic gonadotrophin or dydrogesterone support following in-vitro fertilization and embryo transfer. *Hum Reprod* 1990;**5**(3):271–273.

14. Beckers NG, Laven JS, Eijkemans MJ, Fauser BC. Follicular and luteal phase characteristics following early cessation of gonadotrophin-releasing hormone agonist during ovarian stimulation for in-vitro fertilization. *Hum Reprod* 2000;**15**(1):43–49.

15. van der Linden M, Buckingham K, Farquhar C, Kremer JA, Metwally M. Luteal phase support for assisted reproduction cycles. *Cochrane Database Syst Rev* 2015;**7**:CD009154.

16. Humaidan P, Ejdrup Bredkjaer H, Bungum L, *et al.* GnRH agonist (buserelin) or hCG for ovulation induction in GnRH antagonist IVF/ICSI cycles: a prospective randomized study. *Hum Reprod* 2005;**20**(5):1213–1220.

17. Shapiro BS, Daneshmand ST, Garner FC, Aguirre M, Hudson C. Comparison of "triggers" using leuprolide acetate alone or in combination with low-dose human chorionic gonadotropin. *Fertil Steril* 2011;**95**(8):2715–2717.

18. Engmann L, Romak J, Nulsen J, Benadiva C, Peluso J. In vitro viability and secretory capacity of human luteinized granulosa cells after gonadotropin-releasing hormone agonist trigger of oocyte maturation. *Fertil Steril* 2011;**96**(1):198–202.

19. Shapiro BS, Daneshmand ST, Garner FC, Aguirre M, Thomas S. Gonadotropin-releasing hormone agonist combined with a reduced dose of human chorionic gonadotropin for final oocyte maturation in fresh autologous cycles of in vitro fertilization. *Fertil Steril* 2008;**90**(1):231–233.

20. Humaidan P, Bredkjær HE, Westergaard LG, Andersen CY. 1,500 IU human chorionic gonadotropin administered at oocyte retrieval rescues the luteal phase when gonadotropin-releasing hormone agonist is used for ovulation induction: a prospective, randomized, controlled study. *Fertil Steril* 2010;**93** (3):847–854.

21. Humaidan P. Luteal phase rescue in high-risk OHSS patients by GnRHa triggering in combination with low-dose HCG: a pilot study. *Reprod Biomed Online* 2009;**18**(5):630–634.

22. Humaidan P, Bungum L, Bungum M, Andersen CY. Rescue of corpus luteum function with peri-ovulatory HCG supplementation in IVF/ICSI GnRH antagonist cycles in which ovulation was triggered with a GnRH agonist: a pilot study. *Reprod Biomed Online* 2006;**13**(2):173–178.

23. Seyhan A, Ata B, Polat M, *et al*. Severe early ovarian hyperstimulation syndrome following GnRH agonist trigger with the addition of 1500 IU hCG. *Hum Reprod* 2013;**28**(9):2522–2528.

24. Andersen CY, Fischer R, Giorgione V, Kelsey TW. Micro-dose hCG as luteal phase support without exogenous progesterone administration: mathematical modelling of the hCG concentration in circulation and initial clinical experience. *J Assist Reprod Genet* 2016;**33**(10):1311–1318.

25. Humaidan P, Polyzos NP, Alsbjerg B, *et al*. GnRHa trigger and individualized luteal phase hCG support according to ovarian response to stimulation: two prospective randomized controlled multi-centre studies in IVF patients. *Hum Reprod* 2013;**28**(9):2511–2521.

26. Andersen CY, Andersen KV. Improving the luteal phase after ovarian stimulation: reviewing new options. *Reprod Biomed Online* 2014;**28** (5):552–559.

27. Thuesen LL, Loft A, Egeberg AN, *et al*. A randomized controlled dose–response pilot study of addition of hCG to recombinant FSH during controlled ovarian stimulation for in vitro fertilization. *Hum Reprod* 2012;**27**(10):3074–3084.

28. De Ziegler D, Pirtea P, Andersen CY, Ayoubi JM. Role of gonadotropin-releasing hormone agonists, human chorionic gonadotropin (hCG), progesterone, and estrogen in luteal phase support after hCG triggering, and when in pregnancy hormonal support can be stopped. *Fertil Steril* 2018;**109**(5):749–755.

29. Papanikolaou EG, Verpoest W, Fatemi H, *et al*. A novel method of luteal supplementation with recombinant luteinizing hormone when a gonadotropin-releasing hormone agonist is used instead of human chorionic gonadotropin for ovulation triggering: a randomized prospective

    proof of concept study. *Fertil Steril* 2011;**95** (3):1174–1177.

30. Kang IS, Kuehl TJ, Siler-Khodr TM. Effect of treatment with gonadotropin-releasing hormone analogues on pregnancy outcome in the baboon. *Fertil Steril* 1989;**52**(5):846–853.

31. Skarin G, Nillius SJ, Wide L. Failure to induce early abortion by huge doses of a superactive LRH agonist in women. *Contraception* 1982;**26** (5):457–463.

32. Bar Hava I, Blueshtein M, Herman HG, Omer Y, David GB. Gonadotropin-releasing hormone analogue as sole luteal support in antagonist-based assisted reproductive technology cycles. *Fertil Steril* 2017;**107**(1):130–135.

33. Tesarik J, Hazout A, Mendoza C. Enhancement of embryo developmental potential by a single administration of GnRH agonist at the time of implantation. *Hum Reprod* 2004;**19**(5):1176–1180.

34. Pirard C, Loumaye E, Laurent P, Wyns C. Contribution to more patient-friendly ART treatment: efficacy of continuous low-dose GnRH agonist as the only luteal support – results of a prospective, randomized, comparative study. *Int J Endocrinol* 2015;**2015**:727569.

35. Pirard C, Donnez J, Loumaye E. GnRH agonist as novel luteal support: results of a randomized, parallel group, feasibility study using intranasal administration of buserelin. *Hum Reprod* 2005;**20** (7):1798–1804.

36. Tesarik J, Hazout A, Mendoza-Tesarik R, Mendoza N, Mendoza C. Beneficial effect of luteal-phase GnRH agonist administration on embryo implantation after ICSI in both GnRH agonist- and antagonist-treated ovarian stimulation cycles. *Hum Reprod* 2006;**21** (10):2572–2579.

37. Yıldız GA, Şükür YE, Ateş C, Aytaç R. The addition of gonadotrophin releasing hormone agonist to routine luteal phase support in intracytoplasmic sperm injection and embryo transfer cycles: a randomized clinical trial. *Eur J Obstet Gynecol Reprod Biol* 2014;**182**:66–70.

38. Aboulghar MA, Marie H, Amin YM, *et al*. GnRH agonist plus vaginal progesterone for luteal phase support in ICSI cycles: a randomized study. *Reprod Biomed Online* 2015;**30**(1):52–56.

39. Pirard C, Donnez J, Loumaye E. GnRH agonist as luteal phase support in assisted reproduction technique cycles: results of a pilot study. *Hum Reprod* 2006;**21**(7):1894–1900.

40. Kawamura K, Fukuda J, Kumagai J, *et al*. Gonadotropin-releasing hormone I analog acts as an antiapoptotic factor in mouse blastocysts. *Endocrinology* 2005;**146**(9):4105–4116.

41. Wong KH, Simon JA. In vitro effect of gonadotropin-releasing hormone agonist on natural killer cell cytolysis in women with and without endometriosis. *Am J Obstet Gynecol* 2004;**190**(1):44–49.

42. Kyrou D, Kolibianakis EM, Fatemi HM, *et al.* Increased live birth rates with GnRH agonist addition for luteal support in ICSI/IVF cycles: a systematic review and meta-analysis. *Hum Reprod Update* 2011;**17**(6):734–740.

43. Martins WP, Ferriani RA, Navarro PA, Nastri CO. GnRH agonist during luteal phase in women undergoing assisted reproductive techniques: systematic review and meta-analysis of randomized controlled trials. *Ultrasound Obstet Gynecol* 2016;**47**(2):144–151.

44. Bhurke AS, Bagchi IC, Bagchi MK. Progesterone-regulated endometrial factors controlling implantation. *Am J Reprod Immunol* 2016;**75**(3):237–245.

45. Li S, Li Y. Administration of a GnRH agonist during the luteal phase frozen–thawed embryo transfer cycles: a meta-analysis. *Gynecol Endocrinol* 2018 ;**34**(11):920–924.

46. Janssens RMJ, Brus L, Cahill DJ, *et al.* Direct ovarian effects and safety of GnRH agonists and antagonists. *Hum Reprod Update* 2000;**6**(5):505–518.

47. Cahill DJ. The risks of GnRH agonist administration in early pregnancy. In: Filicori M, Flamigni C, eds. *Ovulation Induction Update'98.* London: Parthenon; 1998:97–106.

48. Marcus SF, Ledger WL. Efficacy and safety of long-acting GnRH agonists in in vitro fertilization and embryo transfer. *Hum Fertil* 2001;**4**(2):85–93.

49. Oliveira JB, Baruffi R, Petersen CG, *et al.* Administration of single-dose GnRH agonist in the luteal phase in ICSI cycles: a meta-analysis. *Reprod Biol Endocrinol* 2010;**8**(1):107.

50. Zhou W, Zhuang Y, Pan Y, Xia F. Effects and safety of GnRH-a as a luteal support in women undertaking assisted reproductive technology procedures: follow-up results for pregnancy, delivery, and neonates. *Arch Gynecol Obstet* 2017;**295**(5):1269–1275.

51. Orvieto R, Kerner R, Krissi H, *et al.* Comparison of leuprolide acetate and triptorelin in assisted reproductive technology cycles: a prospective, randomized study. *Fertil Steril* 2002;**78**(6):1268–1271.

52. Bar-Hava I, Mizrachi Y, Karfunkel-Doron D, *et al.* Intranasal gonadotropin-releasing hormone agonist (GnRHa) for luteal-phase support following GnRHa triggering, a novel approach to avoid ovarian hyperstimulation syndrome in high responders. *Fertil Steril* 2016;**106**(2):330–333.

53. Laufer N, Navot D, Schenker JG. The pattern of luteal phase plasma progesterone and estradiol in fertile cycles. *Am J Obstet Gynecol* 1982;**143**(7):808–813.

54. Lipson SF, Ellison PT. Comparison of salivary steroid profiles in naturally occurring conception and non-conception cycles. *Hum Reprod* 1996;**11**(10):2090–2096.

55. Bouchard P. Understanding endometrial physiology and menstrual disorders in the 1990s. *Curr Opin Obstet Gynecol* 1993;**5**(3):378–388.

56. Smitz J, Devroey P, Braeckmans P, *et al.* Management of failed cycles in an IVF/GIFT programme with the combination of GnRH analogue and HMG. *Hum Reprod* 1987;**2**(4):309–314.

57. Hancke K, More S, Kreienberg R, Weiss JM. Patients undergoing frozen-thawed embryo transfer have similar live birth rates in spontaneous and artificial cycles. *J Assist Reprod Genet* 2012;**29**(5):403–407.

58. Fritz MA, Westfahl PK, Graham RL. The effect of luteal phase estrogen antagonism on endometrial development and luteal function in women. *J Clin Endocrinol Metab* 1987;**65**(5):1006–1013.

59. Vlahos NF, Lipari CW, Bankowski B, *et al.* Effect of luteal-phase support on endometrial L-selectin ligand expression after recombinant follicle-stimulating hormone and ganirelix acetate for in vitro fertilization. *J Clin Endocrinol Metab* 2006;**91**(10):4043–4049.

60. Ghosh D, De P, Sengupta J. Luteal phase ovarian oestrogen is not essential for implantation and maintenance of pregnancy from surrogate embryo transfer in the rhesus monkey. *Hum Reprod* 1994;**9**(4):629–637.

61. Farhi J, Weissman A, Steinfeld Z, *et al.* Estradiol supplementation during the luteal phase may improve the pregnancy rate in patients undergoing in vitro fertilization-embryo transfer cycles. *Fertil Steril* 2000;**73**(4):761–766.

62. Lukaszuk K, Liss J, Lukaszuk M, Maj B. Optimization of estradiol supplementation during the luteal phase improves the pregnancy rate in women undergoing in vitro fertilization–embryo transfer cycles. *Fertil Steril* 2005;**83**(5):1372–1376.

63. Ghanem ME, Sadek EE, Elboghdady LA, *et al.* The effect of luteal phase support protocol on cycle outcome and luteal phase hormone profile in long agonist protocol intracytoplasmic sperm injection cycles: a randomized clinical trial. *Fertil Steril* 2009;**92**(2):486–493.

64. Elgindy EA, El-Haieg DO, Mostafa MI, Shafiek M. Does luteal estradiol supplementation have a role in long agonist cycles? *Fertil Steril* 2010;**93** (7):2182–2188.

65. Var T, Tonguc EA, Doğanay M, *et al.* A comparison of the effects of three different luteal phase support protocols on in vitro fertilization outcomes: a randomized clinical trial. *Fertil Steril* 2011;**95**(3):985–989.

66. Fatemi HM, Kolibianakis EM, Camus M, *et al.* Addition of estradiol to progesterone for luteal supplementation in patients stimulated with GnRH antagonist/rFSH for IVF: a randomized controlled trial. *Hum Reprod* 2006;**21** (10):2628–2632.

67. Ceyhan ST, Basaran M, Duru NK, *et al.* Use of luteal estrogen supplementation in normal responder patients treated with fixed multidose GnRH antagonist: a prospective randomized controlled study. *Fertil Steril* 2008;**89** (6):1827–1830.

68. Kolibianakis EM, Venetis CA, Papanikolaou EG, *et al.* Estrogen addition to progesterone for luteal phase support in cycles stimulated with GnRH analogues and gonadotrophins for IVF: a systematic review and meta-analysis. *Hum Reprod* 2008;**23**(6):1346–1354.

69. Huang N, Situ B, Chen X, *et al.* Meta-analysis of estradiol for luteal phase support in in vitro fertilization/intracytoplasmic sperm injection. *Fertil Steril* 2015;**103**(2):367–373.

70. Pritts EA, Atwood AK. Luteal phase support in infertility treatment: a meta-analysis of the randomized trials. *Hum Reprod* 2002;**17** (9):2287–2299.

71. Gelbaya TA, Kyrgiou M, Tsoumpou I, Nardo LG. The use of estradiol for luteal phase support in

in vitro fertilization/intracytoplasmic sperm injection cycles: a systematic review and meta-analysis. *Fertil Steril* 2008;**90**(6):2116–2125.

72. Jee BC, Suh CS, Kim SH, Kim YB, Moon SY. Effects of estradiol supplementation during the luteal phase of in vitro fertilization cycles: a meta-analysis. *Fertil Steril* 2010;**93**(2):428–436.

73. Wright KP, Guibert J, Weitzen S, *et al.* Artificial versus stimulated cycles for endometrial preparation prior to frozen–thawed embryo transfer. *Reprod Biomed Online* 2006;**13** (3):321–325.

74. Smitz J, Bourgain C, Van Waesberghe L, *et al.* A prospective randomized study on oestradiol valerate supplementation in addition to intravaginal micronized progesterone in buserelin and HMG induced superovulation. *Hum Reprod* 1993;**8**(1):40–45.

75. Fanchin R, Righini C, Schönauer LM, *et al.* Vaginal versus oral E_2 administration: effects on endometrial thickness, uterine perfusion, and contractility. *Fertil Steril* 2001;**76**(5):994–998.

76. Engmann L, DiLuigi A, Schmidt D, *et al.* The use of gonadotropin-releasing hormone (GnRH) agonist to induce oocyte maturation after cotreatment with GnRH antagonist in high-risk patients undergoing in vitro fertilization prevents the risk of ovarian hyperstimulation syndrome: a prospective randomized controlled study. *Fertil Steril* 2008;**89**(1):84–91.

77. Imbar T, Kol S, Lossos F, *et al.* Reproductive outcome of fresh or frozen–thawed embryo transfer is similar in high-risk patients for ovarian hyperstimulation syndrome using GnRH agonist for final oocyte maturation and intensive luteal support. *Hum Reprod* 2012;**27** (3):753–759.

Chapter

30

Ovarian Reserve as a Guide for Ovarian Stimulation

Hassan N. Sallam, Ahmed F. Galal, and Nooman H. Sallam

Ovarian Reserve

Ovarian reserve refers to the number and quality of oocytes present in the ovaries of a woman at a given time and is thought to reflect her ability to respond adequately to ovarian stimulation [1;2]. The term was developed in the context of assisted reproduction to differentiate between poor, normal, and hyper-responders to controlled ovarian stimulation (COS). Although the term is also applicable to anovulatory women treated for infertility with ovarian stimulation, it is mainly used to describe women receiving COS as a part of an in vitro fertilization (IVF) or intracytoplasmic sperm injection (ICSI) stimulation protocol. Attempts were made to differentiate between the "true ovarian reserve" which reflects the resting pool of follicles and which can only be determined accurately by histological examination and the "functional ovarian reserve" which can be measured by the currently available tools [3]. Consequently, in practical terms, the (functional) ovarian reserve can be evaluated by stimulating the ovaries and measuring the response.

Reference Values for Ovarian Reserve

Determining the reference values for ovarian reserve is necessary if this parameter is to be used in clinical medicine. Below these values, the ovarian reserve is considered diminished (and the patient a poor responder) and above them, the response is considered exaggerated (and the patient a hyper-responder). Between these values, the reserve is considered adequate (and the patient a normal responder). Response to COS should therefore be defined by the number of follicles developing and/or the number of oocytes they contain, in response to this stimulation. In the context of assisted reproduction, the determination of the number of oocytes retrieved is more

reliable than the determination of the number of ovarian follicles observed on ultrasonography as these can be confused with other ultrasound artifacts.

In 2005, Sallam et al. were the first to attempt to define the lower limits of ovarian reserve (i.e., poor responders) by determining the number of oocytes retrieved in response to COS [4]. They analyzed 782 fresh IVF and ICSI cycles by constructing receiver operator characteristic (ROC) curves and found that the cut-off number of oocytes retrieved below which the clinical pregnancy rate (CPR) was significantly diminished was five oocytes for women treated with ICSI, six oocytes for women treated with IVF, and eight oocytes for women treated with ICSI/testicular sperm aspiration for non-obstructive azoospermia [4]. This study was followed by that of van der Gaast et al. who analyzed 7422 women and found that the CPR was diminished significantly with the retrieval of less than four oocytes [5]. Similarly, Drakopoulos et al. studied 1099 women and found that the live birth rate (LBR) was significantly diminished when less than four oocytes were retrieved [6]. More recently, Polyzos et al. analyzed data from 14 469 patients and found that the LBR increased steadily with the number of oocytes retrieved and reached a plateau after the recruitment of seven oocytes [7]. There is no universal agreement on the lower reference value for the ovarian reserve, but based on these studies, it is traditionally taken as four oocytes.

Few studies have been conducted to determine the high reference value of ovarian reserve, but in a recent study, Magnusson et al. analyzed data of 77 956 fresh IVF cycles from the National Swedish Registry and found that the incidence of severe ovarian hyperstimulation syndrome (OHSS) increased significantly if more than 18 oocytes were retrieved [8]. Similarly, no uniform agreement on this high reference value has been adopted but traditionally, it is usually taken as 15 oocytes [9].

Markers of Ovarian Reserve/ Predictors of Ovarian Response

Various markers have been studied to determine their ability to predict response to COS (and hence evaluate ovarian reserve) [10]. Strictly speaking these markers should predict the ovarian response in term of the number of oocytes retrieved and not the CPR or LBR as these outcomes are not the mere result of successful stimulation, but are also affected by the laboratory conditions, quality of embryo transfer, any intra/extrauterine pathology, endometrial receptivity, and luteal phase support.

1. Age of the female partner. The quantity and quality of oocytes in the human ovaries are known to decline with age [11]. Consequently, age should be a good marker for ovarian reserve as shown in various studies. In a recent study, Scheffer et al. confirmed that age was significantly correlated with the number of retrieved oocytes and that it was an independent predictor of ovarian reserve and ovarian stimulation outcome [12]. Attempts have also been made to determine the critical age above which the number of oocytes recruited is significantly diminished and Al-Azemi et al., using ROC curves, found that this was 36 years [13].

2. Serum follicle-stimulating hormone (FSH). Measurement of serum FSH levels on day 2 or 3 of the menstrual cycle has been traditionally used as a test for ovarian reserve as high levels of serum FSH are associated with diminished response to COS [1]. Various cut-off points were used for this purpose. For example, Ashrafi et al. found that women with FSH levels ≥ 15 IU/L had fewer aspirated oocytes and a larger number of canceled cycles compared with women with lower levels [14]. Despite its poor sensitivity, FSH is a better predictor of poor response than of high response [15]. With newer tests now available (e.g., anti-Müllerian hormone [AMH] and antral follicle count [AFC]), the value of FSH as a marker for ovarian reserve has dwindled, and, recently, Wang et al. found that AMH was a better predictor of ovarian response and LBR than FSH [16].

3. Inhibin B. Inhibin B is a glycoprotein secreted mainly by the preantral ovarian follicles and is responsible for selective inhibition of the pituitary FSH secretion [2]. Hofmann et al. found that higher numbers of oocytes were retrieved from women with serum inhibin B levels ≥ 45 pg/ml, whereas cancellations were three times as frequent amongst patients with lower levels [17]. Similarly, Steiner et al. found that low inhibin B levels were associated with a poor outcome [18]. However, these findings have not been universally replicated [19]. Inhibin B is not therefore a reliable measure of ovarian reserve [1].

4. Antral follicle count. AFC (2–10 mm follicles) determined on day 2 or 3 of the menstrual cycle is a reliable test for ovarian reserve and for predicting the number of oocytes retrieved with a high specificity (73–100%) but a lower sensitivity (9–73%) [1;20;21]. Popovic-Todorovic et al. compared many markers of poor ovarian reserve and found that AFC was the single most significant predictor of the number of oocytes retrieved [20]. Similarly, Kwee et al. performed a multiple regression analysis of the factors affecting ovarian response and found that the cut-off points for poor response and hyper-response were an AFC of < 6 and > 14, respectively [21].

5. Anti-Müllerian hormone. AMH is a glycoprotein produced by the granulosa cells of small preantral and antral follicles [2]. Its serum level is more or less stable throughout the menstrual cycle and earlier discrepancies between the two available tests have now been resolved with the development of a newer more reliable test (Gen II test) [2]. AMH was shown to be a good predictor of poor ovarian response to COS with a good specificity (78–92%) and a sensitivity ranging from 40% to 97% with a cut-off level ranging from 0.1 to 1.66 ng/ml [1;2]. AMH is also a good predictor of hyper-response and Lee et al. reported a cut-off level of > 3.36 ng/ml for the prediction of OHSS [22].

6. Genetic markers. Genetic markers were also investigated as possible predictors of ovarian response. In a meta-analysis of 16 studies, Tang et al. found that FSH receptor Asn680Ser polymorphism was a significant biomarker for predicting the number of retrieved oocytes,

particularly in Asian subjects [23]. More recently, Motawi et al. found that the frequency of the ESR2 (AA) genotype and the FSHR (Ala307Ala) genotypes were significantly associated with poor ovarian response (less than four oocytes) in Egyptian women [24].

7. Ovarian volume. Ovarian volume measured by ultrasound before the start of ovarian stimulation has limited reliability as an ovarian reserve test [1]. Although several studies have shown that a low ovarian volume (< 3 ml) is a good predictor of poor ovarian response and that its measurement can predict the number of oocytes retrieved [1;21], other studies could not confirm this finding [25]. On the other hand, ovarian volume has been shown to be a good predictor of hyper-response [26].

8. Clomiphene (clomifene) citrate challenge test (CCCT). In this dynamic test, a dose of 100 mg of clomiphene citrate is administered orally to the patient between days 5 and 9 of the cycle. Basal FSH, luteinizing hormone, and estradiol (E_2) levels are determined on days 2 and 3 of the menstrual cycle and again on days 10–12. Poor response is predicted if the sum of basal and post-stimulation FSH levels is higher than 26 IU/L [27]. In a systematic review, Hendricks et al. found that the CCCT did not add any value to the basal FSH level [1;28].

9. Combination of markers. Attempts have been made to combine some of these markers to improve their predictability. For example, Broer et al. found that the combination of age, AFC, AMH, and FSH gave a better prediction for ovarian response over each individual marker (AUC = 0.81, compared to 0.61 for age, 0.68 for FSH, 0.76 for AFC, and 0.78 for AMH) and over other combinations of these four markers [29].

Algorithms for Individualized Dosing

Based on these markers, various algorithms and nomograms were devised to suggest the best stimulation protocol and/or determine the starting dose of FSH stimulation for any individual patient. For example, Nelson devised a chart for suggesting the appropriate stimulation protocol for the patient based on the AMH level and/or the AFC (Figure 30.1) [30].

On the other hand, Popovic-Todorovic et al. devised a simple "bed-side" FSH dosage score nomogram based on ultrasound parameters (AFC, ovarian volume, and Power Doppler score) as well as clinical data (age and smoking habits) to determine the starting FSH dose necessary to recruit the ideal number of 5 to 14 oocytes [31]. Similarly, Olivennes et al. devised a scoring algorithm (CONSORT) based on basal serum FSH, body mass index (BMI), age, and the AFC to determine the starting FSH dose [32]. Two more nomograms were subsequently devised by La Marca and Sunkara based on age and either AMH or the AFC for the determination of the starting dose of FSH (Figure 30.2) [33]. More recently, the POSEIDON group proposed a new stratification for the individualized management of low-prognosis patients [34]. They stratified the patients into four subgroups based on age, AFC, AMH, and previous poor ovarian response [34].

Algorithms were also devised to minimize the risk of hyper-response and incidence of OHSS. Yovich et al. devised such an algorithm based mainly on the patient's age and her AFC but also on day 2 FSH levels, BMI, age, and smoking parameters. They found that the use of this algorithm markedly reduces the risk of OHSS [35].

Comparing Algorithms for Individualized Dosing

Attempts were also made to compare different algorithms to find if any of them was superior in terms of efficiency and safety. In 2013, Lan et al. compared two simple dosing algorithms, one based on serum AMH and the other on AFC, in 348 unselected patients. They found that both algorithms were similarly effective for guiding the starting dose of recombinant FSH (rFSH) to achieve the desired response (8–12 oocytes), with no significant differences in the incidence of OHSS, implantation, CPR, multiple pregnancy, or miscarriage rates [36]. However, they found that AMH level was better than AFC for predicting poor response while AFC was better in predicting hyper-response, confirming an earlier observation by Broer et al. [37].

On the other hand, Magnusson et al. compared two algorithms in 308 unselected women:

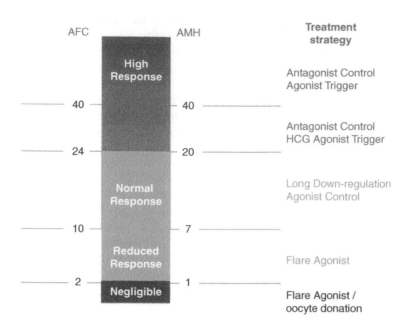

Figure 30.1 Individualization of the stimulation protocol by suggesting the optimal treatment strategy based on the AMH level or the AFC of the patient. From Nelson [30]; with the kind permission of *Fertility and Sterility*.

one based on age, BMI, and AFC and another to which AMH was added. They found that the addition of AMH to the algorithm did not alter the number of patients achieving the targeted ovarian response (5–12 oocytes) and no significant differences in the rate of OHSS [38].

Individualized Dosing for Ovarian Stimulation

Many randomized controlled trials (RCTs) were conducted to evaluate the use of these markers and algorithms to optimize the outcome of IVF by individualizing the stimulation protocol and/or the starting dose. In 2003, Popovic-Todorovic *et al.* conducted a RCT to compare the use of individualized rFSH doses calculated by their dose nomogram with a standard dose of rFSH in 267 patients. They found that the individualized regimen was associated with a higher proportion of appropriate ovarian responses and a higher ongoing pregnancy rate [31]. However, the findings of this single study could not be replicated.

For example, Harrison *et al.* randomized 345 patients undergoing IVF according to their day 3 serum FSH levels and found that in (presumably) normal responders (FSH < 8.5 U/L), the smaller starting dose of FSH stimulation (150 IU/day) was associated with significantly fewer metaphase II (MII) oocytes compared with the higher dose

(200 IU/day). However, in (presumably) hypo-responders (FSH > 8.5 IU/L), no difference was found between the two starting doses of 300 and 400 IU/day [39]. In another study, Klinkert *et al.* randomized 52 patients with a low AFC (less than five) into two equal groups receiving a starting dose of 150 IU or 300 IU of rFSH and found no difference in the number of oocytes retrieved or the ongoing pregnancy rate [40]. In a different study, Berkkanoglu and Ozgur studied 119 (presumably) poor responders (AFC < 12) randomized into three groups receiving 300 IU, 450 IU, and 600 IU of rFSH as the starting dose. They found no significant differences between the studied groups in the number of MII oocytes retrieved, peak serum E_2 concentration, days of stimulation with rFSH, number of embryos available for transfer, CPRs, or cancellation rates [41].

Similarly, Jayaprakasan *et al.* randomized 131 (presumably) normal responders (AFC = 8 to 21) to receive either 300 IU or 225 IU of rFSH as the starting dose of their COS. They found no significant difference between both groups in the number of mature oocytes retrieved, in the incidence of cycle cancellation, in the LBR, or in the prevalence of OHSS [42]. In a different RCT, Levebvre *et al.* studied 356 (presumably) poor responders (FSH > 10 IU/L, AMH < 1 ng/ml, AFC < 8, or a previous IVF cycle cancellation). The patients were randomized into two groups

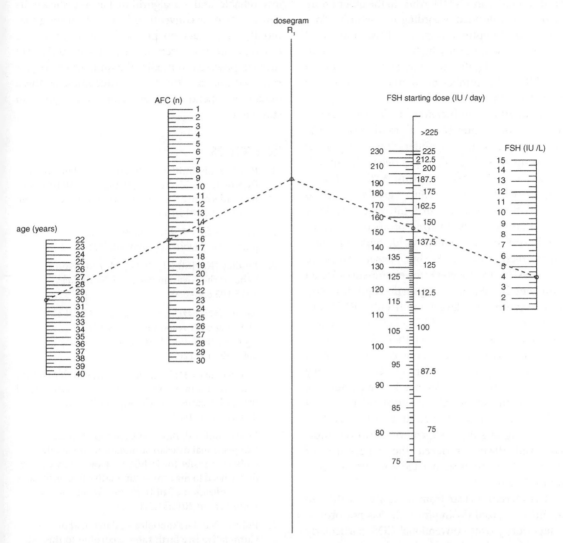

Figure 30.2 Nomograms for the determination of the starting dose of FSH based on the age of the patient and the AFC (left) or the AMH (right). From La Marca and Sunkara [33]; with the kind permission of *Human Reproduction Update*.

receiving 450 IU or 600 IU of highly purified menotropins. There were no significant differences in the number of MII oocytes retrieved, fertilization rate, biochemical pregnancy rate, clinical pregnancy rate, or implantation rate between both groups [43].

Individualized Dosing versus Conventional Protocols

With these disappointing results, RCTs were conducted to find out whether individualized gonadotropin dosing had any benefit over the currently used IVF stimulation protocols in poor, normal, and

hyper-responders. In a multicenter RCT, Olivennes *et al.* studied 200 presumably normal responders treated with IVF and randomized them into two groups receiving follitropin alfa: one group received a standard dose of 150 IU/day while the other group was managed according to the CONSORT algorithm. They found that although a significantly lower number of oocytes were retrieved in the CONSORT group, the CPR was similar in both groups and the incidence of OHSS was lower in the CONSORT group [44]. Similarly, Allegra *et al.* studied 191 unselected patients randomly divided into two groups: in one group the starting dose of FSH was decided according to a nomogram based on

315

age, day 3 FSH, and AMH, while in the other group the dose was decided according to age only. They found that the optimal response of recruiting 8–14 oocytes was significantly higher in the nomogram group, but no significant differences were found in the CPR or the number of embryos cryopreserved per patient [45].

In another multicenter RCT (ESTHER-1 study), Nyboe Andersen et al. randomized 1329 presumably normal responders into two groups: one group receiving follitropin delta with individualized dosing based on serum AMH and body weight, while the second group received a conventional protocol of follitropin alfa. They found that the individualized protocol was associated with similar oocyte yield, ongoing pregnancy rate, and LBR but fewer excessive responses (> 15 oocytes), fewer measures taken to prevent OHSS, and less gonadotropin use [46]. More recently in a larger multicenter RCT, van Tilborg et al. randomized 1515 IVF/ICSI patients into three groups based on their AFC: normal responders (AFC 11–15), poor responders (AFC < 11), and hyper-responders (AFC > 15). They found no significant difference in the cumulative LBR between individualized and standard dosing in the three groups studied and that individualized dosing was more expensive. However, individualized dosing reduced the occurrence of OHSS and the costs associated with its management [47–49].

It is therefore clear from these studies that, so far, individualized dosing for COS has not proven its superiority over conventional COS, particularly in poor responders, but may be of help in preventing problems in the hyper-responsive patients. Indeed, a recently published Cochrane review concluded that tailoring the FSH dose in all ovarian reserve populations (low, normal, high ovarian reserve) did not influence LBR or ongoing pregnancy rates, although, in predicted high responders, lower doses of FSH may reduce the overall incidence of moderate and severe OHSS. The authors added that these conclusions should be taken with caution due to the heterogeneity of the studies [50].

Conclusions

Ovarian reserve can be reliably used as a guide to prevent the occurrence and complications of OHSS in hyper-responders to COS. However, so far, its use as a guide to COS in poor or normal responders is less reliable and no algorithm has yet shown its superiority over conventional COS. Assuming that modifying stimulation protocols can improve the outcome in poor responders, larger RCTs are needed, powered to predict the number of oocytes retrieved and not the clinical outcomes, as these outcomes depend on other factors besides ovarian stimulation.

References

1. Practice Committee of the American Society for Reproductive Medicine. Testing and interpreting measures of ovarian reserve: a committee opinion. *Fertil Steril* 2015;103:e9–e17.

2. Tal R, Seifer DB. Ovarian reserve testing: a user's guide. *Am J Obstet Gynecol* 2017;217:129–140.

3. Findlay JK, Hutt KJ, Hickey M, Anderson RA. What is the "ovarian reserve"? *Fertil Steril* 2015;103:628–630.

4. Sallam HN, Ezzeldin F, Agameya AF, et al. Defining poor responders in assisted reproduction. *Int J Fertil Womens Med* 2005;50:115–120.

5. van der Gaast MH, Eijkemans MJ, van der Net JB, et al. Optimum number of oocytes for a successful first IVF treatment cycle. *Reprod Biomed Online* 2006;13:476–480.

6. Drakopoulos P, Blockeel C, Stoop D, et al. Conventional ovarian stimulation and single embryo transfer for IVF/ICSI. How many oocytes do we need to maximize cumulative live birth rates after utilization of all fresh and frozen embryos? *Hum Reprod* 2016;31:370–376.

7. Polyzos NP, Drakopoulos P, Parra J, et al. Cumulative live birth rates according to the number of oocytes retrieved after the first ovarian stimulation for in vitro fertilization/ intracytoplasmic sperm injection: a multicenter multinational analysis including ~15,000 women. *Fertil Steril* 2018;110:661–670.

8. Magnusson Å, Källen K, Thurin-Kjellberg A, Bergh C. The number of oocytes retrieved during IVF: a balance between efficacy and safety. *Hum Reprod* 2018;33:58–64.

9. Ji J, Liu Y, Tong XH, et al. The optimum number of oocytes in IVF treatment: an analysis of 2455 cycles in China. *Hum Reprod* 2013;28:2728–2734.

10. Broekmans FJ, Kwee J, Hendriks DJ, et al. A systematic review of tests predicting ovarian reserve and IVF outcome. *Hum Reprod Update* 2006;12:685–718.

11. de Bruin JP, Dorland M, Spek ER, et al. Age-related changes in the ultrastructure of the resting

follicle pool in human ovaries. *Biol Reprod* 2004;70:419–424.

12. Scheffer JAB, Scheffer B, Scheffer R, *et al.* Are age and anti-Müllerian hormone good predictors of ovarian reserve and response in women undergoing IVF? *JBRA Assist Reprod* 2018;22:215–220.

13. Al-Azemi M, Killick SR, Duffy S, *et al.* Multi-marker assessment of ovarian reserve predicts oocyte yield after ovulation induction. *Hum Reprod* 2011;26:414–422.

14. Ashrafi M, Madani T, Tehranian AS, Malekzadeh F. Follicle stimulating hormone as a predictor of ovarian response in women undergoing controlled ovarian hyperstimulation for IVF. *Int J Gynaecol Obstet* 2005;91:53–57.

15. Broekmans FJ, Kwee J, Hendriks DJ, *et al.* A systematic review of tests predicting ovarian reserve and IVF outcome. *Hum Reprod Update* 2006;12:685–718.

16. Wang S, Zhang Y, Mensah V, *et al.* Discordant anti-müllerian hormone (AMH) and follicle stimulating hormone (FSH) among women undergoing in vitro fertilization (IVF): which one is the better predictor for live birth? *J Ovarian Res* 2018;11:60.

17. Hofmann GE, Danforth DR, Seifer DB. Inhibin-B: the physiologic basis of the clomiphene citrate challenge test for ovarian reserve screening. *Fertil Steril* 1998;69:474–477.

18. Steiner AZ, Herring AH, Kesner JS, *et al.* Antimullerian hormone as predictor of natural fecundability in women aged 30–42 years. *Obstet Gynecol* 2011;117:798–804.

19. Corson SL, Gutmann J, Batzer FR, *et al.* Inhibin-B as a test of ovarian reserve for infertile women. *Hum Reprod* 1999;14:2818–2821.

20. Popovic-Todorovic B, Loft A, Lindhard A, *et al.* A prospective study of predictive factors of ovarian response in 'standard' IVF/ICSI patients treated with recombinant FSH. A suggestion for a recombinant FSH dosage normogram. *Hum Reprod* 2003;18:781–787.

21. Kwee J, Elting ME, Schats R, *et al.* Ovarian volume and antral follicle count for the prediction of low and hyper responders with in vitro fertilization. *Reprod Biol Endocrinol* 2007;15:5–9.

22. Lee TH, Liu CH, Huang CC, *et al.* Serum anti-Müllerian hormone and estradiol levels as predictors of ovarian hyperstimulation syndrome in assisted reproduction technology cycles. *Hum Reprod* 2008;23:160–167.

23. Tang H, Yan Y, Wang T, *et al.* Effect of follicle-stimulating hormone receptor Asn680Ser polymorphism on the outcomes of controlled ovarian hyperstimulation: an updated meta-analysis of 16 cohort studies. *J Assist Reprod Genet* 2015;32:1801–1810.

24. Motawi TMK, Rizk SM, Maurice NW, *et al.* The role of gene polymorphism and AMH level in prediction of poor ovarian response in Egyptian women undergoing IVF procedure. *J Assist Reprod Genet* 2017;34:1659–1666.

25. Tomás C, Nuojua-Huttunen S, Martikainen H. Pretreatment transvaginal ultrasound examination predicts ovarian responsiveness to gonadotrophins in in-vitro fertilization. *Hum Reprod* 1997;12:220–223.

26. Danninger B, Brunner M, Obruca A, Feichtinger W. Prediction of ovarian hyperstimulation syndrome by ultrasound volumetric assessment [corrected] of baseline ovarian volume prior to stimulation. *Hum Reprod* 1996;11:1597–1599.

27. Loumaye E, Billion JM, Mine JM, *et al.* Prediction of individual response to controlled ovarian hyperstimulation by means of a clomiphene citrate challenge test. *Fertil Steril* 1990;53:295–301.

28. Hendriks DJ, Mol BW, Bancsi LF, *et al.* The clomiphene citrate challenge test for the prediction of poor ovarian response and non-pregnancy in patients undergoing in vitro fertilization: a systematic review. *Fertil Steril* 2006;86:807–818.

29. Broer SL, van Disseldorp J, Broeze KA, *et al.* Added value of ovarian reserve testing on patient characteristics in the prediction of ovarian response and ongoing pregnancy: an individual patient data approach. *Hum Reprod Update* 2013;19:26–36.

30. Nelson SM. Biomarkers of ovarian response: current and future applications. *Fertil Steril* 2013;99:963–969.

31. Popovic-Todorovic B, Loft A, Ejdrup Bredkjñer H, *et al.* A prospective randomized clinical trial comparing an individual dose of recombinant FSH based on predictive factors versus a 'standard' dose of 150 IU/day in 'standard' patients undergoing IVF/ICSI treatment. *Hum Reprod* 2003;18:2275–2282.

32. Olivennes F, Howles CM, Borini A, *et al.* Individualizing FSH dose for assisted reproduction using a novel algorithm: the CONSORT study. *Reprod Biomed Online* 2009;18:195–204.

33. La Marca A, Sunkara SK. Individualization of controlled ovarian stimulation in IVF using ovarian reserve markers: from theory to practice. *Hum Reprod Update* 2014;20:124–140.

34. Haahr T, Esteves SC, Humaidan P. Individualized controlled ovarian stimulation in expected poor-responders: an update. *Reprod Biol Endocrinol* 2018;16:20.

35. Yovich J, Stanger J, Hinchliffe P. Targeted gonadotrophin stimulation using the PIVET algorithm markedly reduces the risk of OHSS. *Reprod Biomed Online* 2012;24:281–292.

36. Lan VT, Linh NK, Tuong HM, *et al.* Anti-Müllerian hormone versus antral follicle count for defining the starting dose of FSH. *Reprod Biomed Online* 2013;27:390–399.

37. Broer SL, Mol BW, Hendriks D, Broekmans FJ. The role of antimullerian hormone in prediction of outcome after IVF: comparison with the antral follicle count. *Fertil Steril* 2009;91:705–714.

38. Magnusson Å, Nilsson L, Oleröd G, *et al.* The addition of anti-Müllerian hormone in an algorithm for individualized hormone dosage did not improve the prediction of ovarian response-a randomized, controlled trial. *Hum Reprod* 2017;32:811–819.

39. Harrison RF, Jacob S, Spillane H, *et al.* A prospective randomized clinical trial of differing starter doses of recombinant follicle-stimulating hormone (follitropin-beta) for first time in vitro fertilization and intracytoplasmic sperm injection treatment cycles. *Fertil Steril* 2001;75:23–31.

40. Klinkert ER, Broekmans FJ, Looman CW, *et al.* Expected poor responders on the basis of an antral follicle count do not benefit from a higher starting dose of gonadotrophins in IVF treatment: a randomized controlled trial. *Hum Reprod* 2005;20:611–615.

41. Berkkanoglu M, Ozgur K. What is the optimum maximal gonadotropin dosage used in microdose flare-up cycles in poor responders? *Fertil Steril* 2010;94:662–665.

42. Jayaprakasan K, Hopkisson J, Campbell B, *et al.* A randomised controlled trial of 300 versus 225 IU recombinant FSH for ovarian stimulation in predicted normal responders by antral follicle count. *BJOG* 2010;117:853–862.

43. Lefebvre J, Antaki R, Kadoch IJ, *et al.* 450 IU versus 600 IU gonadotropin for controlled ovarian stimulation in poor responders: a randomized controlled trial. *Fertil Steril* 2015;104:1419–1425.

44. Olivennes F, Trew G, Borini A, *et al.* Randomized, controlled, open-label, non-inferiority study of the CONSORT algorithm for individualized dosing of follitropin alfa. *Reprod Biomed Online* 2015;30:248–257.

45. Allegra A, Marino A, Volpes A, *et al.* A randomized controlled trial investigating the use of a predictive nomogram for the selection of the FSH starting dose in IVF/ICSI cycles. *Reprod Biomed Online* 2017;34:429–438.

46. Nyboe Andersen A, Nelson SM, Fauser BC, *et al.* Individualized versus conventional ovarian stimulation for in vitro fertilization: a multicenter, randomized, controlled, assessor-blinded, phase 3 noninferiority trial. *Fertil Steril* 2017;107:387–396.

47. van Tilborg TC, Oudshoorn SC, Eijkemans MJC, *et al.* Individualized FSH dosing based on ovarian reserve testing in women starting IVF/ICSI: a multicentre trial and cost-effectiveness analysis. *Hum Reprod* 2017;32:2485–2495.

48. van Tilborg TC, Torrance HL, Oudshoorn SC, *et al.* Individualized versus standard FSH dosing in women starting IVF/ICSI: an RCT. Part 1: The predicted poor responder. *Hum Reprod* 2017;32:2496–2505.

49. Oudshoorn SC, van Tilborg TC, Eijkemans MJC, *et al.* Individualized versus standard FSH dosing in women starting IVF/ICSI: an RCT. Part 2: The predicted hyper responder. *Hum Reprod* 2017;32:2506–2514.

50. Lensen SF, Wilkinson J, Leijdekkers JA, *et al.* Individualised gonadotropin dose selection using markers of ovarian reserve for women undergoing in vitro fertilisation plus intracytoplasmic sperm injection (IVF/ICSI). *Cochrane Database Syst Rev* 2018;2:CD012693.

Index